Functional Morphology

The Dynamic Wholeness of the Human Organism

Functional Morphology

The Dynamic Wholeness
of the
Human Organism

Johannes W. Rohen

Illustrations by Annette Gack,
Marit Budschigk and Jörg Pekarsky

Translated by Catherine Creeger

Scientific editing by Cathy Sims-O'Neil

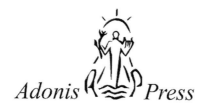

Adonis *Press*

This book was originally published in 2000 under the title *Morphologie des menschlichen Organismus, Versuch einer goetheanistischen Gestaltlehre des Menschen* by Verlag Freies Geistesleben, Stuttgart. In the first edition of the English translation, published in 2007, the original German text was slightly revised. In the present second English edition revisions made by the author in the 2nd, 3rd and 4th editions of the original German book have also been included.

Second, slightly revised edition
Copyright © 2016 by Adonis Press

Published by Adonis Press, 321 Rodman Road, Hillsdale, NY 12529.
www.adonispress.org

The copyright to the illustrations is held by Johannes W. Rohen, Dept. of Anatomy II, Universitätsstrasse 19, D 91054 Erlangen, Germany.

.

ISBN-13: 978-0932776365
ISBN-10: 0-932776-36-1

Cover design by Dale Hushbeck

Copyediting by Jeanne Bergen

*"But far removed from any temporal power
wanders Form—that playmate of all blessed beings—
above in halls of light, a goddess among gods."*

Friedrich Schiller

*"If you wish to grasp the invisible,
delve into the visible as deeply as you can."*

Max Beckmann

*"One will only understand the human body
if one sees it as an expression of the soul and spirit.
If it is seen only as a physical body,
it will remain incomprehensible."*

Rudolf Steiner

Contents

Introduction XIII

Author's Preface XV

BASIC CONCEPTS AND GENERAL PRINCIPLES OF FORM

Introductory Epistemological Remarks 3
  Seeing as an Example of Sensory and Cognitive Processes 4
  Perceiving and Thinking 9
  The Goethean Scientific Method 10
  Branches of Human Morphology 12

General Principles of Form..14
  The Functional Threefoldness of the Human Organism 14
    Basic Functions in the Human Body 16
    The Functional Threefoldness of the Human Body 19
    The Functional Threefoldness of the Cell 22
    Functional Threefoldness and the Human Soul 23
  Structural Principles in the Human Body and Qualitaties of the Dimensions of Space 26
    The Right-Left Dimension 26
    The Up-Down Dimension 28
    The Front-Back Dimension 28
    Functional Differentiations within Dimensional Structural Principles 30
  The Temporal Structure of the Human Body—Qualitative Aspects of Space and Time 35
  Human Embryological Development: Steps in Taking Hold of the Dimensions of Space 37
    Conception 37
    Structural Stages of Embryonic Development 43
    Qualitative Differences in the First Four Stages of Embryonic Development 46
    Human Embryonic Development and Placentation 48
    The Development of Internal Organ Systems in the Body 59
  Spiritual-Scientific Aspects of Embryonic Development 62
    Prior Stages of the Earth's Evolution 62
  A Comparison of Human Embryonic Development and the Earth's Evolution 63

Phylogenetic Processes..64
  Incremental Mastery of the Dimensions of Space in Vertebrate Evolution 64
    Limb Evolution 64
    Head Evolution 65
    Human Consciousness and the Experience of Space 67
    Adaptation and Antiadaptation as Evolutionary Principles 69
    Adaptive and Antiadaptive Processes 71
    The Evolution of the Skull and Head 74
    Antiadaptation and Orthogenesis as Evolutionary Principles 84

THE METABOLIC-LIMB SYSTEM

The Musculoskeletal System 87
   The Structure of the Skeletal System 87
   The System of Active Movement (Muscles and Joints) 100
      Joints and Sutures 100
      Functional Threefoldness of the Muscular System 103
      Muscles as Intermediaries between Blood and Nerves 111
      Movement as a Threefold Psycho-Physical Process 112

The Metabolic System and Digestive Organs 115
   Basic Metabolic Processes 115
      The Functional Significance of Metabolism 119
   Functional Subdivision of the Digestive Tract 120
   The Hepatobiliary System 125
   The Biliary System and Hemoglobin Metabolism 131

The Immune System, Lymphatic Organs, and Spleen 135
   General Organization of the Immune System 135
   The Lymphatic Organs and the Lymph System 137
   The Spleen 140
   Liver, Biliary System, and Spleen: The Organ Trinity of the Upper Abdomen 142

The Urogenital System: The Organs of Excretion and Reproduction 145
   Morphology of the Urinary System (Kidneys) 145
   Ontogeny and Phylogeny of the Urinary System 149
      The Phylogenetic Development of the Kidneys 153
   Morphology and Development of the Reproductive Organs 156
      Development of the Gonads 160

THE ORGANS OF THE RHYTHMIC SYSTEM

Blood and the Organs of Circulation 165
   Functional Threefoldness of the Circulatory System 165
      The Lymphatic Vascular System and the Body's Fluid System 168
   Blood and Bone Marrow 169
   The Heart 174
      The Ontogenetic Development of the Heart and the Dimensions of Space 174
      Cardiac Development and the Dimensions of Space 175
      Development of the Cardiac Tube 176
      Septation of the Cardiac Tube and the Right-Left Dimension 178
      The Heart and the Front-Back Dimension 181
      The Function of the Heart 182
   Phylogenetic Development of the Heart and Circulatory System 185
      Centralization 185
      Concentration 191
      Fetal Circulation 197
      The Empirical Principle in the Evolution of the Circulatory System 199

The Respiratory System 201
    The Connection between the Respiratory and Digestive Systems
              (First Archetypal Phenomenon) 201
        Lung Development and Respiration 204
    Respiratory Rhythm (Second Archetypal Phenomenon) 206
        Human Chronobiological Rhythms 208
    The Organs of Speech and the Faculty of Speech (Third Archetypal Phenomenon) 211
        Evolution of the Speech Organs 211
        The Human Speech Organs 211

THE NERVOUS SYSTEM AND THE SENSE ORGANS

The Functional Threefoldness of the Nervous System 217
    Development of the Nervous System 217
        Basic Morphological Divisions of the Nervous System 221
    Basic Nerve Tissue Functions 223
    General Structure of Reflex Arcs in the Three Functional Domains of the Nervous System 228

The Major Sensorimotor Systems 234
    The First Sensorimotor System (Monosynaptic myostatic reflex arc) 235
    The Second Functional System of the Sensorimotor Systems
              (Complex polysynaptic reflexes) 235
    Cortical Motor Systems (Pyramidal system—the 5th sensorimotor system) 236
    Subcortical Motor System (4th sensorimotor system) 238
    The Vestibular System and the Cerebellum (3rd sensorimotor system) 242

The Sensory Systems 243
    Functional Subdivision and Action of the Sensory Systems 243
        General Functioning of the Senses 244
        Asymmetry of Sensory Reflex Loops 248
    The Organs of Hearing and Balance 249
        The Outer Ear 251
        The Temporal Bone, the Middle Ear, and Pneumatization 252
        The Organ of Hearing 256
        The Vestibular Organ 262
        The Organs of Speech and the Functional Cycle of Hearing and Speaking 263
    The Eye and the Visual System 264
        Morphology and Embryonic Development of the Eye 264
        The Visual Process and the Optic Tract 269
        The Eye's Auxiliary Functional Systems 276
        The Visual System as a Whole 279
    The Chemical Senses (Taste and Smell) 279
        The Sense of Taste (Gustatory System) 280
        The Organ of Smell and the Olfactory System 282
    Surface Sensitivity (The Skin Senses) 286
        The Sense of Warmth or Temperature 287
        The Organs of the Sense of Touch 289
        The Sense of Pain 293

Deep Sensitivity (The Muscle Senses) 293
The Sense of Equilibrium 294
The Visceral Senses (Sense of Life) 297
The Sensory System as a Whole 298

The Autonomic or Vegetative Nervous System 301
   The Peripheral Organizational Level (Intramural System) 303
     How Autonomic Nerves Work 303
     Structure and Function of Autonomic Reflex Loops 304
   The Middle Organizational Level (The Sympathetic and Parasympathetic Systems) 306
   The Upper Organizational Level (Hypothalamus and Limbic System) 310
     The Hypothalamus 310
     The Limbic System 312

The Nervous System and Consciousness 314
   The Brain as the Organ of Consciousness 314
     Lateralization of the Hemispheres 315
     Consciousness and Subconsciousness 317
   The Nervous System as the Foundation of the Human Soul and Spirit 318

The Endocrine System (Hormonal Glands) 320
   Development and Function of the Endocrine Organs 321
     The Pharyngeal Organs: Thyroid, Parathyroids, and Thymus 322
     The Abdominal Endocrine Glands: Pancreatic Islets of Langerhans and Adrenals 326
   The Pituitary as an Endocrine Organ 328
   The Endocrine System and the Reproductive Organs 330
   The Pituitary/Pineal System 330

HEAD DEVELOPMENT AND ORGAN METAMORPHOSES

Head Development and the Integration Principle 335
   Development and Metamorphosis of Bony Elements 337
     Development of the Human Skull 340
     Development of the Torso Skeleton 343
   The Skull as a Metamorphosis of the Torso and Limb Skeleton 345
     Vertebral Metamorphosis 346
     Upper Limb Metamorphosis 351
       The Zygomatic Bone and the Frontal Bone 353
     Lower Limb Metamorphosis 354
       Temporal Bone and Pelvis 356
   The Principle of Formative Integration in Tooth Development 358
   The Threefoldness of the Facial Skeleton and the Physiognomy of the Human Face 362
   The Integrative Arrangement of the Cranial Nerves 364

Organ Metamorphoses 366
   Kidney/Eye Metamorphosis 366
   Upper Abdomen/Labyrinth Metamorphosis 370

Head Development and the Disintegration Principle 373

The Respiratory System of the Head 377
    The Ethmoid Bone and the Paranasal Sinuses 377
        The Paranasal Sinuses 379
    The Olfactory System 380
    The Branchial Apparatus (Branchial or Pharyngeal Skeleton) 381
    Metamorphosis of the Reproductive Organs into the Organs of Speech 382

The Pituitary/Pineal System 385

EVOLUTIONARY ASPECTS OF HUMAN DEVELOPMENT

The Physiological Foundations of Freedom 391
    Rhythms in Human Life 393

Evolutionary Principles and the Genesis of the Modern Human Form 396
    Adaptation and Antiadaptation 397
    The Empirical Principle 498
    Orthogenesis 400
    Human and Animal Evolution 401
    Summary 402

The Future of Human Evolution and the Problem of the Resurrection Body 405

References 411

Index 416

About the Author 425

Introduction
to the First Edition

Morning comes. I arise, don my scrubs, and begin my short walk to the anatomy lab. It is a sunny Saturday morning during my first month in medical school in Maine. As I stroll along, the sound of the waves greets me and the briny smell of ocean air stirs my wakefulness.

The light and warmth of the sun follow me into the anatomy lab, and as I unzip the bag of my cadaver, I meet both the possibility of my own mortality and the mysteries of the human being. It is a physical body that I now see, the signature of humanity. But a spiritual being once inhabited this body, circulating the blood, living in the breath, walking the earth as I now do.

During my first few weeks in gross anatomy at medical school, I was struck by the many wondrous structures under the skin that spoke of the wisdom of our creator: the energetic coursing of the arteries through the body, firm and wavy in their form, whereas the veins seem happy to meander along like a gentle stream.... And the nerves, quiet and still, are unrevealing of the potent power they can assert in pain, pleasure, or in thought. How mysterious it is that the same nerve that allows us to laugh also makes it possible for us to cry! Then there is the melody of the bones, starting in the skull as a stately dome standing guard over the jellylike structure of thinking—the brain. Now as the ribs, they ripple down in the chest, protecting the great organs of rhythm: the heart and lungs. Finally, they come to rest deep in the limbs as radial bones, clothed in spiraling muscle, allowing us to carry our will out into the spatial world!

But it is time to focus on my assignment, so I open my *Rohen* to the page illustrating my dissection, and the day's work begins. The *Rohen* I speak about here is the book almost every medical student in America knows, the *Color Atlas of Anatomy, A Photographic Study of the Human Body.** Professor Rohen pioneered the use of cadaveric photography for illustrating anatomical texts, ushering in a new chapter in the history of anatomical illustration. Now in its 6th edition in English, it is likely the most popular anatomy book in the world, translated into many languages. With excellent photographs of dissections of cadavers and identification of these structures, it is one of our best "friends" during anatomy, the book most of us have open at our side while dissecting. In this way, Dr. Rohen is a professor to us all, anticipating our questions with his illustrations, preparing us en masse for our exams.

The *Color Atlas* is just one of the series of Rohen's books used in European medical schools; his other works include gross anatomy, histologic anatomy, neuroanatomy, and functional/clinical anatomy. This book, *Functional Morphology,* is different. Here, Johannes Rohen invites us into his most penetrating phenomenological studies, into his life's work on human morphology and functional anatomy where he reveals the dynamic threefoldedness of the human organism, opening some surprising new perspectives along the way.

Rohen became most interested in this Goethean approach** to anatomy while a young medical student in Germany. By the age of 20 he had already written the beginnings of this book, commencing with the heart. Inwardly he felt that this organic approach could lead to a more complete understanding of the human being, and he sought to read all he could on the topic. He found the ideas of the threefold human being that Rudolf Steiner first presented in his book *Riddles* of the Soul particularly helpful. However, this was at the time of the Second World War and reading Steiner's works was forbidden by Hitler. So Rohen discretely borrowed Steiner's books from friends, inwardly incubating his ideas and then outwardly giving them birth as he could, first as an anatomical assistant teaching in Mainz and Marburg, then more fully as the head of the Anatomical Institute at the University of Nuremberg in Erlangen, Germany.

There was no anatomy program at Erlangen when Rohen arrived, so he now had the opportunity to put his ideas into practice from the beginning. The program evolved out of long hours spent in study groups with graduate students and faculty. Professor Rohen reversed the conventional method of teaching, which assumes a linear addition of parts to construct a whole. His program unfolds organically: it starts with functional anatomy, moving to topographic or gross anatomy, and from there to functional histology, with functional embryology and neuroanatomy being brought in as independent blocks. The primacy of the Whole remains strong throughout. Thus students are exposed to anatomy as a natural progression from the big picture to the small detail, and the unity of the human being—seen though the window of anatomy and physiology—now becomes palpable instead of implicit. Rohen positioned the anatomy lab on the top floor of the Institute of Anatomy so that his students would have to work a bit harder to reach this destination.

How wide can the heart be, how open the mind, when considering new perspectives on anatomy? This is the question the reader will confront when reading Functional Morphology. Rohen courageously asserts his breadth of insight in this work, ranging from the conventional and materialistic dimensions of anatomy to the far reaches of the most subtle spiritual aspects of the human being. More importantly, he shows how the physical and spiritual aspects are intimately connected.

It follows then that this morphological journey cannot be read as a conventional scientific text. Each anatomical-physiological description can only be fully comprehended in its relation to the whole. One cannot simply grasp at the facts! These dynamic interrelationships become accessible to those who approach them in a mood of quiet reverence and patience and with energetic inner participation. Indeed, Professor Rohen wrote his work in such a state, filled with awe and wonder before the wisdom and potential of the human body. Rightly understood, this book will awaken such a mood in the reader.

As we awaken from our long sleep in the arms of materialism, Rohen's text will serve as a foundational work in the scientific pheno-menological methodology that is emerging in these postmodern times. It is a pioneering work that takes us down a new road of medical education in the 21st century.

Cathy Sims-O'Neil, D.O.
Biddeford, Maine

*The Color Atlas of Anatomy; A Photographic Study of the Human Body, 6th edition, by Johannes W. Rohen, M.D., Chihiro Yokochi M.D., Elke Lutjen-Drecoll M.D., ISBN 9780781790130, published by Lippincott, Williams, and Wilkins, 2006

**The Goethean approach is named after its initiator, Johann Wolfgang von Goethe, 1749-1832. This scientific method is well described in Henri Bortoft's book The Wholeness of Nature, Goethe's Way toward a Science of Conscious Participation in Nature, Lindisfarne Press, 1996.

Author's Preface
to the First Edition

The ideas set forth in this book have occupied me for over fifty years. In late 1948, I completed my first lengthy work, a richly illustrated manuscript entitled *An Attempt at a Goethean Anatomy of the Heart*, which was not published at that time. Its most significant conclusions were incorporated into the current text, as was another unpublished manuscript (begun as early as 1947) on the phenomenology of the ear—specifically, the pneumatization process as it relates to tumor formation. Other individual ideas (on the metamorphosis of vertebrae and bones, the functional threefolding of the nervous system, the qualitative aspects of the dimensions of space, etc.) formed the subject of various lectures over the years. Originally published as short essays, they are now also included in this volume.

During my long career as a scientist and academic teacher I have developed many Goethean ideas, and although much remains unfinished and incomplete, I have finally decided to compile them into a coherent presentation. I do so for two reasons. First, my life is drawing to a close, and I do not know how much more time heaven will grant me for working on a more definitive version. Second, I believe the time has come, even in the scientific community, for alternative schools of thought to slip a word in edgewise. I do not mean to say that the analytical, quantitative way of thinking so prevalent today is wrong and needs to be replaced by its synthetic, qualitative counterpart. I simply mean that quantitative thinking is one-sided and needs to be complemented by holistic attempts to understand functional relationships, living wholes, and qualitative aspects which can unveil a context that comes to impact one's whole life.

Qualitative concepts, however, are often impossible to define as precisely as concepts based on physical systems of measurement; instead, they must be approached through circumlocutions, intuitions, and empathy, just as we would attempt to understand a person's essential character, which also can never be precisely pinned down.

For this reason, critical readers will undoubtedly discover inconsistencies (or even contradictions) in parts of this book and will find it difficult to understand why one fact is taken seriously while another is rejected as inconsequential. Over the years (and after frequent lengthy detours), I have come to understand what Goethe meant when he spoke of an "archetypal phenomenon." As Goethe formulated it, an archetypal phenomenon reveals an idea, a fundamental lawfulness. It manifests this lawfulness directly—and therefore requires no further explanation. Encountering an archetypal phenomenon can be a profoundly moving experience of self-evident truth. We sense the existence of a spiritual reality as it reveals itself in the phenomenon. Without this type of inner experience, all explanations remain merely lifeless words.

Illustrations are important because images are more expressive than abstract words or names. But if we wish to gain access on any deeper level to the immediate reality of living processes, we must learn to meditate on images. Images not only stay with us, they become more and more expressive and penetrating as the years go by. They begin to take on a life of their own, whereas words gradually begin to seem insignificant and relative. Ultimately, images open the door to higher spiritual dimensions.

From a very young age, I have grappled intensively with philosophical questions and studied the works of many great modern philosophers and psychologists (Kant, Nietzsche, C.G. Jung, Husserl, Steiner, and others). When faced with questions arising from my studies in phenomenology, I have most often found satisfying answers in Rudolf Steiner's works. The same has been true with regard to confirmations and/or explanations of my own extremely modest supra-sensory experiences. As a result, I am often more likely to quote Steiner than any other author when I feel the need to complement and expand upon my own ideas. This should not be misunderstood to mean that I take Steiner's statements as "proof" of what I myself am presenting. I point them out simply to add a different but worthwhile dimension that expands and deepens the issues.

I admit to taking a calculated risk in the final chapter, and in fact I hesitated for a long time before deciding to include it in the book. To many, it may seem sacrilegious. If we take St. Paul seriously, however, we know modern human beings have not only the ability but also the responsibility to think about such questions.

Ultimately, humankind's further evolution is an existential problem of concern to us all. Because my thoughts on this subject flowed so effortlessly and logically from the content that preceded them, I felt justified in continuing. Please interpret the result as nothing more than an initial, extremely modest attempt to gain an inkling of these cosmic mysteries.

If I have succeeded in engaging unbiased readers in a more "living" way of thinking, perhaps I will also have contributed one small building block to the edifice of a new and accurately expanded science of the human being that will serve as a foundation not only for many specialized fields such as education and medicine but also for the development of human culture in general. From this perspective, I beg you, the reader, to accept the unavoidable imperfections in this book and to use them not as grounds for destructive criticism but rather as a stimulus for your own creative thinking, so that you can supplant my efforts with better and stronger ones. True creativity lies not in analytical dissection but in grasping the spiritual realities that we must once again access through the tireless efforts of our own thinking.

Johannes W. Rohen
Erlangen, Easter 2007

Author's Preface
to the Second English Edition

Although new illustrations and revised text have been included in some chapters of this second English edition, the overall conception and content of the book remains the same.

Johannes W. Rohen
Erlangen, February 2016

Basic Concepts
and
General Principles of Form

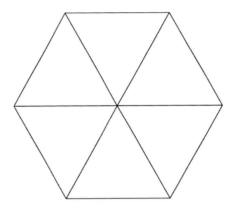

Fig. 1. This hexagon can also be seen three-dimensionally as a pyramid with a hexagonal base, a left-leaning cube, or a right-leaning cube—a striking example of the active, conceptual components of sight.

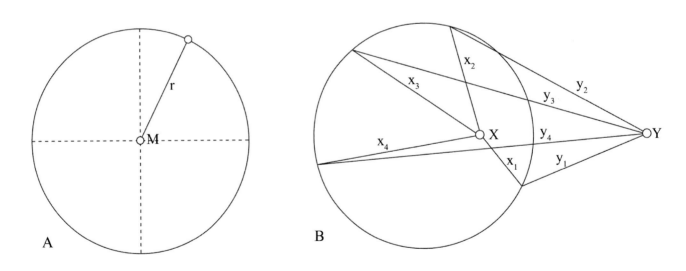

Fig. 2. We cannot see a circle as such; we can only "think" it. Here are two examples of different concepts of a circle:
A: a radial circle, all points of which maintain the same distance "r" from a fixed point (M);
B: an Apollonius or division circle, all points of which are such that the relationship between their distances from two fixed points (X and Y) remains constant. As distance "x" varies while sweeping around the circle $(x_1\text{-}x_2\text{-}x_3\ldots)$, distance "y" increases or decreases proportionally such that the ratio between "x" and "y" remains constant: x_n / y_n = constant.

Introductory Epistemological Remarks

Is our human organism—or any organism for that matter—merely the result of millions of physico-chemical reactions, or are there structural, morphological principles that integrate these individual events into a living, dynamic whole? And if such dynamic principles do exist, how do we apprehend them, and how can we gain scientific insight into their lawfulness? How we relate to and work with living beings will ultimately depend on how we answer these questions. In our endeavor to answer these questions, let us first take a fresh look at the nature of human knowledge itself.

People today usually think of their environment as objective, i.e., as something that is given as a reality, unlike their thoughts and ideas, which they view as subjective and unreal, and therefore as only of personal significance.

Studies in sense physiology, however, tell us that perception is impossible without the active involvement of human thinking and cognition (1). In fact, we cannot experience pure perception without the spontaneous addition of ideas except under exceptional or experimental circumstances. On awakening from anesthesia or after a night of carousing, for example, we may initially not know where we are. For an instant, we see only color fields that differ in size and brightness. Deep-seated anxiety, a moment of despair, a sense of doubt, or a feeling of being lost and helpless may ensue until eventually a thought breaks through, arranging the colored fields into objects and restoring our spatial orientation. Without concepts produced by thinking, the contents of perception are virtually worthless (2).

Even simple but optically ambiguous shapes can illustrate the fact that the activity of perception involves thinking. A group of lines as seen in Figure 1, for example, can be perceived two-dimensionally as a hexagon or three-dimensionally as a pyramid or a cube. The **cube**, in turn, can be "visually grasped" either as leaning toward the

right or toward the left. The spatial appearance of the image shifts, depending on how we see—or better, "think"—the cube. Without the concept "cube," which can also be defined mathematically, we would not see the lines as belonging to a shape at all.

Another example is the **circle** (Figure 2). Purely perceptually, a circle initially appears as merely a number of points. No illustration can be so exact that it truly reproduces the ideal form of a circle, but even a very imperfect rendering conveys the concept "circle" if we are already familiar with it.

As a perceptual experience, therefore, a circle always includes two elements:

1. the optical percept of more or less regularly arranged points or lines (prerequisite: healthy organs of sight), and

2. the formation of the concept "circle" (prerequisite: healthy educated thinking, supported by a normal brain).

These two elements, although they are almost always integrated into a single experience under circumstances of normal ideation, can also be analyzed and brought to consciousness independent of one another. We can mentally increase or decrease the size of the image of a circle, for example, or modify its color. We can change its physical appearance—at least within reason—yet it still remains a circle as long as it meets certain basic requirements. On the other hand, we can also intensify or deepen our consciousness of the concept "circle," even advancing into the realm of higher mathematical ideas. We may realize, for example, that a "normal" or radial circle is the geometric location of all points on a plane that are equidistant from a midpoint (Figure 2A). But we can also see a circle as the geometric location of all points on a plane whose distances from two fixed points maintain a constant ratio (an Apollonius or division circle, Figure 2B). We can experience our usual, radial concept of a circle as static and the concept of such an Apollonius circle as dynamic. If we activate our thinking further, we can even see the circle as a reflective surface that allows shapes external to it to be inwardly inverted in certain regular, lawful ways (circle of inversion). Ultimately, the visual image becomes a symbol of spiritual processes whose reality can be experienced only in thinking, although a perceptual image can serve as a means of visualizing or illustrating them (3).

Someone might object that by following this path, we increasingly lose our firm footing in reality, arriving only at pure abstractions. When we strengthen the "subjective" element of thinking, we then see the only objective element—the physical percept—as a mere symbol of a reality instead of reality itself, somewhat in the sense of the ancient Indian view that everything in the physical world is *maya,* or as Goethe wrote at the end of his *Faust,* "Everything transient is but a parable."

This objection is based on the misconception that either one of the two elements (percept or concept) comprising the experience of perception is inherently capable of constituting a whole. Neither a pure percept nor an isolated concept is whole in itself. Worse still is to declare **one** of these elements subjective and the other objective (2). What is important here is to discover how the two elements are intertwined and **together** constitute reality as we are actually able to experience it, i.e., the reality that lights up in our consciousness.

Our concepts of what is "subjective" or "objective" take their orientation from the over-valuation of sensory perception that shapes our scientific thinking today. In essence, however, this dominance is based on a weakness in our thinking. The flood of sensory impressions to which we are exposed in our contemporary culture has become so overwhelming, and the concepts that accompany them, but that usually go unnoticed, have become so numerous, that we often forget to think for ourselves, to "digest" our perceptions through an independent, unbiased thinking that actually does justice to its objects. Most of what comes toward us is "predigested." Concepts arrive simultaneously with perceptions, and hypotheses (which then replace real ideas) are gradually declared to be facts. The result is a growing sense of the weakness and subjectivity of our thinking, which becomes increasingly lethargic because it is not being roused to any inner activity.

A more exact analysis of the physiological processes of sensory perception, however, readily shows us that the highly valued objectivity of the perceived world has been significantly exaggerated. Perception is sometimes much less reliable than thinking. As we have seen in the examples given above, the concept of a circle is reliable. But our perception of circles is not, as we can realize simply by watching someone ride a bicycle along a street. Although bicycle wheels are circular, at any given moment, depending on our angle of view, they are unlikely to actually look like circles. Yet at no point do we feel that they might "really" be oval, elliptical, or bent, which is how they may appear to our perceiving eyes. As we watch someone ride a bike, the ideational capacity arising out of our power of thinking is so strong that it constantly "corrects" our visual perceptions. The same is true of our perception of size: The bicycle and its rider always seem to be the same size, even though their image rapidly becomes smaller with increasing distance. Something similar is true of spatial perception, the perception of color and brightness, and many other perceptions.

Thus we constantly adjust "wrong" perceptions. As long as we observe the world with our waking consciousness, our cognition "corrects" and objectifies our perceptions. In other words, the sensory world, as we perceive it, is actually a product of our **thinking** (5-7).

Seeing as an Example of Sensory and Cognitive Processes

Now let's consider the process of seeing. The eye is a spherical sensory organ with a diameter of 22 to 24 mm. The retina, with its light-sensitive cells or photoreceptors (cones and rods), is housed in the posterior part of the eye. The point of most acute vision, the fovea centralis, with a diameter

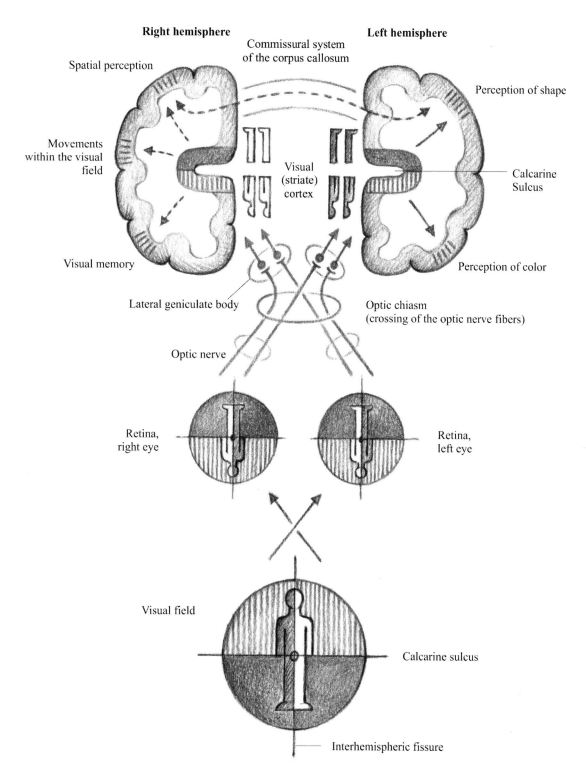

Fig. 3. **The optic tract and the process of seeing.** *The image that appears in the visual field is reversed by the lens. Partial images from different quadrants of the retina are projected "piece by piece" onto the visual cortex in the occipital lobe of both brain hemispheres. From there, image fragments are distributed to different areas of the brain based on their functional values (shape, color, space, movement). Brain centers for resynthesizing the image in its totality, as we experience it, are largely unknown.*

of not more than 0.5 mm, is located in the center of the retina. The entire visual field is centered on this point. What is the significance of the fact that sharp images of the environment can *only* form in this small, pointlike area? How is it that the huge visual space we experience in our surroundings is concentrated and reproduced in this minute point? If you focus your attention even briefly on your peripheral vision, which utilizes the peripheral areas of the retina, you will immediately notice that these images are much weaker, less clear, and less precise.

From the retina, neural stimuli are transmitted to the brain via the optic nerve, which then becomes the optic tract. The optic nerve carries nerve fibers from each half of the retina (red and blue in Figure 3). These two groups of fibers separate, however, in the optic chiasm (the crossing of the optic nerves) so that all those fibers coming from the left side of the retina of each eye (blue) go to the left hemisphere of the brain, and those coming from the right half (red) go to the right hemisphere (Figure 3). Thus the image that forms on the retina of one eye is always projected into the brain twice, once into each hemisphere.

In the cerebral cortex, the projection fields for the visual system lie in the occipital lobe, specifically in the visual cortex (calcarine or striate cortex—area 17 or V_1), which in turn consists of two ridges (gyri) separated by a groove called the calcarine sulcus (Figures 3 and 4). After being routed through the lateral geniculate body, the optic nerve fibers leading from the photoreceptors of the upper right retinal quadrants of *both* eyes end (for example) in the upper gyrus of the right occipital lobe. The fibers coming from the lower right retinal quadrants (also of both eyes) end in the lower gyrus. Similar correspondences apply to the remaining retinal quadrants. This double projection onto the visual cortex occurs because only half of the optic nerve fibers cross in the optic chiasm; specifically, the fibers coming from the inner (medial) quadrants of the retina cross over to the opposite side, while those coming from the outer (lateral) quadrants do not. Thus in a certain sense, our visual images are not only "dissected" but also doubly projected onto the cerebral cortex (Figure 3).

But we experience only a single visual field, not two different ones. Although we have two eyes, we see only one image. And to make matters worse, images are also inverted by the lens, *within the eye itself,* so that all of the points in the upper visual field, for example, are projected onto the lower half of the retina and vice versa.

From the epistemological perspective, what does this unique arrangement mean? Studies in sensory physiology have shown that two images (one from each eye) do indeed exist in the visual system, but *consciously* we experience only one! To put it more simply, the image from one eye becomes dominant (usually the right eye in right-handed individuals) and is perceived consciously, while the other image is suppressed and remains unconscious.

Here we have the first instance of the "intervention" of our thinking in the purely projective "photographic" process that takes place in our eyes. The second ("suppressed") image supplied by the nondominant eye, however, is not totally extinguished. It is carefully separated from the dominant image and transported into higher brain centers where (as we shall see later) it is needed for depth perception.

A second, extremely surprising conclusion is that the perceived image, which remains a coherent whole as far as our consciousness is concerned, is "analyzed," as it were, and distributed to different parts of the cerebral cortex as a result of the idiosyncratic connections described above. Aside from the fact that each point in the visual field is projected into the brain twice, parts of the image that originate in the contiguous quadrants of the retina are systematically "taken apart" in the neural projection process and are "projected" by the nerves into either the left or the right half of the brain and onto either the upper or the lower visual cortex of that hemisphere. If we draw a cross on the visual field to divide it into four parts, the horizontally bisecting arm of the cross corresponds to the groove (calcarine sulcus) in the visual cortex of the occipital lobe, while the vertical dividing line corresponds to the longitudinal cerebral fissure (interhemispheric fissure) between the right and left halves of the brain itself (Figure 3). Partial

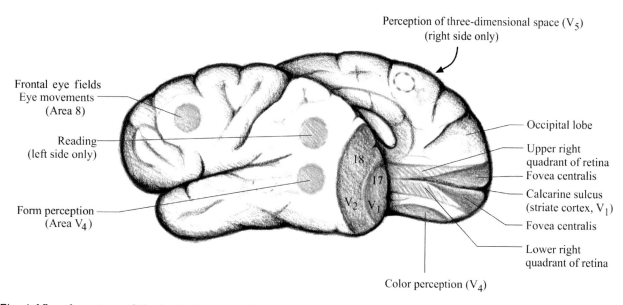

Fig. 4. **Visual centers of the brain.** *Impulses from both eyes stream into the interior of the occipital lobe in the so-called striate cortex (above and below the calcarine sulcus, V_1) of the primary cortical visual center. The greatest amount of space is taken up by projections from the fovea centralis (area of most acute vision). From there, they are distributed to different parts of the cortex (spatial separation of perceptions of color, shape, and movement). Area 18 contains the secondary cortical fields.*

images from the different retinal quadrants are therefore projected onto the visual cortex of the cerebrum in ways that do not correspond at all to the image we perceive. Instead, the image we see of our surroundings is cut apart—it seems almost appropriate to say "shredded to pieces"—by the visual system. If we attempted to piece it back together on the surface of the brain, the result would be a completely distorted, unrecognizable, virtually shapeless thing bearing absolutely no resemblance to the image we experienced, not to mention that it would be the mirror image of its original self and would appear double. And at this stage, physiologically speaking, we are no longer dealing with points on an image but with patterns of action potentials.

Where and how is this dissected, dissolved image of the outer world assembled once again? Resynthesis is often said to occur with the help of the commissural system of the corpus callosum,

which links the brain's right and left hemispheres, including their visual cortex fields. More precise analysis of actual impulses in the cerebrum, however, has shown that this is definitely not the case—in fact, it's quite the opposite! Far from being the last stop before a composite image emerges in areas of the cortex, the projection fields of the visual cortex merely deliver partial information to other areas, each with its own specialized function. Consequently, the projection fields in the visual cortex of the occipital lobe (area 17 or V_1) are viewed as a "**distribution system**" that supplies higher-order integrative cortex fields (V_2-V_6 etc.) or other specific "centers" in the temporal and parietal lobes with the "information" they need for very specialized individual functions such as the perception of shapes, color, movement, or three-dimensional structure. Each of these individual functions has a center lying in a different part of the cerebral cortex (Figure 4). For example, the higher-order center V_5 that assesses impulses projected onto the visual cortex involving the "recogniton" of three-dimensional space is located in the upper portion of the right parietal lobe, while centers which evaluate the form and structure of the perceived image, are located in the left parietal lobe. ***Nowhere in the brain does the image reappear as a whole***. On the contrary, the visual apparatus has "analyzed" the image, broken it down into its component parts, and effectively "destroyed" it as an image. The individual fields of the cortex each tell us something very different about the light-borne coherent "whole" that once approached us as an image from the outside world.

Let's now consider several specific examples. Imagine that an image of a human figure falls on the retina (Figure 3). When this image is projected onto the upper surface of the brain, it is projected doubly (into both hemispheres) and is also split into four parts, with each quarter of the body landing in a different region of the cortex. This human figure is apparently "dissected" and dissolved. It never again appears as a totality. And what if we see a blooming tree against a blue sky? The stimulation pattern of one cortical center allows us to perceive the tree's outline, another center allows us to perceive its three-dimensionality, another center asseses its individual structure (its species, perhaps), and the activity of yet another center conveys its optical values as they relate to emotional components (blue sky/mood/beauty, etc.). A whole catalog of individual functions exists, and while these functions are connected in turn with other parts of the nervous system, there is never a total image produced in the brain that corresponds to our naïve primary visual perception.

As we will discuss later, the left hemisphere is primarily responsible for analytical functions, while the right hemisphere performs functions that are more synthetic or holistic in character. But nowhere do we find anything like an integration center that reassembles all the pieces of the image back into a whole. There is absolutely no scientific basis for the materialistic idea that the brain, when stimulated from outside, "secretes" concepts the way a gland gives off secretions. The human being—that is, the active, thinking "I"—becomes aware of specific elements of a perceived image through the respective brain centers. These "centers of activity," however, do not produce these elements in the form in which we experience them. Instead, the power of thinking must be applied to the individual elements of an image so they can be actively and creatively re-synthesized through the mental process we call conceptualization or "concept formation." Perhaps this dissolution process developed in our sensory organs and nervous system as a sublime "artifice" of nature so that we might have the opportunity and the ability to actively reconstruct the whole through our own spiritual activity. As a result, we initially develop awareness of our perceptions, and then self-awareness. We ourselves are present in the process of image construction—a "subjective" process to be sure, in the sense that it is engendered by a subject, but it is a process with "objective" elements. We cannot make a tree, but on the conceptual level, we can generate its image and all its attendant qualities.

Thus we are granted the ability to recognize the tree as such, not merely superficially but in its essential character. Under normal circumstances, the concept-forming process occurs so rapidly and unconsciously that we no longer notice it at all. For example, we cannot open a door unless many little everyday concepts—such as "doorknob," "distance," "hinge," etc.—are also immediately available to us. This "thinking while seeing" takes place completely as a matter of course, in the flash of a moment. We become aware of it only when it malfunctions, as may happen in certain types of illness: The patient misses the doorknob, seeking it in the wrong place, and so on.

The organs of sight have been described here to exemplify the laws governing a sensory system that focuses on the dissection and analysis of perceptual modalities. This system must be complemented by the active "perceptual will" of a thinking individuality, an "I", in order to reproduce the whole image as it exists externally. We find the same process, however, in any other sensory organ. The "sound image" received by our sound conduction apparatus is also dissected in great detail by our **sense of hearing** in a process called "frequency dispersion." Here, too, downstream centers "dissect" individual elements according to their functional values and distribute them to different areas of the brain. Again, no complete image of the tonal experience—be it a symphony, a sentence, or a melody—ever develops in any specific part of the brain. Although many sensory systems are significantly simpler in structure than the eye or the ear, the lawful patterns described above are always evident in some similar form.

How, then, can we understand this initially mysterious resynthesizing? At this point, we begin to encounter the skepticism of modern philosophy. The analytic aspect of the perceptual process is widely acknowledged, if only because it is based on well-known physiological phenomena, but the synthesizing, soul-spiritual aspect, although no less clear-cut, is generally questioned and more frequently denied.

Perceiving and Thinking

As we demonstrated earlier, any sensory experience consists of concepts on the one hand, and specific phenomena conveyed by the relevant sensory system on the other hand (2, 7). Thus the activity of perceiving and recognizing something includes dissection or analysis by the appropriate sense organ(s) and related portions of the nervous system. But it also includes a "resynthesis" of the perceived object through a more-or-less conscious mental processing of the percept—in other words, through the development of appropriate concepts (2). There is no basis in fact for characterizing one of these processes as objective and the other as subjective. Concepts, although undeniably developed by a subject (i.e., a human being), must correspond to the object—that is, they must be "objective"—if they are to lead to reality-based conclusions about it. Cognition, which is capable of confronting not only the outer, "objective" world but also the thinker's own inner being, is therefore neither objective nor subjective but *transcends*

both. Thus to characterize thinking as subjective is patently wrong (2, 7). The claim that thinking is fundamentally incapable of developing concepts that correspond to reality is easily refuted by the mere existence of technology. A bridge constructed according to correctly formulated architectural laws will not collapse.

To simplify the issue, let's take another look at Figure 1, one of many possible ways of representing a cube. The human sensory apparatus breaks it down into fragmented lines and points. Cognition, meanwhile, reassembles the fragments in a meaningful way, recognizes the whole, and formulates universally valid and immanent concepts—in other words, forms an idea of the cube (resynthesis). Now the sensory image appears as the expression of the idea; the general and the specific once again form a unity. Ultimately, this unity is a trustworthy experience of reality and therefore usable and reproducible.

Any legitimate scientific experience must rest on foundations of this sort. But how are a concept and a percept matched up so that together they represent a reality? Why isn't the concept merely a subjective construct derived by abstraction from an essentially unrecognizable reality, i.e., an entirely personal matter without any claim to universal validity? Through the development and implementation of technology we have proved that the laws recognized by physics and chemistry are indeed realities. The cube, the circle, or whatever other example we choose, contains mathematical laws that can not only be cognitively understood and used but also exist a priori, in the objects themselves. Through thinking, we become conscious of the spiritual lawfulness inherent in the object.

Thus the idea that lights up in a human being stimulated by sense perception is the same spiritual principle that is present in the object itself. Upon closer consideration we realize that we look at each object from two sides: with our sense organs—from outside, and with our cognition—from within.

Just as a straight line disappears into infinity on the right and returns on the left, human beings receive a perception on one side, temporarily relinquish its reality, but then regain its spiritual (cognitive) reality—which returns through infinity on the other side, as it were—in the resynthesizing process. This, then, is how we experience its reality as a whole.

The dual character of the cognitive process has far-reaching implications for understanding the essential nature of the human being. "Dissolution" and "resynthesis" enable us (on a small scale) to repeat the process of the creation of every object we encounter. Consequently, we are able to recognize ourselves and nature (the microcosm and the macrocosm) independently and in freedom. There is indeed a divine element at work in the cognitive process.

In the final stage of evolution, the creator or creators of nature granted human beings the ability to re-create each and every natural object through perception and cognition. As a result, we are always, in a general way, taking part in the process of creation.

Analytic sensory activity is needed to free up space for the subsequent development of ideas so that the experience of freedom can emerge. Cognition becomes reliable, however, only when the ideation process discovers the appropriate patterns and laws for the object in question. Our language characterizes this process quite aptly: "dis-cover" actually means to uncover, to reveal, to make visible something that was hidden within, namely, the inherent idea. Errors and falsehoods occur when the reunion of percept and concept does not take place in the right way.

We modern human beings have achieved a high degree of certainty in recognizing and formulating the laws of physics and chemistry. This certainty is the basis of our virtually unshakable confidence in technological devices. It would never occur to anyone who uses an elevator, an airplane, or a car that these machines might be based on subjective, unreliable ideas or that they do not function according to laws that also prevail in the natural world. Our thinking is very different (and surprisingly inconsistent) when we confront living or animate organisms and the laws that presumably govern their activity. As a rule, ideas acquired from the world of technology have

not proved equally reliable when applied to living things. Living beings—plants, animals, and so on—are not machines. Our exclusive application of technological, physical concepts in our attempts to regulate, alter, or otherwise intervene in the world of living organisms has often led to failure and unforeseen deleterious consequences. In this domain, our thinking has not yet succeeded in developing concepts that are also intrinsic to living organisms (in the form of active forces). We recognize the laws of physics and chemistry with the help of concepts derived from the content of the inorganic, mineral world, but these ideas are not suited to living organisms. The inappropriate application of these laws by humans has often inflicted serious damage or disruption in the living world. Forest dieback and the extinction of species are only a few examples.

At this point, says Rudolf Steiner, modern scientists will again utter Dubois-Reymond's famous "ignorabimus," maintaining that human thinking is denied access to the laws governing living and animate nature (6). But why should it be possible for us to recognize the inherent laws of inanimate natural objects and not those of living or animate organisms? The makeshift solution of many modern researchers and philosophers—namely, to conclude that there is no real difference between these natural kingdoms—is unconvincing. It has become all too apparent that we are incapable of discerning the higher natural processes of living and animate organisms through ways of thinking appropriate only to physics and chemistry.

The Goethean Scientific Method

In the evolution of western culture, Goethe was the individual most successful at developing ways of thinking suited to understanding the organic world (cf. 8 and 9). Goethe was right to take greater pride in his scientific work than in his literary accomplishments, since the former laid the foundation for a new school of scientific thought and opened up a whole new dimension of empirical research. This will allow us in the future (if we understand it and pursue it) to explore the organic world with the precision we already apply to inorganic nature. In the mid- and late nineteenth century, scientists such as Karl Snell, Carl Gustav Carus, and Lorenz Oken—as well as others—initiated a "Goethean" school of scientific thought, although their efforts fell short of any real breakthroughs (10). More recently, Henri Bortoft has given an outstanding account of Goethe's scientific method (11). (For a listing of books in English on Goethean science as well as a list of books in English taking a Goethean approach to medicine, please see p. 415.)

"Do not look behind the phenomena, for they themselves are the theory," said Goethe, meaning that we humans are indeed capable of grasping the creative principles manifested by the phenomena themselves. Because we are able to awaken forces within ourselves that are related to the dynamic, spiritual laws at work in the organic world, we are capable of discerning the laws and patterns of living nature. Rather than attempting to derive explanations from hypothetical forces concealed **behind** natural objects, Goethe's **phenomenological method** seeks to discern the forces at work within these objects by applying a living, receptive, energetically empathic power of discernment. Through our own efforts, we can mobilize active, inner life-forces within ourselves, which are then transformed into reality-based ideas through inner participation in natural processes.

In addition to physical and chemical forces, biological processes are also active in the human body. These are the same processes that allow a plant to become an organism. Growth, regeneration, respiration, and reproduction, are some of the processes common to the bodies of humans and plants. Human bodies, however, are not only alive but also animated and ensouled. Inner sensations such as pain, grief, happiness, love, and anger, appear in our consciousness as primary experiences. These conscious experiences are not secondary or indirect, as in "My brain produces the feeling of sympathy or antipathy." Instead, I experience these feelings as forces that well up within me

and interact according to their own nature. We humans share this world with animals. If we interpret animal behavior correctly, it appears as the manifestation of sentient activity in which pain, joy, excitement, greed, lethargy, and so on are present as they are in us, although generally in exaggerated, one-sided, rudimentary ways.

Unlike animals, however, we human beings each have an "I" that is capable of restraining our soul forces. We can tame our "inner animal" and reduce the impact of the unbridled psyche. For animals, such inhibition occurs only when an urge is satisfied. These differences between man and animal have been comprehensively worked out by Arnold Gehlen (12). A force superior to the purely sentient element is absent in animals but present in humans. This is our "I"-being, the core of our personality, the essence of our individuality.

With appropriate practice and intensification, human cognitive processes are capable of transcending mere physical cognition and reaching the domains of all three types of forces—the domains of life, soul, and individuality. Under normal circumstances, modern human thinking is involved only with the physical-chemical laws and forces at work in the physical body. We feel confident in dealing with physical phenomena because our concepts are fully capable of grasping them. These concepts, however, do not apply to the living world or to soul forces. For example, what does the concept of gravity have to do with a psychological experience of heaviness? How can we possibly hope to explain the rhythmically repeated growth, bloom, and withering of a plant with concepts derived exclusively from physics? Nonetheless, human thinking is also capable of advancing into these "higher" worlds. In other words, we are also capable of developing concepts and ideas that are appropriate to these realms and can be used to grasp their inherent laws and patterns. This process is essentially no different from how we understand physical and chemical phenomena. **Empirical science is also possible in the domains of life and soul because their laws and patterns are also inherent in us** (Figure 5).

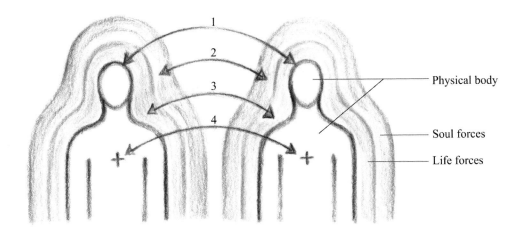

*Fig. 5. **Possible inter-human perceptions** (see text for details). 1: perceiving the physical body; 2: experiencing soul processes; 3: sensing life forces; 4: experiencing personality (perceiving the "I").*

When we succeed in mobilizing the appropriate forces within our own being and raising them to consciousness, we will understand the phenomena of these worlds as surely and certainly as we understand those of the physical world. We cannot merely be content with distinguishing and cognizing the physical world with confidence. We must, in addition, develop a different type of cognition for understanding living phenomena. Often the image itself, the pure phenomenon (Goethe's "archetypal phenomenon"), provides the basis for conceptual understanding, and words are mere circumlocutions. Everything depends upon our ability to mobilize and become conscious of the forces in ourselves that are related to what we are attempting to understand. If trained in this way, our thinking will discover a whole new world of ideas where interconnections with far-reaching consequences are revealed with the same scientific precision that we expect in the fields of physics and chemistry.

Branches of Human Morphology

Essentially, morphology is the study of form (from the Greek *morphe* = form, figure). But whereas anatomy—an analytic, dissecting science—looks at bodies from a more external perspective, morphology is more concerned with their forms as such and attempts to grasp their holistic character, especially in comparison to the forms of other entities. The first conscious use of this more synthetic concept of form occurred in Goethe's scientific writings, although Goethe himself probably did not coin the term "morphology."

In the Goethean sense, it can be said that what lies behind every natural phenomenon is a specific archetypal form—an ***ideal***. In this hierarchical structure, subordinate forms always reflect ideal formative principles.

Analytical research methods have exposed immense quantities of seemingly unrelated individual phenomena whose functional significance within a meaningful contextual whole often remains unexplained if not altogether inexplicable. In contrast, synthetic morphology attempts to describe forms in ways that allow us to recognize their qualitative significance as parts of a whole. There is no hiatus between subject and object, and individual forms reveal their own essential character through the way they reflect the archetype (8, 11-14).

If we disregard distinctions based exclusively on methodological differences, the morphology of the human organism encompasses three main areas:

1. ***Embryology***. Developmental history describes changes in the proportions of the human figure in the course of individual development (embryology, ontogeny). In its broader meaning, the term also describes evolutionary processes and encompasses comparative anatomy and phylogeny. Each individual form thus becomes recognizable as the result of an evolutionary and/or developmental process, that is, as a snapshot of a transitory state within a longer evolutionary or maturational process.

2. ***Systematic anatomy*** (anatomy in the narrower sense) provides descriptions of the current status of individual forms or specific structures. ***Functional anatomy*** emerges only when forms are understood in their connection to related structures, as expressions of specific functional states, and in the context of functional systems—in other words, when details no longer appear in isolation but are understood in the context of the total architecture of interconnected, hierarchically ordered, and functionally nested systems in the organism.

3. Finally, in ***topographical or regional anatomy (clinical anatomy)*** the spatial relationships between organs and parts of organs within an organism are described exclusively in terms of spatial adjacencies, without regard for systemic relationships. By their very nature, regional relationships are especially important in the practice of medicine but are exceptionally difficult to understand on the spiritual level. Initially, it is very difficult from a functionalist approach to see why the thyroid gland should be located in the throat, for example, or the islets of Langerhans in the pancreas, or the pituitary gland in the sella turcica.

General Principles of Form

The Functional Threefoldness of the Human Organism

Seen from the outside, the human body forms a self-contained whole; from the perspective of physics, however, it is an "open system." Energy is added to the system in the form of food and expended on bodily movement, physiological processes, or growth and regeneration. The conversion of food into energy produces wastes that must then be eliminated. In addition to the metabolic system, other systems in the body (such as the nervous system) also interact with the environment. At first glance, therefore, the body's functional systems do not appear self-contained. Closer observation, however, reveals a different picture. The outside world can never intervene directly in the human body but merely stimulates preexisting bodily processes that run their course independent of the outside world. In fact, the body consists of functionally closed systems whose subprocesses are cyclical in character; only at certain points are they open to the outside stimuli that help maintain their homeostatic cycles. This apparent contradiction holds one of the greatest mysteries of human bodily existence.

The nervous system, for example, receives information from the sense organs. Ultimately, however, this information merely triggers the processing and exchange of internal information needed to control organ functions. Instead of "reflecting" the outer world around us, we actually build up our own inner world independent of the world outside.

The material aspect of our life exhibits a similar degree of independence. The body is not a static structure that we can understand once and for all. On the contrary, its substances are constantly being transformed—often at unbelievable rates—and are built up and broken down again in cyclical processes that maintain the body's structure. The surface cells of the intestinal mucosa, for example, have a life span of only 36 to 48 hours. Skin cells live for 10 to 13 days, red blood cells for about 100 days, and so on. From the material perspective, the body is constantly being built up and transformed. Once growth stops, the body's form appears to remain unchanged for a long time, but its material composition changes incessantly. The one constant element is change, not matter.

The substances needed for maintaining the body's structure come from without, but they are digested into their most basic components and are never allowed to infiltrate the body in their original form. By analogy, the same is true with regard to sensory processes and the nervous system. Whether on the material or neural level, the body always maintains its integrity. The decisive point here, however, is that the metabolism recycles the same substances over and over again, with anabolism and catabolism (normally) in a state of

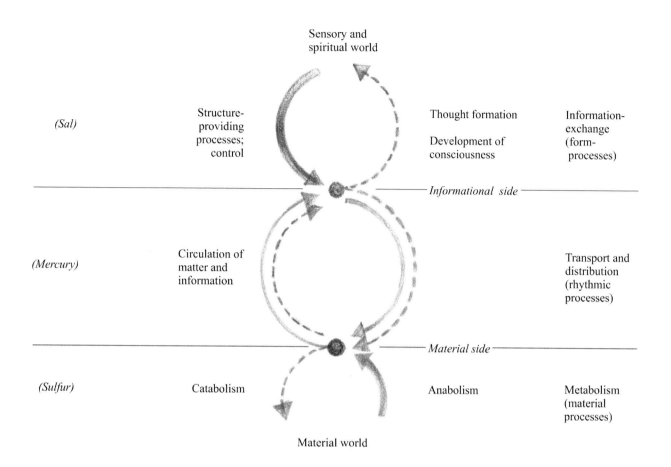

Fig. 6. ***Basic functional processes of the human organism.*** *The body's anabolic and catabolic cycles include two fundamental components, the material component (red), which is derived from the material world (nature, the environment), and the informational (structural) component (blue), which is related to the sensory and spiritual world.*

balance. The compounds in red blood cells, for example—especially hemoglobin with the iron molecule at its center—are largely recycled after being broken down. We know the body is born with almost enough iron to cover the turnover for a lifetime (61)! Cellular protein structures are also constantly being broken down and resynthesized. Life processes, therefore, consist in the constant build-up and breakdown of matter. By and large, this recycling of substances is independent of the outer world (Figure 6). In principle, cyclical

processes of this sort can function completely on their own. They would persist indefinitely were it not for the fact that a small percentage of these substances is always lost in resynthesis and eliminated from the cycle. This small amount must then be replaced from outside. The body is an open system only to this very limited extent.

The dynamics of life's cyclical processes can be altered both by the "pull" of elimination and by the "push" on the supply end. Unusable matter "drops out" of these cycles in a process comparable to entropy in the inanimate natural world, although the waste products that accumulate in the body (especially as we age) generally possess a higher level of organization than the substances still involved in the cycle. If its life processes are arranged in such cyclical systems, why can't the body survive completely on its own? Why is perpetual motion ultimately not possible in this case? This riddle is related to the very nature of our evolution on Earth.

The body consists of many individual systems, each of which incorporates a number of cyclical functions. Each cell controls its own anabolic and catabolic processes, but unless it develops into a cancer cell, it is also integrated into the processes of higher-ranking systems. A hierarchy of smaller and larger systems emerges, with each one concentrating on a single function or group of functions that the overall system performs.

Nowadays we tend to explain all higher-ranking systems in terms of processes that take place in cells, i.e., in terms of the molecular level or the least common denominator. We are satisfied when we are able to identify the molecular or cellular processes that occur even in psychological activity and even see them as viable, fully satisfactory explanations for all processes taking place within the body. Basically, however, we are only describing the mechanisms used to actualize certain functions. Molecules say nothing about the qualitative aspects of these functions. We will arrive at a deeper understanding of life functions only when we learn to assess them with respect to the body in its entirety, that is, when we stop attempting to arrive at the whole by beginning with reductionist minutiae. Let's see what happens when we take the opposite approach: we will attempt to understand the whole before proceeding to the parts. (Hearkening back to Goethe, we will call this path—*from the whole to the parts*—the Goethean approach.) We will discover that the whole is reflected in all subsequent structures in the hierarchy. We will maintain a view of the phenomenon as a whole, regardless of what level we are on, so that mechanical explanations become superfluous. For as we mentioned above, Goethe rightly said, "Do not look **behind** the phenomena, for they themselves are the theory."

In other words, we allow the phenomenon to explain itself and refrain from "taking it apart" in our attempt to find an unknown causative element secretly at work in the darkness "behind" it.

Basic Functions in the Human Body

If we look at the body as a whole, we will be struck by the fact that only three basic functions are present, regardless of whether we are considering the cellular level, the level of organs, or even organ systems. These functions are adapted to suit each level, of course, but always in a way that does justice to their essential character (Figure 6).

The first of these functions involves the body's ability to process information (signals or stimuli). In the body, *exchange of information* is needed to control organ functions and maintain structures. Traffic lights are "signs" that serve the orderly flow of traffic. Although some energy is required to work the lights, their essential feature is the signal (red, green, etc.). Of course a signal must be perceived; in the body, this is done by the appropriate receptors. Thus information processes are largely independent of matter. In this function, exchanges of signals or information rather than exchanges of substances play the primary role. But architecture or structure is also inherently informational. The structures of cells and tissues result in spaces and compartments in which substances are transformed through processes of a completely different type. In the flow of life, therefore, structure is the resting pole, the ordering and form-maintaining principle. The more complex the structure, the higher the degree of order and the greater the amount of information present. Information can be compared to negative entropy, which passes over into entropy when it is lost. Above all, being alive means counteracting entropy, maintaining the structure of organs and tissues right down to the smallest detail. Thus the basic informational function encompasses not only information exchange within the organism (which is needed to control life processes and is accomplished primarily by the nervous system) but also structure-building and structure-maintaining processes in general. These processes shape the internal architecture of the body and its parts and thus make our life on earth altogether possible. In contrast to the material function, we could call this the "structuring function" or "formative function."

Everything having to do with matter, with substance as such, must be seen in utter contrast to the formative function—in fact, as its polar opposite. The best architectural plan is useless if the house is never built. To make a form a reality, the body needs matter for "building blocks." The second major function, therefore, is the transformation of substances, or **metabolism.** The principles that apply to this function are totally different from those governing information exchange. Whereas informational processes always tend to come to rest in forms or structures, material processes manifest in change and transformation. The informational element is the "immaterial" principle, and the metabolic element is the material principle, no less difficult to understand than the first. If information equals order, then matter equals energy. Substance conversion, therefore, always implies energy conversion. To revisit the traffic metaphor, the signals control traffic, but the traffic itself is made up of the movements of individual vehicles, which need energy in order to move. What is surprising about the living body is its use and reuse of matter—anabolism and catabolism are united in a cyclical process that requires energy to remain in motion. Substance conversions, therefore, are primary life processes that exist for their own sake. The image of cars in traffic would be truly apt only if cars not only moved (energy conversion) but also were constantly rebuilt, altered, and restructured (metabolism), with new parts being substituted for old and elements constructed in one place being reused elsewhere. With regard to matter, therefore, the human body is a constantly self-altering structure. Proteins, for example, although constantly broken down into their constituent amino acids, are then immediately resynthesized. This balance is almost always maintained; it is disrupted only in cases of illness such as cancer, which then result in loss of weight. The other substances that make up the body are also constantly transformed through similar cyclical processes. The scope and

speed of these regulatory cycles depends on the amount of energy applied to them. The "wheels turn faster" during the growth spurts of childhood but more slowly with advancing age. Under stressful conditions, the conversion process may accelerate, increasing energy consumption; body mass is then sacrificed to supply energy.

It should be apparent by now that we do not see the metabolic function as restricted to the metabolic system. Like the informational process, it is a capability common to all of the body's cells and organs (15).

The third and final basic function involves **rhythmic or periodic processes.** It is easy to see that the material and informational processes are polar opposite in character. When material processes dominate, structure is lost; when structures harden, material activity is lost. These two basic functions need each other. They appear together in every cell, organ, and tissue. But a third element arises to maintain harmony and balance between them. As a rule, this element is periodic or rhythmic in character. The body's life can be maintained only through an alternation of sleeping and waking, catabolism and anabolism, inhalation and exhalation, systole and diastole— that is, through the rhythmically structured oscillation of form-providing (informational) and materially determined (metabolic) processes. All rhythmic functions, which are most predominant in the cardiovascular and respiratory systems, are inherently healing and ordering. Since antiquity, the organs of breathing and circulation have been considered the prototype of the body's rhythmic system.

As early as the Middle Ages, the alchemists and Paracelsus (among others) were already aware of the significance of these three basic physiological systems, which they called the Sal, Sulfur, and Mercury processes. They understood Sal as the tendency toward hardening, salt formation, and structural definition—the formative, informational element, as it were. Sulfur was understood as chemical conversion, which is always linked to the transformation of matter and the release of energy. Sulfur encompassed not only actual combustion but also the transformation of matter, the metabolic process as such. Mercury,

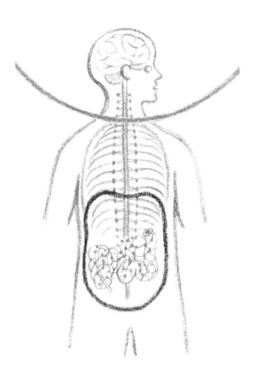

A. The sensory-nervous system

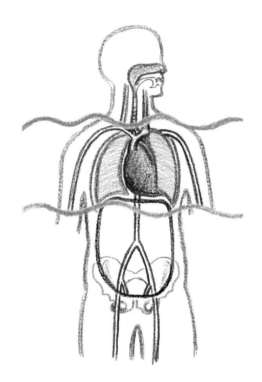

B. The rhythmic system

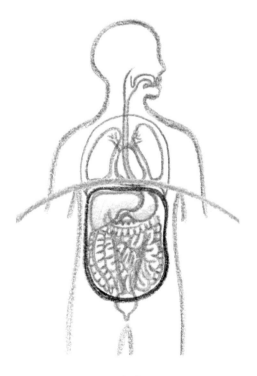

C. The metabolic system

*Fig. 7 A-C. **Functional threefoldness of the human body.** Each of the body's three major functional systems is centered in one of the three body cavities but also extends into other parts of the body.*

Basic functions	Basic physiological processes		
	From the outside in	Internal	From the inside out
1. Information processes	Reception of stimuli (perception)	Processing of stimuli (information exchange)	Response to stimuli
2. Rhythmic processes	Inspiration (inhalation)	Gaseous exchange (respiration)	Expiration (exhalation)
	Influx of blood	Transport and distribution (circulation)	Outflow of blood
3. Metabolic processes	Ingestion (digestion)	Nutrient processing (metabolism)	Elimination (excretion)

Table 1. Basic functions of the organism.
Functional threefoldness of basic processes in the human body.

quicksilverlike and mobile, constituted the middle, rhythmic element in this trinity, inserted between the polar opposites of Sal and Sulfur as a balancing and linking element. Nowadays we have lost all understanding of these more qualitative concepts, but we must admit nonetheless that the scientists of bygone times were essentially accurate in their characterizations of the basic processes of life, even though their thinking was still wholly instinctive and not yet rational.

The Functional Threefoldness of the Human Body

Essentially, the three basic functions described above occur in every cell of the body and are evident even in single-celled living things such as amoebas. Among multicellular organisms (metazoans), the differentiation and specialization of organ systems for these three functions culminates in the functional threefolding of the human body. **Information exchange** takes place primarily in the nervous system. Within this system, we must once again distinguish three basic processes: *intake of information*, for which the sensory organs have been especially developed;

information processing, which is performed by nervous tissue (nerve cells, etc.) concentrated in the brain or other centers; and finally, *response to stimulus*, which occurs with the help of the nerve fibers and sensory terminals that ultimately exercise neural control over all biological processes. In humans in particular, the information exchange system is highly differentiated and is concentrated in the head, which houses not only the major sensory organs (ears, eyes, etc.; see Figure 7A) but also the brain, in the cranial cavity. The brain is connected to the spinal cord, which is encased in the vertebral column. The spinal cord in turn is connected to extensive neural networks that extend into the internal organs (the so-called autonomic nervous system). In this way, the entire organism is pervaded with nerve tissue. But only the central nervous system, which is concentrated in the head, forms the physical basis of our everyday consciousness. The activity of the peripheral (vegetative) networks remains unconscious. Thus we can say that the organ system that specializes in information exchange is located primarily in the head.

In contrast, the organ system that specializes primarily in *metabolic functions* is concentrated in the abdomen and the pelvic cavity. Most notably, the metabolic system includes the gastrointestinal

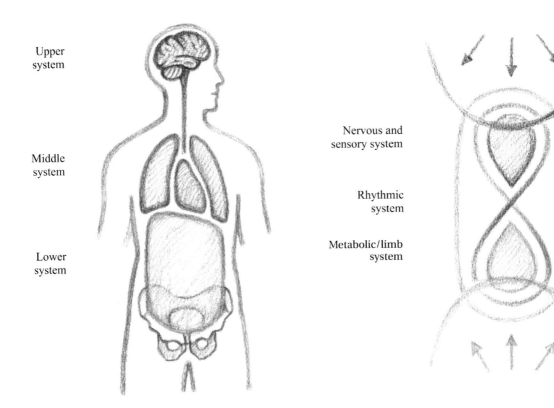

Fig. 7 D. **The functional threefoldness of the human body.** *The two polar functional systems—the information system (brain and sensory organs) and the metabolic/ limb system (abdominal organs and extremities)— are connected, harmonized, and balanced by the organs with rhythmic functions (respiratory system, cardiovascular system).*

Upper system: *nervous system and sensory organs (blue, concentrated in the head);* **middle system**: *rhythmic (cardiovascular and respiratory) system (red, concentrated in the chest);* **lower system**: *metabolism and limbs (green, concentrated in the abdominal cavity and extremities).*

tract and related organs (liver, pancreas, etc.) and also the organs of excretion (kidneys and urinary tract) (Figure 7C). In this system matter is **ingested** and **digested** (oral cavity, digestive tract), **metabolized** (liver, gall bladder) and finally **eliminated** (rectum, renal system). Again, we note three distinct basic functions, as we saw in the nervous system, but with a different emphasis (Table 1). We never become conscious of most of these processes.

The **rhythmic** or **periodically recurrent processes** comprise the third group of basic functions in the body. The circulatory and respiratory systems in particular have specialized

in these processes, and their main organs are housed in the middle of the body, in the chest cavity (Figure 7B). Purely by virtue of location, therefore, these systems occupy an intermediate position between the informational and metabolic systems. Their rhythmically occurring processes are also divided into three basic functions. In the case of the respiratory system, these functions are **inhalation** (air intake), **respiration** (exchange of respiratory gases in the lungs and body tissues), and **exhalation** (elimination of respiratory gases). Three basic functions can also be ascribed to the circulatory system, which is a transport and distribution system that moves fluids rather than air. *Influx* and *outflow* are its polar basic processes. Its central organ is the heart, which manages the *distribution and flow* of blood. The heart's regulatory influence is felt all the way to the peripheral vessels (capillaries) with their influx and outflow functions (Table 1).

How can we sum up this overall situation? We might call the part of the body that specializes primarily in informative functions the "head person," the part that assumes primarily rhythmic functions the "chest person," and the metabolically specialized part the "belly person" (Figure 7D). A nomenclature that refers directly to the systems themselves, however, would be less subject to misinterpretation. Since most energy conversion takes place in the limbs, they belong primarily to the metabolic system, so in very general terms we can speak of a "metabolic-limb system." The "rhythmic system" would consist of the cardiovascular and respiratory systems, and the "sensory-nervous system" of the nervous system, sensory organs, and all other regulatory organs. Referring to the areas of the body dominated by these systems, we might simply call them the upper, middle, and lower systems or functional domains. To be very brief, we might simply refer to the pole of form and the pole of matter. These various nomenclatures cover different aspects of the human body's functional threefoldness as first described by Rudolf Steiner (18).

Surprisingly, this trinity of functions is found not only at the level of the major organ systems but also on the level of individual organs and tissues and even at the cellular level. Thus it appears that threefoldness is a fundamental structural principle of human morphology. The body is not a homogeneous organization of cells but rather a hierarchically structured system, like nesting boxes, whose organ systems are threefold on every organizational level. (In the late 19th century, R.P.H. Heidenhain coined the term "enkapsis" to indicate the relationship between an organism as a whole and its relatively independent organs.) Essentially, there is no such thing in the body as an independent individual cell. Each cell is part of a functionally subdivided cell association and would not survive without the support of the

connective tissue in the surrounding extracellular matrix. Cancer cells, which are the only cells that isolate themselves from the system and initiate an "egotistical" life of their own, become increasingly malignant as their isolation (i.e., dedifferentiation) increases. Cell associations together with affiliated extracellular structures are called tissues. Multiple tissues constitute an organ, and multiple organs are grouped together in organ systems.

If we consider the major *organ systems* from the perspective of threefolding, we find that the basic functions are also reflected in them. Each one is structured in a way that also reflects the same three functional principles. Thus the nervous system, for example, consists of three major functional domains (Table 2). In the *sensorium* (the sensory organs with related areas of the brain), the "form pole" predominates. The segmentally (rhythmically) divided *sensory-motor domain* (the spine and spinal nerves) represents the rhythmic element within the nervous system. Finally, the *autonomic (vegetative) nervous system*, found on the periphery, is functionally associated with the metabolic system. Similarly, the circulatory system is easily divisible into a *peripheral domain* (terminal vessels, capillaries), where exchange of substances predominates; a *middle (rhythmic) domain* (arteries, veins), where transport processes occupy the foreground; and finally, a *central domain* (heart), where regulatory and informational processes (redistribution of blood, etc.) determine physiological events.

Unless we define the respiratory system very narrowly—i.e., as consisting only of the respiratory tract—we also find functional threefolding there. Respiration (gaseous exchange) takes place in every cell and every organ. The lungs and respiratory passages merely mediate and rhythmically organize this all-pervasive respiratory activity. We might say that the lungs are the organizing, regulating "head" of the system as a whole, the respiratory passages its middle domain, and tissue respiration its lower or metabolic domain.

In similar fashion, the metabolic-limb system also exhibits functional threefolding. The

Organ system		Upper domain (form pole)	Middle (rhythmic) domain	Lower domain (substance pole)
1. Nerve-sense system		Brain, sensory organs	Spinal cord	Autonomic nervous system
2. Rhythmic system	Respiratory system	Lungs	Respiratory tract	Gaseous exchange in tissues
	Circulatory system	Heart	Blood vessels (arteries, veins)	Blood, terminal vessels, capillaries
3. Metabolic system		Gastrointestinal tract	Abdominal organs (liver, kidneys, etc.)	Organs of locomotion

Table 2. Functional threefolding of the three major functional systems (cf. Table 1, p. 19).

gastrointestinal tract is the center of this system's physiological activity. This is where the system borders on the outer world (as the sensory-nervous system does in the head). Ultimately, the intestines determine which substances are absorbed and processed and which are not. Metabolism itself (exchange of substances) takes place in all tissues, but especially in the limbs (muscles, blood formation in marrow, etc.). The mediation and regulation of substance flows within the organism occur primarily in the major organs (liver, kidneys). The liver's circadian rhythm, for example, with its rhythmic oscillation between gall secretion and the synthesis of substances, demonstrates how strongly the middle system influences liver functions.

The Functional Threefoldness of the Cell

Even the cell, the body's smallest functional unit, is functionally threefold (Figure 8). Although cells have no nervous, intestinal, or circulatory systems, the three basic functions are still relatively easy to discover (cf. especially reference 17).

Each cell is capable of taking in substances from its surroundings, transforming (even "digesting") them, and eliminating end products.

Complex cellular processes such as endocytosis, exocytosis, and phagocytosis specialize in these metabolic functions. The cell's main "digestive" organs are the lysosomes. Substance exchanges take place in the cytoplasm (Figure 8C). Energy expenditures are required to maintain vital differences in chemical concentrations between cells and their surroundings. At death, these cellular activities cease and concentration differences are equalized. Anabolism on the cellular level is served by the endoplasmic reticulum, where protein biosynthesis occurs in intimate connection with the DNA of the cell nucleus. The cell's movement system consists of the cytoskeleton (which includes a variety of fibrous components), microtubules, centrioles, and contractile elements.

The second major group of functions involves informational processes, that is, the cell's mechanisms of perception and regulation. The cell membranes with their receptor molecules play a leading role in perception (Figure 8A). Intracellular controls originate in the nucleus with its chromosomes (DNA, RNA, etc.), which contain the information that guides protein biosynthesis. The so-called "second messenger system," which conveys signals from the cell membrane to the interior and to the nucleus, plays an important role in integrating individual cells into higher order tissues and organs.

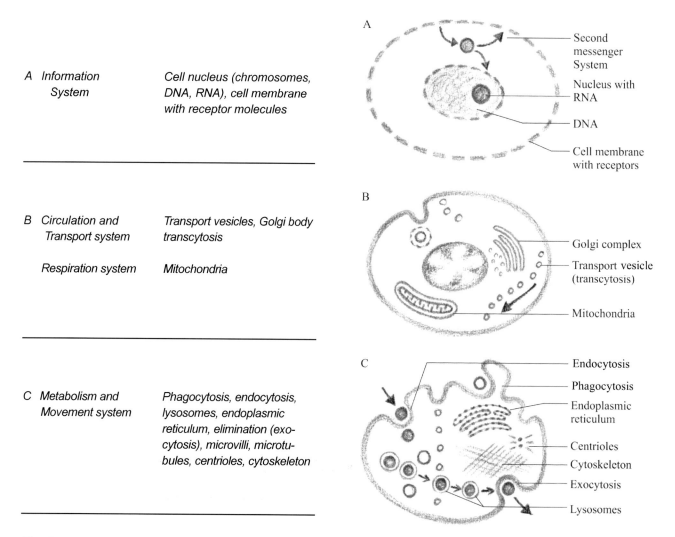

A Information System	*Cell nucleus (chromosomes, DNA, RNA), cell membrane with receptor molecules*
B Circulation and Transport system	*Transport vesicles, Golgi body transcytosis*
Respiration system	*Mitochondria*
C Metabolism and Movement system	*Phagocytosis, endocytosis, lysosomes, endoplasmic reticulum, elimination (exocytosis), microvilli, microtubules, centrioles, cytoskeleton*

*Fig. 8. **Functional threefoldness of the cell.** The cell develops specialized organs for each of the three basic functions (metabolism, information exchange, rhythmical transport and distribution). Thus the threefold functional structure of the organism as a whole is also reflected on the cellular level.*

Within the cell, the organelles mediate between informational and metabolic processes just as the rhythmic system does for the entire body (Figure 8B). In certain respects, the Golgi complex, for example, can be seen as the "heart" of the cellular transport system. Vesicles coming from the membrane or the endoplasmic reticulum accumulate in the Golgi complex; after a period of structural maturation, they are released back into the cell plasma as transport vesicles. The cell's "middle system" also includes the mitochondria (the cell's "lungs"), where biological oxidation and energy production take place.

Functional Threefoldness and the Human Soul

The next question is, how do the three main bodily functions relate to the basic forces of the human soul, namely, thinking, feeling, and willing? Of course the materialistic view maintains that there is no such thing as a human soul and that in "reality" all apparently psychological phenomena originate in matter and are the "epiphenomena" of material processes. Spiritualists, on the other hand, would say that although the psychospiritual component of the human being is supported by bodily processes, it is not identical to them. In recent times, the most commonly held view has been that psychological experiences are made up of subjective phenomena emanating from neural processes in the brain (see, for example, references 6 and 19). But it makes no sense to say that the soul has its seat in the brain and the rest of the body is totally unrelated to it. Nor is it correct to say that with regard to psychological phenomena, the body serves only as an instrument for the activities of the brain. This theory is totally illogical because there are actually only two alternatives: either *all* parts of the body are "ensouled" or *none* of them are. For one organ (the brain, for example) to be ensouled while all other organs are not would be a contradiction in itself and logically untenable. The widespread misconception that the brain is not only the organ of thinking but also of feeling and willing has developed because we confuse feeling and willing with the process of becoming conscious of them. The brain's physiological processes do indeed allow us to become aware of our own psychological activity, but that activity, far from being based exclusively on brain functions, is based on organ functions throughout the entire body.

As we have already seen, the body as a whole is functionally threefold. In the early twentieth century, this fact had already begun to be associated with specific constitutional types and behaviors. For example, French scientists described three constitutional types that correspond surprisingly well to the three great functional systems described above. These three constitutional types were: the metabolic type (*type digestif*), the nerve type (*type cérébral*), and an intermediate type (*type respiratoire*) dominated by respiratory functions. Kretschmer subsequently elaborated on this theory and was the first to include emotional and mental attributes in addition to body types (20). Kretschmer also recognized three basic types:

1. The *pyknic* type, in which metabolic functions predominate and a tendency toward obesity appears. On the psychological level, joviality, flexibility, and taking pleasure in telling stories are attributes that correspond to the comfortably padded shapes of the pyknic body.

2. The *asthenic* type, characterized by a slender, angular build. Functionally, the nervous system and sensory processes predominate. Ideologies offer these lean types something to sink their teeth into, and asthenics easily become fanatical.

3. The *athletic* type, an intermediate type supported primarily by the rhythmic system. The athletic type tends to have a powerful ribcage and well-developed muscles. As the name suggests, representatives of this type are often athletes with resilient respiratory and circulatory systems (cf. 15).

Kretschmer believed that the psychological idiosyncrasies of each of these three body types were related to a characteristic one-sidedness in organic processes (metabolism, neural regulatory functions, etc.) and that such one-sidedness might also contribute to typical psychopathological phenomena (e.g., psychiatric disorders).

In 1917, (after more than thirty years of work, as he repeatedly emphasized), Rudolf Steiner published his first elaboration of these efforts, offering a more precise description of the connections between bodily and psychological processes (18). According to Steiner's account, *willing* is based primarily on metabolic processes, *cognition* (thinking) on nerve processes, and *feeling* on rhythmical (i.e., circulatory and respiratory) processes in the body. Here are Steiner's own words:

"In looking for the soul's connection to the body, we cannot base our search on Brentano's...classification of psychological experience.... We must take our departure... from the division of psychological experience into cognition, feeling, and willing....

The physical counterparts of the soul activity of cognition are the processes of the nervous system as it extends into the sensory organs on the one hand and the interior organization of the body on the other....Just as cognition relates to nerve activity, we must also relate feeling to the rhythms of life that center on, and are related to, respiration. For our present purposes, we must trace the rhythms of respiration and everything related to them to the body's outermost periphery. ....The soul dwells in feeling when it bases its

Information exchange	Structural and informational processes	Nervous system	Thinking
Rhythm, transport, balance	Rhythmical processes	Circulatory system Respiratory system	Feeling
Metabolism	Substance processes, exchanges of matter and energy	Metabolic system	Willing

Table 3. Basic functional processes of the human body and their relationships to soul functions (18, 23, 24).

activity on the rhythms of respiration, just as it bases its conceptual activity on neurological processes. And with regard to willing, we find that it in turn is supported by metabolic processes. Once again, we must take into account all of their branches and offshoots throughout the body. When we "conceive" of something, the soul's consciousness of this conception is based on a neurological process. Similarly, when we "feel," a modification of the respiratory rhythm occurs, by means of which the feeling is enlivened in the soul, and when we "will," a metabolic process occurs and constitutes the bodily basis for what the soul experiences as will. [Of these three types of experiences,] only the cognition conveyed by the nervous system is present in the soul in full waking consciousness. Ordinarily, our consciousness of everything conveyed by the rhythm of respiration (including all feelings, affects, passions, and so on) is only as strong as our consciousness of dream images. Willing, which is supported by metabolic processes, is not experienced with any greater degree of consciousness than the very dull level of consciousness that is present during sleep. After closer consideration of these issues, we will notice that we experience willing very differently from cognition. We experience the latter as if we were seeing a painted surface, but we experience willing as a black surface within a colored field. What we "see" on the black surface is the absence of color impressions in contrast to its surroundings. Likewise, we "conceive of" willing because within the soul's cognitional experiences there are certain places

where an absence of cognition inserts itself into our fully conscious activity, similar to the way sleep interrupts the conscious course of our life. The full variety of soul experience in cognition, feeling, and willing results from these different levels of conscious activity."

To materialists who attribute soul phenomena exclusively to the workings of matter, we must point out something that is easily ascertained from careful self-observation, namely, that soul activity functions according to laws of its own, which are fundamentally different from those evinced by inanimate matter. A stone falls to the ground because matter is subject to gravity. In the psychological realm, however, gravity has no significance. In thinking, feeling, and willing, human beings can opt out of the Earth's gravitation field at any time, or in other words, "abolish" space. (Think here about the effects of falling in love, or of other joyous experiences on one's inner being.) Furthermore, the "I"-being, the thinking individual, is even capable of influencing—strengthening, weakening, or even completely suppressing—psychological processes. Simply by concentrating on a specific thought, one can enhance psychological excitement to such an extent that physiological processes appear (increased blood pressure, flow of tears, etc.). Conversely, intense thinking can curb or even banish emotional excitement. These observations, which are simply a few examples among very many, prove nothing less than that forces emanating from the "I" outrank psychological and bodily processes and that psychological events are not unconditionally linked to bodily (i.e., material) processes. On the contrary, physiological processes are subject to "higher" forces, and material processes in the human body can even be altered by emotional and mental activity.

The three basic functions of bodily life (metabolism, information exchange, and rhythm or periodicity) have been rediscovered only recently and are gradually being applied to technical ends. In technologies based on pure mechanics, we see the application of laws hidden in the human **metabolism and limb system**. In electronics, which has undergone explosive development in recent decades, technology tackles the opposite dimension, that is, it taps the world of **informational processes**. Although at present they are becoming destructively one-sided, technological advances cannot be restrained. Crises are already looming on the horizon, and technology will transcend them only if it also incorporates the principles governing the human body's third system. Only **rhythmic forces** with their balancing, harmonizing, and healing effects are capable of relieving technology of its destructive one-sidedness, but even they will fail to have a beneficent impact unless we can overcome the fundamental self-serving tendencies and boundless egotism that are omnipresent in our technological culture today.

Structural Principles in the Human Body and Qualities of the Dimensions of Space

Since time immemorial poets and artists have viewed the upright human figure as a symbol of royal dignity and beauty. With its head that appears to float weightlessly atop the slightly S-curved spinal column, its rhythmically segmented ribcage, and its radially extended limbs, the human form seems to embody a sense of grace and harmonious balance. And in fact, the human body is inserted differently into the three dimensions of space than the body of a four-footed mammal, for example. In each of the three dimensions, the human figure reveals a different formative principle related to the qualitative aspects of that dimension (Figures 9 and 10).

The Right-Left Dimension

The plane separating the human body into right and left halves is called the median plane (or, more precisely, the median sagittal plane, from the Latin *sagitta*, arrow). It divides the body into two identical or at least similar halves, which are mirror images of each other. The structural principle at work here is **bilateral symmetry**. The shapes of many invertebrates, such as radiolarians and sea urchins, are based on radial symmetry. As a result, instead of being fully involved in three-dimensional earthly space, they perpetuate a spherical, more unitary structural principle. In contrast, all vertebrates from fish to mammals incorporate bilateral symmetry into their bodily structures. This is the right-left dimension.

It is not easy to grasp the essential character of this structural principle. Basically, anything present on one side is mirrored or repeated on the other without any changes or additions. But the accuracy of any reflected image depends on a static, unchanging reflective surface. A lake can reflect the face of someone bending over it only as long as the water's surface is smooth and motionless. In antiquity, the goddess Athena was usually depicted carrying a shield that reflected the head of Medusa. For the Greeks, the goddess who sprang from the head of Zeus was the image of thoughtful, reflective consciousness. Her reflective shield allowed her to ward off the demonic forces of the subconscious, depicted by the head of the Gorgon Medusa.

Essentially, our sensory organs and nervous system create a reproduction of the outer world through a reflective process. The more we are able to capture the object in the mirror of our consciousness, the truer the resulting image is to the object's essence. Cognition is based primarily on accurate reflections of the outer (or inner)

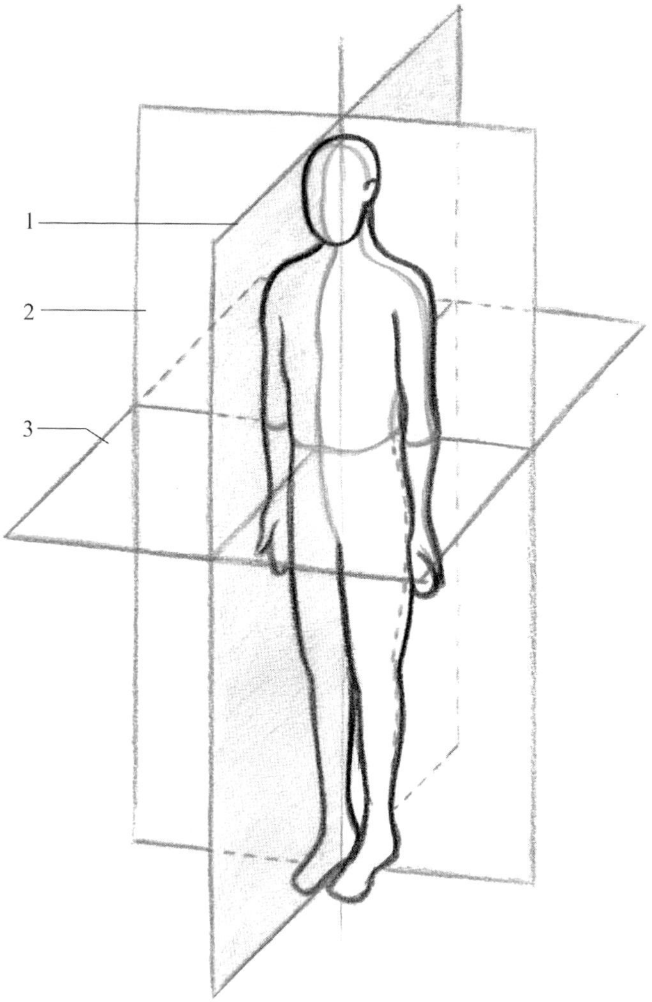

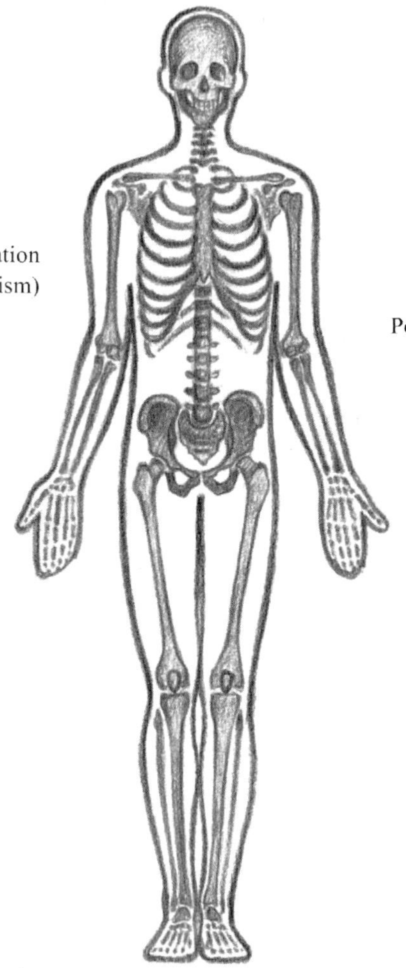

Fig. 9. **The three planes that separate the human body into halves** *(1, 2, 3) subdivide it according to three fundamental structural principles that reappear in the psychological domain.*
1: sagittal (median) plane: the plane separating the body into right and left halves (bilateral symmetry)
2: frontal (coronal) plane: the plane separating the body into anterior and posterior (ventral/dorsal) halves (segmentation principle)
3: transverse or horizontal plane: the plane separating the body into upper and lower halves (polarity principle).

Fig. 10. **The human body and its skeletal system.** *The three fundamental structural principles of the space surrounding the upright human being are revealed most impressively in the skeletal system.*

world. We then take hold of these reflections with our thinking and pin them down with concepts.

On the soul-spiritual level, therefore, we might associate the right-left dimension with reflective cognition.

Of the three constitutional types, the asthenic or *type cérébral* is most strongly related to the forces at work in this dimension.

The Up-down Dimension

The up-down or vertical dimension reveals a fundamentally different structural principle. The human being enters the vertical dimension by standing upright, with the spherical head directed toward the cosmos above and the radially structured limbs toward the Earth below. In the upper part of the body, the sphere is the dominant shape. The skull that encloses the brain is approximately spherical. The rounded eye socket encloses the spherical organ of sight and its appendages, and the oral and nasal cavities also form spherical enclosures for soft tissues. In contrast, radial shapes dominate in the limbs, which are characterized by linear sequences of elongated forms that become smaller, more polymorphic, and more numerous toward the periphery (Figure 10). In functional terms, immobility predominates in the head and movement in the limbs. We become conscious of the activity of our nervous system but remain largely unaware of our limbs. (Although we become aware of our movements through cognition, the actual processes that take place in our limbs during movement never become conscious.)

By standing upright, we insert ourselves vertically into the Earth's gravitational field. Our lower limbs are fully subject to this gravitational field, but the head is relatively independent of it, a condition that creates the prerequisite for thinking. In the vertical dimension, therefore, the principle of *polarity* dominates. This is the domain of tension between opposites such as gravity and levity, Earth and cosmos, and centrifugal and centripetal forces. It is also the dimension of material processes. Whereas animals live in the horizontal dimension for the most part, the

growth of many plants unfolds primarily in the vertical dimension. Their roots shoot into the ground and develop radial branching patterns, while their flowers, which are often complex in shape and incorporate "headlike" hollow spaces, develop upward into the light and air. In the plant kingdom, therefore, a polarity exists between roots and flowers.

The forces we humans develop in coming to grips with matter are different from those we learned about in connection with the right-left dimension—that is, in the informational domain. On the soul-spiritual level, the force most actively involved with the material world is the will. Our will forces work in the polarity between our experiences of gravity (through the movements of our limbs in three-dimensional space) and of "levity" and freedom in our sense perceptions and ideas. The will aspect of this dimension is clearly apparent in the will-emphasis of stamping our feet or our sense of being released from the Earth in flight. In Goethe's *Faust*, when Mephisto (albeit reluctantly) tells Faust the secret of how to enter the underworld, the realm of the Mothers, he lists three forces that correspond in some ways to our characterization of the three dimensions, namely:

1. the "key"—the informational element, cognition, thinking, etc.;

2. courage, or feeling;

3. will—"stamping descend and stamping rise again." Earlier, Mephisto says, "Sink down, or—I could also tell you—rise, it's all the same." This is the up-down or vertical dimension, in which the will is the primary element at work. Of the three constitutional types, the pyknic or *type digestif* is especially related to the forces of this dimension.

The Front-Back Dimension

Once again, a completely different structural principle is revealed in the third and final dimension, the front-back aspect. Surprisingly, there are no further dimensional structural principles, a fact that can provoke the most profound astonishment and contemplation. Here, we are dealing with one of the mysteries of the universe.

The human torso takes shape primarily in the front-back dimension (Figure 11). Here the corresponding structural principle is most clearly expressed. The torso consists of a number of uniform or similar elements or *segments*. In each section of the spine, the segments are essentially similar in structure. For example, in the chest we find twelve pairs of ribs that correspond to twelve thoracic vertebrae in the back. On either side, each vertebra is attached to a rib that curves around to the front. Each segment also includes a bundle of blood vessels and nerves as well as a muscular component. The intercostal muscles run between the ribs and are arranged in more or less the same way in each segment. So are the spinal nerves that emerge from the spinal cord, which is also segmental in structure. The neck and the lumbar region also consist of segments that are basically similar in structure. A frontal plane (plane 2 in Figure 9) divides each segment into front and back sections (Figure 12). The back section forms the neural space enclosing the spinal cord; the significantly larger front section forms the ribcage, which houses the internal organs in the chest and abdominal cavities.

The repetition of identical or similar segments is called *metamerism*, a structural principle that is especially pronounced in reptiles such as snakes. In humans, who walk upright, the principle of polarity significantly modifies the structure of the segments closer to the body's poles (head and limbs). Toward the top of the ribcage, for example, the shape of the bones becomes increasingly closed and more "headlike." Toward the bottom, the ribs open up and become more radial or "limblike" in shape. The lumbar vertebrae preserve mere rudiments of ribs in the form of short transverse processes. The five vertebrae of the sacral region fuse into a single structure (Figure 11). In the area of the abdominal wall, the intercostal muscles also lose their segmented character and fuse into broad muscle plates (the oblique and transverse abdominal muscles). Thus metamerism acquires aspects of the upper pole as the segments

approach the head and of the lower pole below. The structural tendencies that appear in the upper torso are more headlike in character, while in the lower torso the tendencies of the limbs and metabolic region come to the fore. In other words, the metameric structural principle occupies an intermediate position between the two other principles. At the same time, it incorporates the archetypal rhythmic or periodic element that unites space and time.

A polarity also exists between the front and back portions of each segment, which are separated by the frontal plane (Figure 12). The neural space at the back encloses the spinal cord and the roots of the spinal nerves. Functionally, it is still part of the head pole. The internal organ cavity in front (the ribcage) houses the metabolic organs as well as the heart and lungs. In contrast to the up-down dimension, in which sphere and radii or neural space and metabolic space are quite far apart, in the front-back aspect of the torso the polar portions of each segment form a structural unity in a single plane. As an image for this situation, we might choose the lemniscate, a special form of Cassini curve (Figure 12). The lemniscate is perhaps the most rhythmical of all geometric forms. The essential aspect of the body's structure in the front-back dimension consists in uniting the polar structural principles into a single functional entity in the same plane, i.e., in the same segment. Consequently, the metamerically segmented torso includes all three structural principles—bilateral symmetry, polarity, and metamerism—and can therefore be considered the core of the human body's structure.

The corresponding soul element is feeling, which lies between will and cognition and always abuts on one of these two poles. Semi-conscious, dreamlike feeling oscillates between the unconscious world of pure will and the conscious activity of cognition.

Of the three constitutional types, the athletic type or *type respiratoire* develops this aspect of human existence to the greatest extent.

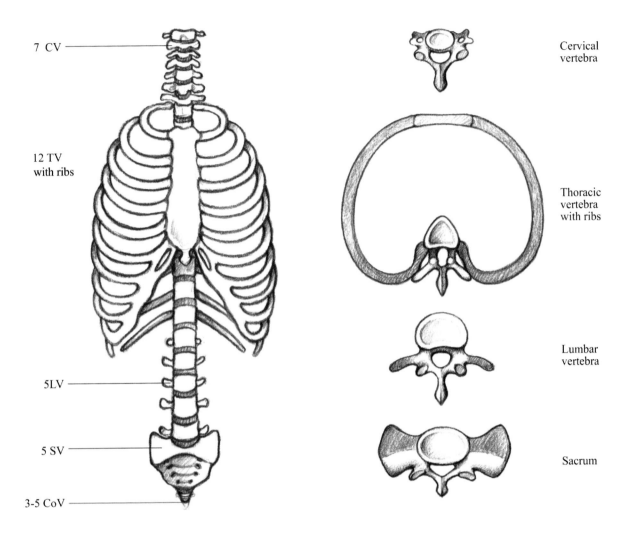

7 CV

12 TV
with ribs

5LV

5 SV

3-5 CoV

Cervical
vertebra

Thoracic
vertebra
with ribs

Lumbar
vertebra

Sacrum

*Fig. 11. **Metameric organization of the torso.** Toward the top, the ribcage assumes a more "headlike" (closed) form; toward the bottom, it is more "limblike" (open). In the neck and the lumbar region, the ribs are mere rudiments (red). In the sacrum, five vertebrae fuse into a single bone.*

CV :   *cervical (neck) vertebrae*
TV :   *thoracic (chest) vertebrae*
LV: *lumbar vertebrae*
SV: *sacral vertebrae*
CoV: *coccygeal vertebrae*

Functional Differentiations Within Dimensional Structural Principles

In the human body, neither the rhythmical segmentation nor the polarity that prevails between above and below nor the mirror-image similarity between right and left halves is ever realized in pure form. All three structural principles always work together; each one is merely dominant in its respective plane, as described above. Ultimately, the lively interaction of these three principles is what creates the great variety of phenomena encountered in the structure of the human body.

For example, **bilateral symmetry** is not realized with equal consistency throughout the body. It is clearly apparent in the skeletal system but less prominent in the organs that occupy the three body cavities. In the skull, the brain is largely symmetrical in structure (left and right hemispheres), and the major sensory organs (eyes, ears) are also symmetrically arranged. In the mouth, however, this symmetrical arrangement is partially abandoned in favor of a single central cavity with no dividing wall. In the chest, the lungs are roughly symmetrical in structure, but the heart falls out of the plane of symmetry because it tilts and is displaced slightly to the left, although the organ itself is bilaterally symmetrical in structure (right and left chambers).

In the abdominal cavity, the major organs of the metabolic system (gastrointestinal tract, liver, pancreas, spleen) are bilaterally symmetrical during embryonic development. Later, however, organ-specific rotations and displacements create asymmetries. In adults, the liver is ultimately located primarily on the right side, the spleen and stomach in the left half of the abdominal cavity. Only in the urogenital system (kidneys, ovaries, testes, etc.) is the original bilateral symmetry largely preserved.

Moving from top to bottom, we see that bilateral symmetry is increasingly abandoned. What is the deeper meaning of this phenomenon? In functional terms, the two halves of the body are very different, not merely mirror images of each other. In several respects, a polarity also exists between right and left. Thus the limbs of the right half of the body are usually stronger and more active, at least in right-handed people, who tend to perform skilled activities with the right hand, while the left hand aids and supports it. We turn inward on the left but outward, toward the world, on the right.

The brain also exhibits a distinct polarity between right and left. In right-handed people, the left hemisphere (which is associated with the right side of the body due to the crossing of major nerve tracts) is the dominant, outward-directed side. It makes possible analytical, detail-oriented cognition related to the world around us. Since the speech centers are located in the left hemisphere, our outward-directed ideas are often verbal in character, with definitions and verbal concepts playing a

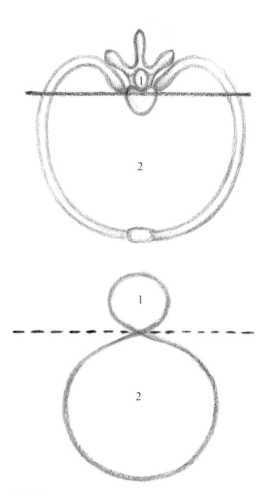

Fig. 12. **Structure of a complete torso segment.** *Anteriorly, the interior cavity (e.g., ribcage) is surrounded by the ribs (2); posteriorly, the laminae of the vertebral arch form the vertebral canal for the spinal cord (1). Thus each torso segment assumes the form of a lemniscate, the archetypal image of the rhythmic element.*

decisive role. In contrast, the right hemisphere (which belongs to the left side of the body) makes possible a more pictorial, holistic, synthesizing cognition that is nonverbal in character and delves more deeply into the essence of things. The left half of the brain counts the trees, so to speak, while the right half experiences the forest as a whole. This phenomenon is known as the dichotomy or lateralization of the brain. Clearly, the two sides of the brain must work together if we are to understand

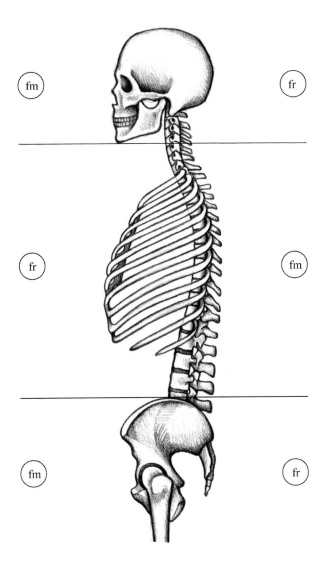

Front ←— ‖ —→ Back

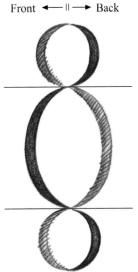

the world in its essential character. The inherent differences between right and left give rise to a tension that creates a differentiated consciousness and thus also allows us to experience ourselves in the world in an active, living way that could not be achieved through a purely reflective (and therefore dead) process.

Now we understand why the level of consciousness with which we experience bodily functions declines from top to bottom as bilateral symmetry is increasingly abandoned (as in the abdominal cavity, for example). The urogenital system, whose organs are mostly arranged in bilateral symmetry, seems to constitute an exception. In the events of procreation, however, consciousness again appears, although it is not centered on the individual organs themselves. In the metabolic domain we find ourselves in the realm of the unconscious or subconscious. But the more we move upward (toward the head), the brighter our consciousness becomes and the more strongly the structural principle of bilateral symmetry emerges.

Because the segmented torso is located between the head and the limbs in the vertical dimension, characteristic variations also develop among the front-back planes of the segments. Toward the top, the segments become more headlike—that is, the influence of the spherical structural principle increases. Toward the bottom, the impact of the radial principle of the limbs increases: the ribs become limblike rods, and muscles fuse into larger entities.

The principle of polarity, however, also expresses itself in the front-back dimension of each segment in a variety of ways. As we have already described, the segmented anterior wall of the torso encloses the internal organs, where metabolic processes take place, whereas the neural space at the back houses the spinal cord,

*Fig. 13. **Side view of the skeleton.** The qualitative aspect of the forces of form reverses itself twice in the front-back dimension (for details, see text). Blue: form at rest (fr); red: form in motion (fm).*

which is part of the information system (Figure 12). Thus each lemniscate-shaped torso segment mediates between the body's two polar processes. The portion of each segment that belongs to the neurological system can be seen as the more structured and highly organized part, whereas the front portion, which is more closely associated with the internal organs, is less formed (Figure 13). The ventral (front) side presents the body's softer, more sensitive, and less structured aspect. Even though the rhythmic movements of respiration take place here, the morphological differentiation is relatively slight. In contrast, the posterior aspect of the torso is inherently more highly formed and organized simply by virtue of the back's many muscular and bony components.

If we consider the head-limbs relationship from this perspective, we discover a double reversal of structural principles in the body (Figure 13). In the head, the less divided, more enclosed portion that corresponds to the rounded, protective abdomen lies in back, not in front, while the face, which lies in front, is more similar to the back in its level of complexity and expressiveness. The same is true of the limbs: the dynamic, constantly changing forms that bring about movement are more evident in front, in our field of sight, where grasping occurs. In the posteriorly located pelvic girdle, very little movement is possible. Thus, within the three main regions of the body (head, torso, and limbs), two reversals of the front-back polarity occur—once in the transition from head to torso and once in the transition from torso to limbs (Figure 13).

This phenomenon leads us to still another important connection. The right-left dimension is virtually static. Internally, the body's two sides are somewhat morphologically differentiated, but on the exterior they are mirror images of each other. As has been indicated, this reflecting quality is related to the development of consciousness. The up-down dimension is also not truly dynamic, since we seldom move vertically. Its dynamic lies more in the long-term metamorphosis of inside to outside, in the materialization and dematerialization of substance, i.e., in the processes of incarnation and excarnation and thus in the totality of evolution.

In contrast, the front-back dimension is the actual dimension of human activity. In front of us lies our active domain, which we perceive through our sensory organs and grasp with our limbs. In the head, sense organs and apertures are located in front. This is where we are open to the world around us and communicate with it through speech and mimicry. In contrast, the posterior aspect of the head consists of the enclosed skull and, in a somewhat animallike gesture, is still covered with hair. With the help of our brain, we process sense impressions, plan our actions, and become self-aware. In the head's front-back dimension, therefore, the outer (foreign) world and the inner (personal) world are polar opposites. Our cognitive activity takes place between these two poles.

The situation is very different in the torso, where the protected cavity that houses the internal organs lies anteriorly. The rhythmical movements of the ribcage serve respiration and (indirectly) circulation. The chest and abdominal cavity house almost all of the organs of metabolism, circulation, and respiration, without which we would be unable to maintain our earthly existence. In the torso, the midsection of the body, life processes occur rhythmically. Here we find the actual human domain, where the rhythmical processes of the heart and lungs create space for our feelings in which we experience our autonomous sense of self. The posterior aspect of the torso is quite different, i.e., much more highly structured. Its many small muscles move highly differentiated little vertebral joints and thus provide the foundation for limb movements, which always originate in the torso. In a certain respect, therefore, the back is the torso's "face."

In the limbs, a second reversal occurs. Here, the relatively undifferentiated and immobile forms corresponding to the dome of the skull are once again posterior, namely, the pectoral and pelvic girdles, which support the mobile limbs. The limbs' primary field of movement and activity lies anteriorly, in the visual field, where we can effectively use gestures and signs to support mimicry. Thus the "face" of the limbs is in front, where our hands and feet move and interact. In contrast, the dorsally located pectoral and

	Dimension	Plane of separation	Structural principle	Functional domain	Psychological domain*
1.	Right-left	Median sagittal	Bilateral symmetry	Information processes	Cognition
2.	Front-back	Frontal, through the vertebrae	Metamerism, segmentation	Rhythmical processes	Feeling
3.	Up-down	Horizontal, through the body's center	Polarity	Material processes	Willing

*Table 4. Structural principles governing the human organism, with their relationships to the three dimensions of space and the basic soul forces. * cf. Steiner (22).*

pelvic girdles are more comparable to the less differentiated, resting form of the back of the head. The posterior aspect of the pelvic area is almost "headlike" in the spherical forms of the buttocks, while the more differentiated shapes of the pubic bone and reproductive organs are located anteriorly.

In the polarity between front and back lies the contrast between movement and rest, day and night, extroversion and introversion. It is almost symbolic that we take to the horizontal position—the dorsal side of existence, so to speak—when we sleep but revert to uprightness on awakening so that our limbs and sense organs have access to the space of their daily activity, which lies in front of us. This rhythmic alternation of waking and sleeping reveals their "metameric" character. Our consciousness, like our activity, is discontinuous. Thus our life is centered on a "segmental" or rhythmic structure that ensues quite naturally from its mediating position between the forces at work in the two other dimensions.

The double reversal of structural relationships in the front-back dimension was already known to Plato (21). In a quasi-mythological account, he describes how human beings once possessed a more spherical form, but when they became too powerful for the gods, the gods cut them down the middle, from top to bottom. But for humans to be able to make love and procreate, their heads and genitals had to be turned to the front so that the two halves would fit together again and form a whole.

The Temporal Structure Of the Human Body— Qualitative Aspects of Space and Time

In connection with our discussion of the concept of space and how the human body is inserted into its three dimensions, we must also briefly consider the concept of time and human life within it.

In space, we experience the *impenetrability* of material objects: each body occupies a space that no other body can occupy at the same time. Where one body is, no other body can be. In contrast, time—which has to do with changes in space—falls into the category of movement. All growth and development (and ultimately, all life processes) take place in time and come to rest in space (23). In morphology, time and space reappear as function and form. In a functional process, a static, "coagulated" form becomes dynamic. In other words, it becomes involved in a time process, which then enables us to understand it in its living context. The human body's shape, size, and structure change over time. Development, aging, and death proceed according to specific temporal rhythms. Spatial structures move in time.

If space and time exist, it follows logically that there must also be nontime and nonspace, or counterspace (128). We can describe this condition as "eternity." In the corporeal world, we extrapolate time from spatial changes in our surroundings (the movement of the sun, the expansion of particles of matter, etc.). The resulting linear concepts, however, apply only to the spatial world, where time is quantified. Here, we are subject to the illusion that time consists of measurable and reproducible equal parts (time quanta). But even in the plant and animal kingdoms, this linear arrangement is inadequate. In the realm of living processes, periods of longer and shorter duration alternate, and rhythms, repetitions, and reversals appear. Rapid evolution may be followed by phases of involution or metamorphosis—in other words, by stages of apparent rest that conceal a great deal of activity. The temporal rhythms (rhythmical time) analyzed by the modern branch of science known as chronobiology have their own laws and can no longer be measured according to linear benchmarks (23, 24).

Earlier cultures often had concepts of time that were fundamentally different from ours. For example, Robert Aaron writes:

> For the Romans and all subsequent technocrats who became their highly visible, virtually omnipotent progeny, culture's justification for existing is the conquest of space or its subjugation to time. For the Jews of Jesus's time, the purpose of every spiritual deed was to sanctify time. "We all live in time," writes Abraham Heschel, "and very nearly identify with it to such an extent that we almost do not notice it at all. The spatial world surrounds our life, but it brings us nothing that is indispensable to us and that we could not do without. We are even free to change our location in space. Existence does not necessarily imply a spatial fortune, but the years of our life are of absolute importance to us. Time is the only possession that we really use, and we use it so naturally that becoming aware of it at all requires an effort. Spatial things lie on the shore, but our journey takes place in time. (25)

On the *soul level*, time ultimately loses its identity (dynamic time); under certain circumstances, it can be suspended completely. On this level, therefore, our experience of time can no longer be measured linearly. We may experience a great deal in a split second of intense experience or have very few significant experiences (or even none at all) for hours on end. In decisive moments of our life, our experience of time may be extremely compressed. The soul realm, therefore, represents a transition between the earthly categories of space and time and the spiritual category of "eternity."

Just as space has three dimensions, time also has three qualitatively different stages: past, present, and future. We live in the present and cannot directly observe either the future or the past. As St. Augustine astutely acknowledged, we recognize the past only through images that exist in the present ("the past in the present") and the

Spirit	"Eternity" Duration					
Soul	Dynamic time	?	?	Cognition	Feeling	Willing
Life	Rhythmical time	Function	Movement	Past	Present	Future
Inanimate world	Space	Form	Extension	Right/left	Front/back	Up/down

Table 5. Elements of space and time as they relate to body, soul, and spirit.

future through ideas and assumptions about what may eventually appear ("the future in the present") (26). The past is finished and has hardened into form; it is closed and cannot be brought back. The future is a mere sprout, the anticipated emergence of something as yet undetermined; it is highly planned and endowed, yet receptive to the new. On the soul level, therefore, the future corresponds to the will element. The past, which reflects things as they have become, is related to cognition; here, everything is reduced to an image. With our will, however, we grasp the future, sowing the seeds of new life and new destiny (27).

How can we characterize the connections between time and space more exactly? We have already recognized a cognitional element in the right/left dimension. Bilateral symmetry, which is based on mirror-image duplication of a phenomenon, represents a process similar to cognition, which reflects and depicts reality. Something similar is true of the character of the past. We might say that when the forces at work in the element of the past become space, the right-left dimension appears. Likewise, will processes, which have to do with the future, find their expression in the up-down dimension of space. And in the living evolution of events, our life in the front-back dimension, as described above, is our "present," in which becoming and passing away, sleeping and waking, evolution and involution alternate rhythmically.

Novalis beautifully characterized the stages of space and time in terms of point, line, plane, and space (see Table 6 below) (28). The four stages in the development of space "emerge simultaneously" with their correspondences in the element of time. The point, or moment, is not-time or not-space, the seed from which the three subsequent stages develop. Human embryonic development is a wonderful reflection of the stages from point to surface (the embryonic disc) and eventually to three-dimensional space (the embryonic body).

d	g	b	a
Space	Surface	Line	Point
δ	γ	β	α
Period of time [Expansivenes *rhythmical* time]	Area of time [Resistance *dynamic* time]	Stream of time	Moment

Table 6. d and δ—g and γ—b and β—a and α appear simultaneously.

Human Embryological Development: Steps in Taking Hold of the Dimensions of Space

Unlike building a house, where one building block is placed on top of another in a quantitative, additive process, human embryological development is a qualitative, internally differentiated process in which the individuality takes hold of the dimensions of space one after the other. Thus development of the embryo proceeds from the whole to the parts and not the reverse. Individualized, specialized cells are actually the end product of this process.

Conception

Embryonic development begins with conception, when an egg cell and a sperm cell unite. Actually, it is incorrect to apply the term "cell" to these gametes. If we consider how the gametes differentiate during the processes leading up to impregnation, we find that as the original primitive germ cells develop into elements capable of fertilization, they lose their cytological integrity, i.e., their cell-like character, and become increasingly one-sided. In the end, they are incomplete entities that are no longer capable of surviving on their own.

Sperm cell maturation (spermatogenesis). Male sperm cells are derived from primitive germ cells (spermatogonia) that are found in the testes and multiply there throughout a man's lifetime. At regular intervals, a germ cell singles itself out from the pool of spermatogonia and moves inward, from the basal layer of the germinal epithelium to the next layer, the adluminal compartment. The blood-testis barrier separates the adluminal compartment from the basal compartment. In the adluminal compartment, isolated from the rest of the organism and not directly accessible

from either the interstitial stroma (connective tissue) or the vascular system of the testis, further stages of differentiation occur (Figure 14). Step by step, the germ cell loses its organelles and becomes extremely one-sided. It loses almost all of its cytoplasm, and the nucleus becomes highly concentrated. Through two maturational divisions (meioses), half of its genetic material is discarded and excluded from further development, reducing the chromosome number from diploid to haploid. The centrioles, however, multiply and form a complex flagellum (threadlike tail) that allows the sperm to move.

If the ***spermatogonium*** is a complete cell that still has all the organelles a cell needs to survive, then the differentiated sperm is a "half cell" with only half of the original genetic material and a portion of the necessary organelles. Since a sperm cell in this form is not capable of surviving on its own, it is supported and nourished by helper cells, the Sertoli cells that line the seminiferous tubule. The largely "naked" heads of the sperm cells are embedded in the spaces between the supporting Sertoli cells (Figure 14).

Egg cell maturation (oogenesis). During egg cell maturation in the ovaries, a similar reduction takes place (Figure 15). Female primordial germ cells multiply in the ovarian cortex approximately until birth, after which they gradually die off. At regular intervals, female egg cells (oocytes) develop from the remaining primordial germ cells (oogonia). Unlike sperm cells, however, they do not discard cytoplasm but instead acquire large amounts of it. With each meiotic division, one of the polar bodies is discarded and its share of cytoplasm is added to the egg cell. Due to this great increase in cytoplasm, the egg cell gradually becomes incapable of maintaining its own metabolism. Without the help of other cells, the egg's metabolic processes would quickly weaken, eventually killing the cell. Like the Sertoli cells that support the immature sperm, the squamous epithelial or follicular cells, which surround the egg cell in a wreathlike arrangement (corona radiata), keep

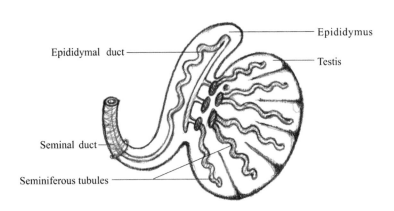

Epididymal duct

Epididymus

Testis

Seminal duct

Seminiferous tubules

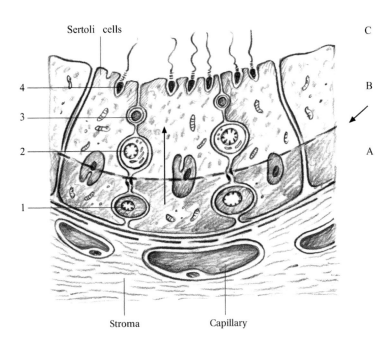

Sertoli cells

C

B

A

4

3

2

1

Stroma   Capillary

Fig. 14. **Sperm cell development in the male gonad (testis).** *Primitive germ cells (spermatogonia) multiply in the basal compartment (A) of the germinal epithelium. The basal compartment is separated by the blood-testis barrier from the adluminal and luminal compartments (B, C), so that toxins circulating in the vascular system cannot disrupt the sperm's further development. In the maturation process, each sperm's nucleus is reduced so that it contains only half of the original number of chromosomes (haploid form), and its cytoplasm is discarded and "digested" by the Sertoli cells.*

Cross section of the epithelium of a seminiferous tubule.

A : Basal compartment with spermatogonia (1)
B: Adluminal compartment with primary spermatocytes (2) and secondary spermatocytes (spermatids) (3)
C: Luminal compartment with immature spermatozoa (4) with their heads buried in the cytoplasm of the Sertoli cells.
Arrow: blood-testis barrier

Stages of germ cell development:

1: immature germ cell (spermatogonium, diploid)
2: primary spermatocyte (diploid)
3: secondary spermatocyte (spermatid, haploid)
4: immature sperm cell

the egg cell alive (Figure 15). As the female egg cell differentiates, it also loses half of its genetic material, which is discarded along with the polar body; ultimately, only a haploid number of chromosomes remains.

From a phenomenological perspective, the wholeness of a cell is "torn apart" during the maturation of a gamete. Both sperm cells and egg cells possess only a portion of the organelles present in a "whole" cell. They have differentiated into polar opposite forms (Figure 16).

Fertilization (conception). Fertilization restores wholeness on the cytological level. The two fragmentary half cells—which had survived on the very edge of biological existence only with help from the Sertoli and follicular cells—merge to form a complete cell (Figure 17). Furthermore, when the sperm penetrates the

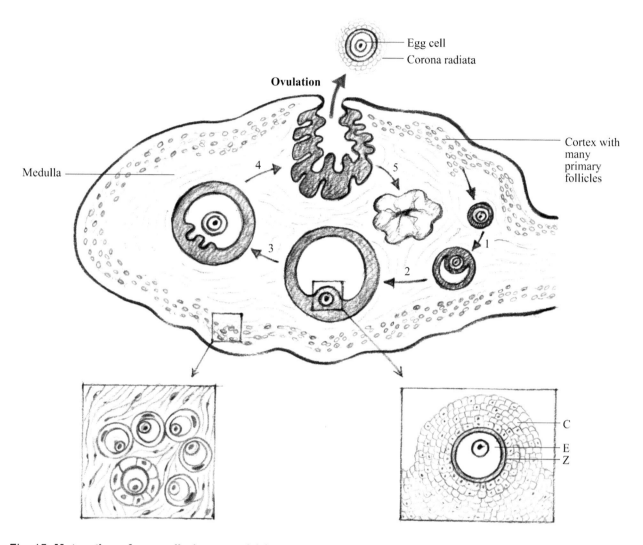

Ovulation

Egg cell
Corona radiata

Cortex with many primary follicles

Medulla

C
E
Z

*Fig. 15. **Maturation of egg cells (oogenesis) in the human ovary, to the point of ovulation** (red arrow).*
1: Development of a secondary follicle from a primary follicle in the cortex; migration into the medulla of the ovary.
Detail, left: Cortex with several primary follicles (immature egg cells or oocytes)
2: Transition to the maturing Graafian follicle
3: Tertiary (Graafian) follicle. Detail, right: the cumulus with the egg cell (E), corona radiata (C), and protective layer (zona pellucida, Z)
4: Ovulation (ejection of the egg cell together with the surrounding corona radiata)
5: Development of the corpus luteum, which is then resorbed, leaving behind the corpus albicans (scar).

ovum at conception, the ovum's formerly greatly reduced metabolism is reactivated. Cellular respiration intensifies abruptly, and metabolic processes (as markers of biological activity) increase significantly. The support cells are no longer needed and are eventually discarded (Figure 18).

On closer consideration, however, the result of fertilization is much more than "just" the reestablishment of a viable cellular whole; it is a whole **new organism.** The **fertilized ovum**, or zygote, which is the physical germ of this new organism, is not just an ordinary cell of the sort seen in later developmental stages. Transition

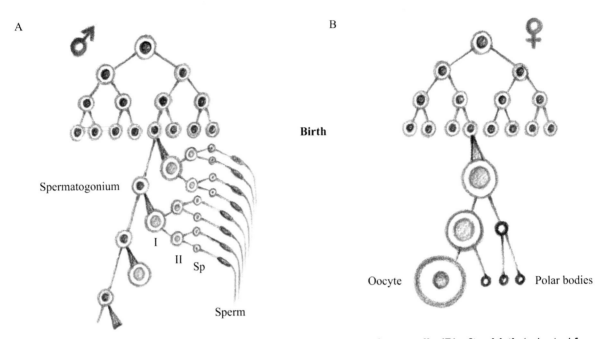

Fig. 16. **Differentiated development of sperm cells (A) and egg cells (B) after birth** (adapted from Rollshoven). I: primary spermatocytes; II: secondary spermatocytes; Sp: spermatids.

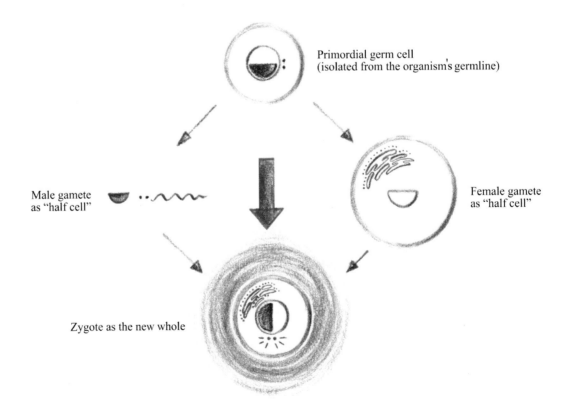

Fig. 17. **The conception process.** A new element (red arrow) creates a new whole (organism) out of two cellular "halves."

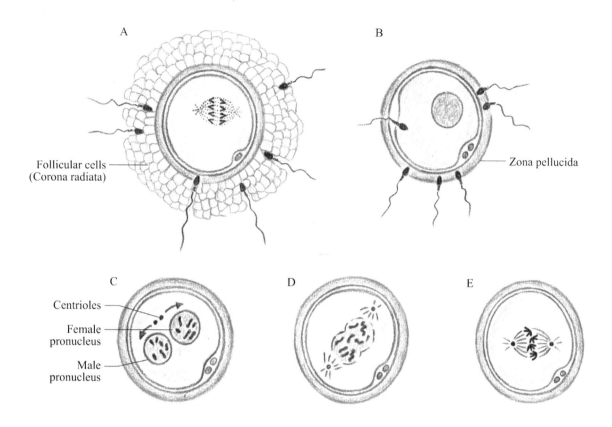

Fig. 18. **The fertilization process** *(adapted from 36).*
A: Egg cell surrounded by follicle cells, shortly before fertilization. The second meiosis begins;
B: Sperm penetrates the zona pellucida; second meiosis is complete;
C: Development of male and female pronuclei, separation of centrioles;
D: Fusion of the two pronuclei, formation of a mitotic spindle;
E: Chromosome pairs (now a diploid number again!) line up on the equatorial plate. The genome has been reconstituted. The spindle is completed and the first mitosis begins.

through an almost lifeless, chaotic stage prior to fertilization—when the chromosomes undergo significant structural changes during meiosis and the genetic material is mixed and rearranged—appears to be the single most important prerequisite for the incarnation of a new individual (29). During meiosis, the chromosomes lie closer together than they do in ordinary cell division (mitosis). They form so-called **tetrads** (groups of four chromosome filaments or chromatids). In this close proximity, exchanges, crossovers, and displacements occur. In addition to being completely rearranged, the genetic material is

also given a thorough "spring cleaning," i.e., the chromosomes are repaired, eliminating all the disruptions and errors that develop in the course of an individual life. According to Hayflick, research with cell cultures has shown that each cell in the human body is capable of only about fifty successful divisions (30, 31). If the aging cells of a mature or dying organism were passed on unchanged to the germ cells, the cells of the resulting embryo would be "old" even before development began. The "cellular timer" needs to be reset to zero. We do not yet know exactly how this happens, but we do know that by the time

Cell organelles	(sperm)	(egg)
Nucleus (chromosomes)	½	½
Mitochondria	0	++
Cytoplasm (endoplasmic reticulum, etc.)	0	+++
Centrioles	++	0

Table 7. Differing distribution of cell organelles in the maturation of egg and sperm cells.

conception occurs, a completely new, unique, young, and "clean" complement of chromosomes is available. The cytoplasm with its organelles has also been renewed. It is quite possible, therefore, that outside forces participate in transforming and renewing the genetic material and cytoplasm during preparation for conception. What forces these are has not been explained by sciences limited to knowledge produced by physical cognition, but the phenomena described here speak emphatically in favor of the preexistence of the human spirit, because the cellular fragments arbitrarily thrown together at conception cannot entirely account for the new, organizing element that reveals itself after fertilization (cf. especially reference 29).

The father (sperm cell) contributes not only half of the genome but also the centrioles, which play a role in cell division and in the cellular organizational processes of the developing organism. In addition to the other half of the genome, the mother (egg cell) contributes metabolic organelles, cytoplasm, and mitochondria (Table 7). The fertilized egg (zygote) is no ordinary cell; it is the archetypal cell, the germ of a total organism that is not yet recognizable but is already completely present as a potential. If such a whole were not present, the embryo would die off, and in fact this does happen in somewhat less than half of all cases. (According to American studies [115], approximately 40 percent of all fertilized eggs die in the uterus *before* implantation.)

The significance of the fertilization process.
To truly understand the essence of the fertilization

process, there is still one more thing we must make clear: Egg and sperm cells are isolated and independent "cells" that exist nowhere else in a comparable form. In the body, there are no other single cells of this sort; there are only cell associations. Even where individual cells are present (blood, connective tissue), they belong to more highly organized cellular tisues that are always embedded in specific surroundings.

The **gonads** (testes, ovaries), however, are areas that have been separated off from the organism as a whole; they have no direct significance for the body's life processes. Their very isolation, however, makes the one-sided differentiation of germ cells possible. The gonads are "empty spaces," so to speak, where the cellular whole can be "torn apart" without interference from the life processes in the rest of the organism. The uterus and fallopian tubes are also "spare rooms" where the fertilization and embryonic development of a new organism foreign to the mother's body can occur, independent of the rest of the body.

Fertilization, or the union of an egg cell and a sperm cell, generally takes place in the ampulla, the widest section of the fallopian tube. If germ cells essentially consist of "dying" cell fragments, what causes the abrupt revitalization of cellular elements and the immediate inception of embryonic development after conception? Today it is postulated that the sperm activates the egg through molecular mechanisms. However, such activating factors cannot ultimately explain early embryogenesis.

Since the mother's body simply makes a "spare room" available for the new organism's development, the causes cannot be found there. Embryonic development takes place in four major stages that cannot be compared to any other processes in the human body. In all the "normal" organ processes in the mother's body, there is no precedent for the cleavages that take place after conception or the developmental processes that set in after the embryo implants in the endometrium. This raises a question of greatest importance for understanding the essence of the human being, and it must remain an open question at this point. Meanwhile, let's take a closer look at the steps in embryonic development itself.

Structural Stages of Embryonic Development

The first cell divisions after conception, which are cleavages rather than mitotic divisions, make it clear that the fertilized egg or zygote is no ordinary cell. Cleavage, unlike normal cell division, is not associated with growth or differentiation and simply leads to an exponential replication of the cleavage cells (blastomeres). Exponential division (1-2-4-8-16, etc.) is otherwise unknown in the body except under pathological conditions— in tumors, for example. Embryonic development begins when the fertilized egg divides in half without further differentiation, producing two blastomeres. In amphibians, if one of these halves is killed, the other half continues to develop into half a body (Figure 19), as proved by a famous experiment conducted by Wilhelm Roux, who punctured one blastomere to prevent it from developing (32). Hans Driesch subsequently proved that the remaining half is still capable of developing into a complete body if the two halves are separated and shaken lightly (33). Therefore, the developmental fate of the two cleavage cells is not predetermined. Roux's experiment does demonstrate, however, that the plane of the first cleavage later becomes the body's median plane. In other words, the first cleavage determines the right-left dimension (Figure 20 A1). The second cleavage plane is perpendicular to the first (Figure 20A2). The third cleavage plane is perpendicular to both of the other planes; in amphibians, for example, it separates the primordium into vegetative (ventral) and animal (dorsal) poles (Figure 20A3). Thus the first three cleavage planes divide the embryo into the three dimensions of space with almost mathematical precision. But "space" is not yet internalized; it remains external to the embryo.

Subsequent cleavages then create ever-smaller cells. The end result is a globular mass of cells (the **morula**, Figure 20B1) that is no larger than the original fertilized egg. No growth has occurred; the original material has simply been partitioned into smaller units.

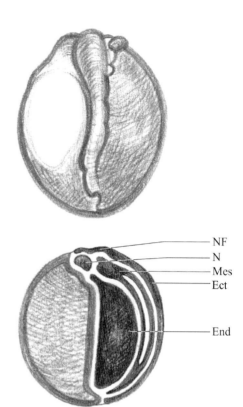

Fig. 19. **Development of a frog** *(Rana)* **half-embryo** *after the left blastomere has been destroyed by puncturing it (37).*
NF: neural folds
N: notochord
Mes: mesoderm (somites and lateral plates)
Ect: ectoderm
End: endoderm

The developmental steps of the next stage have been especially well researched in amphibians. The blastula (Figure 20B2 and B3) is characterized by fluid accumulation, which causes a hollow space to develop in the interior. This space, the blastocoel, is surrounded by a layer of cells that is the prerequisite for later cell movements.

Gastrulation. Next, in a dramatic moment, the first cell movements (migration and displacement of cells) occur, causing cells to be displaced inward, so that a process of invagination or gastrulation begins. These movements begin in one specific location (the blastopore).

In *Amphioxus*, a chordate that foreshadows the evolution of the fishes, the sheet of invaginated tissue becomes the endoderm; in amphibians, it becomes the dorsal mesoderm and the ventral endoderm. The sheet remaining on the outer surface then becomes the ectoderm (Figure 20C). Thus gastrulation gives rise to the germ layers. For the first time, the embryo now has a distinct inside and outside. The interior space, which develops through invagination and is accessible through the blastopore, is called the **archenteron** or primitive gut. Interior spaces and internal structures are the most important features distinguishing animals from plants. Thus we can say that gastrulation is the beginning of animal development as such.

The gesture of invagination as we have described it, however, represents only the outer aspect of the process. In 1926, Spemann discovered that transplanting a bit of tissue from the dorsal blastopore lip (Figure 20C2, BL) to another location sets a gastrulation process in motion there, too (34). Because this bit of tissue is capable of organizing invagination and all subsequent processes up to and including the development of a second embryo, Spemann called the dorsal blastopore lip the **organizer** of the developing organism.

How does this organization take place? Experiments have shown that "impulses" emanating from the invaginated cells in the roof of the archenteron (i.e., the mesoderm plate in amphibians) also trigger invagination processes in other parts of the embryo: First, the neural tube is separated from the ectoderm that lies above it, forming the basis for development of the nervous system. Later, the intestinal tube develops, and the primitive segments (somites) and the lateral plates develop from the mesoderm. At this stage, therefore, the primordia are already present for the development of all future organ systems (40).

With the enclosing of the neural tube, the fourth stage (**neurulation**) of early embryonic development begins, and the embryo is now called the **neurula** (Figure 20D) to distinguish it from the earlier gastrula.

Developmental perspectives: organizing impulses issuing from the notochord and prechordal mesoderm induce the overlying ectoderm to form the neural plate. Tissues that induce organ development in adjacent, still undifferentiated tissue are called inducers. **Induction** not only determines developmental direction but also limits the omnipotence of cells, which formerly allowed them to develop into almost any type because their fate was not yet determined. Experimental transplants have resulted in a "fate map" of the blastula's surface, showing areas that will subsequently give rise to particular types of cells. At this stage, however, cell areas can be interchanged through transplantation without causing developmental disorders. Although a plan exists, it is not yet "fixed" or pinned down in tissue. Induction and determination only begin with gastrulation, after which arbitrary transplantation has significant consequences. If neural tube tissue is transplanted, it continues to develop as nerve tissue and no longer takes its cue from its surroundings. In other words, development is governed by origin rather than location. At this stage, cells have largely lost their adaptability and are no longer omnipotent but only pluripotent or even unipotent.

Thus determination occurs in stages rather than all at once. Initially, the determining fields are relatively large and even overlap in places. Metaphorically speaking, the "commands" issued by embryogenetic fields are initially more general (for example, "make nervous system") but later become increasingly detailed and specialized (for example, "make neural tissue," or later still, "make neurons"). The induced fields thus become ever smaller and more subdivided.

It is currently assumed that these "commands" are issued by specific genes that cause the development of the structures in question. A whole hierarchy of genes, working together with relevant structures in the cytoplasm, sets in motion a chain of reactions that ultimately leads to the development of the organ in question. Although the molecular biological mechanisms of such

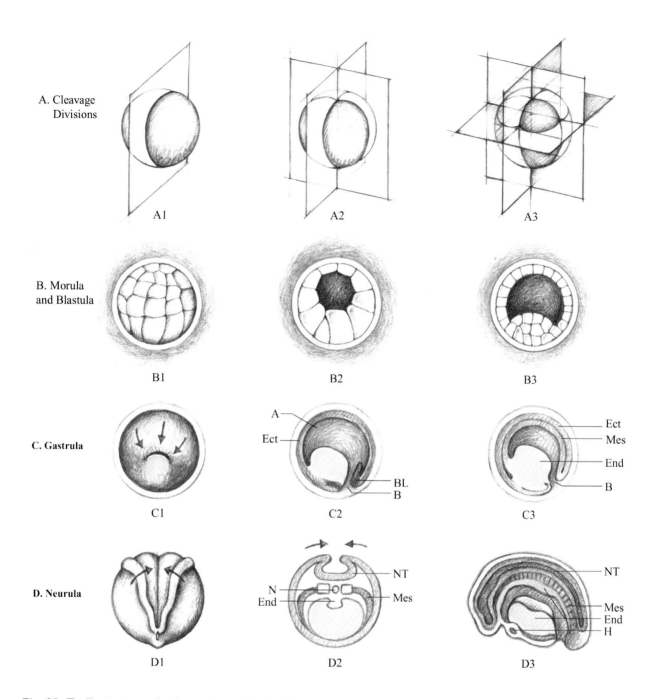

Fig. 20. **Earliest stages in the embryonic development of lower vertebrates** *(amphibians).*
A: The first three cleavage divisions (A1, A2, A3); **B1**: *The* **morula** *stage;* **B2** *and* **B3**: *Cross sections of the* **blastula** *stage;* **C**: *Invagination (the* **gastrula** *stage);* **C1**: *Development of the blastopore begins (arrows); **C2**: Cross section of an early gastrula, showing the beginning of invagination of the ectoderm and the development of the archenteron (Ect: ectoderm; A: archenteron; B: blastopore; BL: blastopore lip);* **C3**: *Cross section of a late gastrula. Development of the germ layers is complete (Ect: ectoderm; Mes: mesoderm; End: endoderm; B: blastopore);* **D**: *The* **neurula** *stage;* **D1**: *The neural folds begin to appear (development of the neural tube, arrows);* **D2**: *Cross section through an early neurula. The primordia for the three great functional systems develop from the three germinal layers: the nervous system from the ectoderm (the neural tube (NT) begins to develop, arrows), the intestinal system from the endoderm tube (End), and the circulatory organs, notochord (N), and connective tissue from the mesoderm (Mes).* **D3**: *Longitudinal section through a late neurula. NT: neural tube; Mes: mesoderm with somites; End: primitive intestinal tube with yolk remnants; H: heart primordium.*

reaction sequences are becoming known with ever-increasing precision, the forces that ultimately set them in motion and synchronize them remain mysterious. An inducing substance (inducer) has only a very narrow window of opportunity for inducing a differentiation process in another tissue. In other words, the tissue must be "receptive" to the induction stimulus. Thus embryonic development is based on a highly complex temporal organization ("time structure"), without which a normally formed body cannot develop. Consequently, a system of forces of a higher order must be responsible for the organism's structural design. Genetic processes represent only the form-actualizing mechanisms within this system.

At this juncture, if not already earlier, we need to ask about the source of the forces that rearrange genetic material during meiosis, revitalize the "dying" ovum, and trigger the formative processes that begin after conception. There can be no doubt that the genome contains the code for a specific developmental program. But how is this program accessed and what are the forces that make it a reality?

Perhaps these phenomena suggest that the incarnating individuality itself unites with the zygote at conception. Could it be that the individuality initiates further developmental steps from the periphery, from the outside in, retracing the major evolutionary stages of the human race in principle (although not in detail) in the process of incarnating or "becoming flesh"?

This perspective allows us to see conception in an entirely new light. We see why the fertilized ovum (zygote) cannot be a "cell" in the usual sense. At this point, the entire future individuality is present, if only as a "sphere" of peripheral forces (Figure 17). All later manifestations are already present, at least as potentials; nothing more will be added. We cannot say that human existence actually begins only after the first, second, or even third month of gestation. The new human being exists from the very first moment. Of necessity, therefore, the idea of the preexistence of the human spirit provides a totally new and different perspective on all questions related to termination of pregnancy.

Qualitative Differences in the First Four Stages of Embryonic Development

The four developmental stages described above are of fundamental importance. Morula, blastula, gastrula, and neurula signify steps in the history of development; each step achieves a qualitatively new level of existence.

In the *morula*, the "force field" as a whole is not yet united with the embryo but still surrounds it like a sphere. Only the dimensionality of space as such (right-left, up-down, front-back) has been realized, as we see from the fact that if one of the two cleavage cells is destroyed, only half of the body develops. To represent this stage, we might choose the mathematical image of a point surrounded by a circle or sphere (cf. Novalis, p. 36, reference 28). In a certain respect, the morula is only a point around which future development begins to crystallize. Cell growth and differentiation are still nonexistent. This state is comparable to inanimate organizational forms in the natural world. It is the "mineral" stage, so to speak, because as yet the embryo has no inner space of its own and therefore no real vitality.

The *blastula* stage is characterized primarily by the development of surfaces. If we trace the fate of individual cell areas, a map or plan for their development is apparent on the blastula's surface. This plan, however, has not yet become fixed or determined. At this stage, growth cannot occur from the inside out, and the growth that does occur can be compared to a mirroring or reflective process. This is the embryo's "plant" phase. Of course a plant is alive and grows, but its existence as an organism is still characterized primarily by the development of surfaces. Goethe's archetypal plant consists essentially of metamorphoses of the leaf. The development of surfaces, however, is also characteristic of blastulation.

The development of an animal body as such begins only with *gastrulation*, when an inside and an outside appear for the first time. Invagination produces an "inner world" that previously did not exist in this form. The ectoderm

Stage	Amphibian	Human	Processes	Forces	Mathematical comparison (see Novalis)	Comparable level of existence
1.	Morula	Morula	Cleavage divisions	Peripheral (sphere)	Point	Mineral
2.	Blastula	Blastocyst (embryoblast + trophoblast), embryonic disc	Formation of surfaces (germ layers) (ecto- + endoderm)	"fate map"	Plane	Plant
Invagination						
3.	Gastrula	Primitive streak, notochord process	Cell movement, invagination (mesoderm-mesenchyme	Induction, determination	Space (polarity of inner and outer)	Animal
4.	Neurula	Neurulation	Growth (organ systems, organs, cells)	Segregation of embryo-genetic fields	Time + space	Vertebrate, human

Table 8. The four basic developmental stages of early embryonic development in vertebrates and humans. The time factor of course plays a role at the animal level as well, but only in humans does the passage of time result in higher development.

shuts the embryo off from its surroundings, and the archenteron and mesoderm develop in the interior. Now the embryo begins to organize all aspects of the developing physical body from the inside out. In the gastrula stage, the first major inductions take place. Organ systems are determined, but initially no appreciable growth or cell differentiation occurs.

Actual growth begins only in the **neurula** stage, when peripheral forces relocate from the surrounding sphere into the embryo and its tissues. Now these forces work not from the outside but from within, in an increasingly specialized direction, ultimately driving the process of differentiation and specialization into the development of individual cells, until finally intestinal cells, nerve or glial cells, and muscle, blood, and bone cells are present. The specialized cell, therefore, represents the end rather than the beginning of the developmental process. **Development proceeds** **from the whole to the parts.** The fertilized ovum represents the whole. The germ layers are the primordia of the basic major functional systems, out of which in turn the primordia of individual organ systems develop. But instead of containing "cells" in the usual sense, these organ systems contain only the potential to develop them. Only after neurulation, when growth and differentiation set in, do individual organs and tissues develop within the organ systems. Cells with specialized structures and functions appear later still, at the very end.

In functional terms, the blastula is still all surface, and the new organism's first interior space develops only at gastrulation, when the third dimension is added. Through invagination, the organism develops an independent interior space which is then further configured in subsequent stages. Repeated reworking of the interior spaces constantly increases the internal surface areas of organs such as the lungs and circulatory organs, making them more complex and varied in shape. Higher development of this type occurs not only in individual development (ontogeny) but also in vertebrate phylogeny (the evolution of species). The gesture of gastrulation or invagination, which transforms external surfaces into internal ones, is the archetype of all animal development and continues to shape it in later stages. The multiplication of internal surface area through invagination is a theme that recurs throughout vertebrate evolution. Present from the very beginning, it later becomes one of the most incisive developmental factors in phylogeny.

As we mentioned earlier, differentiated growth begins only after neurulation. The body begins to divide into ever-smaller functional units. With the addition of rhythms of growth and differentiation, *time* is added to *space* as an active formative factor. In this context, Bautzmann speaks of the embryo's "time structure" (35).

Table 8 summarizes the most essential characteristics of the first four major developmental stages, which can also be found in early human development, although they look somewhat different in humans than in amphibians, birds, and mammals. The main difference is that in the human embryo, the dramatic invagination that transforms part of the periphery into the body's interior is visible in a much more elemental or archetypal way. Nonetheless, the results of experimental research on amphibians and chicken embryos can help us better understand qualitative differences among individual stages of human embryonic development. There is no longer any need to imagine the "sphere" of peripheral forces; it materializes in early human development in the form of the protective chorion. The concepts formulated above can be considerably deepened by shifting our view from lower vertebrate to human embryonic development.

To summarize, embryonic development is not an additive progression from a single cell to a "nation of cells." Instead, it proceeds *from the whole to the parts* (cf. Table 2, p. 22). The organism as a whole is already present in po-

tential form in the zygote, which subsequently subdivides into ever smaller functional units. Only at the very end does the individual cell appear as such. Thus the sequence of steps in the differentiation process is:

1. Total organism
2. Germ layers
3. Functional systems
4. Organs
5. Tissues
6. Cells with associated extracellular matrix.

Human Embryonic Development and Placentation

Morulation. After fertilization, which in humans usually occurs in the ampulla of the fallopian tube (Figure 21), the *cleavage divisions* that produce the morula begin. In humans, however, these divisions are not as regular as they are in amphibians. As a result, odd numbers appear in the exponential series of cell-replication numbers (1, 3, 5, 7, 13, etc.). This is due to the fact that one group of cells, the future embryoblast, falls behind in its growth at a very early stage, while the adjacent trophoblast develops more rapidly (Figure 22).

Blastulation. As development continues, the mass of cells, now differentiated into *embryoblast* (inner cell mass) and *trophoblast* (outer cell mass), becomes bubblelike as the result of fluid accumulation in the interior (see *blastocyst*, Figure 22). In humans, this vesicle buries itself in the endometrium (*implantation*) anywhere from five to six days after fertilization (Figures 21 and 23). Inside the endometrium, the blastocyst immediately begins to increase in size very rapidly, with most of the increase occurring in the trophoblast (36-38).

In contrast, the embryoblast continues to develop slowly. Instead of compact masses of cells, it develops only two small, fluid-filled vesicles known as the amnion and the yolk sac.

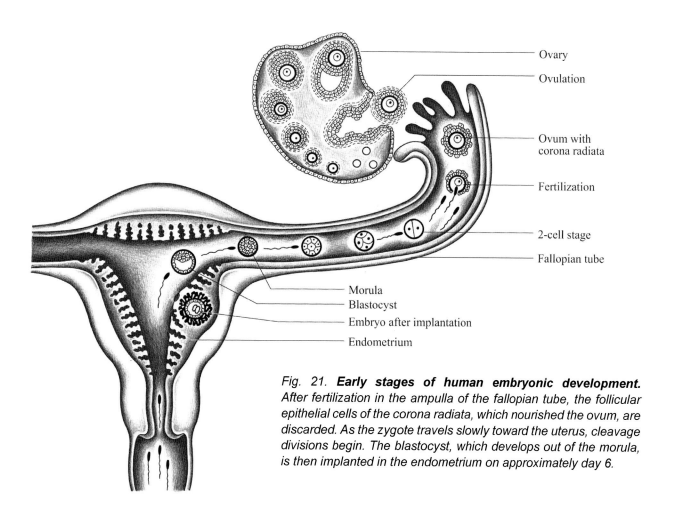

Ovary

Ovulation

Ovum with corona radiata

Fertilization

2-cell stage

Fallopian tube

Morula
Blastocyst
Embryo after implantation
Endometrium

Fig. 21. **Early stages of human embryonic development.** *After fertilization in the ampulla of the fallopian tube, the follicular epithelial cells of the corona radiata, which nourished the ovum, are discarded. As the zygote travels slowly toward the uterus, cleavage divisions begin. The blastocyst, which develops out of the morula, is then implanted in the endometrium on approximately day 6.*

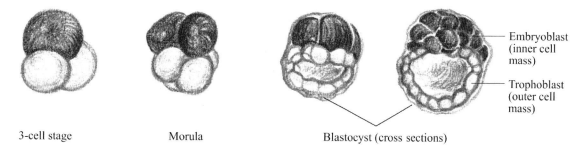

Embryoblast (inner cell mass)

Trophoblast (outer cell mass)

3-cell stage   Morula   Blastocyst (cross sections)

Fig. 22. **Development of the human blastocyst.** *Differences in the timing of cleavage divisions in the early blastocyst lead to two distinct cell masses, the slower-growing embryoblast (dark) and the more rapidly dividing cells of the trophoblast (light).*

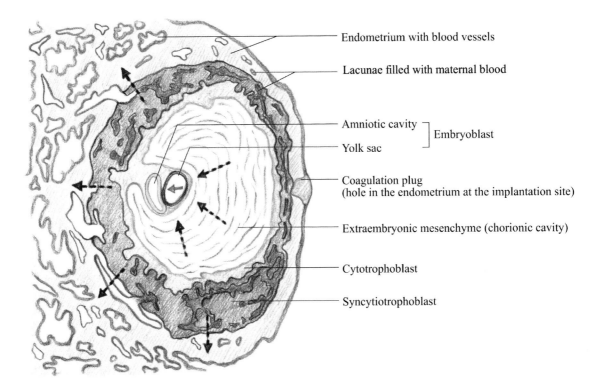

Endometrium with blood vessels

Lacunae filled with maternal blood

Amniotic cavity ⎤
Yolk sac ⎦ Embryoblast

Coagulation plug
(hole in the endometrium at the implantation site)

Extraembryonic mesenchyme (chorionic cavity)

Cytotrophoblast

Syncytiotrophoblast

Fig. 23. **Human embryo after implantation** *(day 16, from reference 38). The trophoblast (dark) sends irregularly branched villi (arrows) into the endometrium. The embryoblast remains delayed in its growth (centripetal growth tendency, broken arrows) but forms two thin-walled vesicles, the amnion and the yolk sac. The embryonic disc lies where these two vesicles meet (red arrow). The amniotic layer of the embryonic disc develops into the epiblast (the future ectoderm), the yolk sac layer into the hypoblast (the foundation for the development of the endoderm).*

The future body of the embryo will develop where the surfaces of these two vesicles meet, in the area called the embryonic disc (Figure 23).

Thus the second major phase of human embryonic development, which follows cleavage, ends with the development of an embryogenetically potent surface. The cleavage stage, or morulation, was still more or less pointlike or elongated in character, and the three-dimensionality of space was reflected on the surface of the embryo but did not take possession of it. At the blastula stage, with the development of the embryonic disc, the second dimension (surface area) is added. A three-dimensional body is achieved only in the next stage through the formation of the primitive streak in the embryonic disc and the development of a middle germ layer (mesoderm).

Gastrulation. The part of the amniotic vesicle that borders on the yolk sac forms the epiblast (later the ectoderm); the neighboring yolk sac epithelium forms the hypoblast (the foundation for the future endoderm, although not the endoderm itself) (Figure 23). In the epiblast, around day 15, cells begin to move toward the middle to form the **primitive streak** (Figure 24A). In the primitive streak, cells force their way under the epiblast and sideways between the epiblast and hypoblast. The primitive streak marks the future center of the body, establishing the right-left dimension. Soon thereafter (around day 17) a groovelike invagination (**primitive groove**) appears at the anterior end of the primitive streak as an expression of the invagination that leads to the development of the notochord process (Figures

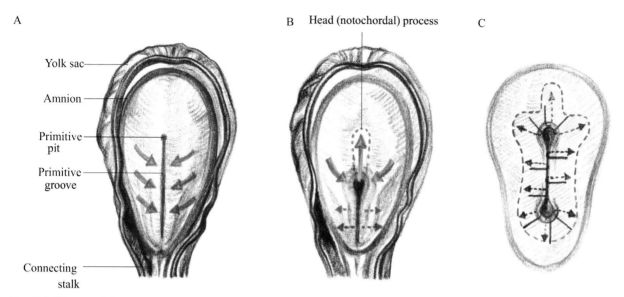

Fig. 24. **Views of the human embryonic disc after the opening of the amniotic cavity.**
A: Embryo at day 15. Development of the primitive groove (arrows) and establishment of the right-left dimension.
B: Embryo at day 17. Development of the notochord process. From the primitive pit, cellular matter forces its way to the front under the epiblast (the future ectoderm) to form the notochord process, the future notochord. The emergence of the notochord process establishes the up-down dimension. Cellular matter also grows toward the sides from the primitive groove (broken arrows).
C: Schematic view of the invagination processes in the embryonic disc that form the third germ layer (mesoderm: dotted red line). As the mesoderm develops, the primitive streak (the primitive pit and groove) becomes shorter and finally disappears completely.

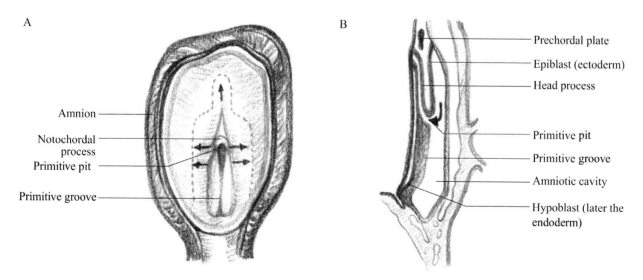

Fig. 25. **Development of the Mesoderm. A**: *View of the embryonic disc of a human embryo, day 17. The amniotic cavity has been opened. Red dotted line: third germinal layer (mesoderm) formed through invagination and proliferation of the two primary layers (epiblast and hypoblast).*
B: Longitudinal section through the middle of the embryonic disc in A. Invagination of the notochord process, which emerges from the primitive pit (arrow), is clearly recognizable (from 39).

24B and 25). The notochord process is a strand of tissue growing between the epiblast and the hypoblast; it later develops into the **notochord**, the embryo's axis, which lies in the exact center of the future embryonic body and induces the first endogenous organ primordium (the neural tube) in the adjacent ectoderm, thus establishing the second dimension (up-down). The notochord process grows from below upward (i.e., in the direction of the future head) between the epiblast and the hypoblast (Figure 25). The notochord, which emerges from the notochord process, later ends at the base of the embryonic skull. Actual head development, which obeys developmental laws of its own, manifests in the so-called prechordal plate (Figure 25B), which lies directly *in front of* the tip of the notochord. We will have more to say about the mystery of head formation later (see p. 65).

Through the invagination process described above, a third germ layer (the **mesoderm**) forms between the outer and inner germinal layers. Initially, the mesoderm is also a thin layer (Figures 24 and 25). Near the body's axis, however, cube-shaped structures (the **somites**) appear in rhythmic succession next to the notochord, which has separated from the notochord process. Although somewhat greater in volume, they are still cellular (epithelial) in character (Figure 26). This marks the first appearance of the third structural principle, metamerism or rhythmic subdivision, which later becomes the basis of the torso's organization.

Next begins a dramatic process that leads to the actual development of the embryonic body (36-38): **Somite disintegration** initiates mesenchyme development. The original epithelial arrangement of somite cells suddenly begins to loosen, and the cells swarm out into their surroundings. They remain in contact with each other, forming a loose network of cells that fills with intercellular substance. The resulting **embryonic connective tissue**, or mesenchyme, is the first actual connective tissue to develop. It eventually surrounds all the organ primordia, thus establishing the three-dimensional character of the embryonic body. The mesenchyme gives

rise to the primordia of all organs of movement (cartilage, bone, muscles, vessels, and blood), the tissues that make up most of the mass of the mature organism's torso and limbs.

In a process somewhat comparable to gastrulation in lower vertebrates (although it does not result in an archenteron), the mesoderm develops, through invagination, in the primitive node (Hensen's node) and primitive groove. As soon as this process is complete, the primordium of the nervous system develops through a separation of the neural tube from the ectoderm (neurulation); similarly, the primordium of the digestive tract develops out of a fold in the yolk sac. The further development of the resulting embryonic body is characterized by the expansion and differentiation of these primordia (Figure 27). The neural tube is the primordium of the entire information system, the primitive intestinal tube that of the metabolic system, and the mesoderm (from which the cardiovascular system and organs of locomotion emerge) that of the "rhythmic" system. Although the three germ layers cannot be strictly equated with the three major functional systems, it can be said nonetheless that the essential structure of the threefold organism is present at the conclusion of this gastrulationlike invagination process.

Elementary developmental phases of the human embryo. In humans, therefore, as in lower invertebrates, the embryonic body develops in four basic stages. We might follow Novalis in describing their sequence as point, line, plane, and space (see Table 6). Cleavage is the pointlike stage, the primitive streak is linear, the germ-layer stage emphasizes surfaces, and mesenchyme development represents the emergence of three-dimensional space.

Applying our previously developed concepts of the three dimensions, we see that the embryo successively conquers each dimension. The first recognizable dimension is that of bilateral symmetry, which appears when cell movements begin to the right and left of the primitive streak marking the future median plane. With the appearance of Hensen's node and the primitive groove, the up-down orientation develops. The notochord process, which grows toward the

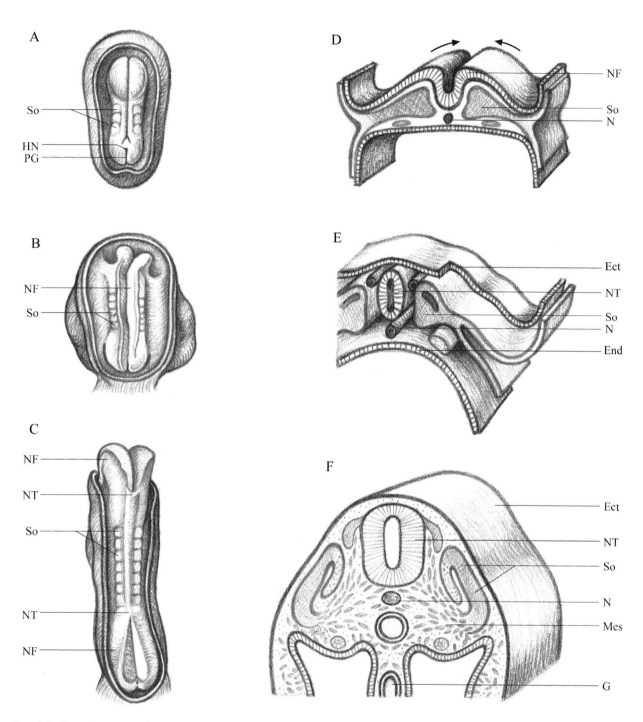

Fig. 26. **Developmental stages of the mesoderm and development of the embryonic body** *with the primordia of the three basic functional systems. The nervous system develops out of the ectoderm, the intestinal system out of the endoderm, and the circulatory and motor systems out of the mesoderm. Through disintegration of the somites (F), embryonic connective tissue (mesenchyme) develops, establishing the three-dimensional character of the embryonic body through addition of the front-back dimension.*

Ect: ectoderm, End: endoderm, Mes: mesenchyme, HN: Hensen's node or primitive node (disappears at the end of invagination), G: primitive gut tube (develops out of the endoderm), N: notochord, NT: neural tube, NF: neural folds (fold together—see arrows in illustration D above—forming the neural tube, which is the primordium of the entire nervous system), PG: primitive groove (grows shorter and disappears), So: somites (disintegrate, forming mesenchyme).

A

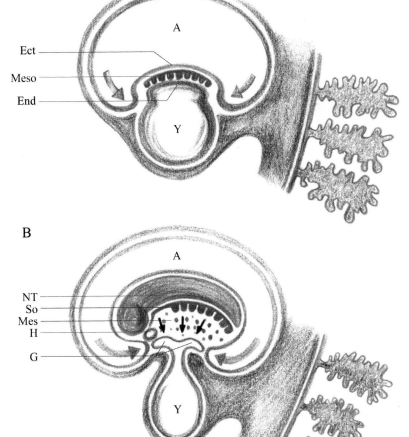

Ect

Meso

End

A: Amniotic cavity
Ect: Ectoderm
End: Endoderm
Y: Yolk sac
Mes: Mesenchyme
Meso: Mesoderm
G: Primitive gut
NT: Neural tube
H: Heart primordium
So: Somites

B

NT
So
Mes
H

G

Fig. 27. **Development of the embryonic body through disintegration of the somites** (So) and subsequent development of mesenchyme or embryonic connective tissue (Mes, red), which expands (arrows) in the space between ectoderm (Ect) and endoderm (End). As a result of mesenchyme development, the initially flat embryonic disc (Figure A) rises above its base (large arrows) and becomes a three-dimensional body (embryo).
A: approx. day 18
B: approx. day 20

front, represents the head end, and the shrinking primitive streak represents the tail or caudal end of the future embryo (Figures 24 and 25). The last to develop is the middle germinal layer (mesoderm), whose segmentally arranged somites mark the first appearance of the principle of metamerism. With the embryonic body's subsequent development, the final (front-back) dimension comes into play. Three-dimensionality emerges only when the somites disintegrate and mesenchyme develops. The human individuality now has an interior space of its own, i.e., a body (Figures 26 and 27). This body floats weightlessly in the amnion until

it enters the outside world at birth, when it begins to develop into a self-reliant individual capable of movement within the Earth's gravitational field.

As we see, the four basic stages of primitive development are also recognizable in human development. Cleavage division is almost the same in humans as in vertebrates. The second stage, the development of surfaces (blastulation), takes place in two substages in humans (as in other mammals). Except for the fact that it is implanted in the endometrium, where it undergoes specialized development to adapt it to intrauterine life, the mammalian

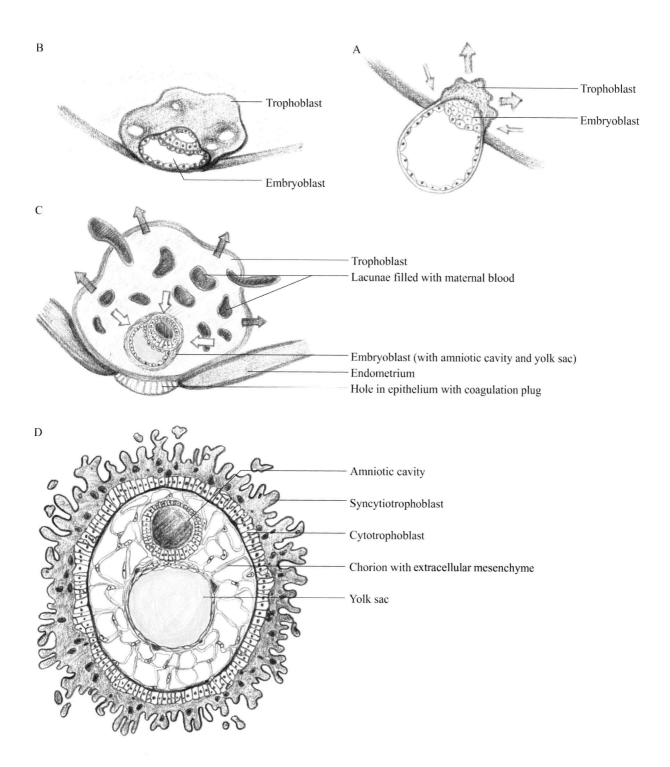

B

Trophoblast

Embryoblast

A

Trophoblast

Embryoblast

C

Trophoblast
Lacunae filled with maternal blood

Embryoblast (with amniotic cavity and yolk sac)
Endometrium
Hole in epithelium with coagulation plug

D

Amniotic cavity

Syncytiotrophoblast

Cytotrophoblast

Chorion with extracellular mesenchyme

Yolk sac

Fig. 28. **Early stages of human embryonic development.** *A – C: implantation in the uterine endometrium (A: day 6, B: day 7.5, C: day 12, D: day 16). Development of the embryoblast (C, light arrows) is delayed while the trophoblast, which penetrates the endometrium during implantation, undergoes rapid centrifugal growth, forming a heavy ring of many villi (dark arrows). The trophoblast develops a surface layer of plasma that is not divided into cells (syncytiotrophoblast); it performs virtually every function that the embryo will later assume. The cellularly structured cytotrophoblast constantly adds to the syncytiotrophoblast.*

blastocyst largely corresponds to the blastula of amphibians and reptiles. Before development of the embryo continues, the trophoblast penetrates the endometrium in a centrifugal gesture and develops into the organ that will nourish the embryo. For a true understanding of this initially mysterious organ, however, deeper-reaching concepts are required.

Placentation and the fetal membranes. We have already described how the **trophoblast** rapidly develops from the blastocyst after implantation (Figures 22 and 23), growing in a centrifugal direction into the endometrium, which it dissolves to form a spherical covering for the embryoblast (Figures 28 and 29). Amphibians do not need this protection because they develop in water; they absorb nutrients from their immediate environment and release wastes into it. The protective sphere that develops in humans, however, is not an ersatz natural outer world for the future embryo but develops out of part of the embryo itself.

Two different groups of cells emerge from the trophoblast. The superficial layer that comes into contact with the endometrial stroma becomes the syncytiotrophoblast, which is constantly regenerated by the underlying cell layer, the cytotrophoblast (Figures 23 and 28). The cytotrophoblast is cellular in structure and increases through very rapid mitosis. The syncytiotrophoblast, however, is not partitioned into separate cells but is a single large mass of protoplasm with irregularly distributed nuclei. This syncytium, however, is by no means functionally undifferentiated. On the contrary, all the functions characteristic of the future organism (nutrition, respiration, elimination or excretion, regulation, defense) take place here, although they are not served by specialized organs (cf. references 38-40). Eventually, the placenta emerges from this mass of protoplasm through the development of villi and the consolidation of distinct structures (40). The syncytiotrophoblast performs all the functions of the future body's organs (lungs, kidneys, gastrointestinal tract, etc.), an astonishing phenomenon. If we see the embryo as constituting a whole from the very beginning, this means that all the organ functions of the entire organism are already present and active. Initially, however, they occur on the periphery (sphere) without any organs to support them. In human as opposed to lower vertebrate early development, the embryo's immediate environment is a concrete reality generated by the embryo itself.

How can we characterize the further development of the embryonic disc, the transition from the surface-forming stage (blastula) to three-dimensional space (gastrulation)? Within the embryonic body's internal space, which comes about through mesenchyme development, each of the functions initially localized in the trophoblast (periphery) acquires an organ system of its own, although initially only in the form of a nonfunctional primordium. ***This is multilevel invagination on a grand scale***, working from the periphery of the protective organ into the future embryo. At first, the protective sheath consists only of the villi-forming syncytiotrophoblast, the cytotrophoblast, and a loose network of extraembryonic mesenchyme (Figure 28), tissue that surrounds the embryonic disc with the amnion, yolk sac, etc. Soon, however, the part of the trophoblast that borders on the endometrium differentiates into a specialized organ (the **placenta**), while the part facing the uterine cavity becomes thinner and thinner, forming the so-called fetal membranes (Figure 29).

As functional invagination continues, we see the actual embryonic body begin to develop as a three-dimensional organism with an inside and an outside as well as internalized functions that are associated with specialized organs consisting of differentiated cell systems (Figure 30).

The fourth stage of embryonic development, which begins with neurulation, involves more development on the interior surface between the amnion and the yolk sac (embryonic disc)—in other words, a development of organ systems and organs *inside* the growing embryonic body, for which the amnion (which is also growing) serves as a place-holder. With the beginning of growth, exchanges begin to take place between peripheral placental functions and the growth processes in the embryonic body's internal space. The extracellular mesenchyme, a loose network of cell tissue and extensive protein-rich intercellular substance (the chorion, Figures 23 and 28), lies between the cytotrophoblast and the embryo. It differentiates to serve these various exchanges. Until the embryo develops a vascular system of its own (which also serves the placenta), all substances moving from the periphery to the embryo and back again pass through this "sponge." The vessels sprouting from the embryo, along with the blood they contain, and the heart (which is initially located completely outside the embryo), comprise the first organ system the embryo develops to mediate between its own growth processes and peripheral placental functions. This early circulatory system forms a functional bridge between these two domains (Figure 31).

After the beginning of the fourth stage, functional invagination increasingly becomes an accomplished fact as more individual organs and specialized tissues develop within the embryo. Intraembryonic structures become available to serve peripheral functions, which are then able to "make the leap" from the periphery to the inside of the body. As a result, the placenta dies off very slowly, a process that is completed at birth. Ultimately, therefore, birth means slipping out of an initially all-encompassing functional periphery and taking hold of a body that has assumed these functions step by step, in a specific time sequence.

This is a major transformation. Neither in the trophoblast nor in the later placenta is there any spatial or regional differentiation of individual functions. All the life processes are still one great, almost incomprehensible unity. In contrast, in the newborn body, each of the three basic processes (which we described as a threefolding of functional systems in the adult organism) is served by a specialized organ system. *The unity has become a trinity.* Information processes (the nervous system) and metabolic processes (the metabolic system) are polar opposites. The organ systems with rhythmic functions (cardiovascular system, respiration, etc.) constitute a mediating, balancing middle element. It is important to grasp

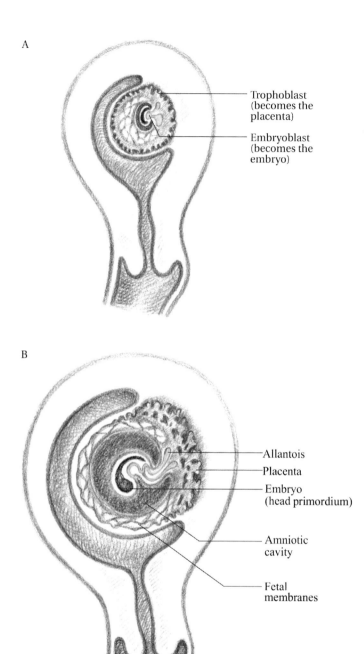

Fig. 29. ***Further development of the trophoblast*** *(which initially surrounds the embryoblast on all sides) is concentrated on the side facing the wall of the uterus, where the trophoblast differentiates into the placenta. The remaining portions of the trophoblast, together with the decidual uterine mucosa and the amnion, form the fetal membranes.*
A: embryo at day 21;
B: embryo at approximately 4 weeks.

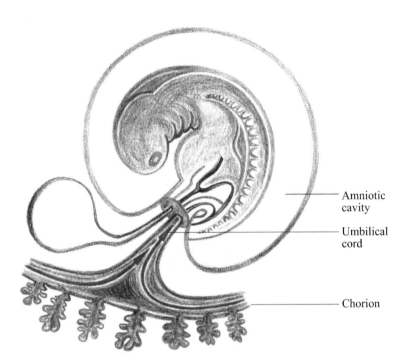

Amniotic cavity

Umbilical cord

Chorion

Fig. 30. **Development of the human embryo** *through transfer of functions from the chorion via the umbilical cord to the embryo body floating in the amnion (approx. day 41, 10 mm). For details, see text.*

the meaning of the reorganization that occurs as the result of functional invagination during embryonic development. But we must become aware of still another element before we can even attempt to solve this profound mystery.

As mentioned earlier, differentiated growth—and hence also the **element of time**—come into play only at the fourth stage of embryonic development (neurulation).

Looking back on the **time factors** in early development, we notice a distinct seven-day rhythm, like the weekly rhythm inherent in many generative processes. The first stage (morulation) lasts five or six days in humans. Implantation occurs on the sixth or seventh day after conception (fertilization) when the blastocyst penetrates the endometrium.

The second week is characterized primarily by growth of the trophoblast, which forms a protective sphere around the embryo-to-be. Meanwhile, the embryoblast forms the two primary vesicles (amnion and yolk sac). This second stage in human embryonic development is blastulation in the narrower sense.

The third stage (gastrulation or invagination with the emergence of a rudimentary interior space) begins on day 14 and leads to the development of the three germ layers (ectoderm, mesoderm, and endoderm). Between day 18 and day 21, the neural groove stage is reached. As a result of this process, and the prior development of the mesenchyme, a three-dimensional embryonic body appears for the first time.

Only in week 4 is the development of the primordia of all the basic organ systems completed, so that the body's entire basic structure is present as potential. This point marks the beginning of the fourth stage (neurulation), which lasts until birth and serves to develop organs, tissues, and (finally) specialized cells (Table 9). Once functional differentiation **within** the embryonic body begins, subsequent structural processes also take place in a specific time sequence rather than simultaneously (Figure 32).

Stage	Days after conception	Phase	Qualities	Corresponding element of the human constitution
I	1-3	Cleavage (morula)	Warmth envelope	←—1
	3-6	Blastocyst	Sphere, still no growth	
	6-8	Implantation		←—2
II	8-12	Amnion and yolk sac	Plantlike sprouting	
	12-14	Primitive streak	Invagination	←— 3
III	14-17	Mesoderm formation (axial organs)	Animal development, internal organs	
	18-21	Mesenchyme formation (neural groove)	Induction processes	←—4
IV	22 +	Development of the embryonic body	Human development as such begins ("I"-development)	

Table 9. The seven-day rhythm in early human embryonic development and its relationship to the elements of the human constitution (40, 42, 48).

1: The physical body finds a foothold
2: Entrance of the life body
3: Entrance of the soul
4: First anchoring of the "I-organization."

The Development of Internal Organ Systems in the Body

Blood and vessels constitute the first primordium of an actual endogenous, functioning organ system. The **vascular system** starts to develop as early as day 13-15, beginning with the so-called blood islands on the yolk sac and in the surrounding chorion (Figure 31). At the end of week 3, the first primitive tubes of the heart develop (still outside the embryonic disc) and connect to blood vessels in the yolk sac, body stalk, and fetal membranes. Through the tension that develops between the centrifugally expanding "sphere" of the fetal membranes and the more centripetal processes of the embryonic disc, a flow of blood develops between the center and the periphery (Figure 31) around day 31. Next, the heart primordium begins to contract regularly, inserting an ordering element into the flow. Thus the **cardiovascular system** is the first embryonic

organ system to become functional. It forms a bridge between periphery and center, between the fetal membranes and the embryonic disc, between the functions of the "undivided sphere" (trophoblast) and the differentiated organogenetic processes in the embryonic disc and embryo. The body stalk, which persists until birth in the form of the umbilical cord, provides a physical bridge for this transition, i.e., for the functional invagination of peripheral processes into the embryo's internal space (Figures 30 and 31).

Although the cardiovascular system is the first to develop and begin working, it becomes fully functional only after birth. The transfer of functions is complete only when respiration shifts from the placenta (periphery) to the lungs (interior). The circulatory and respiratory systems do not become capable of working in ways adapted to life on Earth until immediately after birth. A newborn can only survive when the heart and circulatory system have shifted from fetal to adult mode, i.e., when the lungs begin

Superior view of the embryonic disc in Figure A. The heart
primordium still lies in front of the neural folds in the head region.

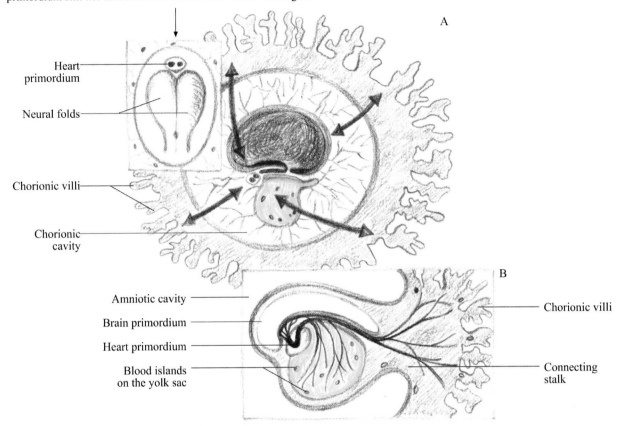

A

Heart
primordium

Neural folds

Chorionic villi

Chorionic
cavity

B

Amniotic cavity

Brain primordium

Heart primordium

Blood islands
on the yolk sac

Chorionic villi

Connecting
stalk

Fig. 31. *Development of the cardiovascular system.* *The circulatory system is the first functioning organ system to create a connection between the periphery (chorion) and the primordial embryo. Arrows indicate the first streams of fluids, which result from functional tensions between the two domains. The body stalk, which later becomes the umbilical cord, forms the bridge. Blood islands on the yolk sac and in the chorion are the source of blood. Initially lying outside the embryonic disc (Figure A, day 18), the heart primordium then shifts position until it lies under the brain primordium in the area of the neck.*

Developmental stages:
Days 13-15: Blood islands develop on the yolk sac, in the body stalk, and in the chorion.
Day 17: The first vessels form.
Day 20: The first primitive endocardial heart tubes develop.
Day 21: The heart primordium is connected to the vessels, and circulation begins.
Day 22: The heart begins to beat.

to breathe air and the aperture in the heart's interatrial septum (foramen ovale) is sealed. As such, therefore, human life on Earth is made possible by the two middle organ systems (heart and lungs).

The next systems to become functional are the **nervous system** and the **metabolic organs**. Both are largely mature before birth, especially the nervous system. The first reflexes can occur before birth, anytime from the third month onward. The nervous system's rapid, early development makes possible not only the timely development of vital reflexes (grasping reflex, sucking reflex, etc.) after birth but also higher mental development (Portmann's "cerebralization," reference 56), which begins later. During the first few months of life, the major sense organs are not yet fully functional. The motor centers of the central nervous system mature only gradually—i.e., in the first few years of life—in connection with the limbs' motor functions. Children become ready for school only around age 6, when they lose their baby teeth and the first stage of physical development comes to a close.

The gastrointestinal tract slowly becomes accustomed to earthly food and takes a relatively long time to become fully functional.

The **organs of excretion** (kidneys, etc.) begin to function immediately after birth, but it takes a long time for the baby to learn to control urination and bowel movements. The **organs of reproduction**, which are part of the urogenital system, assume their specific functions only after puberty, which sets in between ages 12 and 14 (Figure 32).

The defense organs of the **immune system** (thymus, spleen, lymphatic organs) differentiate only after birth. The lymph organs begin to "learn" specific defense processes immediately after birth (assuming that they come in contact with foreign matter), but the thymus (unlike the organs of reproduction) begins to atrophy as early as the mid- to late teens, which means that this aspect of the immune system's functional activity gradually begins to decline (Figure 32).

Finally, the **musculoskeletal system** is the body's youngest organ system. At birth, it is relatively undeveloped and suited only to awkward crawling movements. The first major step in the development of this system occurs 12 to 16 months later, when the child first stands upright. Subsequently, the limbs grow in rhythmic spurts (one growth spurt in each of the first three seven-year periods) until growth ceases in the person's early to mid-twenties (59, 117, 118).

Thus, taking hold of body-based functions occurs in **three major phases**:

Phase 1: Directly after birth, the organs of the middle system (cardiovascular and respiratory systems) assume their definitive functions, which they retain until life ends.

Phase 2: The functionality of the polar organ systems (nervous system and metabolic system) gradually increases as they take up their earthly tasks.

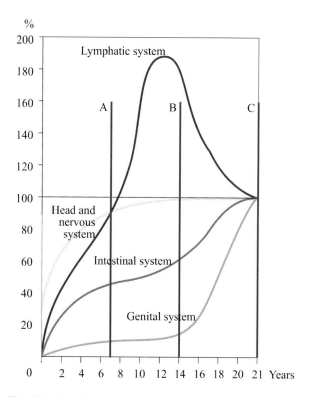

Fig. 32. **Relative rates of growth of different human organ systems after birth.** *100% = weight in adults. The nervous system and sense organs develop early, achieving almost their adult weight by the end of the first seven-year period (A). The lymphatic organs undergo a growth spurt in the second seven-year period (B), while the development of the organs of reproduction lags behind. The intestinal system takes relatively longer to achieve complete maturity. The growth of the body is completed only at the end of the third seven-year period (C). (Adapted from Tanner, in Rohen, 15).*

Phase 3: Numerous individual functions within the three major superordinate organ systems of the threefold human body—functions supported by organs and cell systems that gradually mature postnatally—begin to become active, thus completing the process of becoming human. In this phase, the immune system, which is uniquely related to the individuality itself, also gradually becomes functional (40).

Spiritual-Scientific Aspects of Embryonic Development

Prior Stages of the Earth's Evolution

In biology, the four great stages of embryonic development are repeatedly associated with the so-called "fundamental biogenetic law." According to Haeckel, von Baer, and others, all higher stages of development achieved in phylogeny are repeated in principle—that is, at least in abbreviated or simplified form—in the ontogenetic development of each individual. Thus human embryonic development includes a "fish" stage in which the potential to develop gills is present, although the human embryo ultimately develops neither true gills nor a fishlike body. Only the **principles of structural design** that governed this early stage of vertebrate development become manifest. Ernst Haeckel repeatedly emphasized that the early stages of embryonic development are similar in all animals (the gastraea theory, reference 41). Haeckel pointed out that gill development invariably begins at the cleavage-division stage (morulation), which is always followed by blastulalike and gastrulalike developments. Many lower animals remain at such primitive stages of development, but vertebrates pass through them and go on to achieve more complex configurations.

In this connection, it is interesting to note that Rudolf Steiner also spoke of four great stages in the evolution of our solar system (14). According to Steiner, three planetary stages preceded the development of the Earth as such:

1. **Ancient Saturn**: During Ancient Saturn evolution, the human physical body took shape but remained as yet without life or internalized soul life. "To get a picture of this, imagine how a mulberry or a blackberry is made up of small individual fruits. To those with supersensible perception, Saturn at this period in its evolution was likewise made up of individual Saturn beings, which, although they did not yet possess individual lives and souls, reflected the lives and souls of the beings that lived in them." (14, p.142)

2. **Ancient Sun**: On the Ancient Sun, human beings achieved a higher level in that the "physical body, already seminally formed on Saturn," became "the vehicle for an etheric or life body." "The first signs of inner vitality also entered the germinal human being. Life began." If the Saturn stage saw only mulberrylike, unenlivened "eggs of warmth," the Ancient Sun had animate, living forms capable of "inner movements that can be compared to the movements of sap in a present-day plant." (14, pp. 154-55)

3. **Ancient Moon**: On the Ancient Moon, the "influx of the astral body" began. Along with the astral body, human beings acquired their "first soul characteristics." As a result, "processes that took place in the astral body because it possessed a life body—processes that had still been plantlike in character during the Sun phase of evolution—began to be accompanied by sensation, and the astral body began to experience pleasure and displeasure because of these processes." (14, p.167)

On the Ancient Moon, therefore, animallike sentient life began for the first time within the germinal human being, whose plantlike, outward-directed existence was replaced by an independent, internal life in which feelings and drives appeared. In other words, a functional invagination had occurred.

The substance present on Ancient Saturn resembled warmth or fire, and something related to air and light was present on the Ancient Sun. On the Ancient Moon, matter condensed to a "watery" substance of sorts, although admittedly only in qualitative terms, since this matter did not correspond to water as we know it today.

4. **Earth evolution**: The fourth planetary stage is that of the Earth. Earth evolution as such, however, did not begin immediately but only after a recapitulation of the three earlier planetary stages. During the actual Earth stage of evolution, further densification occurred and matter achieved the mineral, solid, or "earthly" state (14).

Stage	Stage of embryonic development	Potential present in the germinal human being	Planetary stage	Cosmic state of matter	Corresponding natural kingdom
1. (Point)	Morulation	Physical body	"Ancient Saturn"	Warmthlike	Mineral
2. (Surface)	Blastulation	Life body	"Ancient Sun"	Air/lightlike	Plant
3. (Space)	Gastrulation (development of the embryo)	Soul (astral body)	"Ancient Moon"	Waterlike	Animal
4. (Space and counterspace)	Birth of the fetus	"I"	Earth	Solid	Human

Table 10. Stages of human embryonic development and their relationship to prior planetary stages (adapted from Steiner, reference 14).

A Comparison of Human Embryonic Development with the Earth's Evolution

It is completely possible to see human embryonic development as reflecting the four stages of planetary evolution as described above (Table 10). In that case, the morula would correspond to the Saturn stage. After implantation, a plantlike kind of life begins in the human embryo as streams of fluids and blisterlike hollow spaces (yolk sac, amnion) appear. No inner life is present as yet; the essence of the human being is still present on the periphery, in the embryonic sheaths, and is reflected on the surfaces of the vesicles. The embryonic disc with its germ layers is a surfacelike structure and represents an "archetypal leaf" or "archetypal plant" of sorts, since it still lacks any internal organization with interior surfaces and organs.

The third (Moon) stage would correspond to gastrulation, which begins in humans with the development of Hensen's node and the primitive groove. This stage, which includes somite disintegration and mesenchyme development, is the first to produce a three-dimensional embryonic body. In a certain respect, therefore, it represents the development of life on the animal level.

The actual Earth stage would then be achieved only at birth, when the human being emerges onto solid ground and breathes the air of the Earth's atmosphere for the first time, leaving behind the "sphere" of the membranes that supported life in the womb. The placenta is expelled in the form of the afterbirth. At this stage, the "I" slowly begins to move into the body, one step at a time.

Phylogenetic Processes

Incremental Mastery of the Dimensions of Space In Vertebrate Evolution

If we take our introductory sketch of the human being as evolution's endpoint and thus as our standard for the evolutionary process as a whole, then we might say that the vertebrates—the only group of animals we will consider here—master the dimensions of space one at a time. Two incisive events occurred in vertebrate evolution: first, the transition from aquatic to terrestrial life (i.e., from fish to amphibians); second, the development of the ability to stand upright among primates, which ultimately led to the emergence of the upright human form.

Through uprightness, human beings gain a totally new relationship to space, new options for moving within its dimensions, and a free space in which to exert their will extensively and independently. In contrast, animals' organs of locomotion are typically very one-sided structures and significantly limit what they are able to do.

Friedrich Schiller once expressed this phenomenon as follows: "In animals and plants, Nature not only provides the goal but also undertakes its achievement. In the case of human beings, however, Nature sets only the goal, leaving its achievement up to us....Of all known beings, only we have the prerogative to apply our will to given circumstances, which remain inalterable

for merely natural beings, and to initiate a whole new series of phenomena within ourselves."(43) Herder says, "No longer infallible machines in the hands of Nature, human beings become the goal and purpose of their own striving." (44)

The unique status of human beings in the animal kingdom is not only evident in brain development but also impressively apparent in the phylogeny of the limbs.

Limb Evolution

Primitive vertebrates (***Acrania and fish***) lived in water and had no real extremities, although bilateral symmetry and segmental subdivision of the torso (metamerism) were clearly developed. Because their heads and limbs were still in the early stages of evolution, we are somewhat justified in seeing these early vertebrates as "torso creatures." Actual limb development began only with the transition to terrestrial life, i.e., when animals touched solid ground. It is interesting to note that the head began to be reshaped at the same time, becoming more clearly differentiated from the torso (119).

Initially, ***amphibians and reptiles*** evolved limbs that stuck straight out sideways. Because these limbs were used primarily to provide lateral leverage for torso movements, the functionally most important muscle groups were still located in the torso itself (Figure 33). These laterally extended limbs worked primarily in the right-left dimension.

Unlike birds, which evolved separately, **mammals** derived from the earliest reptiles, or perhaps directly from amphibians. Mammalian extremities now shifted to a location **under** the torso, i.e., into the front-back dimension as seen from the animal's perspective. As a result, the limbs' capacity for self-movement increased significantly. Muscles and motor mechanisms located near the torso but in the limbs themselves increased in importance relative to the torso's motor system. Differentiated self-movement of the terminal sections of the limbs (hand, foot), however, was still not possible.

In the transition to the **upright human being**, the limbs again rotated ninety degrees. As a result of this final major rotation, the limbs conquered the last of the three dimensions of space, namely the up-down dimension. The lower limbs were then fully integrated into the Earth's gravitational field and completely took over the tasks of standing and walking, while the upper limbs were released from direct involvement in these functions and became available for use in practical and artistic activities. Only at the human level did hands and feet develop specific, distinctly different motor capabilities, a sign that polarity (the typical structural principle in the up-down dimension) was also being applied to the limbs. Although front and hind extremities are somewhat differentiated in the vertebrates, they represent a true polarity only in human beings. Essentially, therefore, the true qualities of the three dimensions of space appear for the first time in human beings.

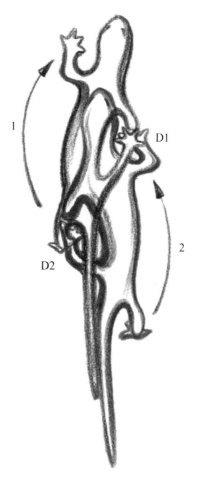

Fig. 33. **Crawling motion of a salamander**. From the initial position (red), the left forefoot swings in an arch (arrow 1) around the pivot point in the right forefoot (D1). In a corresponding gesture, the right hind foot then swings forward (arrow 2) around the pivot point of the left hind foot (D2). The limbs are used as "crutches" for the snakelike motion of the torso (adapted from stills from motion pictures, H. Braus, Anatomie des Menschen, Vol. 1, 1929).

Head Evolution

Similar evolutionary processes occurred in the head pole. In fish, the head is a part of the torso. The relatively hard, scaly exterior serves only to enclose the torso and to protect the sense organs, nervous system, and gills. The head became structurally distinct from the torso only in amphibians and reptiles, i.e., after the transition to terrestrial life and the beginning of

limb development. A true neck developed for the first time in mammals. The mammalian head is tubelike in shape and is characterized by a linear arrangement of different functional areas. The nose, mouth, and skull cavity lie roughly one behind the other, and the snout with its powerful jaws is much larger than the brain and sensory portions of the skull. The head still looks as if the

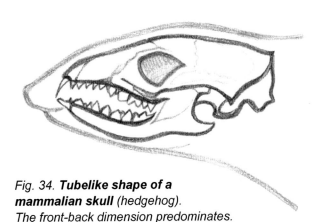

*Fig. 34. **Tubelike shape of a mammalian skull** (hedgehog). The front-back dimension predominates.*

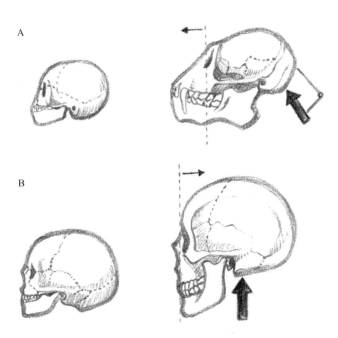

A

B

*Fig. 35. **Postnatal changes in skull shape in higher apes** (gibbon, A) **and humans** (B). Skulls of newborns (left) are still similar in apes and humans and are basically spherical in form. Postnatal growth of the facial skull is significant in the ape, whereas in humans the growth of this part is restrained while the brain cavity continues to grow (arrows; adapted from 48). The human skull, which balances on the spinal column (broad arrow), is freely mobile; the adult ape skull, which is weighed down in front by the disproportionate size of the facial skull and chewing apparatus, can no longer balance on the torso and must be held in place by powerful neck muscles.*

torso had simply been extended forward, in the body's main direction of movement.

Limb specialization is reflected in the head, especially in corresponding differentiations in the chewing apparatus. In the tubelike mammalian skull as well as in the limbs, the front-back dimension predominates (Figure 34).

In the evolution of humans, the body's new vertical orientation brings the up-down dimension into play. Among primates, the head becomes increasingly spherical. Functionally distinct spaces within the skull (oral, nasal, and brain cavities) are now stacked **vertically** instead of being arranged in a front-to-back sequence. The tubelike shape of the mammalian skull is abandoned, the growth of the snout is restricted, and the head assumes a spherical form so that it can balance freely at the top of the spinal column (Figure 35).

Thus the head of the vertebrate, like the limbs, traverses the dimensions of space during its evolution. Among lower vertebrates, especially in fishes, bilateral symmetry (right-left) still largely dominates the structure of the head. In mammals, the front-back dimension is added, elongating the head (Figure 34). In humans, an approximately spherical head that fully incorporates all three dimensions appears for the first time. In contrast to the limbs with their radial structure, the ideal sphere is a body that does not actively take hold of the three dimensions but instead inverts and encloses "radial space." The sphere's surface does not reach out, it encloses (Figure 36). Thus we must see head evolution and limb evolution as a developmental polarity that has led to completely opposite results in human beings (i.e., at the end of the evolutionary sequence). Our radial, many-jointed limbs reach out and insert themselves fully into space, enabling us to experience it. The human head is the exact opposite of the limbs. It has withdrawn from space, and its spherical surface encloses a kind of counterspace in which we grasp the dimensions of space on the mental level (through perception and cognition) instead of taking hold of them directly. Matter, like space, is altered whenever it enters the head. The act of chewing, for example, physically breaks down the three-dimensional structure of food and initiates its chemical breakdown through digestion. Similarly, the major sense organs located in the head take the surrounding world apart through perception so that it can re-appear in our consciousness. Within the head's "counterspace," the nervous system provides the basis for mental processes such as cognition and memory to take place freely, unaffected by the spatial world of colliding bodies.

Human Consciousness And the Experience of Space

When we focus our waking consciousness on our experience of space, we notice that the way we experience space in the head (i.e., in the domain of the senses and nervous system) is diametrically opposed to how we experience it in our limbs. In fact, we experience the three dimensions of space in three different ways in our lower-limb activity, upper-limb movements, and sense organs (45).

When we walk, we experience all three dimensions in the same way. Our will submerges itself into the spatial world, so to speak; with the help of our lower limbs, it becomes active in all three planes of space, although we remain unconscious of them as such.

The situation is somewhat different in the body's middle structural domain—for example, in upper limb movement (Figure 37). We move our arms primarily in the horizontal plane. Bringing our hands together allows us "grasp" the spatial world, both literally and figuratively. In the body's middle domain, in the experience of symmetry and in our expressive or working gestures, we experience primarily the horizontal dimensions (front-back and right-left). The third dimension, the vertical dimension of up and down, is experienced differently. Although we

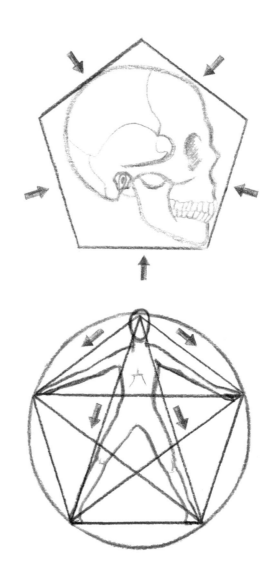

*Fig. 36. **Polarity between head formation and limbs**. The head can be seen as a spherical structure shaped from outside, the limbs as organs that radiate outward from within and become active.*

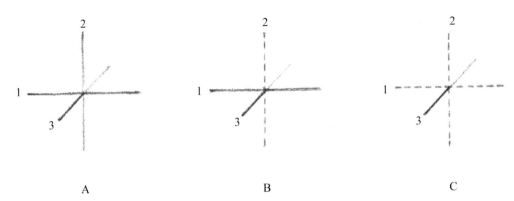

Fig. 37. **Experiencing movement in space** *(adapted from Steiner, 45).*
Dimensions: 1: right-left; 2: up-down, 3: front-back.
A. In the domain of the lower limbs (walking), movements in all three dimensions are experienced through the will.
B. In the domain of the upper limbs, we carry out conscious movements especially in the horizontal plane (dimensions 1 and 3).
C. In our visual field, we mainly experience the dimension of depth (dimension 3).

may walk on our hands or lift an object, our will lives differently in the vertical element than it does in the horizontal. The vertical dimension becomes a "given," present from the very beginning (45).

In the head, two dimensions (right-left and up-down) become "givens" that are no longer fully accessible to the will (Figure 37). In the act of seeing, the dimension of depth (front-back) is the only dimension we still take hold of actively and therefore experience as space. There is a big difference between depth perception and perceiving an image as surface. Consciously experiencing three dimensions in seeing requires a deliberate act of will in which the brain is involved.

Steiner's account of these phenomena is based primarily on will experience (45). It is also possible, however, to consider them from the opposite perspective, namely, from the thinking side. In our lower limbs, we submerge ourselves completely in the world of space. This is how we become convinced of the reality of space, although the experience does not become conscious on the mental level. In the middle (rhythmic) domain, our will withdraws from one dimension—the vertical dimension of height—so that we can acquire the forces we need for cognitive activity. And finally,

in the sense organs of the head, an additional dimension is released, and our will remains active only in the dimension of depth. Here, an image of the three-dimensionality of space develops, but we cannot experience the reality of the corporeal world itself. Ultimately, supported by the nervous system, we free ourselves even from this third dimension. Through our faculties of abstraction and creativity, we can bring all the forces of space to manifestation in our cognition, memory, or creative ideas, without being involved in real space at all. Here we see an internalization of all the dimensions, an "invagination" that transforms space into nonspace, or counterspace, on the mental level.

Because animals have not completed the passage through the dimensions that culminates in upright posture, they also cannot achieve human levels of mental development. Arnold Gehlen offers an impressive account of the unique status of human beings in contrast to the animal kingdom (46, 47). He writes about a "reduction of instincts" and the "freeing of human sense organs from animal functional cycles." He also points out that "all true use of symbols (such as language) rests on the ability to separate behavior from the immediate situational context, because the essential character of any symbol is that it points to **something that is not given**, to something inaccessible from this context." Almost all animals, says Gehlen, are to a great extent "bound to specific regional environments to which they are adapted. Consequently, observing their organic structure—right down to the very details of their sense organs, defensive and offensive weapons, organs of digestion, etc.—allows us to draw conclusions about their lifestyles and habitat, and vice versa."

"Human beings alone are capable of independent action. They are not predetermined," In other words, "They themselves are still their own work-in-progress.... It is part of their physical nature to be unfinished." They are "beings at risk; the chance of meeting with failure is inherent in their physical constitution" (46).

Adaptation and Antiadaptation As Evolutionary Principles

In considering the qualities of the three dimensions of space, we addressed the question of evolution for the first time. We assumed that a process of higher development does exist in which human beings represent at least a provisional end-stage.

But before we ask about the principles at work in evolution, two preliminary questions must first be clarified: First, can vertebrate species be classified in an evolutionary series ranging from lower to higher stages of development, or do they simply represent variations on a theme at essentially the same level? The second incisive question has to do with the temporal sequence of these developmental stages. If more highly organized forms really do represent higher evolutionary stages that build on previous levels, they must have emerged later, and the paleontological sequence of fossilized animals must reveal these evolutionary stages. Without such a sequence, true evolution (from simpler to higher forms of organization) would be inconceivable.

With regard to the first question, if we compare the **structural models** (not the individual traits) of the six major vertebrate classes, we do indeed

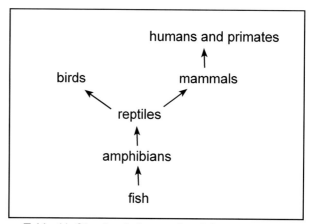

Table 11. Structural stages of vertebrate evolution (adapted from Portmann, 48).

discover a clear sequence, which forms the basis of most zoological studies. First in the sequence are forms such as Amphioxus, followed by fish, amphibians, and reptiles. After the reptilian stage, birds and mammals must be seen as parallel developments. Primates (including humans) represent a further development of the mammalian branch, whereas the development that began with birds has not yet achieved a next step. If we consider birds a side branch in vertebrate evolution, **five different vertebrate structural models** remain. From the perspective of functional morphology, these basic models also represent stages of increasing complexity and perfection.

But do they also represent a time sequence of steps toward higher development? Portmann answered this fundamental question in the affirmative (48). He writes,

If we trace the appearance of fossilized animal forms in the fauna of past epochs and record (for simplicity's sake) only the layers of the Earth's crust in which representatives of the major systematic groups are observed for the first time, we note an important correspondence between the structural stages outlined above (Table 11) and the earliest geological appearances of animal groups. In other words, **the order of appearance of vertebrate groups in geological layers is the same as their classification in terms of morphological**

Geological Era	Period	Epoch	Duration in millions of years	Millions of years elapsed since its beginning	First appearance of vertebrate groups
Cenozoic	Quarternary	Present	0.025		
		Pleistocene	1	1	
	Tertiary	Pliocene	10		
		Miocene	13		Hominids
		Oligocene	14		
		Eocene	20		
		Paleocene	13	70	Primates
Mesozoic	Cretaceous		65	135	
	Jurassic		45	180	Birds
	Triassic		40	220	Mammals
Paleozoic	Permian		50	270	Reptiles
	Carboniferous		80	350	
	Devonian		50	400	Amphibians
	Silurian		40	440	Agnatha, fish
	Ordovician		60	500	
	Cambrian		100/110	600	

Table 12. Geological periods and the first appearance of vertebrate groups (adapted from Portmann, 48).

complexity.... The fact that the systematic classification of vertebrates according to their structural relationships corresponds to the order of their appearance in the history of the Earth deserves considerable attention. It is one of the most fundamental arguments that this vertebrate series is the image of a real and coherent relationship, i.e., that more highly organized species emerged from more simply organized forms in the course of geological time.

The human beings who appear at the end of this series as the last and most highly developed living things must therefore have passed through all the preceding levels of organization (i.e., structural models, not individual animal forms) during their bodily evolution. Incremental progress in the direction of higher development, however, is inconceivable unless there is a goal inherent in evolution itself (theory of orthogenesis). Consistent, incremental development from one structural model to the next is impossible unless each stage represents another step in the direction of the endpoint of evolution, namely, the human species.

In our discussion of limb evolution, we discovered evidence of an immanent "goal" of evolution in that each vertebrate structural model masters a new dimension of space and all three dimensions appear in their primal quality for the first time in the human model.

But how can we characterize the forces underlying these evolutionary processes more precisely to permit a better understanding of evolution as a whole?

Most evolutionary biologists dismiss any possibility of an orthogenetic thrust in evolution and accept only adaptation (i.e., natural selection of the forms best suited to the corresponding environmental conditions) and mutation (changes that occur as the result of completely random coincidental mutations) as effective forces in evolution. The "struggle for survival" is assumed to select mutations in such a way that the best-adapted organism survives to reproduce, and less than optimally adapted species die out. Nature "does not learn from her failures but only from her successes" (49). These successes are presumed to be exclusively the product of coincidental processes.

Macbeth offers a formidable critique of the logical inconsistencies and one-sidedness of these views (50). That current theories of evolution are still hypothetical in many important points is often overlooked (cf. 51-54). In particular, the orthogenetic principle—i.e., the possibility that evolutionary events are all directed toward a common, immanent goal—is seldom discussed seriously any more.

The principle of adaptation can no longer be questioned now that we are aware of so many examples of it, but is it the only principle at work? Haven't other processes played a role in evolution? Recently, this question has again been raised repeatedly (52, 54, 55). In the next section, we will consider it from the perspective of macroscopic phenomena, disregarding issues of molecular biology.

Adaptive and Antiadaptive Processes

There are countless examples of the way adaptation has occurred over the course of evolution, but we will mention only the often-cited developmental sequence of the horse. The oldest form of horse, the *Eohippus* of the Eocene epoch, was very small and still had four-toed extremities and a complete set of teeth. The larger *Mesohippus*, which had three-toed limbs, appeared during the Oligocene epoch. The modern horse has only a single, highly developed third toe; its remaining digital rays— the so-called splint bones—have degenerated. Its teeth have also become differentiated in a one-sided way and the snout has become much larger in proportion to the cranium. A great variety of horselike forms occur together in the fossil record (50). Thus this famous horse series cannot be seen as a line of descent but only as a sequence of stages in an increasingly one-sided process of

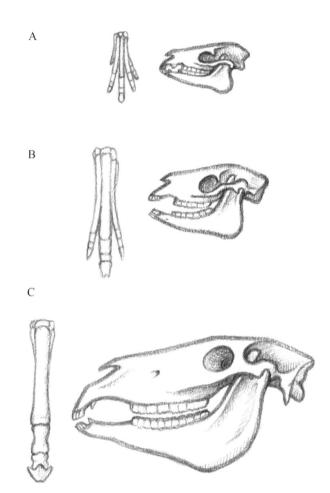

Fig. 38. **Evolutionary series of horselike forms** *(skull and foot). Types A – C represent a geological series whose stages are separated by millions of years (adapted from Portmann, 48).*
A: Eohippus, *the smallest, most ancient (Eocene) form of horse, which had four-toed extremities;*
B: *three-toed horse of the Oligocene period (e.g.,* Mesohippus, America);
C: *Species of large horses with strongly developed third toes (solidungulates) became increasingly common beginning with the Miocene period (e.g.,* Equus, *the modern horse genus, which has been in existence since the Pliocene period).*

differentiation. Clearly, however, the overall trend resulted in an extremely one-sided end product (Figure 38). In the evolution of equine limbs, an originally versatile structure was abandoned in favor of a single function, namely, speed in running. The limbs of recent horse species are extremely well adapted to rapid locomotion but have sacrificed all other possibilities. Similarly, the equine head has become dominated by highly specialized structures adapted to a very one-sided diet.

We cannot talk about adaptation in the same way with regard to **human limbs**, even though the process of acquiring an **upright** stance is crucial to human limb evolution. Most apes still exhibit numerous limb specializations: their arms are unduly long, their legs relatively short. Many have feet that can be used for grasping, which is useful for tree-dwellers but not well suited to walking upright on the ground. But the human foot is certainly not one-sided in its adaptation to upright walking. On the contrary, the complex architecture of its arch has evolved so as to be flexible rather than rigid. The human foot is elastic enough to adapt to uneven ground—a quality that is enhanced by the foot's ability to rotate (pro/supination). In humans, the lower limbs are capable of supporting the body in an upright position without any unsteadiness. As a result, the head and upper limbs are totally relieved of the burden of supporting and moving the body and become available for other functions. The space accessible to the upper limbs is increased enormously; the hands can be used for grasping and thus also for practical and artistic activities— one of the most important preconditions for human culture.

Logically, it cannot be said that the freeing of the upper extremities in the process of acquiring uprightness constitutes an adaptation. On the contrary, it is a process of the opposite kind, which we will simply call **antiadaptation** for the moment. In the case of the human upper limbs, increased opportunities for movement do not serve primarily specialized functions or signify any new specialization or one-sidedness for the body as a whole. Rather, they open up a new spatial dimension in which new forms of movement and new possibilities for the expression of the human soul and spirit can be freely developed.

Arnold Gehlen formulated these connections as follows:

The thrust of natural evolution is to adapt highly specialized structures and organs to very specific environments and thus to exploit the many different "milieus" that exist in nature as niche habitats for adapted life forms. Shallow edges of tropical waters, ocean depths, barren mountain cliffs, and the underbrush of sparse mixed forests are all specific environments for animals that can live only there, just as certain parasites can survive only on the skin of warm-blooded animals, to name one of countless unique examples. In contrast, from the morphological perspective humans have almost no specialized organs. The human being consists of a series of **unspecialized** attributes that appear primitive from the perspective of evolutionary biology. Human teeth, for example, show a primitive absence of spaces between them and a generalized structure, which suggests neither a vegetarian nor a carnivorous diet. The great apes, as highly specialized tree-dwellers, have overdeveloped arms for swinging from branch to branch and feet adapted to climbing; they have coats of fur and massive canine teeth. In contrast, human beings are hopelessly maladaptive by the standards of the natural world. Biologically speaking, humans are uniquely ill equipped and unspecialized. The only feature that makes up for these deficits is the human capacity for work or dexterity, i.e., our ability to use our hands and intelligence. This is why we are upright and conscious of our surroundings and our hands are free (46).

Somewhat later, Gehlen describes human beings as subject to a very unanimallike and burdensome overstimulation of the senses. For humans, "relieving themselves of this burden, independently and through their own means, i.e., transforming the deficits of their existential situation into opportunities for life, is a vitally important and physically necessary task" (46).

It has often been said that the prehensile human hand is an adaptive specialization rather than a "primitive" or primordial feature that has avoided any animallike adaptation to specialized functions. While it is true that the human hand with its five digital rays still preserves some of the primitive traits of primordial limbs, there can also be no doubt that it has achieved a high degree of differentiation with regard to prehensile ability. Think about the structure of the thumb joints and related musculature, major finger joints, or muscles between the carpal bones, to name just a few examples. The decisive point, however, is that all this differentiation is directed toward versatility rather than one-sidedness, toward universality rather than specialization and adaptation. In other words, no single individual function predominates here. Instead, a higher degree of functional potential is achieved, although its meaning becomes apparent only through the actual activities it permits, which are not predetermined. Thus this is a case of **antiadaptive** (rather than adaptive) **differentiation**.

A very similar process also occurs in the head. The evolution of the vertebrate brain, for example, is characterized by the constantly increasing size of the neocortex. Especially among primates, the size of the cortex increases so much that the surface of the brain develops more and more convolutions (gyri and sulci). Ultimately the endbrain/telencephalon expands so much that the other parts of the brain (the midbrain/ mesencephalon, interbrain/diencephalon, and cerebellum) are covered by the cerebral cortex (Figure 39). Portmann calls this phenomenon the constantly increasing "**cerebralization**" of the brain over the course of evolution (56).

In the transition between humans and apes, brain size often serves as the only reliable criterion of the human or nonhuman character of fossil finds. It is commonly said that increased brain capacity gave the first humans an enormous adaptive advantage, because they could apply their increased communication ability to the struggle for existence. This conclusion,

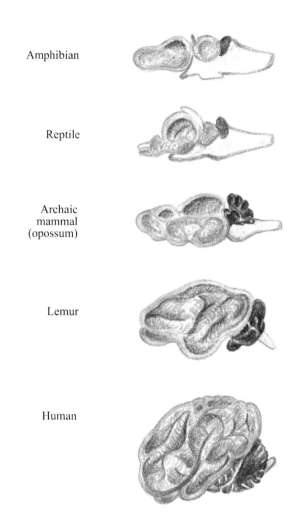

Amphibian

Reptile

Archaic mammal (opossum)

Lemur

Human

Fig. 39. **Phylogenetic series of increasing cerebralization** *(adapted from Portmann, 56). The cerebrum develops vigorously, increasingly covering and displacing the other sections of the brain. Formation of furrows and ridges (gyrification) intensifies as evolution proceeds.*
Cerebrum (neocortex): blue;
Rhinencephalon (olfactory brain): red;
Cerebellum: black;
Brain stem and midbrain (in amphibians and reptiles): green.

however, is completely unfounded. If we study the development of the cerebral cortex, both as it appears to have evolved and as it is repeated in ontogeny, we will be surprised to discover that undifferentiated cells "swarm" out from the interior of the brain primordium and settle in the surface zones of the cortex to form new groups of neurons. For the most part, the functions of these groups of nuclei are not predetermined. Although they outrank "older," subordinate areas of the brain, they initially have no fixed functions in the body's adaptive field. The specialized functions of the emigrant cerebral cortex cells, which in humans number between 14 and 16 billion, are only gradually determined during a person's life. The location and scope of these cell groups determine a person's ability to learn, but their functional connections are not predetermined. They are independent and "impressionable." A person learning a new language, manual activity, or pattern of behavior, no matter how late in life, can always count on the enormous, un-predetermined and un-adapted potential of cerebral cortex cells. **Human beings remain capable of learning all their lives**, whereas animals remain impressionable only for a short time after birth and then become inflexible for the rest of their existence. Thus the cerebralization of the human brain is also a process that does not increase adaptation. On the contrary, it increases an individual's scope, universality, and versatility. In other words, it represents an antiadaptive process.

With increasing cerebralization, evolution is aiming for an organism that can free itself from the immediate constraints of its environment and its own biological instincts (Portmann, 56). The goal is an organism capable of inventing, mastering, and permanently remembering functions that are not primarily intrinsic to the nervous system but are present only as potentials and possibilities, as is also the case with regard to the use of our human hands.

The Evolution of the Skull and Head

The transformation of the **skull** from lower to higher vertebrates is protracted and complex.

In fish species, the skull consists of a mosaic of bony plates that make up the relatively "expressionless front end of a swimming body" (Portmann, 48). It consists of three parts that evolved relatively independently of each other (Figure 40):

1. The **dermatocranium**, which consists of many small bony plates that develop directly out of the connective tissue of the skin, forms the skullcap.

2. The **neurocranium**, whose bony elements develop out of cartilaginous preliminary stages, surrounds primarily the brain and the sensory organs (the eye, organ of smell, and labyrinth). Later, it forms the base of the skull.

3. The **viscerocranium** or **splanchnocranium** consists of several segmentally arranged, jointed, cartilaginous branchial arches separated by so-called branchial grooves. In fishes, the visceral skeleton serves the processes of taking in food (jaws) and oxygen (gills).

After the transition to terrestrial life and the development of pulmonary respiration, a radical transformation of the skull occurs in amphibians and reptiles. The gills degenerate and are partially incorporated into the newly emerging organs of hearing and vocalization. In mammals, what was the primary jaw joint in fish is transformed into the joint between the hammer and anvil of the middle ear; the joint that now serves mastication (the joint between the lower jaw and the base of the skull) is a new formation (secondary temporomandibular joint).

Evolutionary changes in the chewing apparatus and jaw muscles are accompanied by a dissolution of the original, compact skullcap to make room for the enlarging brain. Flat, scalelike bones developing directly out of connective tissue then form a new skullcap and, together with the

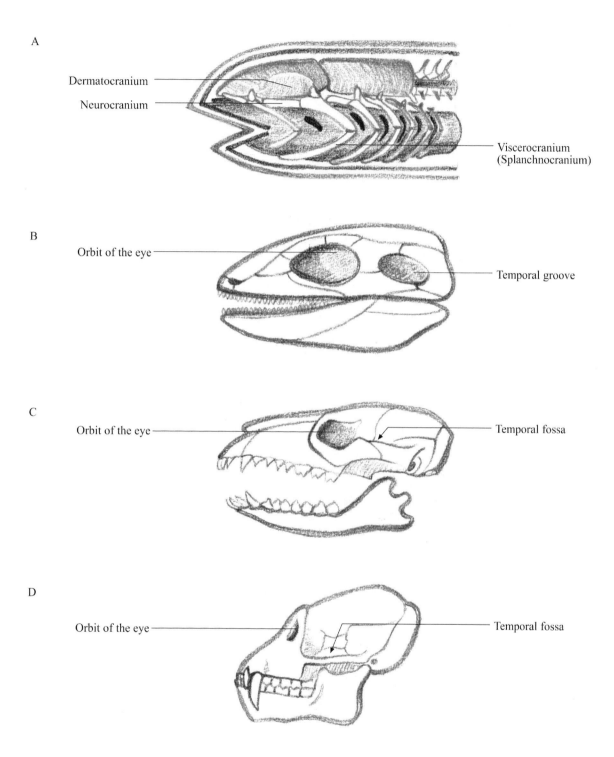

Fig. 40. **Evolution of the skull in vertebrates** *(from Portmann, 48).*
A: Basic structural model of the vertebrate skull. The neurocranium, which develops from cartilage, forms the base of the skull. The bones of the roof of the skull, which develop directly out of connective tissue, form the dermatocranium, and the viscerocranium or splanchnocranium provides the basis for the facial skeleton.
B: Skull of a mammallike reptile (theriodont) with a temporal fenestra.
C: Skull of a primitive mammal. The eye orbit and the temporal fossa are continuous in the same structure.
D: Ape skull. The eye orbit and temporal fossa are separated, and the jaw bones are more differentiated.

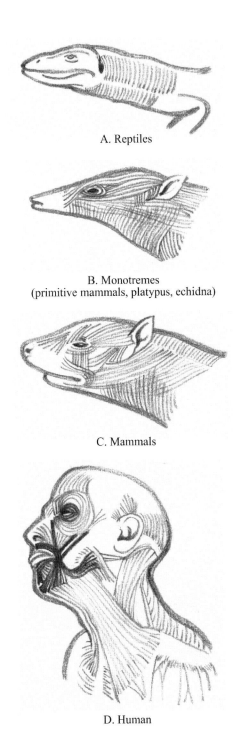

A. Reptiles

B. Monotremes
(primitive mammals, platypus, echidna)

C. Mammals

D. Human

Fig. 41. **The evolution of the muscles of facial expression** *becomes possible when the skin muscles of the torso shift toward the front and become concentrated around openings in the skull (A-C from Portmann, 48).*

cartilage-derived bones of the base of the skull, form a new protective covering for the brain (the dermatocranium). These developments explain why a number of bones contain portions of both the primary dermatocranium and neurocranium—for example, the squama and os petromastoideum of the temporal bone or the squama and basal portion of the occipital bone.

Lateral dissolution begins at the reptilian stage with the development of the temporal fenestrae. This process continues in mammals, where the eye socket and the lower temporal fossa are continuous. Below them, a pronounced zygomatic arch marks the former lower edge of the skull (Figure 40).

Beginning with the tetrapod stage, the occipital joint clearly delineates the back of the skull from the spinal column. A neck develops, and the head becomes independently mobile as a result of unique muscular and bony structures. The second branchial arch gives rise to skin muscles, which in mammals are increasingly displaced toward the front, into the area around the major body openings (palpebral fissure, mouth, nasal opening). Ultimately, they develop into the mimetic musculature, completely transforming the expressionless faces of fish and lower vertebrates and creating entirely new and varied possibilities for soul expression, especially in primates and humans (head gestures, mimicry; see Figure 41).

Contrary evolutionary directions in the dermatocranium and viscerocranium. To superficial consideration, evolutionary transformations in the skull could be seen as adaptive necessities triggered by the transition from aquatic to terrestrial life, i.e., from gills to pulmonary respiration. It is undoubtedly true that the earliest terrestrial vertebrates would not have survived if their gills had not developed into functional jaws for chewing and their foregut into organs for breathing air. Clearly, these are adaptations to a new environment and new lifestyles. But the same principles fail to explain the noteworthy fact that jaw development in primates, for example, is increasingly retarded as species approach a more humanlike form.

Why would a highly differentiated adaptation of the chewing mechanism be developed and then abandoned?

Today it is universally acknowledged that the human jaw remains retarded. Its numbers of molars are reduced, and the upper and lower jaws stop growing once the milk teeth emerge. As unbelievable as it may seem at first glance, the arch of the first dentition is the same size as the corresponding section of the adult dental arch (cf. Kipp, 54; see Figure 42). Since the adult jaw holds 32 teeth and the juvenile jaw only 20, there is no room for three additional adult molars on each side. The back of the human dental arch grows (by adding bone) to accommodate them. In apes, but not in humans, the front of the dental arch also expands. The part of the human jaw that formerly held the milk teeth remains completely unchanged in both size and shape. Prognathism (growth of the jaw in a forward direction), which is so characteristic of nonhuman primates and leads to the development of a pronounced jaw that can also serve as a weapon, appears to be inhibited in humans through an early ossification of the epiphyseal plates between the bones in the facial skull. This inhibition applies not only to the jawbones themselves but also to all other viscerocranial elements. Their epiphyseal lines, the areas of actual growth, all ossify shortly after birth.

The human viscerocranium (face) does not undergo the elongation so characteristic of mammals and primates; the related specialization of jaw and head structures (chewing apparatus, temporomandibular joint, lips, teeth, palate, nose, etc.) is also absent. Human facial development avoids specialized adaptation to any specific, one-sided function. Like the hand in the domain of the extremities, the human facial skull remains primitive, "juvenile," relatively unadapted, and suited to many purposes.

It is interesting to note that the facial skull of juvenile nonhuman primates is still spherical and "undifferentiated" in shape. As postnatal development continues, however, the juvenile shape is soon abandoned, and differentiation in the direction of one-sided, specialized structures

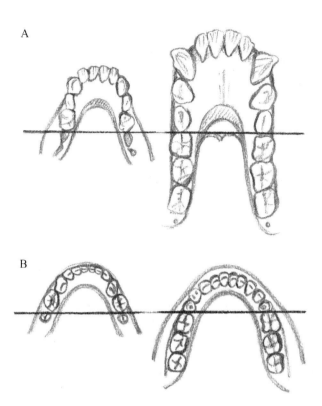

Fig. 42. **Dental arch of the orangutan lower jaw** (A) **and human lower jaw** (B), showing milk teeth on the left and the adult teeth on the right. In contrast to the development in apes, the part of the jaw in which the milk teeth are set is not enlarged in human adults (from Kipp, 54).

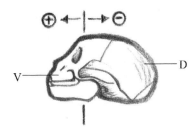

Newborn

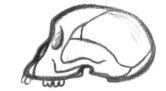

Juvenile with the first dentition complete

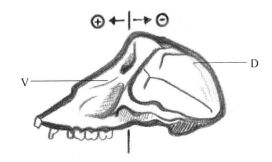

Adult animal (female)

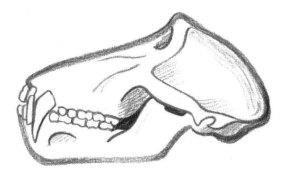

Adult animal (male)

*Fig. 43. **Differences in postnatal growth of the braincase** (dermatocranium, D) **and facial skull** (viscerocranium, V) **in apes** (baboon). Especially in males, a powerful mastication mechanism develops postnatally. Through early ossification of the cranial sutures, postnatal growth of the braincase is increasingly retarded.*

occurs by leaps and bounds (Figure 43). This is the same process that we described above: an undifferentiated, initially universal juvenile form encompassing many possibilities is transformed into a highly specialized form unique to its species.

The specializations thus achieved are often astounding (Figure 44). In **rodents**, for example, the incisors grow constantly, becoming long and chisellike, and in the temporomandibular joint, the orientation of the head of the mandible is nearly longitudinal, resulting in almost exclusively gliding movements. In **carnivores**, almost all the teeth are pointed and look like canine teeth. The head of the mandible becomes a transversely oriented cylinder, so that the jaw moves almost exclusively like a hinge. This joint is extremely strong and allows considerable force to be applied to catching, dragging, or tearing apart prey. The proportions of the jaw are very different in **ruminants**, where none of the teeth resemble fangs. The dominant element here is the molar type, with a broad crown and a horizontal chewing surface. Canine teeth are often totally absent. The jaw joint is especially adapted to lateral chewing motions. Thus a ruminant's mastication apparatus reflects its digestive tract as a whole, which has become specialized in breaking down cellulose (indigestible for humans) through repeated mechanical and chemical assaults (Figure 44).

Many nonhuman primates have developed powerful jaws with specialized functions. The jaw may serve as an active weapon of offense or defense, or may have very prominent canine teeth that are used to threaten or frighten enemies, in which case psychological gesturing becomes more important than actual use.

In contrast, **human** teeth are exceptionally harmonious and not restricted to a single function. The different tooth types (incisors, canines, molars) that are selectively emphasized in other mammal species are incorporated into a uniform, harmonious row of teeth with no gaps, and all types are represented more or less equally (Figure 42).

Humans, therefore, maintain an undifferentiated, quasi "preadaptive" condition that probably represents the point of departure for all mammalian specializations. Instead of adaptive processes, nonadaptive processes have prevailed in humans, preventing all of the many possible specialized differentiations.

This lack of specialization is also evident in the structure of the human ***temporomandibular joint***, which is not used one-sidedly as it is in animals. In the human jaw, all three motions (gliding, hinge, and grinding) are equally represented and readily usable. Furthermore, this joint is one of the most mobile in the entire human body. The head of the mandible easily slides out of its socket; it can move back and forth as well as from side to side. This phenomenon, which we would call a dislocation in any other joint, has become a normal physiological feature in the jaw. It's easy to demonstrate the range of movement in this joint. Simply touch the skin in front of your ear and move your jaw in all directions. It's astonishing to note how freely the head of the mandible moves. (Of course, a pathological dislocation of the jaw is also possible, which in no way contradicts this conclusion.)

The temporomandibular joint's exceptional flexibility and freedom of movement depends on a number of anatomical features unique to humans. For example, the capsule/ligament apparatus is very resilient, and the chewing muscles are relatively delicate in structure. The chewing muscles do not reach all the way to the braincase (dermatocranium) as they do in apes, some of which develop huge bony combs on the skullcap to serve as attachment points. Furthermore, the ascending branch of the human lower jaw is longer than it is in most animals and almost forms a right angle. Studies in photoelasticity (120) confirm that as a result of this structure, almost all the pressure of chewing is limited to the teeth and joint capsule and ligaments. Almost no pressure is placed on the joint itself.

These and many other structural idiosyncrasies all point in the same direction: The less dominant the mechanical functions of mastication

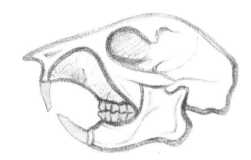

A. Rodent (squirrel)

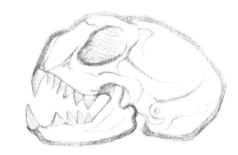

B. Carnivore (meat diet, cat)

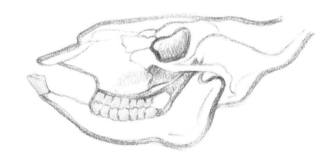

C. Ruminant (plant diet, cow)

Fig. 44. **One-sided dental development in different mammalian groups**.
A: Rodent (e.g., squirrel): incisors dominant
B: Carnivore (e.g., cat): canines dominant
C: Ruminant (e.g., cow): molars dominant

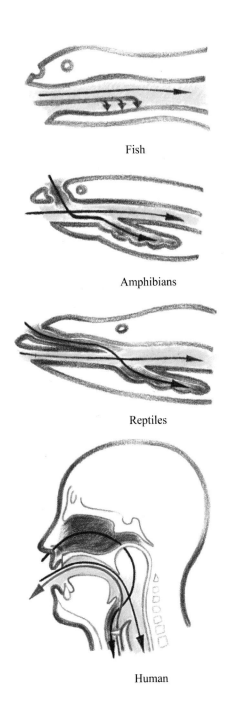

Fish

Amphibians

Reptiles

Human

Fig. 45. **Evolution of the oral and nasal cavities** *in relationship to the human capacity for speech. In lower vertebrates (e.g., fish) the respiratory and alimentary passages run parallel, but in animals with legs (amphibians, reptiles) these passages cross in the pharynx, preparing the way for the possibility of developing speech. The fact that air can be forced into the oral cavity via the pharynx (red line) makes it possible for humans to produce articulated sounds (speech).*

become, the more another functional context emerges, namely, the **development of speech**. Closely spaced teeth with no gaps; harmonious, relatively unspecialized tooth shapes; a highly mobile temporomandibular joint; delicate chewing muscles that are richly supplied with nerves and no longer rely on sheer force; reduced pressure on the head of the mandible due to elongation and angling of the lower jaw—all of these are unique structural features whose functional importance becomes clear only when seen in the context of phonation and articulation. We might mention many other structural attributes of the facial skull whose functional purpose is revealed only in the human ability to speak—for example, the development of a domed palate, a mobile uvula, highly differentiated tongue musculature, a closed, specially shaped oral cavity, and the descent of the larynx and its ability to slide back and forth in the loops of differentiated hyoid muscles (15, 57). Many details of the structure of the human jaw, oral cavity, and larynx no longer have very much to do with their original chewing function and make sense only in terms of the newly acquired capacity for speech.

At this point, materialistic evolutionists generally present arguments similar to those on brain development: At some unknown stage in the transition from apes to humans, a species emerged whose retarded, "embryonic" chewing apparatus made it unfit for the struggle for survival. This species would have died out if it had not suddenly discovered that this "underdeveloped" feature could be "exploited" for communication among individuals (speech), thus giving rise to new adaptive possibilities that allowed it to survive the "remorseless" process of natural selection.

For the moment, we will disregard the fact that this new capacity for speech, far from being the result of a single structural change in the head or throat, depends on the prior development of a number of structural features that appeared almost simultaneously. The human capacity for speech is not the result of a new functional possibility that appeared suddenly in our hominid ancestors due to a variety of structural changes (mutations). It is the result of a gradual, single-minded, coordinated process of transformation in the head and throat. The beginnings of this transformation, which affected almost all structures in this region of the body, are apparent even in lower vertebrates, although the process achieves its "functional goal" only in human beings (Figure 45).

After the transition to terrestrial life, *amphibians* developed a dorsal nostril while the related respiratory passages (trachea, bronchi, lungs) developed ventrally (Figure 45). As a consequence, the respiratory and alimentary passages had to cross in the back of the oral cavity. From a biological perspective, this crossing made little sense. In fact, it required the development of many auxiliary features, such as protective sphincter muscles and neural reflex mechanisms, to prevent food from getting into the respiratory tract and air into the gastrointestinal tract. In the context of the basic amphibian model, this crossing was a "bad design." According to the principle of natural selection, we would expect it to be eliminated in the further course of evolution, but the exact opposite happened. The crossing of the respiratory and alimentary passages was maintained, developed, and perfected from one level to the next. In *reptiles*, for example, the primary palate was elongated and a secondary palate formed, shortening the crossing area and concentrating it in the back of the oral cavity, where the pharynx developed. At the same time, the organs of the larynx and the sphincter mechanisms at the entrance to the air passages were perfected. In *mammals*, a movable soft palate appeared, but the primates were the first to develop the uvula and the specialized muscles that play a major role in forming consonants as well as allowing humans to close off the oral cavity during speech.

A further decisive step in transforming the mouth into a speech organ occurred when the base of the skull curved downward and the larynx descended to a position under the oral cavity. This allowed for an advantageous positioning of the pharynx within the general topography of these organs. The most important prerequisite for the development of the bend in the base of the skull was the formation of a spherical head. This could only be completely achieved when the body was able to stand upright. As a result, the "long-pursued goal" of the capacity for speech became attainable only after uprightness was achieved. As a result of laryngeal descent, the pharynx elongated downward and the epiglottis was also displaced downward, producing a gap between the palate and the base of the tongue. Through this gap, air from the respiratory passages could then be forced into the oral cavity, and the teeth, lips, palate, tongue, etc., could be used to shape sounds.

These new functional possibilities of the oral cavity, pharynx, larynx, etc., gave functional meaning to the crossing of the respiratory and alimentary canals in the pharynx, which had first appeared in amphibians. These new possibilities did not develop coincidentally or randomly. They were achieved through deliberate, complex, and incremental transformations of a number of very different tissues in a process that may have taken millions of years and certainly occurred long *before* the actual capacity for speech appeared. This fact offers convincing evidence that we need to see evolution as a deliberate, goal-directed process of *orthogenetic development.*

Many other examples exist, but we will mention only a few that will be important for our later discussions.

We have already described the *transformation of the jaws and teeth*. Speech can emerge only when the teeth form a closed, harmonious arch and the facial portion of the skull forgoes any one-sided adaptations related to chewing. This evolutionary transformation was also not a sudden, coincidental event. It too was achieved gradually, i.e., deliberately. In primitive placental mammals, the skull is still tube-shaped and the dental formula is 3143:3143. Among prosimians, the facial skull is somewhat less pointed (prognathic) and therefore contains fewer teeth (dental formula 2133:2133). Among more highly evolved simian species, the facial skull is smaller and the dental formula reveals only eight

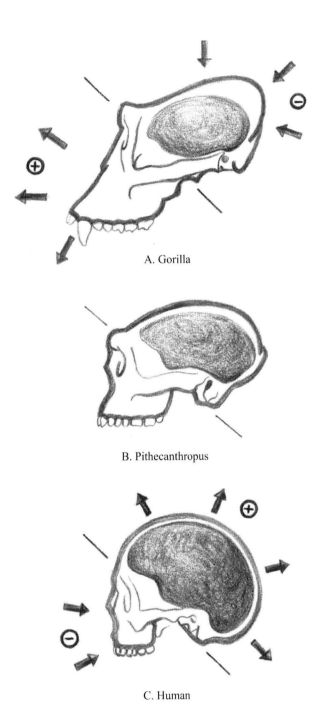

A. Gorilla

B. Pithecanthropus

C. Human

*Fig. 46. **Shape of the cranium and brain size** in higher apes (A), fossil hominids (B), and modern humans (C, from Weidenreich). Massive development of the brain (and especially of the frontal lobe) reshapes the frontal portion of the facial skull (forehead). Arrows: direction of predominating growth.*

teeth on each side (2123:2123). In humans, there is often no room for the third molar; as a result, the dental formula tends to become 2122:2122. Here again—as emphasized above with regard to skull evolution—we are not dealing with an incremental process of reduction from a primitive to a more highly evolved form, i.e., from an adapted to a nonadapted form. Rather, human teeth remain at an earlier developmental level, while the jaws and teeth of apes and various other mammals actively expand in a forward direction to make room for more teeth. The human mouth preserves its original, juvenile proportions and does not become as one-sided and differentiated as the mouths of other primates and mammals.

Transformation of the cranium (dermatocranium and neurocranium). In terms of tissue mechanisms, evolutionary retardation in the area of the facial skull, as described above, is due to the early ossification of facial sutures, which are actually "growth points," comparable to the epiphyseal plates of the long bones. In humans, the forward thrust of growth in the upper and lower jaw stops after the first dentition. This is also why the human intermaxillary bone grows together with the two maxillary bones at an early stage and is often difficult to identify after birth, whereas in animals (including apes) it is still quite evident. A sense that this phenomenon conceals a profound biological issue was undoubtedly what prompted Goethe to search for the human intermaxillary bone. As with his vertebral theory, Goethe probably suspected a more comprehensive problem whose solution might provide a key to understanding the entire process of human evolution. But the time was not yet ripe for understanding such evolutionary relationships, since the idea of evolution itself was only beginning to be explored, and no well-founded theories of evolution existed. Goethe, however, was one of the first to clearly formulate the idea of evolution and to recognize its significance for a new understanding of human beings and the natural world.

In humans, the epiphyseal lines of the facial skull ossify at an early stage. In contrast, the sutures between the flat bony plates forming the roof of the skull, as well as the fontanelles (which are actually only enlarged epiphyseal lines), continue to exhibit growth for years after birth. It is well known that the fontanelles persist postnatally for a year to a year and a half. The sutures of the skullcap and cranium, however, retain some proliferative ability until age 18 or 20 and ossify only in middle age or later, and sometimes never. As a result, the skull cavity can continue to expand after birth and the brain can continue to grow (Figure 46).

In contrast, a pronounced growth of the facial skull and chewing muscles commences immediately after birth in higher apes. The major chewing muscles (such as the temporalis) push forward over the skullcap, and huge sagittal crests develop. The head becomes heavy and falls forward. The arms elongate and are often used solely for support, with the fingers bent to provide a weight-bearing surface (knuckle-walking, Figure 47). The skull sutures, unlike those in humans, ossify early; consequently, the interior of the skull cannot expand and brain growth ceases. The bones of the skullcap become very thick, developing bony crests and hollow spaces to increase the size of the attachment surfaces for neck and chewing muscles. Adaptive processes dominate this picture, and antiadaptation loses significance (Figures 46 and 47).

In humans, skullcap growth and continuing brain development are not isolated processes that would have "suddenly" conferred a selective advantage on more highly evolved species with enhanced intelligence. In fact, these developments must be seen in connection with the other processes described above, especially the evolution of speech organs, which are useless so long as the brain is incapable of managing the informational aspect of speech and does not possess centers to help with more advanced speech processing, including memory and the creation of language. Higher apes have brains that are relatively highly developed and may even include the beginnings of speech centers (scientists are divided on this point), but the head and neck structures belonging to the speech apparatus have not developed. Their absence makes it

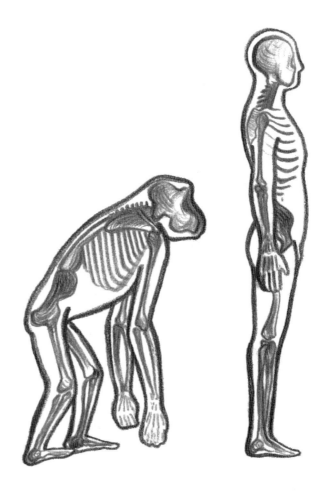

Fig. 47. **Differences in posture and body proportions in humans and apes.** *In apes, the arms are greatly elongated, the legs shortened, and the head inclined toward the front.*

impossible for apes to develop into individualities that free themselves from their environment and express themselves through speech. For them to do so would have required greater retardation through antiadaptive processes (Figure 48).

Based on everything we have considered so far, the next section presents a preliminary overview of the process of evolution.

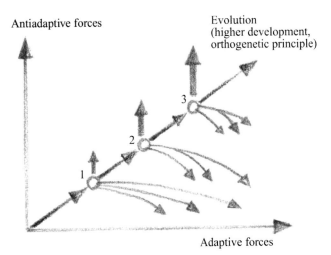

Fig. 48. *Countereffects of adaptive and antiadaptive forces in vertebrate evolution*. *1, 2, 3: three successive stages of higher evolution, which always emerge from fetal states that remain capable of development.*

Level 1: lower evolutionary stages. Strong tendency toward adaptation; little actualization of antiadaptation.

Level 2: middle evolutionary stages. Antiadaptive forces become more effective in organ formation. "Juvenile forms" appear.

Level 3: higher evolutionary stages. In "advanced" forms, adaptive tendencies are suppressed and the "degree of freedom" (red arrows) increases.

Antiadaptation and Orthogenesis As Evolutionary Principles

We have seen that the well-adapted shapes of the tubelike skull were abandoned in favor of less specialized spherical forms. Furthermore, the cranium and brain increased in size and the chewing apparatus and head and neck structures involved in speech evolved incrementally from forms present in lower vertebrates. How can we possibly imagine that the laws of probability and natural selection were the only forces at work in these transformations? The problems that result from this assumption will not be resolved as long as we apply only the classic principles of evolution. As we saw earlier, nonadaptive or antiadaptive processes also played a role. Including these processes in our definition of evolution makes it possible to understand why newborns of lower species resemble adults of more highly evolved species. Verhulst, basing himself on earlier studies by Bolk, covers this phenomenon more thoroughly in a recent book (52). Multiple fossil finds support hypothetical evolutionary series showing the progress from apelike to increasingly humanlike skull forms. These series also demonstrate that infantile or juvenile skulls usually look much more humanlike than adult skulls of the same species (cf. Figures 35 and 43).

From the biological perspective, it is almost unimaginable that new, "less adapted" structures could evolve from markedly well-adapted forms. Therefore antiadaptation can affect only embryonic or juvenile forms, preventing increased specialization (adaptation) of individual functions. Once an initial degree of retardation is achieved (for example, in the chewing apparatus), a second degree can prevent stronger adaptation and preserve more embryonic, undifferentiated conditions during early developmental phases when bodily forms are still flexible. A more highly evolved form could thus be achieved by repeatedly "applying the brakes" on adaptive tendencies and activating antiadaptive processes—assuming that the individual stages are parts of a coordinated and coherent "program"; in other words, that final (orthogenetic) and antiadaptive processes work together (Figure 48).

The Metabolic-Limb System

The Musculoskeletal System

The Structure of the Skeletal System

No animal achieves the independent, fully upright posture found in the human body; the human being is the only organism that is effectively integrated into all three dimensions of space (Figure 49). This "dimension-compatible" stance is possible primarily because of the human skeleton. In its many individual bony elements, we can recognize two fundamentally different shapes, one long and tubelike and the other broad and flat. The general threefold functional division of the human body is also reflected in the skeletal system (15, 58).

The **head** is primarily spherical in shape and is dominated by the flat bony plates enclosing the cranial cavity. This entire structure has hardened into a fixed form, and, with the exception of the jaws, the joints (sutures) in the head permit very little movement. Active movement is concentrated in the mimetic musculature, which permits highly expressive facial expressions and remains independent of the body's movements in space.

The opposite structural principle is evident in the **limbs**, which consist of sequences of long, tubelike bony elements that are quite mobile because they are connected by joints. This mobility means that human beings can express a soul content not only through facial expression but also through movements of the limbs. In the limbs, however, such expression is very brief; gestures change constantly and never manifest completely.

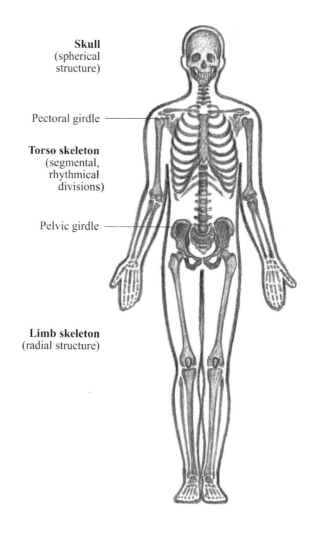

Skull
(spherical structure)

Pectoral girdle

Torso skeleton
(segmental, rhythmical divisions)

Pelvic girdle

Limb skeleton
(radial structure)

*Fig. 49. **Morphological divisions of the human body based on the skeletal system** (15).*

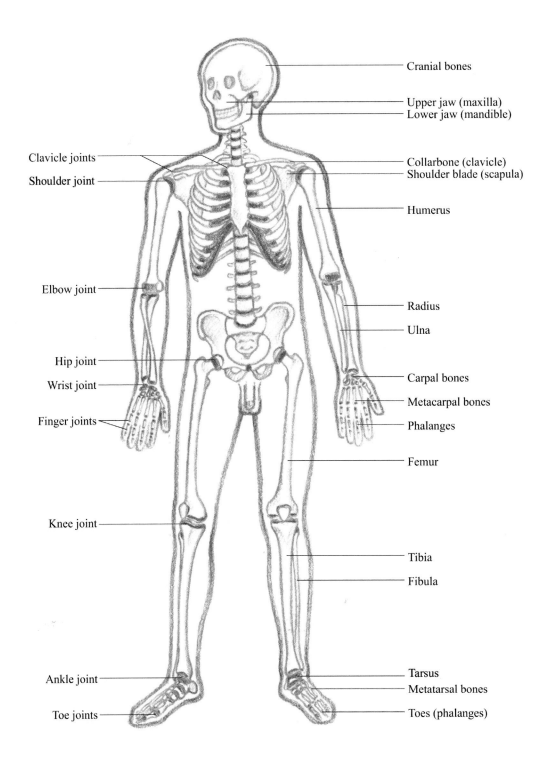

Cranial bones

Upper jaw (maxilla)
Lower jaw (mandible)

Clavicle joints

Shoulder joint

Collarbone (clavicle)
Shoulder blade (scapula)

Humerus

Elbow joint

Radius

Ulna

Hip joint

Wrist joint

Carpal bones

Metacarpal bones

Finger joints

Phalanges

Femur

Knee joint

Tibia

Fibula

Ankle joint

Tarsus
Metatarsal bones

Toe joints

Toes (phalanges)

*Fig. 50. **Structure of the human skeletal system and location of the most important joints**.*

The *torso*, where segmental division prevails, is inserted between the head and limb poles and is characterized by the rhythmical repetition of relatively similar structural elements such as the vertebrae or ribs. These are intermediate in form between the platelike and tubelike bones of the two poles. Although both ribs and vertebrae include structural elements of both types, the ribs more closely resemble the tubelike skeletal elements of the limbs, and the vertebral neural arches the platelike bones of the skullcap.

This basic threefold division, however, needs elaboration in order to account for the entire miraculous structure of the human skeleton, which Husemann analyzed in terms of sculptural and musical laws (59). The limbs (arms and legs) emerge from the *pectoral* and *pelvic girdles*, which serve as fulcrums for moving the long limb bones. These girdles are not tubelike in shape but are made up of flat bones (shoulder blade, hip bone, etc., Figures 49, 50), which represent the resting pole or "head element" in the dynamic domain of the limbs. A similar quality is evident in the hand's carpal bones and the foot's tarsal bones. These individual bones are short and relatively shapeless rather than flat. However, they are arranged into flat, mosaiclike wholes, which again form stable bases for movement, in this case for the fingers and toes. In the sequences of mobile limb bones, these structures again characterize a headlike element.

Conversely, even the head pole (especially the facial skeleton) contains limblike structural elements in addition to the flat, platelike bones of the skullcap. The same is true of the entire midsection of the skeletal system, the metamerically divided torso, whose segments include both tubular, limblike bones (ribs) and short, headlike flat bones (clavicle, vertebral body). We will return to this phenomenon later, in connection with a discussion of developmental processes.

Each mobile *limb* (arm, leg) consists of three sections (upper arm/forearm/hand or thigh/calf/foot), which are connected by joints (Figure 50). In each case, the number of bony elements increases toward the periphery. The upper arm with its single bone (humerus) is followed first by the two forearm bones (ulna, radius), then by three upper and four lower carpal bones, and finally by five metacarpal bones and five fingers, each of which (with the exception of the thumb) consists of three phalanges. The leg is similarly structured, beginning with the single bone (femur) of the thigh, followed by the two lower leg bones (tibia, fibula). In the foot, however, the progressive increase in the number of bones toward the periphery is not as clear because the tarsal bones (which correspond to the carpal bones in the hand) have fused together for the sake of stability.

Peripheral increases in the number of bones enhances mobility and flexibility and thus also the limbs' expressive possibilities. Movement begins in the large joints near the torso (shoulder joint, hip joint), where the humerus and femur form large, spherical "heads." In contrast, the humerus has a cylindrical bulge (trochlea) in the elbow joint that looks like a clenched fist; it anticipates gestures that become realities in the hand. The shapes of the forearm bones also reflect gestures that become fully recognizable only on the periphery. The "hand" of the radius is located at its lower end, where it forms a solid basis for wrist movements. The ulna opens its "hand" above, to receive the cylindrical end of the humerus (Figure 59). In the hand, the two gestures of opening/receiving and closing/clenching appear in actual movements for the first time, made possible by the thumb's two phalanges and the movable saddle joint that connects the first metacarpal bone (unlike the others) to the carpus.

In contrast, the leg has become specialized primarily for support and locomotion functions (Figure 59). The foot forms a right angle with the axis of the leg. The big toe has sacrificed mobility to become the supporting element for the arch of the foot. The supporting girdle, where the limb meets the torso, has also been transformed; together with the sacrum, it forms the solid ring of the pelvis. It has also developed an arch on each side to accommodate the lateral head of

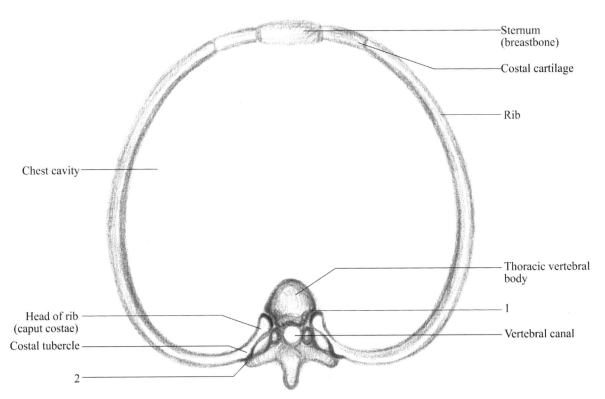

Sternum
(breastbone)

Costal cartilage

Rib

Chest cavity

Thoracic vertebral
body

1

Head of rib
(caput costae)

Vertebral canal

Costal tubercle

2

Fig. 51. **Structure of a bony segment in the chest.** *The ribs surround the chest cavity, the vertebral arches surround the neural space. The overall image is that of a lemniscate (compare Figure 12, p. 31). 1: superior costal facet joint; 2: transverse costal facet joint.*

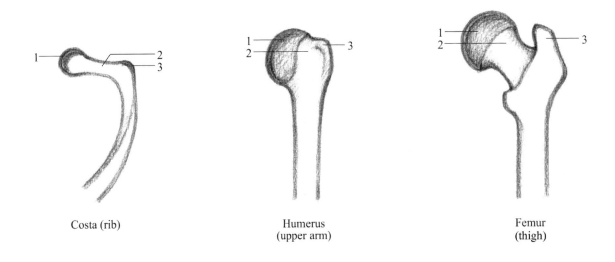

Costa (rib)

Humerus
(upper arm)

Femur
(thigh)

Fig. 52. **Structural relationships among rib** (costa), **humerus, and femur.** *Blue: articular cartilage surfaces.*
1: caput; 2: neck; 3: tubercle or trochanter.

the femur, forming a secure base for almost all body movements. As a result, the pectoral girdle (scapula and clavicle) of the upright human being is freed from support functions and achieves an astonishing degree of mobility because it is connected to the ribcage only by the inner clavicle joint.

The limbs' many-jointed, differentiated sequences of long (hollow) bones and the spherical, almost immobile head are polar opposites that can coexist harmoniously in a single organism only because they are connected by the vertebral column and ribcage, i.e., the skeleton of the torso. The S-shaped spine consists of seven cervical, twelve thoracic, and five lumbar vertebrae (for a total of twenty-four) together with the five sacral and three-to-six coccygeal vertebrae. At its upper end, the spine supports the head; in the middle, the pectoral girdle and arms (with the help of the ribcage); and at its lower end (via the sacrum), the body's weight, which is carried by the legs (Figure 50).

The fundamental features of all the structural elements noted above already reveal themselves in the torso segments. In the chest, the central section of the skeletal torso, each segment consists of one vertebra, one pair of ribs (costae), and the corresponding portion of the breastbone (sternum), which connects the two ribs, resulting in the fundamental form of a lemniscate. The small loop of the lemniscate is the vertebral arch, which encloses the neural space (vertebral canal and spinal cord); the large loop is formed by the ribs, which surround the chest cavity with the heart and lungs (cf. Figures 11, 12, and 51). The cartilage-covered head of each rib (caput costae) articulates with the vertebral body. Moving outward, the caput costae is followed first by the neck of the rib (collum costae) and then by the costal tubercle (tuberculum costae), which rests on and articulates with the transverse process of the corresponding thoracic vertebra (Figure 51). Next is the flattened body of the rib, which curves around the chest cavity and is intermediate in form between a cylindrical long bone and

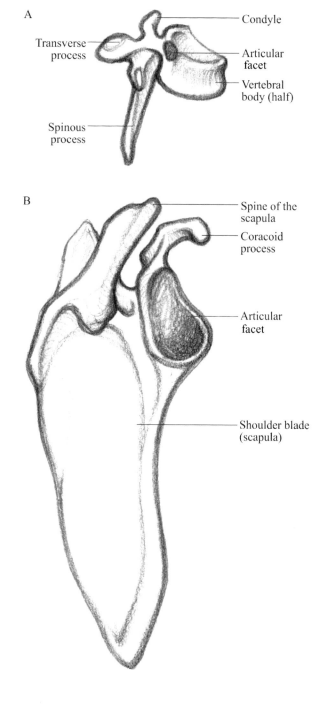

Fig. 53. **Comparison of one half of a thoracic vertebra (A) with a shoulder blade (B).** *In each case the bone from the right side of the body is shown, as viewed diagonally from in front.*

a platelike skull bone. Thus the ribs already suggest the structural principle active in the limb bones. The head and neck of the rib correspond to the head and neck of the femur or humerus, while the costal (rib) tubercle corresponds to the much more prominent epicondyles of limb bones. The body of the rib corresponds to the shaft of a long bone (Figure 52). Obviously, the ribs lack any peripheral bony elements such as those in the hands or feet. Figuratively speaking, the ribs limit their "hands" to an undifferentiated mass in the breastbone in order to form a closed ring (Figure 51). In the limbs, this ring is "broken open," the long bones elongate, and the terminal structures (hands and feet) undergo further configuration in connection with newly emerging functions.

The unique structural features of both pairs of human limbs are easier to understand if we imagine separating a rib segment in half and allowing each half to develop into one limb: Each half-vertebra becomes a platelike girdle, and the rib itself becomes a tubular limb bone. For example, if we imagine cutting a thoracic vertebra in half, the resulting piece of bone is clearly the structural counterpart of the flat bones of the pectoral or pelvic girdle (Figure 53). In addition to its flat section, the shoulder blade also has two pronounced processes, the coracoid process and the spine of the scapula, which are connected by taut ligaments and form the "roof" of the shoulder, which supports the humerus when the arm is lifted, similarly to the way the vertebral transverse processes support the ribs. The point where the head of the rib articulates with the vertebral body would then correspond to the shoulder joint's articular cavity. The spinous process would become the spine of the scapula and the transverse process its coracoid process (Figure 54).

As we see, this transformation entails a reversal in the front-back dimension. The vertebral body, originally located in front, spreads out in back and becomes a platelike bone, while the processes connected to the vertebral arch shift forward in order to serve as attachment points

for muscles (Figure 54). The vertebral articular processes disappear because connections comparable to the intervertebral articulations no longer exist in the arm. The bones of the arm arrange themselves vertically or horizontally. Through a newly formed membrane bone (the clavicle or collarbone), the pectoral girdle connects with the sternum and thus with the bones of the torso.

The pectoral girdle maintains considerable freedom of movement and almost "floats" atop the torso. The pelvic girdle and the legs, however, sacrifice much of this freedom in order to provide a stable means of support during locomotion. Consequently, the hip joint's bony elements are significantly more differentiated than the corresponding parts of either an upper extremity or a rib segment (Figure 55). The hip joint becomes a ball-and-socket joint, the articular cavity deepens, the neck of the femur becomes more pronounced, and the epicondyles (which are not especially pronounced even in the humerus) develop into powerful trochanters in the femur. The platelike bony element of the pectoral girdle (the shoulder blade or scapula) reappears in the pelvis in the form of the ala of the ilium (Figure 55). The scapula's bony processes are significantly elongated in the pelvic bones, extending forward to the pelvic symphysis and surrounding the obturator foramen. In this metamorphosis, the coracoid process becomes the pubic bone, the spine of the scapula the ischium, and the scapula's articular cavity the acetabulum (Figure 55).

This transformation can be further substantiated by considering that arms bend forward but legs backward. To transform a lower human limb into an upper limb, the leg would not only have to be shortened and its structure refined, it would also have to be rotated 180 degrees so the angle of the knee joint would lie in back, the flexors in front, and the extensors in back. As a result of these changes, the knee would become the elbow joint and the hollow of the knee the bend in the elbow. The thigh extensor muscle (quadriceps) would become the upper

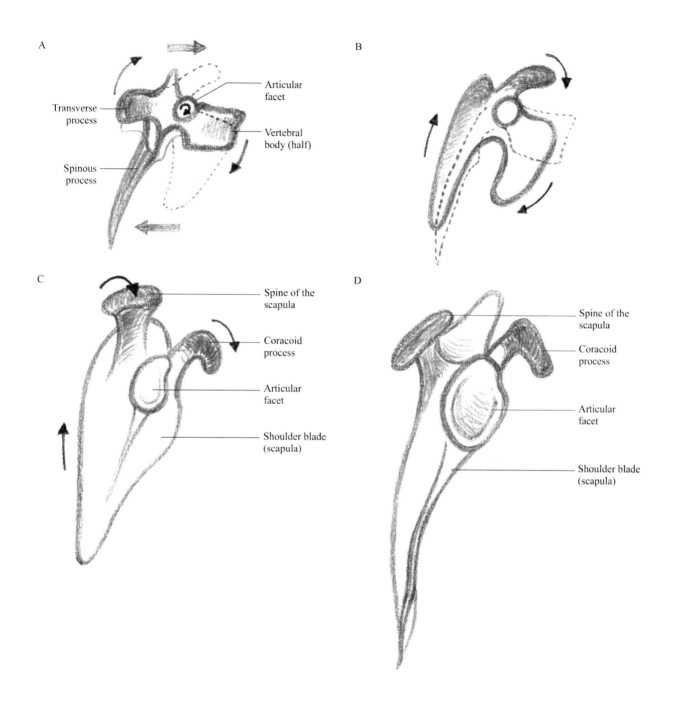

A

Articular
facet

Transverse
process

Vertebral
body (half)

Spinous
process

B

C

Spine of the
scapula

Coracoid
process

Articular
facet

Shoulder blade
(scapula)

D

Spine of the
scapula

Coracoid
process

Articular
facet

Shoulder blade
(scapula)

Fig. 54. **Incremental transformation of half of a thoracic vertebra into a scapula.**
A: *half of a thoracic vertebra as seen from the side;*
B and C: *intermediate stages;*
D: *scapula as seen from the front.*
The articular facets of the vertebral body become the articular cavity of the shoulder joint. The transverse process becomes the coracoid process (blue); the half of the spinous process becomes the spine of the scapula (red), and the half of the vertebral body becomes the scapula (shoulder blade, dotted line). Arrows indicate the direction of movement of the changes.

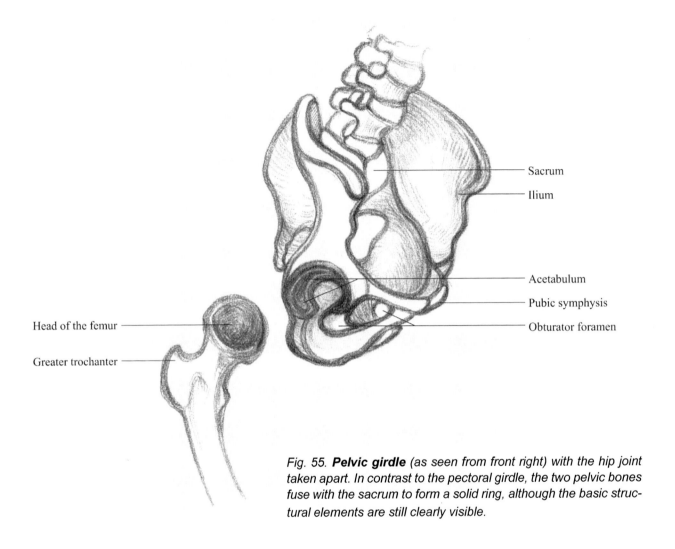

Sacrum

Ilium

Acetabulum

Pubic symphysis

Obturator foramen

Head of the femur

Greater trochanter

Fig. 55. **Pelvic girdle** *(as seen from front right) with the hip joint taken apart. In contrast to the pectoral girdle, the two pelvic bones fuse with the sacrum to form a solid ring, although the basic structural elements are still clearly visible.*

arm extensor (triceps), which sometimes even develops a little kneecaplike bone (patella) in its tendon. The coracobrachialis muscle of the upper arm corresponds to the group of adductor muscles in the leg.

The assumption that these metamorphoses are related to the evolution of uprightness sheds new light on the emergence of the membranous bone (clavicle) in the pectoral girdle. Let's look again at these transformations from the opposite direction. That is, how could the pectoral girdle be transformed into the pelvis? If we rotate the shoulder's articular cavity inward by 180

degrees, the coracoid process shifts inward and to the front. If we then strengthen and lengthen this process diagonally (forward and downward), the result is what appears in the pelvis, where the two branches of the pelvic bone serve as attachments for the adductor muscles (Figure 56). These muscles, which are powerful and complex in the lower limbs, are present in the upper arm only in the form of the relatively small coracobrachialis, but the relationship is clear in that the coracobrachialis attaches to the coracoid process. To connect with the pubic bone and enclose the obturator foramen, the spine of the

A

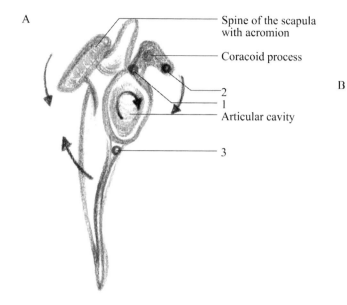

Spine of the scapula with acromion

Coracoid process

2

1

Articular cavity

3

B

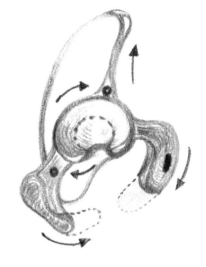

C

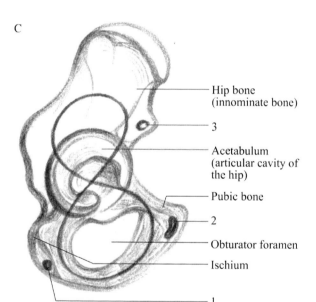

Hip bone (innominate bone)

3

Acetabulum (articular cavity of the hip)

Pubic bone

2

Obturator foramen

Ischium

1

*Fig. 56. **Transforming the shoulder blade into the hip bone.***
A: right shoulder blade (front view);
B: intermediate stage;
C: right hip bone (side view).
The coracoid process (blue) becomes the pubic bone, and the spine of the scapula (red) the ischium. In the hip bone, the coracoid process and spine of the scapula develop into a second framework that surrounds the obturator foramen. The result is a double bony framework that forms a lemniscate (red line) whose crossing point lies in the acetabulum (articular cavity of the hip).
1-3: origins of the chief muscle groups:
1: flexors (biceps femoris and brachii);
2: adductors (coracobrachialis in the arm, adductor muscle group in the leg);
3: extensors (triceps, quadriceps).

scapula must be elongated downward and to the back to form the ischium. As the muscles that attach to the outer side of the shoulder blade and to the spine of the scapula (e.g., the deltoid muscles) are transformed into the buttocks muscles, the epicondyle of the humerus becomes the greater trochanter.

Through elongation of the shoulder blade's processes, the innominate bone becomes a double or hollow framework that can be understood as a lemniscate (Figures 56 and 57). At the lemniscate's crossing point lies the articular cavity, in which the three bones of the pelvis (ilium, pubis, ischium) come together in a

A

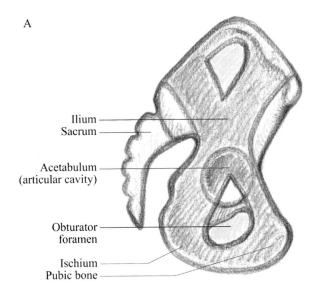

Ilium
Sacrum

Acetabulum
(articular cavity)

Obturator
foramen

Ischium
Pubic bone

B

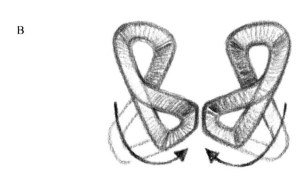

C

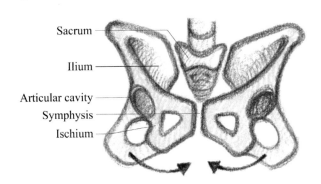

Sacrum

Ilium

Articular cavity
Symphysis
Ischium

Fig. 57. ***Development of the pelvis into a three-dimensional structure*** *(from Mollier).*
A: lemiscatic structure of the right hip bone (side view);
B: The lower branch of the lemniscate must bend inward at a 90-degree angle (arrows) to create the shape of the pelvis. Transition from a two-dimensional form to a three-dimensional one.
C: Incorporation of the wedge-shaped sacrum completes the pelvis and transforms it into a three-dimensional structure that encloses a hollow space.

Y-shaped suture. The pelvis itself, however, as the three-dimensional structure enclosing the pelvic cavity, comes about only because the two surfaces of the lemniscate are bent toward each other at a 90-degree angle. In other words, the front scaffold, which surrounds the obturator foramen, is turned inward toward the upper back framework (the ilium), so that the two pubic bones meet in front in the pelvic symphysis (Figure 57). The three-sided wedge of the sacrum fills in the gap in the back to complete the solid ring of the pelvis. The necessary foundation for standing and walking upright in three-dimensional space becomes available only at this point.

In mentally picturing the transformation of the pectoral girdle into the pelvic girdle, it is impressive to experience how the pectoral girdle's more-or-less two-dimensional platelike structures, which are not only relatively independent of each other but also quite freely mobile, sacrifice their independence in the pelvic girdle, where they are "forced" into a three-dimensional structure. From the opposite perspective, to achieve the structure of the upper limbs, the pelvic girdle must be "torn apart" and the legs turned outward—a dramatic change that clearly reveals the essential character of the upper limbs and the ability to "step outside of space" that their development sets in motion.

Hands and feet. As a result of the evolution of uprightness, the functions of the terminal portions of the arms and legs are no longer remotely similar, and their anatomical structures have diverged (Figure 58). In the hand, the fingers have become greatly elongated, increasing their flexibility and mobility. The relatively small and undifferentiated carpal bones of the hand form a flat surface for supporting objects when the hand is used for grasping. In contrast, the corresponding (tarsal) bones of the foot are heavily differentiated and overlap to form a strong arch that supports the body, while the toes remain small and barely mobile. Originally, the distal row of carpal or tarsal bones contained five small bones corresponding to the five digital rays, but bones 4 and 5 have become fused, forming the hamate bone in the

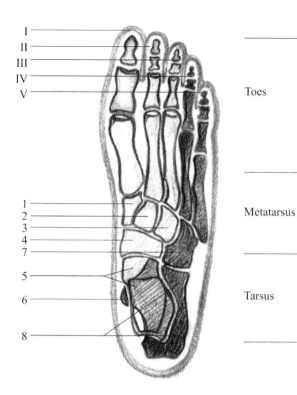

I
II
III
IV
V

Toes

1
2
3
4
7

5

6

8

Metatarsus

Tarsus

Fig. 58. **Polar differentiation of the human hand and foot.**

A: skeleton of the foot (view from above). The medial portion of the foot includes the first three digital rays (I-III), the three cuneiform bones (1-3), the navicular (scaphoid) bone (4), and the talus (5). The lateral portion consists of the fourth and fifth digital rays (IV and V), the cuboid bone (7), and the calcaneus (8). The longitudinal arch of the foot develops as a result of the overlap of the talus and calcaneus (diagonally shaded area) and the formation of the sustentaculum tali, a medial process of the calcaneus, which supports part of the talus. The wedge-shaped arrangement of the three cuneiform bones is the most important factor in the development of the transverse arch.

1, 2, 3: cuneiform bones
4: navicular bone
5: talus
6: sustentaculum tali (process of the calcaneus)
7: cuboid bone
8: calcaneus (heel bone)

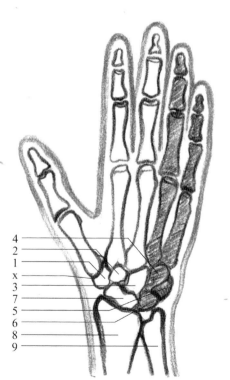

Fingers

4
2
1
x
3
7
5
6
8
9

Metacarpus

Carpus

B: skeleton of the hand (view from above). In contrast to the tarsus of the foot, the bones of the carpus of the hand are small and only slightly arching. The fingers are elongated and highly mobile. The first digital ray (thumb) is much more mobile than the big toe. It has only two phalanges. A biaxial saddle joint (x) in the carpus allows it to move freely. The hand shows only traces of a structural arch.

1: trapezium
2: trapezoid
3: capitate
4: hamate
5: triquetrum
6: lunate
7: scaphoid
8: radius
9: ulna

hand and the cuboid bone in the foot and thus reducing the number to four. In the proximal row, the bony elements have been further reduced to three. The hand's scaphoid and lunate bones are fused in the talus of the foot, while the triquetrum of the hand is enlarged in the foot to form the calcaneus.

In general, more primitive or less-specialized proportions persist in the hand. In the foot, fusion of primary bony elements and differentiation of individual bones results in two overlapping segments and the subsequent development of a longitudinal arch. The foot's lateral segment includes the fourth and fifth digital rays, the cuboid bone, and the talus. This lateral portion maintains contact with the ground and provides firm support for the inner (medial) segment, which connects with the bones of the lower leg. From the three cuneiform bones through the navicular and talus, the medial portion is raised off the ground by the overlap of the talus and calcaneus (Figure 58). The radius and ulna of the arm correspond to the tibia and fibula of the leg. Only the radius is involved in the wrist joint, but in the foot the tibia and fibula form a fork that clasps the head of the talus allowing the ankle joint to be located on the upper side of the foot.

Forearm and lower leg. In keeping with the overall structural model of the arm, the two forearm bones are oriented in different directions. The radius is directed downward, toward the hand, and is thicker at its lower end. It is the only bone that articulates with the carpal bones in the wrist joint. In contrast, the ulna is thicker toward the top and articulates with the humerus in the elbow joint. At the bottom, it ends in a small head similar to the top of the radius. The ulna, which is separated from the wrist joint by a cartilaginous disc, does not move significantly when the hand moves. It represents the resting element around which the radius rotates in the movements known as pronation and supination, which turn the hand. Thus the radius is the more hand-oriented forearm bone. From the functional perspective, it belongs to the grasping dynamic that is fully expressed in the human hand's opposable thumb, powerful

grip, and dexterity, which are usually associated with pronation (turning inward). In contrast, the ulna is directed away from the hand. Its bowl-shaped upper end receives the trochlea of the humerus to form the hingelike elbow joint. The ulna's direction is away from the Earth, toward the upper, nonearthly element. This direction is also expressed in the motion of supination (turning outward), which emphasizes the lateral portion (little-finger side) of the hand and reveals the receptive palm.

In the foot, this dynamic is reduced to the dual functions of support (served by the arch of the foot) and movement (served by the angled lever of the foot and leg). The lower limbs lack the forearms' multiple expressive possibilities, which are based on free alternation between up and down. In the leg, the radius becomes the tibia and is forced into service within the support apparatus. The lower leg does not rotate. Pronation and supination are possible only in the foot itself—specifically, in the lower ankle joint. In the leg, the fibula (the counterpart of the ulna) also loses its upward orientation. It forms part of the upper ankle joint but not part of the knee joint. Fibula and tibia are parallel (Figure 59). The possibility of turning and crossing has been sacrificed for the sake of stability, and the lower leg's range of motion is reduced. Its bones and tendons are larger and stronger, in keeping with the leg's support function. The gesture of the lower extremity is a 90-degree bend. The inner side (sole) of the foot has turned completely earthward, but its arch frees it from gravity to a certain extent. The upper extremity's characteristic gesture is the alternation between supination and pronation, between turning upward (to reveal the palm turned away from the earth) and turning downward (toward the earth and earthly activity), with the palm oriented toward the objects that the hand grasps, shapes, or manipulates. This dynamic is possible only because the forearm bones and all of the arm's other structures have accommodated this dual orientation. In addition, the carpus has avoided further specialization and remained a direct continuation of the lower arm.

A

B

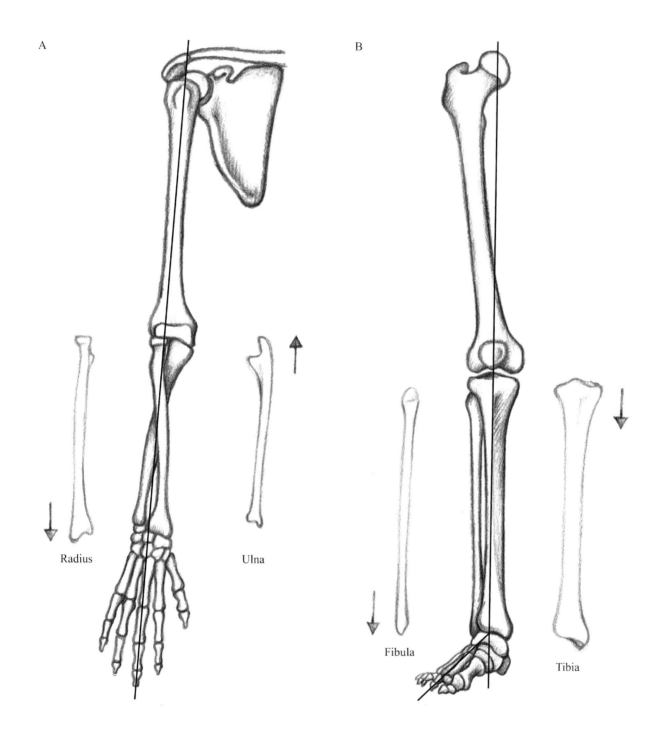

Radius

Ulna

Fibula

Tibia

*Fig. 59. **Comparison of arm and leg skeletons.** The arm (A) is shown turned inward (pronation). Its primary axis runs through the third digital ray, i.e., through the middle of the hand. The forearm and lower leg bones have evolved divergently. The ulna's functional thrust is upward, while the radius is oriented downward (arrows). In contrast, the tibia has become the leg's main supporting column, while the fibula plays a secondary role in support and also helps form the ankle joint. In the leg (B) the main axis runs through the middle of the joints and through the second digital ray of the foot. The foot forms a right angle with the lower leg.*

The System of Active Movement (Muscles and Joints)

Joints and Sutures

The skeleton can be seen as a movement system hardened into form. Bone shapes reflect the living, constantly changing shapes of limb movements. Through muscles that attach to bones, the limbs produce an array of "movement pictures" that are recognizable in the skeleton itself only as shapes that have permanently come to rest. But these movements are possible only because the limbs' series of bony elements are interrupted by joints.

The *joints* of the human body are not static, mechanical hinges. They are somewhat malleable and move in individually very different ways, depending on the plasticity of their joint cartilage and ligaments and especially on the activity and flexibility of associated muscles. Each joint is a miniature body cavity of sorts and is even slightly depressurized.

Articulating bony elements are covered with a layer of cartilage that contains no blood vessels. Instead, this articular cartilage is nourished by the synovial fluid of the joint cavity, which is completely enclosed in the articular capsule. The capsule's inner layer, the synovial membrane, is richly supplied with blood vessels and with villilike protrusions that extend into the joint cavity. These protrusions are *not* covered with epithelium. They secrete oxygen, hyaluronic acid, and other chemicals important for maintaining joint cartilage and preserving its flexibility (Figure 60B). In a certain respect, therefore, the joint cavity is a specialized connective tissue "space" that is only supplied with blood vessels from the outside. The dense covering of vessels concentrates warmth in the interior; cooling is often associated with sclerotic processes such as arthritis, which restrict movement. In the bloodless interior joint space,

however, different forces prevail. The mucuslike synovial fluid allows the nonvascularized, flexible articular cartilage surfaces, which exert a slight attraction upon one another, to slide across each other freely.

In the *skull sutures*, unlike the joints of the extremities, the "joint space" is completely filled with immature connective tissue, which proliferates vigorously as the body develops (Figure 60A). Thus the skull sutures are also epiphyses. In the true joints of the limbs, growth also proceeds constantly from the epiphyseal plates as a result of cell division in the cartilage. This is the basis of longitudinal growth in the bones and joints. A calcification zone, in which the fibrous elements of cartilage are anchored, develops on the boundary between cartilage and bone only when growth is complete. The proliferative tendency that works from the inside out then gives way to a gradual dying-off that can even intensify into degeneration (arthritis, articular rheumatism) with advancing age. This process is counteracted from outside by the up-building (anabolic), nourishing forces of the richly vascularized articular capsule and synovial membrane (Figure 60B).

Inside the joint, therefore, one can say that a process comparable to inflammation (under pathological conditions) occurs, only here it represents a normal physiological event. In this process, as everywhere in vascular and connective tissue, tissue dissolution releases forces (fluid secretion and warmth) that are then bound up again in subsequent proliferation and tissue formation.

Thus the joints represent a "middle ground" or intermediary between the skeletal system's hardened forms and the muscular system's constant movement.

The *limbs* develop as jointed sequences of bony elements. The joints near the torso are more mobile than peripheral joints (Figure 61). The scapula and humerus form the shoulder joint, which permits movement in all three planes of space. In contrast, the elbow joint permits only two types of motion (flexion/extension and rotation). The wrist also permits motion in two planes only

A

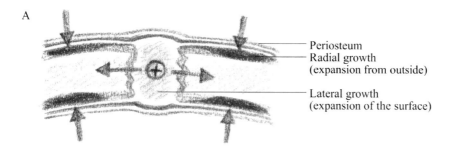

Periosteum
Radial growth
(expansion from outside)

Lateral growth
(expansion of the surface)

B

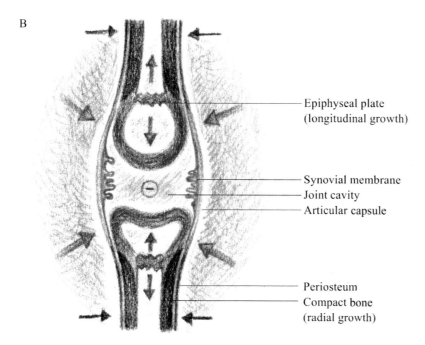

Epiphyseal plate
(longitudinal growth)

Synovial membrane
Joint cavity
Articular capsule

Periosteum
Compact bone
(radial growth)

Fig. 60. **Structure and growth dyamics of joints in comparison to skull sutures.**
A: suture between membranous bones in the skull.
In the bones of the cranium, expansion of the surface (lateral growth) proceeds from the sutures, increase in thickness (radial growth) from the periosteum (see arrows).

B: joint between endochondral bones in the limbs.
Longitudinal growth in the long bones proceeds from the epiphyseal plate; radial growth from the periosteum of the compact bone.

(flexion/extension and lateral movement). And finally, the middle and terminal finger joints move only in a single plane.

The same pattern of joint mobility is also evident in the lower limbs, although overall, they are generally less mobile. The hip joint (formed by the hip bone and the head of the femur) allows motion in all three planes of space, although the range of motion is much smaller here than in the shoulder joint. The lower leg (which consists of two bones, like the forearm) articulates with the femur in the knee joint, but the fibula does not participate. Rotation is possible, but only when the knee is bent.

In contrast to the biaxial connection between the forearm and the hand, the joint between the lower leg and the tarsus has only one axis. The ankle joint consists of a bony fork (formed by the fibula and tibia) that articulates with the trochlea of the talus in a hinge joint. The structure of the lower ankle joint in the tarsus, however, still permits rotation of the foot itself to a certain degree. In the arm, such rotation occurs in the forearm.

To move these joints, the body possesses a highly differentiated system of muscles that not only perform movements but also hold the joints together and regulate tensions within the skeletal system.

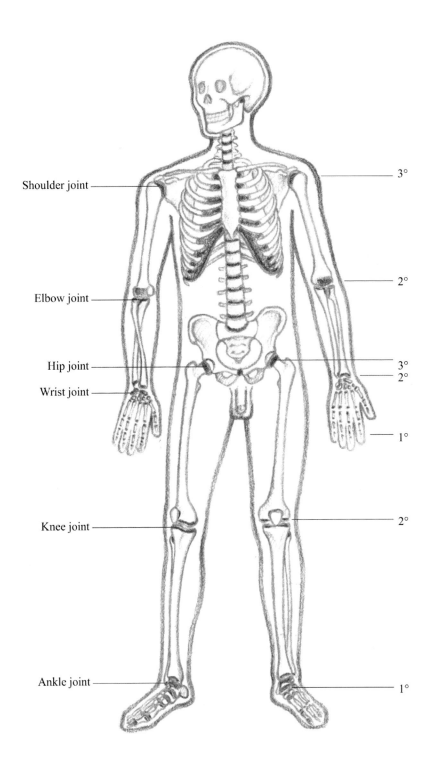

Shoulder joint

Elbow joint

Hip joint

Wrist joint

Knee joint

Ankle joint

3°

2°

3°
2°

1°

2°

1°

Fig. 61. **Overview of the location of major joints in the limbs.** *Ball-and-socket joints (such as the shoulder and hip joints) with their three degrees of freedom (3°: ability to move in three directions) lie close to the torso. Toward the periphery, the degree of freedom decreases (2° in the elbow and knee joints, 1° in the joints of the fingers and toes). Red: cartilage tissue.*

Functional Threefoldness of the Muscular System

Our many different movement possibilities are directly determined by the shapes of our joints and the arrangement of our skeletal muscles. Due to the inherent limitations of three-dimensional space, muscles can only work in their respective planes, and their action requires two antagonistic muscle groups that work in opposite directions. For example, if a flexor contracts, the corresponding extensor must be relaxed.

But muscles serve static as well as dynamic functions. Since they always connect two or more skeletal parts, they function like elastic belts that pull on the bones. By itself, the human skeleton would have to be much more robust in order to effectively support and move the body. Our bones can be relatively slender and delicate only because a great deal of compressive and tensile stress is dispelled by the pull of the muscles. Thus the entire human musculature functions as a bracing system that relieves strain on the joints and therefore allows a richly varied array of movements and expressive possibilities.

The evolution of uprightness means that our **lower limbs** have specialized almost exclusively in support and locomotion. Each leg constitutes a weight-bearing column on which the body's entire weight can balance. The pervasive structural principle that allows the legs to serve this function is the **arch**. The pelvis and sacrum constitute an arch with its bases in the hip joints, which in turn are braced horizontally by the pubic bone (Figure 62). The two femurs with their angled necks also form an arch, albeit one that is interrupted by the pelvis. An additional arch at the lower end of each femur is supported by the tibia's wide bearing surface. The foot has evolved an especially important arch. Its wonderfully harmonious longitudinal arch, together with the transverse arch in the tarsus, is the most important prerequisite for upright human walking. But instead of being a static vault, this arch is

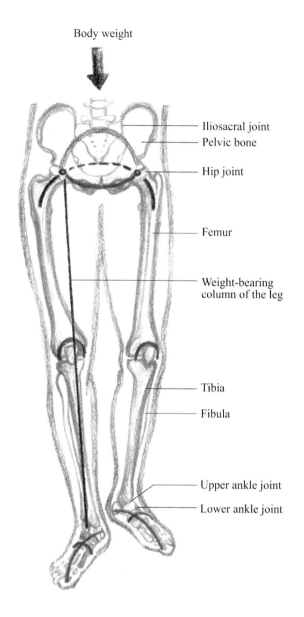

Body weight

Iliosacral joint
Pelvic bone

Hip joint

Femur

Weight-bearing column of the leg

Tibia

Fibula

Upper ankle joint

Lower ankle joint

Fig. 62. **Functional arches in the pelvis and legs** *(red). Right: supporting leg; left: moving leg. The architecture of the arches becomes much more differentiated toward the periphery. Because the foot has both a longitudinal and a transverse arch as well as rotational ability in the lower ankle joint, it can adapt flexibly to all static and dynamic demands.*

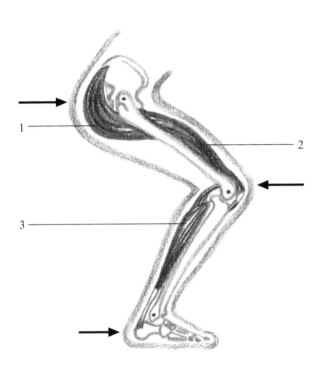

Fig. 63. **Extensor muscles of the leg and their function in uprightness.** *In humans, the long extensors of the leg are exceptionally strong because they work against the weight of the body to maintain an upright stance (from Benninghoff). 1: gluteus maximus; 2: quadriceps; 3: gastrocnemius/soleus.*

a mosaic of bony elements that even permit rotation (pronation/supination) around a diagonal longitudinal axis whenever the leg is freed from support functions.

Rotation is also possible in the knee joint when it is bent. Although the leg has made the sacrifice of totally submerging itself in three-dimensional space (in order to give the arm more freedom), it retains an astonishing freedom of movement, which, however, must be safeguarded by the muscular system. That is why the leg is dominated by the long extensor muscles, which return the leg to the vertical position after it has

been bent. These muscles are exceptionally strong because they always work against the weight of the body (Figure 63). Mephistopheles, the devil with the horse's hooves, had to have artificial calves made for himself so he could pass as human. The extensor muscles of the upper and lower legs are among the strongest muscles in the body and are unique to the human muscular system, since only humans truly walk upright (Figure 63).

Foot muscles, too, serve more to secure the structure of the arch than to move toes. For example, the foot's equivalent of the superficial flexor in the lower arm is located in the sole, where it braces the longitudinal arch (Figure 64).

In contrast, the **upper limbs**, which uprightness has relieved of the burden of supporting the body, possess the potential for a great variety of movements. The carpal bones are relatively small, but the fingers are long and shaped like little isolated limbs. The metacarpus forms a shallow dome, and the mobile, opposable thumb can selectively touch each of the other fingers. The human hand has become a grasping hand—a natural work of art that is adapted not only to practical and creative manual activities but also to a multiplicity of expressive possibilities on the soul level.

The muscles that move the fingers, unlike the corresponding muscles of the foot, are located for the most part in the lower arm and connected to the finger bones by long tendons. The arm's axis of movement passes through the third finger (i.e., the middle of the hand), not—as in the foot—through the second ray with a bend in the tarsus (Figures 59 and 64). But "relieving" the upper limbs of support functions results in several other noteworthy gains: The lower arm rotates independently, and the pectoral girdle is mobile in relationship to the torso. Specialized muscles have evolved to turn the lower arm inward (pronation, which positions the hand for the work of grasping, holding, touching, etc.) and outward (supination, which positions it for receiving or carrying objects). The pectoral girdle's mobility expands the hand's range of action considerably, allowing it to reach almost any point within our

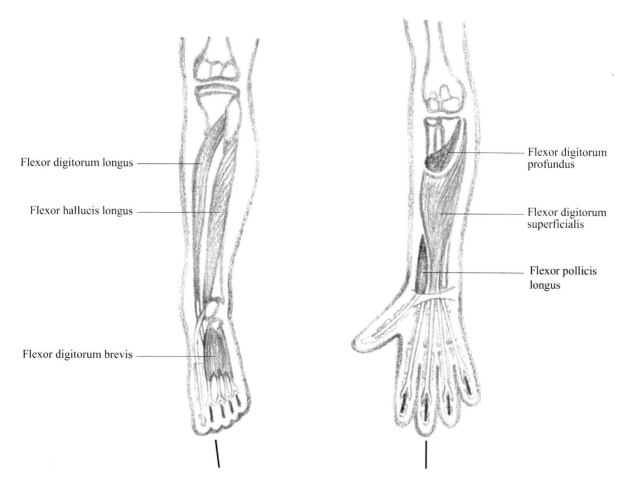

Fig. 64. **Comparison of the flexor muscles of toes and fingers.** *The two finger flexors are located in the lower arm. Consequently, there are no muscles in the palm. In the foot, however, the flexor digitorum brevis is located in the sole to support the arch of the foot. The dynamic axis runs through the second ray of the foot but the third ray of the hand.*

field of vision (Figure 65). This wide range of motion is possible because the scapula (shoulder blade) is connected to the torso (ribcage) only through the clavicle (collarbone); powerful muscle loops (especially the serratus anterior and the trapezius) move it in all directions (Figure 66).

Another unique feature of the upper limbs is that some of their muscles (e.g., latissimus dorsi, pectoralis major) extend well onto the torso, whereas the leg muscles end at the iliac crest in the pelvis. Thus the shoulder musculature is functionally very closely linked to the midsection

of the torso (ribcage, spine), and in fact some of these muscles can also assist in respiration.

The **muscles of the head** have taken a further step in freeing themselves from the static and mechanical imperatives of three-dimensional space. The muscles of facial expression consist of ringlike sphincter muscles that close the seven body openings in the head and radial dilators that open them. These two muscle types are most readily apparent around the mouth. The ring-shaped sphincter muscle (orbicularis oris) contrasts clearly with several groups of radial

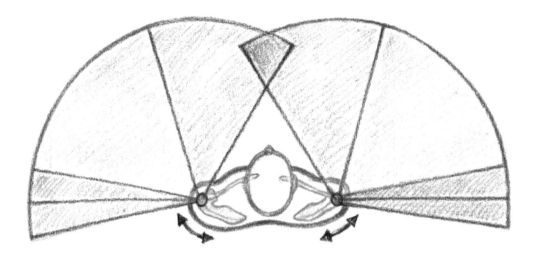

Fig. 65. **The arm's range of motion in the shoulder joint** (gray area) can be significantly expanded (red areas) by adjusting the position of the pectoral girdle (arrows). It is obvious that our "field of grasping" largely corresponds to our field of vision.

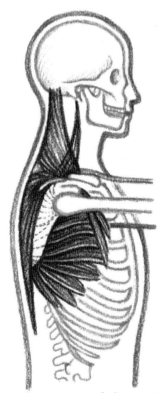

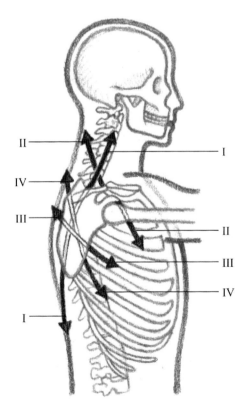

Fig. 66. **The muscle loops of the pectoral girdle** move the scapula both horizontally and vertically in relationship to the ribcage. With each movement, the articular cavity of the shoulder joint acquires a new base for arm movements. For example, for the arm to be raised above the horizontal (so-called elevation), the scapula must move forward and rotate.

I: levator scapulae-trapezius loop;
II: pectoralis-trapezius loop;
III: serratus-trapezius loop;
IV: serratus-rhomboideus loop (15).

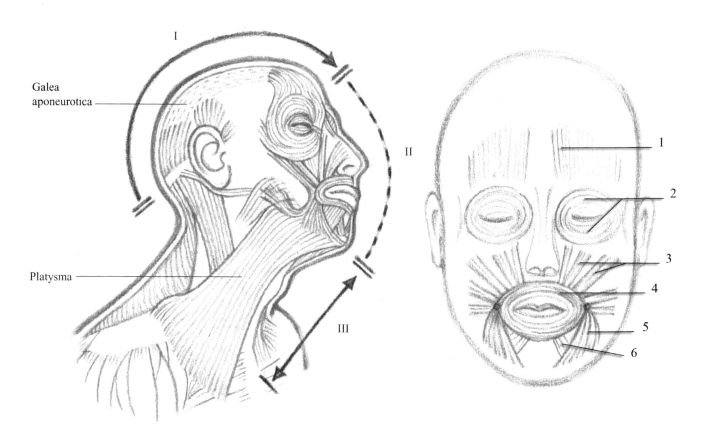

Galea
aponeurotica

Platysma

Fig. 67. **Structural principles governing the mimetic musculature** *(II), which lies between the platysma (III) and the galea aponeurotica and epicranius (I). Compensatory contractions of muscle groups I and III make facial expressions possible by preventing the shifting of facial skin that would otherwise inevitably result from all bodily movements.*

Fig. 68. **Facial apertures, especially the mouth and eyes**, *are surrounded by circular and radial muscles capable of producing tremendous variation in the movements of opening and closing. These movements then assume the new function of expressing soul content.*
> 1. *Occipitofrontalis*
> 2. *Orbicularis oculi*
> 3. *Zygomatici*
> 4. *Orbicularis oris*
> 5. *Depressor anguli oris*
> 6. *Depressor labii inferioris*

muscles that attach to the lower lip or the corners of the mouth. These muscles open or widen the mouth (Figures 67 and 68). Similar structures are evident in the eyelids but less apparent around the ears and nostrils, which barely move in humans.

The **mimetic muscles** are skin muscles capable of acting in relative independence of other bodily movements. The platysma, a thin layer of skin muscles at the front of the neck, prevents displacement of facial skin that would otherwise occur whenever the limbs or torso move (Figure

67). In back, skin displacement is kept from continuing into the head by the fact that the neck muscles end at the occiput. A separate layer of muscles (the epicranius and galea aponeurotica) has evolved to cover the top of skull and move freely over it (see Figure 67). Thus the skin covering the skull and face can move relatively freely, relieved of the bracing function of the skin that covers the rest of the body. In addition to serving the physical needs of opening and closing body openings in conjunction with food intake and

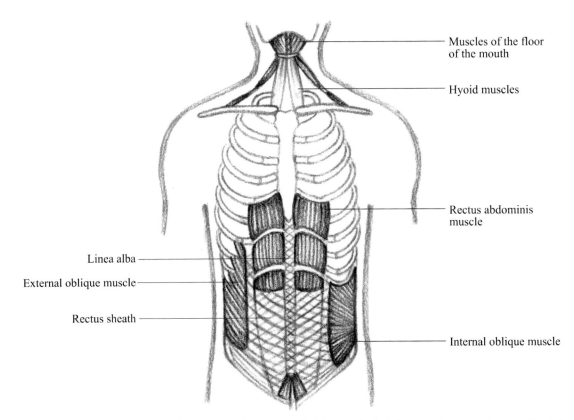

Fig. 69. **Straight muscle system of the ventral torso wall.** *A band of straight muscles runs the length of the torso from neck to pelvis. The rectus abdominis is encased by the rectus sheath, which is made up of the aponeuroses of the oblique abdominal muscles. The tendon fibers form a double spiral brace and cross in the midline (linea alba).*

eye movements, the facial skin can also become an organ for soul expression.

It is interesting to observe how this functional reorganization occurs. For example, when the gesture of opening the mouth or eyes no longer necessarily serves a practical purpose, it can express a soul gesture such as attentiveness, extroversion, etc. Conversely, closing a body opening signals introversion, turning away from the outer world, depression, and so on. In this connection, we must keep in mind the overall threefoldness of the face. In the area of the forehead and eyes, "upper" human processes prevail (thinking, perception), while the nasal area is dominated by middle or rhythmic processes (feeling, breathing) and the lower part of the face (mouth, cheeks) by metabolic will processes. Thus psychological processes rooted in the domain of

the will are expressed in the mimetic musculature surrounding the mouth. A few examples are the compressed lips of a person who is desperate or depressed, or the broad smile (open mouth) of a sanguine temperament enjoying life. At the other pole, eyelid movements say a lot about the momentary movements of our thoughts and reveal our degree of attentiveness, whether we are turning toward or away from the outer world, or whether we are happy or sad in relationship to our mental activity of the moment. The face is the mirror of the soul, but only because it has evolved a muscular system that is largely freed from constraining natural functions and can therefore be used for symbolic expression or signaling.

In the lower limbs, the forces of movement (i.e., will forces) are largely bound up with the mechanics of movement. Toward the head, however, these same forces become increasingly independent, as is already clearly apparent in the upper limbs. Here movements are increasingly used to express soul processes. Raising our hands can mean pleading, begging, or praying; clenching our fists can signal anger or a threat; folding our hands can suggest concentration, reverence, or self-absorption. We have at our disposal an endless variety of hand positions and arm movements suitable for the symbolic expression of psychological contents. The hand positions in statues of the Buddha, for example, offer an interesting study.

The same principle underlies all shifts in the functions of limb movements. Released from practical necessities, they can be placed in the service of soul processes. Without changing their character, they become signs or symbols of events on the psychological level. This process is especially impressive in the head—specifically, in the chewing muscles and the muscles of the mouth and larynx, where the freedom acquired through human uprightness is put to use in developing speech. Words, which become symbols of expressive movements of the human psyche, are carried on the stream of the breath and shaped by the larynx and oral cavity.

The release of movement forces to serve psychological expression increases from bottom to top in the three major areas of the human musculoskeletal system (pelvis and legs below, arms and pectoral girdle in the middle, and the head with its jaw joints, chewing muscles, and mimetic musculature). All three areas are united in a functional whole by the **torso and its musculature**. The spine and ribcage are connecting elements that also provide the basis for movement, whether in the lower, middle, or upper parts of the body. Each limb movement originates from the spine, i.e., from the torso. The torso is a safe platform for all of our movements. As a result, the spinal column is easily affected by errors in peripheral movements.

The torso has two major muscle systems that are responsible for bracing our entire movement apparatus. The first is a vertical (caudal-cranial) system of straight longitudinal muscles that connect the torso segments, often in manifold

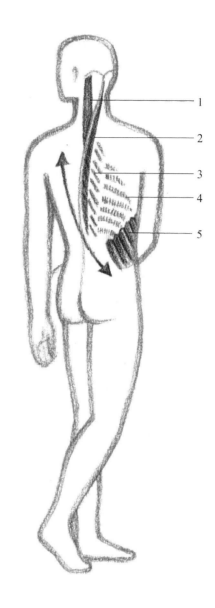

Fig. 70. **Spiral loops of dorsal muscles spanning the torso.** *Multiple muscle systems that run in the same direction create an elongated spiral of muscles. The spiral running in the opposite direction is not shown.*
1: neck (splenius) muscles;
2: transversospinal group of the autochthonous (indigenous) back musculature;
3: levatores costarum;
4: external intercostal muscles;
5: external oblique muscle (15).

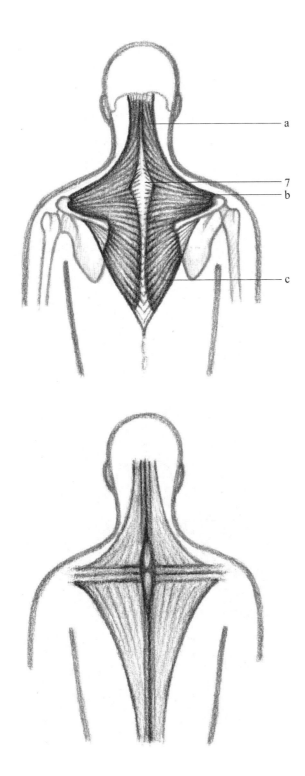

Fig. 71. ***The trapezius muscle*** *connects the pectoral girdle, head, and spinal column. Its three major parts (a, b, c), whose aponeurosis is located on the level of the dorsal process of the seventh cervical vertebra (7), form a crosslike shape (lower illustration).*

and very complex ways (Figure 69). This system consists of the rectus abdominis and the straight neck muscles of the floor of the mouth, hyoid, and larynx in front (Figure 69) and of the many individual autochthonous (indigenous) m *the spinal cord* uscles of the back. The second is a spiral system of two large, crossing series of muscles that run from the pelvis to the head and span the entire torso (Figure 70). This system includes the oblique abdominal muscles, the transversospinal muscle group of the back, and the oblique neck (splenius) muscle.

In ancient times, the spinal column with its spiral loops of muscles was experienced as a serpent (Kundalini) that rises out of the pelvis and genital area and extends its head into the forehead, where it can either bestow powers of supernatural consciousness or plunge human beings into the dark abyss of emotional disorientation.

In the area of the chest, these muscle spirals lie beneath the pectoral girdle, which moves back and forth above them with astonishing freedom. As a result, the shoulder joint (whose glenoid cavity serves as the basis for all arm movements) can assume a great variety of positions, and the arm can move in almost all directions, including high above the horizontal to a vertical position. The trapezius muscle, which connects the pectoral girdle and moves it in relationship to the torso, is of crucial importance here. Seen from the back, this muscle looks almost like an angel's wing attached to the spinal column (Figure 71). Its crosslike shape derives from the attachment of muscle bundles to the horizontal shoulder blade and from vertical (ascending and descending) strands of muscle fiber that leave a rhombic tendon window open around the dorsal process of the seventh cervical vertebra. Is this the cross that we have to bear as a consequence of being human? For Siegfried, who failed to complete the process of giving birth to his higher being, the center of this cross was his vulnerable spot, covered by a linden leaf when he bathed in dragon's blood. In any case, the pectoral girdle lies in the body's middle, transitional domain, where forces of movement that are bound up in metabolism in the lower body are released to be transformed into psychologically expressive gestures or cognitive abilities.

Muscles as Intermediaries between Blood and Nerves

The actual activity of movement takes place unconsciously. Although we move our limbs deliberately and our sense organs perceive their movement from the outside, we remain unconscious of what is actually going on in our muscles. Nonetheless, our motor system is "trainable." We can alter the forces applied in any given instance, and we can consciously practice and eventually perfect the specialized interplay of specific muscle groups for specific purposes (such as a sport or playing an instrument). All of this would be inconceivable without a nervous system that from a functional point of view is intimately connected to the motor system. But even in the motor areas of the nervous system, many processes run their course reflexively, and we are fully conscious only within a very narrow range—when we are practicing new forms of movement, for example. The process of "imprinting" these movement patterns on our motor system is long and often arduous (think of learning to play a musical instrument). How does it happen? How can nerves and muscles work together so closely? Does the nervous system "know" anything at all about what is going on in the muscles? And what role does our will play in all this?

These questions and our views on them are centrally important not only to our understanding of what it means to be human but also to our social interactions. Whether we see the human being as a machine with movements directed by the nervous system or as a spiritual entity endowed with free will makes a fundamental difference in how we live together in society, a difference that is reflected even in legislation.

It has long been known that the nervous system is very closely connected to the muscular system. Skeletal muscles are not only organs of movement but are also kinesthetic and proprioceptive sense organs that constantly inform us of the location of our limbs in space and the tension in our muscles relative to outside forces

(gravity, weight, etc.). With surprising precision, we can estimate the weight of objects held in our hands. We know the position of our limbs (for example, whether our fingers are straight or bent) even when we can't see them. This is possible because the skeletal muscles contain specialized sense organs (muscle spindles) that constantly inform us about muscle tension. The spindles are primarily stretch receptors. Striking a tendon, for example, causes a brief contraction of the associated muscle (monosynaptic reflex) because the muscle spindles are stretched abruptly, sending stimuli to the spinal cord via an afferent nerve. From the spinal cord, an efferent stimulus is sent out, reaching the muscle via a motor nerve (proprioceptive reflex).

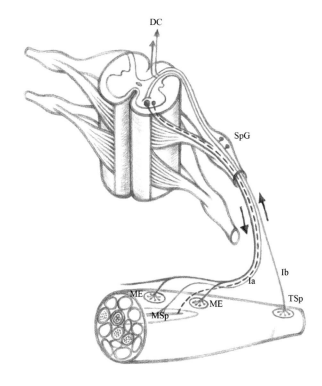

Fig. 72 A. **Innervation of muscle fibers** *from the spinal cord. Each segment of the spinal nerves consists of an afferent neuron (blue) and an efferent (motor) neuron (red). DC = Dorsal column of spinal cord; ME = Motor end plate; MSp = Muscle spindel; TSp = Tendon spindel; SpG = Spinalganglion; Ia = Muscle spindel afferences; Ib = Tendon spindel afferences.*

The "information" that reaches the spinal cord via afferent nerves may also be transmitted to the brain by way of long, afferent nerve tracts, in which case the event in the motor system becomes conscious. These afferent tracts, however, carry information not only to the cerebral cortex but also to deeper-lying subcortical centers that are important for learned, automatic, or unconscious movements.

Muscle activity, however, requires intact connections not only to the nervous system but also to the circulatory and respiratory systems. Blood vessels transport oxygen and nutrients (especially glucose) to the muscles and remove carbon dioxide and metabolic wastes such as lactic acid. Ultimately, movement always involves all three major functional systems: cytoplasmic metabolic processes within the muscle fibers; the circulatory system's rhythmic processes, which permit exchanges of respiratory gases and metabolic substances; and informational processes guided by the nervous system through changes in cell membranes. In other words, *all three functional systems must be intact*. Until relatively recently, the role of the nervous system was often overemphasized at the expense of the other two systems.

Movement as a Threefold Psycho-Physical Process

Each muscle fiber (a gigantic multinucleate cell) contains contractile fibrils (myofibrils) consisting of two different types of filaments (myosin and actin) that can shift position in relationship to each other. Their shifting causes a contraction or relaxation of the muscle fibers. The central processes in contraction are the release of Ca^{++} ions (induced by the motor end plate) in muscle fiber cytoplasm and the conversion of ATP to ADP, which makes energy available. Calcium concentrations increase abruptly by a factor of 100, the myofibrils contract, and the muscle becomes hard (Figure 72B). The same thing happens after death, when the muscles initially become stiff and immobile in rigor mortis. From the qualitative perspective, therefore, muscle contraction represents hardening and dying off— in other words, a form process. Not surprisingly, it is triggered by nerve processes similar to those involved in informational and stimulatory events elsewhere in the nervous system. To put it simply, action potentials always develop whenever Na^+ ions move into the nerve fibers and K^+ ions flow out of them, that is, whenever and wherever the negative charge on cell membranes breaks down briefly (depolarization). The same ion displacements also occur after death, when the nerves become unresponsive to stimuli and die off in the absence of energy to run the recharging process.

Skeletal muscle fibers are transversely striated and characterized by close, synapselike membrane contacts between nerve and muscle fibers. As a result, the negatively charged muscle fiber membrane can be rapidly depolarized via the efferent ("motor") nerve fiber in the motor end plate. In other words, Na^+ ions flow into the muscle cell while K^+ ions flow out. This shift mobilizes the Ca^{++} ions present in the muscle fiber, channeling them into the cytoplasm so that energy can be released through the conversion of ATP to ADP, causing the myofibrils to contract (Figure 72B).

For the muscle to relax, this "death process" must be counteracted by some sort of reenliving process, i.e., by adding energy. And in fact the "hardening" of the muscle can be reversed only by applying energy to make the muscle fibrils mobile again. Rebuilding ATP requires energy, which comes primarily from the "combustion" of sugars (glucose) in the presence of oxygen (aerobic glycolysis). Although muscle fibers usually have large stores of glycogen (animal starch, from which glucose is then formed), they always need adequate additions of sugars and oxygen in order to become flexible again after contraction. The vascular system, which must also carry away

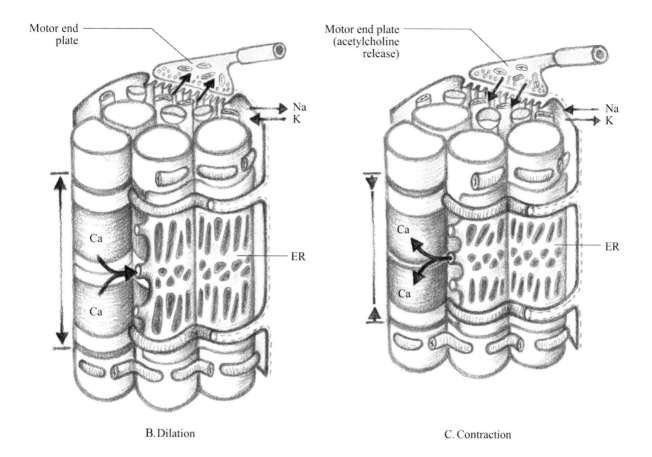

*Fig. 72 B and C. **Basic processes in muscle contraction** (17). During contraction (C), influx of Na++ ions and outflow of K+ ions (initiated by the motor end plate) results in depolarization of the cell membranes of the muscle fiber. As a consequence, Ca++ ions are released (broad arrows) from the sacs of the endoplasmic reticulum (ER), causing the contractile muscular fibrils (myofibrils) to shorten. During dilation (relaxation, B), energy is used to pump Ca ions back into the sacs (broad arrows). The calcium concentration in the cytoplasm drops and the muscle fibrils lengthen.*

the breakdown products of intracellular "combustion" (carbon dioxide, lactates, etc.), therefore represents the reenlivening, regenerative element. Its functions are diametrically opposed to the catabolic processes of the nervous system. We must also realize that movement can happen only when the counterparts of contracting muscles relax **simultaneously**. Antagonists must expand as much as agonists contract, and at exactly the same time. This process is regulated by the nervous system.

Most of the basic processes underlying contraction and relaxation, therefore, are intracellular metabolic processes (changes in Ca++ concentrations, energy conversion, etc.). In contrast, shaping the movement (the image of the movement as an informational element) takes place through membrane processes triggered by the nervous system (Na+, K+ ion exchange, etc.). And finally, balancing these inherently polar processes is the responsibility of respiration and related substance transfers mediated by the vascular system. The result is a threefold process that reflects the overall functional threefoldness of the human body.

First and foremost, muscle movements are expressions of the will that work all the way into the metabolic processes of muscle fibers. Regulating the streams of forces involved, i.e., harmonizing individual contractions and reconciling them with the Earth's gravitational field (compensatory movements to maintain equilibrium, etc.), are the task of the nervous system, which therefore also allows us to actualize a "movement concept." A third, generally disregarded component is supplied by the rhythmic system, which forms the physical basis for feeling. Via respiratory and circulatory processes, psychological sensations can exert balancing and modifying effects on movement. All artists and athletes know how much their performances depend on their momentary emotional state. Unconscious respiratory and circulatory processes in and around muscle fibers—i.e., rhythmic alternations between contraction (hardening) and relaxation (reenlivening), which are made possible by intertissue exchanges of solids and gases—are of central importance to accom-

plishing movement. The related sensations that appear in our consciousness ("I'm feeling in good shape/bad shape") are ultimately only concomitant phenomena. For the most part, therefore, will processes related to movement are unconscious, while rhythmic processes are semi-conscious (on the feeling level), and neurological processes more or less conscious to the extent that we develop concepts about our own voluntary motor activity. The organic tissue processes in all three components obviously remain unconscious.

As Rudolf Steiner emphasized repeatedly, if we see the activity of movement as a threefold psycho-physical process, we cannot logically consider the somatomotoric (sensorimotor) nerves as the "will" nerves, giving rise to movement (18, 27, 60). These nerves, which are linked to the skeletal muscles by motor end plates, are efferent nerves; they regulate contractile processes in the cytoplasm and regulate and harmonize the muscular system as a whole. They have nothing to do with will processes as such. We will return to this issue when we discuss the so-called sensorimotor systems of the nervous system (see p. 234 ff.).

The Metabolic System and Digestive Organs

Rarely have contemporary ideas about the human body aroused as much controversy as the concept of the metabolic system as a combustion engine. Foods are imagined as fuels that are "burned" in the body, releasing energy for work and cellular activity. Food values are measured in calories, which indicate how much heat per unit of time is produced by burning the material in question in a test tube. Other aspects of the metabolic and digestive system have also repeatedly triggered speculation, not to mention mystification. Even apart from commercial interests, nutrition has often been the subject of vehement debate on the value (or lack of value) of specific foods for human health or spiritual development. (Vegetarian and vegan practices are only two examples.) But the "combustion theory" does not adequately explain various astonishing phenomena, such as the body's (relative) independence of the type and amount of food consumed. Some saints, such as Switzerland's patron saint Nikolaus von der Flüe, were known to eat nothing or very little for years. Some people eat a lot and stay slim while others eat little and gain weight. Like the sensory and cognitive activity that takes place in the nervous system, human metabolism is a mysterious process that presents many riddles.

Basic Metabolic Processes

Let's begin by considering several fundamental processes involved in ingesting and processing foods (Figure 73). According to current thinking on this subject, we would expect food to be taken into the body "as is" and then transformed ("burned") directly, but this is not the case. In the digestive tract, solid food is not simply chewed and mixed with fluid but is **completely** broken down into its basic building blocks. This is the first archetypal phenomenon of digestion. Proteins are broken down into amino acids, fats into glycerin and fatty acids, and polysaccharides into monosaccharides (glucose, fructose, etc.). These constituents then pass through the intestinal wall and into the body. But what does this disintegration signify? Obviously, any natural compounds (whether preprocessed or not) that are suitable for food possess intrinsic qualities, specific "energetic," vital, or even spiritual potentials that enable them to produce specific effects in their original context. For example, proteins can work as enzymes, hormones, or neurotransmitters. By breaking foods down, the digestion that follows ingestion destroys these functional potentials. In other words, it eliminates intrinsic qualities and creates "neutral" building blocks that express nothing and do nothing. The body then creates **its own** substances out of these building blocks, imbuing them with new and different qualities of its own. The result of this resynthesis, which

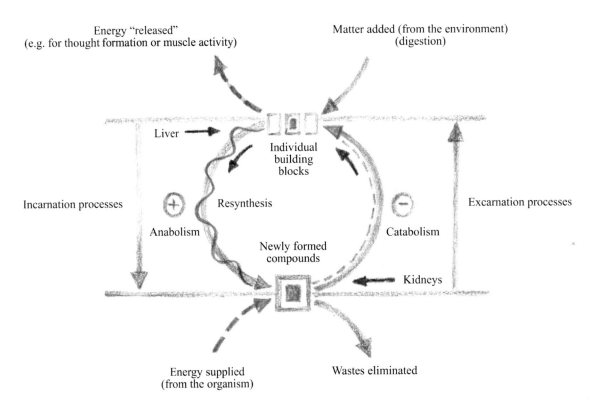

Energy "released"
(e.g. for thought formation or muscle activity)

Matter added (from the environment)
(digestion)

Liver

Individual
building
blocks

Incarnation processes

(+)

Resynthesis

Anabolism

Newly formed
compounds

Catabolism

(−)

Excarnation processes

Kidneys

Energy supplied
(from the organism)

Wastes eliminated

Fig. 73. **Basic metabolic processes.** *Anabolic (+) and catabolic (-) processes are integrated into a cycle.*

takes place inside the body, is that the newly created substances acquire specific qualities determined by the organism itself; they do *not* retain their original qualities.

A similar disintegration and resynthesis of substances take place constantly in all cells and tissues. From the material perspective, therefore, the body is always being broken down, rebuilt, and renewed. ***These functions are collectively known as metabolism.*** In human blood, for example, the concentration of amino acids (3 mmol/l) is held constant. If too many amino acids are absorbed from the intestines (due to a high-protein diet, for example), they are synthesized into proteins and stored in the liver or other tissues so that blood levels remain the same. If blood levels sink and more amino acids are needed (during fasting, for example), tissue proteins are broken down and the resulting amino acids are released

into the bloodstream. The body always attempts to maintain a balance between anabolic and catabolic processes and to eliminate outside influences (through immune responses, if need be).

Within the body, therefore, compounds are broken down and resynthesized in a constant, self-equilibrating cyclical process (Figure 73). From this perspective, the body actually should not need food, because its own amino acids, for example, are always recycled as building blocks for protein synthesis. Strangely enough, however—and this is the second archetypal phenomenon of metabolism—a certain amount of matter always falls out of this cyclical process and cannot be reused. This (and only this) matter is then eliminated and must be replaced through food. If this phenomenon, which is so typical of life on Earth, did not exist, our metabolism would be an example of perpetual motion.

As we see, metabolism always includes two basic types of processes:

1. Absorption of qualitatively neutral building blocks and their subsequent transformation into endogenous substances with specific (vital and spiritual) properties. Through these anabolic processes, the soul-spiritual element "incarnates" into the material world.

2. Breakdown of endogenous matter, which yields building blocks for resynthesis. Through these catabolic or "excarnation" processes, "qualities" are released from their association with matter.

When building blocks resulting from catabolic processes are reused in life's cyclical processes, life forces and related soul-spiritual forces re-engage in the material world. But when matter is eliminated as unusable, the forces (potentials) associated with it are set free. Excretion, therefore, regardless of where it appears in the body—although it is associated primarily with the kidneys, of course—always means that life forces are released to serve soul-spiritual processes. Ultimately, the availability of forces for cognitive and sensory activity depends on elimination processes.

Energy conversion. The processes taking place in the body include not only material cycles of synthesis and breakdown (which would produce only states of equilibrium, not changes) but also conversions in which "energy" is bound up or released, work is performed, and matter is moved. Energy is different from dead substance. Ultimately, the agent that applies energy, converts it, and activates it, is our will. The release of energy enables our will to intercede in our metabolism so that development can occur and something new can emerge. Energy conversions enable our muscles to perform work and transform our will impulses into deeds. It is interesting to note that the material processes involved in releasing energy are always the same. The building blocks absorbed from foods in the intestine are resynthesized in the liver and stored in fat deposits or in the liver itself. But none of the three basic nutrients (proteins, fats, and carbohydrates) can be used

directly for energy conversion. This is the third archetypal phenomenon of the metabolic process. As a result of complex catabolic processes, all three sources yield a single (very unspecific) basic building block (acetyl-CoA). Through the citric acid cycle, the hub of the metabolism, acetyl-CoA releases H^+ ions. With the help of respiratory enzymes (cytochromes), these H^+ ions are brought into contact with oxygen (O_2) through the many incremental steps of the process known as biological oxidation. This process takes place primarily in specific organelles (mitochondria) within the cells. When hydrogen and oxygen combine, water is produced and energy is made available, as also happens when a combustible gas burns. But instead of being released directly, as in a gas boiler, the energy is "packaged" and stored in ATP (adenosine triphosphate) molecules (Figure 74).

The most astonishing aspects of these processes, however, are:

1. that the initial substance (acetyl-CoA) is always the same, regardless of whether it is derived from proteins, fats, or carbohydrates;

2. that the final reaction in the respiratory chain (the combining of hydrogen and oxygen molecules to form water), is very unspecific and merely produces "energy," which is stored in energy-rich phosphate molecules and thus becomes available wherever energy is needed in the body. It is interesting to note that there is also an inefficiency in this "internal combustion" in that part of the energy released is lost in the form of heat.

In summary, we have ascertained that the metabolic process as a whole takes place on three interconnected levels (Figure 74):

1. Purely material conversions, i.e., the cyclical processes of anabolism and catabolism. These

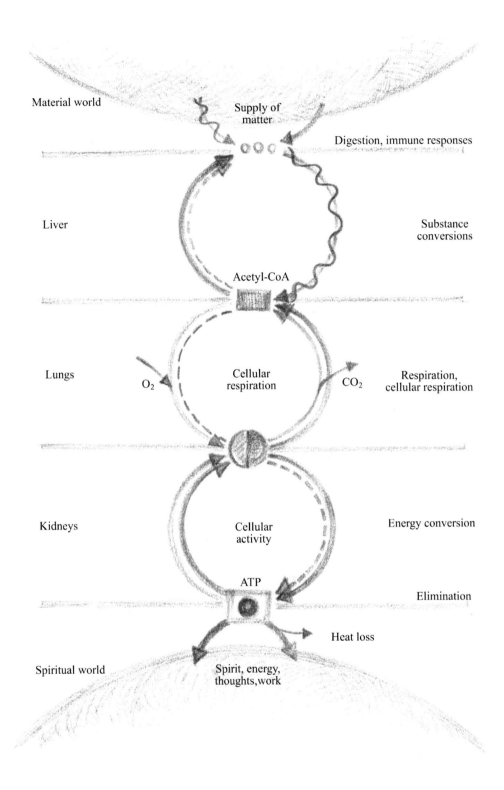

*Fig. 74. **Three stages of metabolic processes in the body** and their connections to three major organs (liver, lungs, kidneys).*

processes are centered in the liver and connected to the environment through the intestinal tract.

2. Cellular respiration, in which acetyl-CoA produces hydrogen ions and respiratory enzymes, makes oxygen available so that water and energy are produced. These processes are basically rhythmical in character, and the lungs, as the primary organ of respiration, play a role in them.

3. The intracellular cycle of ADP+P and ATP. At any time and anywhere in the body, the appropriate enzymes (ATPases) can make energy available by removing a phosphorus atom from ATP. Conversely, energy can always be stored by converting ADP to ATP. This third level is the level of the will. Energy transformations may involve heat (warmth), light, chemical, or life energy, depending on the organs in which they occur (61 and 62).

The Functional Significance of Metabolism

From the purely material perspective, it should make no difference which nutrient class supplies the source compounds for energy conversion, since the end products (hydrogen ions, ATP) are always the same. Let's remember, however, that we are attempting to make the transition from a purely quantitative, chemically and physically oriented way of thinking to a more process-oriented, functional thinking. While it is true that digested nutrients lose their "qualities," or essential (living) nature, the human body learns about the material world by destroying these qualities. It learns through the forces this destruction requires, and through the resistance encountered in "foreign" matter from a different organism. Breaking down ingested foods becomes an "inner experience" of their inherent qualities. In rebuilding similar substances on the other side of the intestinal wall, the organism can assesses the expenditure of energy required to create compounds of its own, i.e., to raise these foreign building blocks to the level of human existence. Unconsciously,

the body experiences which forces of its own must be mobilized for resynthesis. Compounds from the mineral kingdom require the greatest "expenditure of energy" because they must pass through the plant and animal levels on their way to being transformed into human substance (three stages). Plant matter requires only two stages, animal matter only one, and human matter none at all. In metabolic terms, cannibals are the "laziest" eaters. Meat-eaters, too, can indulge in a degree of digestive comfort. Plant and mineral food sources stimulate the most internal forces and are therefore especially enlivening and stimulating for endogenous life processes. We take the outer world into ourselves; in breaking down foreign matter, we experience qualitative and therefore essential aspects of natural substances from the world around us.

It is interesting to note that the endless variety of possible foods can be reduced to **three** qualitatively very different **nutrient categories**, namely, proteins, fats, and carbohydrates (plus water and salts). Carbohydrates play the primary role in energy conversions. One can easily understand glucose, which can be made available rapidly and at any time for use in cellular respiration, as a substance of the will. Proteins serve primarily regulatory, structure-forming, and structure-maintaining functions and therefore represent an informational element in the material realm, comparable to the nerve element in the body as a whole. Fats represent a middle element. They sometimes contribute to structure formation, as they do in the joints or as stabilizing components (cholesterol) of cell membranes, but they can also serve as energy sources. Adipose tissue develops out of reticular connective tissue, which has the ability to differentiate and dedifferentiate, i.e., the potential to develop in both directions. As "mediating" compounds, fats play a role in many locations within the metabolic system. In general, therefore, they can be ascribed to the body's middle (rhythmic) system (cf. 62).

Functional Subdivision of the Digestive Tract

In early embryonic development, the intestinal tube develops out of a fold in the yolk sac (Figure 75). As development of the three-dimensional body proceeds (cf. Figure 27), this tube continues to elongate and to separate from the shrinking yolk sac until the connection is reduced to a narrow canal (the omphalomesenteric duct). The embryonic intestinal tube is initially closed off by the pharyngeal membrane in front and the cloacal membrane in back. Both membranes eventually rupture and disappear, leaving the intestinal tube (secondarily) connected to the outer world. This process is the opposite of the development of the neural tube, which is initially open at both ends but later closes.

Already at a very early stage, *five sections of the intestinal tube* are apparent:

1. The pharyngeal gut with the pharyngeal pouches, which are part of the branchial/pharyngeal apparatus or system. The primitive pharynx develops into the oral cavity and pharynx. 2. The esophagus, which forms a passage through the chest area. 3. The stomach. 4. The upper branch of the umbilical loop, which later forms the small intestine; its first section gives rise to the two major digestive glands (liver and pancreas, Figure 75). 5. The lower branch of the umbilical loop, which later develops into the large intestine.

In the mature human body, the intestinal tract forms a much-convoluted tube that begins in the oral cavity and ends in the rectum. Its total average length is four to five meters (see Figure 76). Because it is open-ended, it is actually a part of the outer world that runs through the body. In theory, a probe could be inserted into the intestinal tract through the mouth and guided all the way through until it comes out the anus. The intestinal wall constitutes the boundary between the interior of the body and the outside world. This boundary is secured by multiple immunological barriers. The most important section of the gastrointestinal tract is the small intestine, where most digested nutrients are absorbed into the blood. This critical

event, however, requires careful preparation so that it happens in a relatively germ-free (although not totally sterile) milieu. For this reason, the small intestine is preceded by the stomach, which produces bactericidal hydrochloric acid. The lower end of the small intestine also contains immunologically active tissues—specifically, the Peyer's patches—which are clusters of lymph follicles. Germs arising from the large intestine can be warded off by immune responses at the local level.

From the functional perspective, therefore, the gastrointestinal tract consists of five different sections (cf. Figure 76):

1. The *oral cavity*, most of which develops out of the embryonic ectodermal stomatodaeum (out of an invagination of the skin primordium). This is where foods begin to be broken down through chewing, mixing with saliva, and tasting, which serves as an initial sensory "safety check."

2. The adjacent *pharynx* and its continuation in the esophagus transport bites of swallowed food through the throat and chest to the stomach. This is where food actually enters the body. As mentioned in an earlier chapter, the crossing of air and food passages in the pharynx is a definitive prerequisite for the development of speech (cf. Figure 45).

These first two sections of the digestive tract constitute the "foregut," in contrast to the small intestine (midgut) and large intestine (endgut). By taking in food and tasting and touching it (and also through close association with the respiratory system's organs of speech), this section assumes the more "informational" functional character typical of the upper part of the body. No actual digestive processes take place here, although the salivary glands do secrete starch-digesting enzymes (amylases).

3. Digestion actually begins in the *stomach*, which connects with the outside through the esophagus and oral cavity and with the interior through the duodenum. It occupies the center of the entire system and represents a rhythmic element, as is evident in its motor activity. The body of the stomach (fundus and corpus), which

A

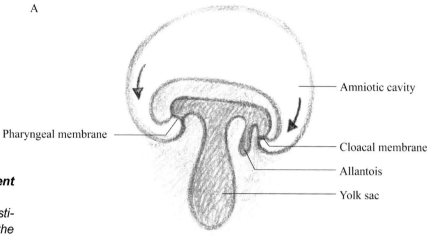

Pharyngeal membrane

Amniotic cavity

Cloacal membrane

Allantois

Yolk sac

B

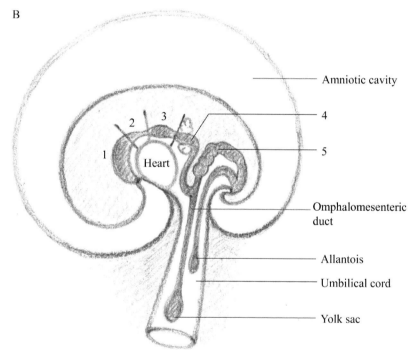

Amniotic cavity

4

5

Omphalomesenteric duct

Allantois

Umbilical cord

Yolk sac

Heart

*Fig. 75. **Embryonic development of the primitive gut.***
(A: day 26; B: day 35). The intestinal tube develops out of a fold in the yolk sac. Initially, it is closed off by the pharyngeal membrane in front and the cloacal membrane in back (tail fold). It shifts inward as a result of the folding of the embryonic disc (head fold, arrows) and development of the embryonic body. It becomes open to the outside as the two membranes disintegrate. The yolk sac also degenerates, as does the allantois, which persists only inside the embryo, where it forms the primordium of the bladder. The five functional sections of the digestive tract (1-5) are recognizable at an early stage:

1: oral cavity, foregut;
2: esophagus;
3: stomach;
4: small intestine (upper portion of the umbilical loop);
5: large intestine (lower portion of the umbilical loop), endgut.

serves as an expandable reservoir, has three muscle layers instead of two and does not develop true peristalsis, which begins only in the stomach's pylorus section. (The pylorus has a normal two-layered musculature that moves semiliquid food into the duodenum in batches.) Digestion of protein begins in the body of the stomach, which produces hydrochloric acid and protein-digesting enzymes (pepsin). The absence of peristaltic mixing allows the gastric juices to take full effect. The fundus expands as additional masses of newly swallowed food (boli) accumulate from the center outward.

The digestive tract's unique rhythm commences only in the stomach's second section, the pyloric antrum, which does not produce hydrochloric acid. Here, semiliquid food is neutralized and then transferred in small boluses through the pylorus into the duodenum. Thus the stomach adjusts imbalances in the arhythmical, random timing of food intake and provides a transition to the unconscious digestive and

Functional Subdivision		Foods		
Section	General functions	Carbohydrates	Proteins	Fats
1. Oral cavity, pharnyx	Chewing, tasting	0/+	0	0
2. Esophagus	Transport	–	–	–
3. Stomach	Reservoir, initiates digestion	+	++	0
4. Duodenum plus liver and pancreas	Secretion and absorption	+++	+++	+++
5. Large intestine	Reabsorption, elimination	–	–	–

Table 13. Functional subdivision of the digestive tract with regard to the digestion of foods.

absorptive processes of the small intestine, which for the most part obey laws of their own. High concentrations of hydrochloric acid in the gastric juices also destroy pathogens and toxins in food.

4. Digestion is actually accomplished in the *small intestine*, where—especially in its first section, the *duodenum*—all three types of nutrients are broken down into their basic building blocks by the corresponding enzymes (amylases, peptidases, and lipases). The pancreas, whose main exit duct empties into the duodenal papilla, is the source of most of these enzymes. The liver participates in fat digestion by secreting bile, which also flows into the small intestine through the duodenal papilla. Bile acids emulsify fats, allowing them to be attacked by enzymes (Table 13).

Absorption, which begins only after foods have been completely "destroyed" or broken down through digestion, is facilitated and accelerated by the many folds, villi, and microvilli that greatly increase the surface area (approximately 200 m²) of the small intestine's mucous membrane. To digest and absorb semiliquid food (chyme), the small intestine secretes large quantities of fluid. This fluid, along with compounds important for the body (bile acids, bile pigments, trace elements, salts, etc.), is almost completely reabsorbed in subsequent sections of the intestinal tract, especially the ileum (the last part of the small intestine) and large intestine.

5. The function of the *large intestine* (colon) is to store and concentrate the intestinal contents and to reabsorb water and important compounds. Surprisingly, foreign organisms (bacteria) play an important part in this process. Bacteria make up 30 to 50% of the dry weight of stools.

Storage and processing are primarily the task of the colon's ascending section (cecum and ascending colon), where chyme is kept for up to twelve hours or longer and is often held in place by antiperistaltic waves of contractions originating in the transverse colon. This pause in the passage through the intestine provides opportunities for "internal perception" of the small intestine's digestive activity and reabsorption of important substances based on what the body needs. (K⁺ reabsorption, for example, is adjusted entirely according to the body's needs.) Typically, 80 to 90 percent of the water and 95 percent of the salts in the large intestine are reabsorbed.

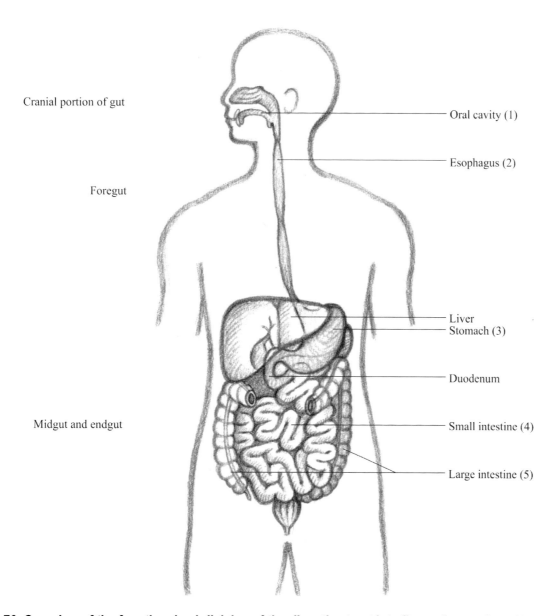

Cranial portion of gut

Foregut

Midgut and endgut

Oral cavity (1)

Esophagus (2)

Liver
Stomach (3)

Duodenum

Small intestine (4)

Large intestine (5)

*Fig 76. **Overview of the functional subdivision of the digestive tract into five major sections** (1-5). The small intestine is 2.5 — 4 meters long, the large intestine 1.2 — 1.65 meters. The large intestine forms a garlandlike frame around the convolutions of the small intestine. Functionally, the liver belongs to the duodenum.*

A surprising and unique feature of the large intestine is the enormous number of bacteria (close to 400 different species) that populate it. These bacteria help with processing what remains of digested food and decomposing compounds secreted into the small intestine (along with bile, for example). Bacterial activity allows the body to retain important compounds (bile pigments, vitamins, etc.) that would otherwise be eliminated.

Some bacteria also synthesize nutrients such as vitamin K, which plays a role in synthesizing coagulation factors in the blood. Coli bacteria are involved in making cobalamin (vitamin B_{12}). The short-chain fatty acids that many bacteria produce from fiber (cellulose, etc.) supply part of the colon's energy needs. As we can see, the colon supports a balanced, stable microbial ecosystem that is very important to the metabolic system as

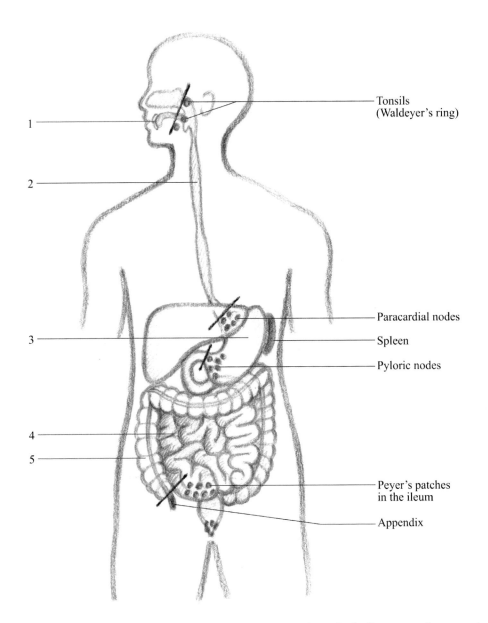

1

2

3

4

5

Tonsils
(Waldeyer's ring)

Paracardial nodes

Spleen

Pyloric nodes

Peyer's patches
in the ileum

Appendix

Fig. 77. **The gastrointestinal tract and associated lymphatic organs.** *Lymphatic tissues and organs (red) are heavily concentrated around the transitions between the five major functional sections (1-5) of the gastrointestinal tract. 1: oral cavity, pharynx; 2: esophagus; 3: stomach; 4: small intestine; 5: large intestine.*

a whole. Its biological activity differs significantly from the chemical activity of the small intestine.

This **fivefold subdivision** of the gastrointestinal tract is not arbitrary. A specific function can be ascribed to each of the five sections. In digestion—an **incremental process** of coming to grips with the outside world—the major functional processes of preparation, rhythmicization,

secretion, reabsorption, and excretion follow a logical, consistent sequence. The intestinal wall is the boundary between inside and outside, and the body invests heavily in multiple safeguards to prevent the uncontrolled penetration of foreign elements. In the intestinal wall itself, complex immune responses fend off antigens. Furthermore, concentrations of lymphatic tissue appear at the transition from each intestinal section to the next, so access to each section is safeguarded by a specific immunological protective zone. The four major tonsils (palatine, pharyngeal, tubal, and lingual), for example, are located at the transition from the oral cavity to the pharynx in Waldeyer's lymphatic ring (Figure 77). Numerous lymph follicles appear in the mucosa at the stomach's entrance (cardia) and exit (pylorus). At the end of the small intestine, before the transition to the large intestine, we find huge aggregates of lymph follicles (Peyer's patches, mentioned above). The appendix, which has been called the "tonsil of the intestines," develops at the beginning of the large intestine (Figure 77). These immune barriers support the defensive functions of the mucous membranes as a whole and safeguard the digestive functions of each section. Approximately fifty percent of all lymphatic tissue is located around the gastrointestinal tract. It is interesting to note that the intestines are involved in all immune responses and always function as a whole in this capacity. For example, when an antigen penetrates the intestinal mucosa at a certain point, B-lymphocytes (after differentiating into plasma cells) do not begin to produce antibodies locally but first migrate into the bloodstream via the lymphatic vessels and lymph nodes of the intestines and thoracic duct and are then distributed throughout the intestinal area via the blood (Fig. 78). This roundabout route allows the immune response, rather than remaining narrowly localized, to be extended to the entire intestinal tract, since any antigen originating in the outside world could already be present in many parts of the digestive tract.

The Hepatobiliary System

Contrary to what we might expect, the basic building blocks derived from foods taken in from the outside world do not pass directly into the bloodstream for distribution throughout the body. Instead, they are channeled into the liver through a dedicated major vessel, the portal vein (Figure 78). Thus the liver serves as the gateway to the body's three-dimensional structure. In the liver, food-derived substances are resynthesized: Amino acids are converted into proteins, and monosaccharides into polysaccharides (especially glycogen). Once again, fats constitute an exception. Almost all of the substances used to build up the body are produced in the liver, where anabolic processes dominate. In the liver, compounds such as proteins are enlivened and animated (that is, imbued with qualities characteristic of the human organism) and transformed into endogenous substances. In the gastrointestinal system, foods are "chopped up" and "killed off," but in the liver they are reenlivened (in a unique incarnation process, cf. Figures 73 and 74) and made usable for the soul-spiritual element occupying a specific body.

It makes sense, therefore, that the *liver* should retain a quasi-embryonic status for the entire life of the body. Like the body as a whole during embryonic development, the liver is pervaded with mixed (venous/arterial) blood, and most of its capillaries are fenestrated sinusoids that allow plasma to wash freely around its cells. Between the rows of hepatocytes and the sinusoids lies the space of Dissé, a lymph-filled gap that collects plasma from the sinusoids. The plasma flows toward the liver's peripheral lymph vessels and then into the cisterna chyli and on into the lymphatic circulatory system (Figures 78 and 79).

The liver consists of lobules that are hexagonal in shape when viewed in cross section. Portal vein blood, which carries "nutrients" from the intestine to the lobules, flows centripetally, i.e., from the periphery toward the center (Figure 79). The plasma that filters into the space of Dissé flows in the opposite direction, from the center toward the

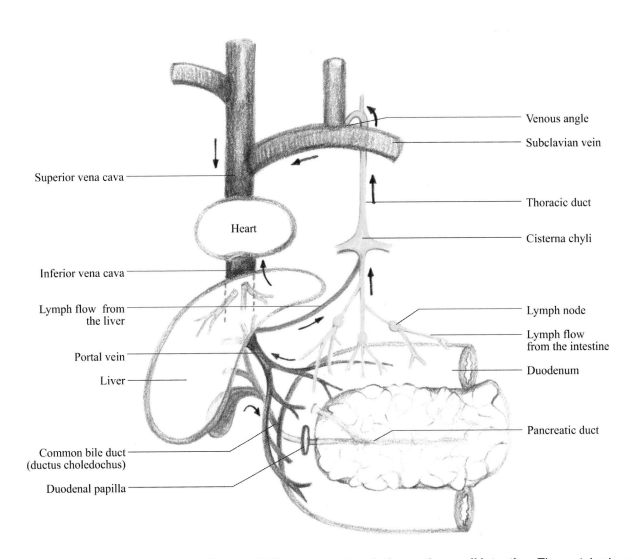

Fig. 78. **The portal vein system, liver, and biliary system in relation to the small intestine.** *The portal vein carries blood enriched with nutrients (especially carbohydrates and amino acids) from the intestine to the liver. The fats absorbed from the intestine, however, do not pass through the portal vein. Most of them flow from intestinal lymph vessels and nodes into the cisterna chyli and then into the thoracic duct, which empties into the left subclavian vein. Bile, which is formed in the liver, flows through the common bile duct (ductus choledochus) into the duodenum. Lymph from the liver reaches the cisterna chyli via liver-specific lymph vessels.*

periphery, into the hepatic lymph vessels. These flows are associated with anabolic processes and serve to enliven and renew the body.

The liver's second major function is related to **bile formation**. In this instance, the liver functions more like a gland. Bile flow within the lobules is centrifugal (Figure 80). It begins far from the bloodstream, in small gaps (bile canaliculi) **between** the hepatocytes. The canaliculi (canals of Hering) increase in diameter as they approach the periphery of the lobule, where they become bile ducts. The small bile ducts merge into the hepatic duct, which then joins the gallbladder duct (ductus cysticus) to form the common bile duct (ductus choledochus), which empties into the duodenum through the duodenal papilla together with the pancreatic duct (Figure 78). This system, which carries bile (liver secretion) into the duodenum of the small intestine, is a typical glandular ductal system.

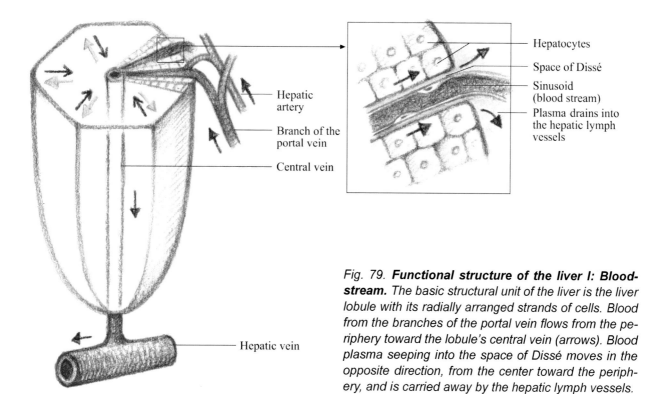

Hepatic artery

Branch of the portal vein

Central vein

Hepatocytes

Space of Dissé

Sinusoid (blood stream)

Plasma drains into the hepatic lymph vessels

Hepatic vein

Fig. 79. **Functional structure of the liver I: Bloodstream.** *The basic structural unit of the liver is the liver lobule with its radially arranged strands of cells. Blood from the branches of the portal vein flows from the periphery toward the lobule's central vein (arrows). Blood plasma seeping into the space of Dissé moves in the opposite direction, from the center toward the periphery, and is carried away by the hepatic lymph vessels.*

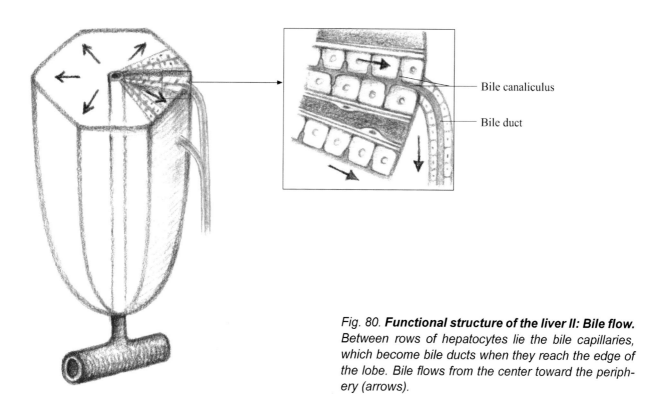

Bile canaliculus

Bile duct

Fig. 80. **Functional structure of the liver II: Bile flow.** *Between rows of hepatocytes lie the bile capillaries, which become bile ducts when they reach the edge of the lobe. Bile flows from the center toward the periphery (arrows).*

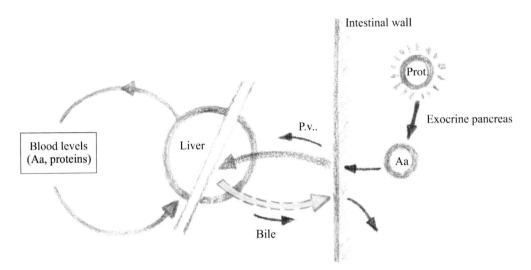

*Fig. 81. **Basic liver functions I: Protein metabolism.** Aa: amino acids, Prot.: proteins, P.v.: portal vein. Metabolic wastes and detoxified substances are excreted into the intestine along with bile.*

These two great flows of substances in the liver—the centripetal flow of blood and the centrifugal flow of bile—play different roles in processing each of the three major nutrient classes (protein, fat, sugar). In each of these three instances, the liver serves a different function and works together with a different organ.

First, let's consider ***protein metabolism*** (Figure 81). As mentioned earlier, enzymes secreted by the pancreas and the intestinal mucosa break the proteins in foods down into amino acids, their basic building blocks. These "qualitatively neutral" components pass through the intestinal wall and are carried to the liver by the blood of the portal vein (Figure 78). This blood, however, is not yet truly human blood. It is a pre-blood of sorts, still "contaminated" with substances from outside. It must first be reconfigured by and in the liver before it enters general circulation as the body's own, individually specific "life blood."

Thus the liver represents a threshold and serves as a gatekeeper. It has a tremendous ***capacity for detoxification***; foreign matter, toxins, and so forth cannot pass through it. The liver has three different detox mechanisms available.

The first targets foreign substances directly. In the hepatocytes, exogenous substances (toxins, etc.) carried into the liver by the portal vein are metabolized and detoxified, usually by combining them with glucuronic acid. Together with bile, these compounds are then excreted into the intestine. The liver itself cannot develop antibodies against foreign proteins (antigens), since that function is specific to the immune system. But as soon as antibodies (primarily IgA) have been produced by immune responses in the intestinal wall's lymphatic tissue, the liver demonstrates a remarkable ability to extract them from the blood, concentrate them, and excrete them into the intestine along with bile fluid. This second mechanism provides immunological protection for the entire surface of the intestine and keeps it "clean," preventing foreign substances from infiltrating the organism. A third defensive mechanism is available in case substances do penetrate the intestinal wall. The walls of the liver sinusoids have many star-shaped Kupffer cells that consume (phagocytize) and break down foreign matter. Only when this barrier is also breached does the immune system itself come into play, and the spleen then either

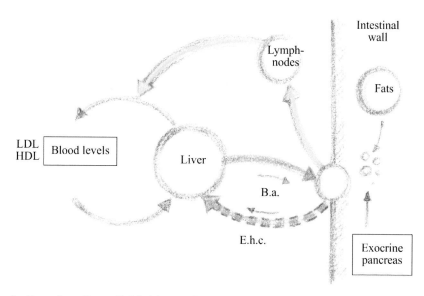

Fig. 82. **Basic liver functions II: Lipid metabolism.** *The liver "transfers" the digestion of fats to the intestine by secreting bile salts (bile acids), but up to 80 percent of bile acids (B.a.) are reabsorbed and reused (E.h.c.: entero-hepatic circulation). Lipids absorbed from the intestine flow into the blood via the lymph vessels and lymph nodes (LDL, HDL: blood lipids).*

eliminates foreign substances by filtering the blood or renders them harmless through antigen-antibody reactions (see below).

The liver is a large organ weighing 1,500 to 2,000 grams. It presents a solid bastion of defense against the material onslaught of the outside world. Under cover of this protection, synthesis of endogenous proteins, especially blood proteins (albumins, etc.), can occur safely. In the liver, "dead" nutrients extracted from their living contexts by the intestine are reenlivened and made suitable for use in processes guided by the human soul and spirit. The qualities that these reenlivened components regain are no longer those of the outer world; they are unique to the individual body. In protein metabolism, therefore, we are dealing with an "upper" world where the formative processes representing the "informational" element in the metabolic domain are at home (Figure 81).

The situation is totally different in **fat metabolism** (Figure 82). The liver has "shifted" the digestion of fats outside of itself to the intestinal wall, where fats become vulnerable to attack by pancreatic enzymes (lipases, etc.) only after being emulsified by the bile acids secreted by hepatocytes. Only then can fats be broken down enough to pass into the intestinal epithelium, where they are immediately resynthesized (not in the liver, as other basic nutrients are). The microscopic fat droplets produced in the intestinal epithelieum are coated with protein to form chylomicrons and then move directly into the intestinal lymph vessels. Here we confront an astonishing fact: Already in the intestinal wall, digested nutrients are separated into two streams, with fats entering the lymph stream and carbohydrates and proteins the bloodstream of the portal vein. Fats never inundate the blood; when available in excess, they are captured and phagocytized in the abdominal lymph nodes, then released in batches via the thoracic duct into the blood and transported to the liver for further processing.

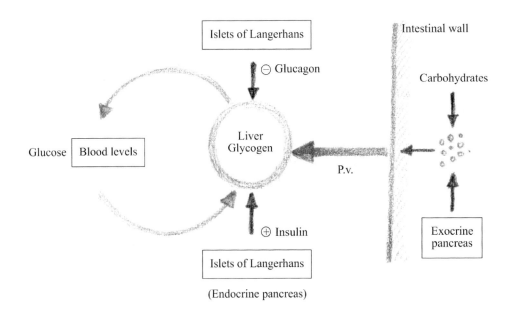

Fig. 83. **Basic liver functions III: Sugar metabolism.** *The pancreas works to regulate sugar metabolism on both sides of the intestinal wall—within the intestines, through its exocrine functions; in the bloodstream, through insulin secreted by the islets of Langerhans. P.v.: portal vein. In the liver, glucagon triggers the breakdown of glycogen, insulin its synthesis.*

Up to 90 percent of the **bile salts (bile acids)** are reabsorbed into the blood in the ileum (the lower portion of the small intestine) and especially in the colon, where the process is aided by coli bacteria. The liver absorbs bile salts from the blood and secretes them into the intestine again via the bile ducts in a cycle known as **enterohepatic circulation**. Bile salts formed in the liver are reused repeatedly and may be recycled ten to twelve times after a single fatty meal. In the end, however, approximately ten percent of the bile salts are not reused and are eliminated in the feces. This is another example of a phenomenon mentioned earlier: A small percentage of the substances reused repeatedly in metabolic cycles become unusable and must then be eliminated. We will return to this issue in the final chapter.

The liver is involved in the absorption of fats in the intestinal wall only because it produces bile acids, but this does not mean it has nothing further to do with fat metabolism. Just as the liver balances blood levels, uptake from the intestine, and conversions in the body in amino-

acid metabolism, it also maintains constant blood levels of fats and plays a role in metabolizing these energy-rich compounds. Fats can be stored in adipose tissue or serve as structural elements, but they can also be mobilized at any time to serve as energy supplies. Because of these two possibilities, fats occupy an intermediate position among nutrients, as is also expressed in all of their activity within the metabolic system (cf. 62).

The third complex of functions involves the "lower" level or energy conversion as such, i.e., **carbohydrate metabolism** (Figure 83). In this instance, the liver no longer functions as an independent organ but relies on the endocrine portion of the pancreas, the islets of Langerhans. Enzymes secreted by the intestinal mucosa and the exocrine pancreas break the carbohydrates in food into their basic components (monosaccharides), which then pass through the intestinal wall and are carried by the blood through the portal vein to the liver. There they are synthesized into polysaccharides, especially glycogen. Unlike proteins and fats, glycogen is stored in hepatocytes. Depending on the need, it can be broken down into glucose and funneled into the bloodstream or resynthesized from glucose and withdrawn from the bloodstream. These anabolic and catabolic processes are regulated by two hormones produced by the islets of Langerhans—insulin, which stimulates glycogen synthesis, and glucagon, which stimulates the release of glucose (Figure 83). As a result, *blood sugar levels* can remain constant. Because sugar is the chief source of energy for all metabolic processes in the body and also supplies energy for muscle contraction and brain activity, the liver is the most important organ for all will and thought activities. For example, unconsciousness sets in if blood sugar levels rise above normal (diabetic coma). Disrupted liver functions are associated with depression (will paralysis). The liver manages the body's sugar "bank account" and can make withdrawals at any moment to cover sudden increases in activity.

The liver's work rhythm. The flow of bile secretion in the lobules is centrifugal, the anabolic stream centripetal. The former is associated with a decrease in the size of hepatocytes as a result of excretion of bile fluid, the latter with an increase in cell size due to synthesis of substances. Expansion and contraction of the organ, however, are polar processes that can occur only in alternation, not simultaneously. The result is a 24-hour or circadian work rhythm that conforms to the position of the sun (i.e., local time) and is relatively independent of food intake. The liver's weight increases by 15 to 20 percent during the substance-forming, anabolic (assimilatory) phase, which peaks at night (around 2:00 or 3:00 a.m.), and decreases again during the secretory, catabolic (dissimilatory) phase, which reaches its maximum between 2:00 and 3:00 p.m. Anabolic processes dominate at night, excretory and catabolic processes during the day. Thus the liver resonates with the universal, sun-defined rhythms of life. The liver is like an "internal sun" that integrates us into the material world. Through it, we participate in nature's growth rhythms. In this context, it makes sense that the liver also possesses significant regenerative ability. When

three-quarters of the organ are removed from a laboratory animal, the liver regenerates almost completely.

The arterial system. The liver not only has its own supply of venous blood (via the portal vein coming from the intestine), it also has its own artery, which supplies it with oxygen and connects it to the rhythmic system (heart and blood circulation, Figure 79). The branches of the hepatic artery empty either into the periphery of the lobule or more toward the center. Sphincterlike restrictive mechanisms selectively support anabolic or catabolic processes in the hepatocytes by concentrating oxygen-rich blood either centrally or peripherally. This hepatic arterial system introduces a rhythmicizing (middle) element of internalized respiration into the liver's metabolic processes.

The rhythm of anabolic and catabolic processes in the liver is clearly symbolized in the Greek legend of *Prometheus*, who stole fire from the gods and was punished by being chained to a rock. An eagle ate away at his liver by day, but it regenerated each night. The rock symbolizes the material world to which earthly human beings are bound, while the eagle symbolizes intellectual thinking, which consumes life forces. But the growth forces of the material world regenerate the liver at night, when consciousness is extinguished. As a result, Prometheus was able to survive until he was finally rescued by Hercules, the representative of the higher "I".

The Biliary System and Hemoglobin Metabolism

The biliary system is also related to other processes involving not only the liver but also the spleen. As described above, nutrient building blocks from the intestine are carried by the portal vein into the liver, where they are resynthesized, i.e., reenlivened with the organism's own forces and integrated into the body. With the liver's help, we constantly incarnate into our bodies on the

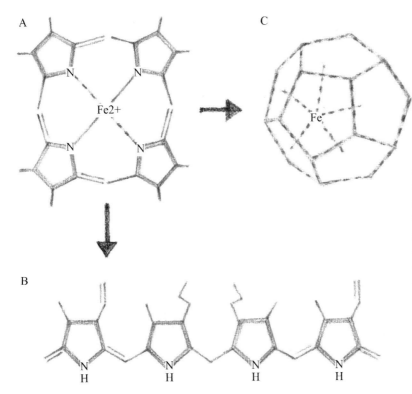

Fig. 84. **Structure of heme (A) and bilirubin, a bile pigment (B).** Hemoglobin, the red pigment in blood, is a chromoprotein consisting of four polypeptide chains (globins), each with a heme group (pigment). Each heme molecule (A) consists of four pyrrole rings surrounding an iron atom in the center. Bile pigments (e.g., bilirubin, B) are produced when hemoglobin breaks down. The Fe atom is either transported in a pentagon-dodecahedron-shaped protein (transferrin) or stored in ferritin (C) (121).

material level. The flow of substances is made possible by the blood and depends heavily on the blood's transport function with regard to respiratory gases. With the help of oxygen, we bind forces and kindle metabolism (incarnation); through CO_2 elimination, these same forces are then released from the material world (excarnation). Ultimately, these processes are made possible by the blood's content of hemoglobin, the iron-containing pigment concentrated in red blood cells (erythrocytes). Hemoglobin, therefore, is a key molecule in anchoring the "I" in its physical vessel.

Hemoglobin is a chromoprotein consisting of four subunits, each with a heme and a protein (globulin) component. The iron molecules anchored in hemoglobin's porphyrin rings bind oxygen and release it again in the tissues (Figure 84). Transport of respiratory gases by the iron molecules of red blood cells thus becomes an essential physical foundation for actualizing the individuality's will activity, either within the body or in the outer world.

Novalis offers a very telling depiction of this connection in his parable of Eros and Fabel (63). For the babe Eros lying in his cradle, the birth of the "I" begins at the moment he takes possession of a sliver of iron that falls from heaven. He soon grows into a handsome youth who thirsts for action and sallies forth into the world, with the iron sliver serving as a compass to orient him in space.

But the red blood cells with their high concentration of iron-bearing hemoglobin have life spans of only 100 to 120 days. This means that approximately 2.5 million new red blood cells must be formed every second (or 150 million per minute). This tremendous turnover, which occurs primarily in the bone marrow, can be maintained only because cell components (especially hemoglobin and iron) are repeatedly reused. And in fact the iron released through hemoglobin breakdown is jealously guarded in the body. Each iron molecule is immediately incorporated into a molecule of transferrin (a protein with its 24

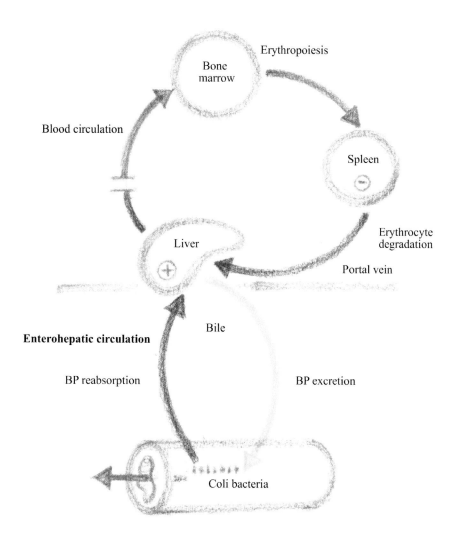

*Fig. 85. **The biliary system and hemoglobin metabolism.** In the spleen, erythrocytes are broken down (-). Bile pigments (BP) formed through hemoglobin breakdown are resynthesized (+) into hemoglobin in the liver and incorporated into new erythrocytes in the bone marrow. The bile pigments (BP) are secreted into the intestine along with bile and partially reabsorbed, so they can be reused by the liver (enterohepatic circulation).*

identical peptide chains arranged in the shape of a pentagon dodecahedron) and then transported to the bone marrow, where it is integrated into a developing erythrocyte (Figure 84). The body's reserves of iron at birth are almost sufficient for a whole lifetime. Only small amounts need to be supplemented through nutrition intake (61)!

The liver and the spleen collaborate in breaking down and regenerating hemoglobin and red blood cells. Hemoglobin breakdown takes place to some extent in specialized liver cells (Kupffer cells) but especially in the spleen (Figure 85). The spleen "recognizes" and breaks down aging erythrocytes that have outlived their usefulness. In this process, hemoglobin is broken into its components (iron, porphyrin, and globin). Until it is incorporated into new hemoglobin molecules, the iron may be stored in the liver, but it can also be stored in other tissues in large protein molecules (ferritin) that hold up to 4,300 iron molecules each. The protein component (globin) is broken down and later resynthesized. Porphyrin breaks down into **bile pigments** (biliverdin, bilirubin, etc.). Bilirubin combines with glucuronic acid in the liver and is excreted (along with bile fluid) into the small intestine via the bile ducts. It then moves into the colon and is eliminated along with the rest of the colon's contents. Approximately 10 to 20 percent is reabsorbed, however, and carried back to the liver via the portal vessels in another example of enterohepatic circulation. Bilirubin is an antioxidant that protects against water-soluble peroxides (oxygen radicals). It is interesting to note in this context that reabsorption of bile pigments in the large intestine is possible only through the cooperation of coli bacteria, normally harmless saprophytes that colonize the large intestine (Figure 85).

As befits a process related to anchoring the "I" in its physical vessel, the physical scope of the hepatobiliary cycle is exceedingly great. It extends from the lungs (where oxygen is inhaled) through the spleen (where red blood cells are broken down) to the marrow of the bones (where hemoglobin with its iron molecule is recycled and incorporated into newly developing red blood cells). The cycle of iron-bearing hemoglobin and bile pigments, which even extends to the outside world inasmuch as intestinal bacteria are involved, occupies a central position in human incarnation.

The Immune System, Lymphatic Organs, and Spleen

General Organization of the Immune System

The immune system safeguards the body's material integrity. In other words, it ensures that compounds (especially proteins) produced by the liver are allowed to retain their individualized character. Within the immune system, we must distinguish between the two basic functions of cellular and humoral defense (Figure 86). Macrophages serve as a mediating element or bridge between these two mechanisms. When an exogenous compound (antigen) penetrates tissue, it is phagocytized, i.e., broken into fragments by macrophages or related cells. Antigen-specific fragments are then presented to the so-called T lymphocytes (cells that have become immunocompetent in the thymus). The T lymphocytes then attack and destroy the antigens. In the case of invading microorganisms, T lymphocytes function as "killer cells" and destroy entire cells. This is the mechanism of *cellular defense.* But antigen-presenting cells also stimulate the other major lymphatic cell population, the B lymphocytes, which are thought to achieve immunological maturity in the bone marrow. Thus stimulated, B lymphocytes develop into plasma cells that synthesize specific antibodies. These antibodies unite with the antigens to form harmless antigen-antibody complexes. Since antibodies, usually immunoglobulins, circulate in the blood, this mechanism is called *humoral defense*. The B cells and their descendants, the plasma cells, do not take direct action against foreign matter.

Instead, they send out their antibodies to fight antigens "in the field." In contrast, T lymphocytes actively circulate in the blood until they encounter foreign microorganisms or antigens. T lymphocytes "patrol" the body at regular intervals to find invaders and destroy them on the spot (cellular defense, Figure 86).

But before any foreign element reaches the blood, the innermost and most uniquely human part of the body, it must breach several successive barriers, as in a military defense system. The first barrier is the body's boundary with the outside world (either the skin or the intestinal wall). The intestinal wall, which represents the first line of defense, possesses an extensive system of lymphatic tissue with numerous lymphocytes, macrophages, etc. Antigens that succeed in breaching this barrier enter the lymph stream via the intestinal lymph vessels. Regional *lymph nodes* are inserted into these vessels at regular intervals. This is the second level of the body's defense system (Figures 87 and 88).

Lymph flows into each lymph node from the periphery via numerous vessels and then flows out again from the central hilus area (Figure 87). This characteristic filtering system processes lymph from the corresponding section of the intestine, trapping any antigens that may be present. Because the cortex of each lymph node not only houses lymph follicles—nodular aggregations of lymphocytes—but also stores many other immune cells, an effective immunological defense can be mounted immediately. Regional lymph nodes associated with each section of the intestine are

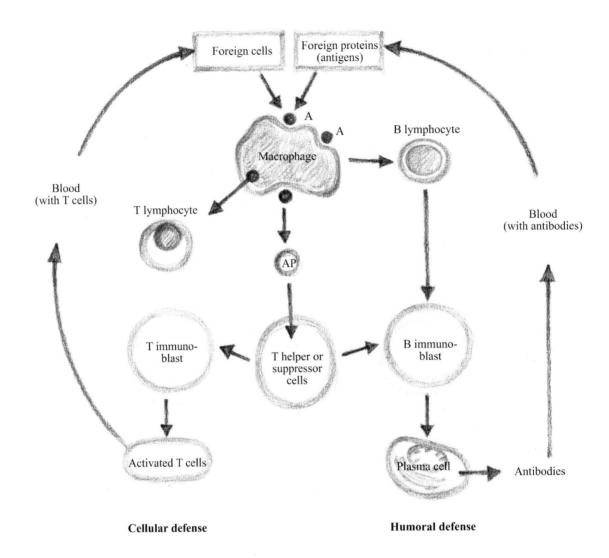

Fig. 86. **Cells of the immune system.** *Schematic representation of the most important connections between the cellular (T cells) and humoral (B cells) defense systems. Macrophages serve as intermediaries between these two systems. A: antigen; AP: antigen-presenting cell.*

arranged in multiple rows and form an effective barrier against any foreign elements that succeed in infiltrating the body through the intestinal wall.

Antigens that manage to pass this second barrier are eventually carried on the lymph stream into the blood via the thoracic duct (Figure 89). The resulting "blood poisoning" can have deadly consequences. The blood is the body's inner sanctum, its most precious and functionally most

important organ system. Here the spleen serves as the final bastion of defense (Figures 88 and 89). Unlike lymph nodes, the spleen filters blood, not lymph. The spleen's immunological defenses are powerful. Because it also breaks down red blood cells and eliminates many substances from the blood, the spleen is the counterpole to the liver, which is totally dedicated to synthesis, blood regeneration, and metabolic detoxification.

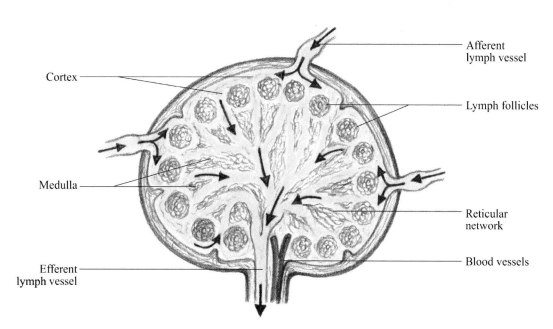

Fig. 87. **Structure of a lymph node** *(17). Immune reactions occur as lymph (yellow) flows from the periphery toward the center through the medulla's filtration network (arrows). The most essential structures in this process are the lymph follicles, located in the cortex of the node.*

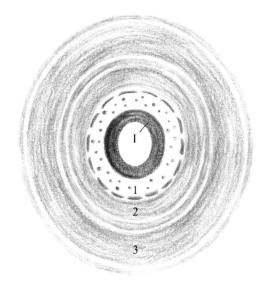

Fig. 88. **Subdivision of the immune system into three successive stages of defense.** *I: intestinal wall or skin as the surface bordering the outside world;*
1: First zone of defense, a layer of connective tissue (with scattered lymphocytes and lymph follicles) that borders the covering epithelium;
2: Second zone of defense, the lymphatic vessel system with its series of (regional) lymph nodes;
3: Third zone of defense, which consists of the spleen and circulating blood.

The Lymphatic Organs and the Lymph System

The lymphatic system occupies an intermediate position between blood and tissue. Lymph forms when tissue fluid flows into the gaps in intercellular connective tissue and collects in delicate lymph vessels. All exchanges between blood and cells take place via this intercellular matrix. The matrix is the source of lymph, a largely cell-free fluid that flows through the body in its own vascular system (Figure 89). The larger lymphatic vessels are contractile and exhibit intrinsic rhythmicity; some of them are valved. The intestinal lymphatic vessels merge into the larger intestinal trunk, which

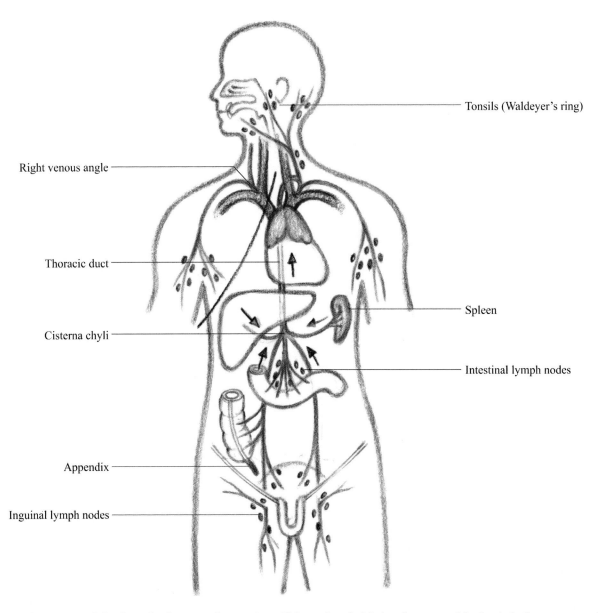

Right venous angle

Thoracic duct

Cisterna chyli

Appendix

Inguinal lymph nodes

Tonsils (Waldeyer's ring)

Spleen

Intestinal lymph nodes

Fig. 89. **Structure of the lymphatic vascular system.** *This system is bilaterally symmetrical only in the upper part of the body (above the curved diagonal line). Lymph from the lower body (abdominal cavity, legs, etc.) accumulates in the cisterna chyli and then flows through the thoracic duct into the left jugular angle. The lymphatic ducts (red) include regional clusters of lymph nodes that serve various parts of the body.*

empties into the cisterna chyli at the approximate level of the first lumbar vertebra (Figure 89). But before entering the cisterna chyli, the lymph must pass through several groups of lymph nodes, which trap any foreign substances or microorganisms that may be present and eliminate them through immune reactions. Droplets of fat (chylomicrons) that enter the lymph stream from the intestine are also filtered out in the intestinal lymph nodes. This protects the blood from becoming inundated with fat. As mentioned earlier, fat absorption in the intestines occupies a unique position in that it utilizes the lymph stream rather than the blood, which takes a considerable burden off the liver.

Lymph flowing vertically from the lower limbs, pelvis, and genitals also empties into the cisterna chyli, as do more horizontal streams coming from the liver (on the right) and the spleen (on the left). The cisterna chyli is the largest lymph-collecting basin in the lower half of the body and is located in the area of the solar plexus. Lymph leaving the cisterna chyli passes through the chest cavity via the thoracic duct and empties into the bloodstream at the left jugular angle. Just before this junction, however, the thoracic duct also receives lymph from the jugular trunk, a major lymphatic vessel that collects lymph from the left half of the head and neck. Lymph from the left arm also pours into the veins of the left jugular angle. It is interesting to note that the lymphatic system is bilaterally symmetrical in the upper part of the body (head and the limbs) but not in the lower part. The right jugular angle receives lymph from the major lymphatic duct of the right half of the head and neck as well as from the lymphatic vessels of the right arm and the right half of the chest (Figure 89).

All lymphatic ducts include lymph nodes that serve as filtration and monitoring stations. These nodes serve specific regions of the body and are clustered at important intersections such as the mandibular angles, throat, armpits, and groin. Swelling of the lymph nodes develops when inflammation occurs in associated organs. As such, however, inflammation is more characteristic of the blood's vascular system, whereas malignancies more typically occur in the cellular and lymphatic systems. Strangely enough, tumor cells spread preferentially through the body's lymphatic vessels. A finding of cancer cells in a regional lymph node is therefore an important indicator of a primary tumor in a related organ. If cancer cells breach the lymphatic barrier and reach the blood, metastasis has usually achieved its final stage.

Lymph streams and the movement of substances in the intercellular matrix are closely related to the organism's life processes as such. In a person weighing about 70 kilos or 150 pounds, the volume of *intra*cellular fluid, which is linked to cell plasma, amounts to approximately 30 liters, while *inter*cellular fluid amounts to only ten to twelve liters, and the total volume of blood is only

four to five liters. Clearly, the flow of fluid between cells is very important for the life processes of the organs it bathes and pervades. All exchange processes must pass through extracellular space. Preserving acid-base balance and maintaining constant concentrations of chemicals (to mention just a few factors) depend on the movement of fluids in this "internal milieu." Because malignant, "egotistical, self-centered" proliferating cells have fallen out of the organism's life processes, it makes sense that they should spread primarily in this dimension, in the borderland between solid and liquid, which in some respects is also the borderland between life and death.

If we understand the totality of lymphatic space as consisting of intercellular connective tissue (matrix), intercellular fluid, and lymph, we discover two designated areas where this space connects with other spaces, namely:

1. The lymphoepithelial organs such as the tonsils of the oral cavity, where the system meets the outside world, and

2. The spleen, where it meets the body's interior. Blood is filtered into the spleen's peri-articular lymphatic vessels and monitored for possible antigens, which are then eliminated. As a result, "clean" lymph constantly flows from the spleen back into the system.

Lymphatic defenses take a different form in the transition from the oral cavity to the throat, where multiple **tonsils** are concentrated in a small area. The tonsils, which are richly supplied with lymphatic tissue, are capable of setting immune responses in motion. Around the tonsils, the surface epithelia of the oral mucosa is loose (loose junctions); this allows germs (antigens) from the oral cavity and from semiliquified food to infiltrate the tissue (at the subepithelial level) and initiate an immunological reaction. Thus, at the very beginning of the digestive tract, the organism has installed an opening that allows the lymphatic system to contact the outside world directly, thus providing the immune system with "learning opportunities." Of course such contacts are also possible at various points in the lower digestive tract (lower small intestine, appendix, etc.). But in the oral cavity, where the epithelium actually ceases to be a tight asso-ciation of self-contained cells and enters into an intimate functional connection with lymphoreticular tissue (hence the name "lymphoepithelial organs"), the places of contact with the outside world are especially well differentiated.

The brain, the eyes, and a few other major sense organs have no lymphatic system of this sort, and normal immune responses are suppressed there. The brain has no lymphatic vessels, although it floats in cerebrospinal fluid, which is lymphlike in that it is free of cells and proteins. Cerebrospinal fluid drains into the head's venous system. Unlike the lymph in the rest of the body, this fluid does not collect in extracellular space because the brain has no extracellular space in the usual sense. Instead, the cerebrospinal fluid protects the sensitive, floating brain and endows it with buoyancy. Among others, Rudolf Steiner in particular emphasized the exceptional psychological importance of the resulting "sensa-tion of lightness" for the development of thinking in the upright human being (64). With regard to the lymphatic system, therefore, the head occupies an exceptional position to which we will later return.

The Spleen

The spleen is the last major line of defense against foreign substances that have reached the bloodstream. The spleen is tucked away in the upper left portion of the torso, under the diaphragm and behind the stomach. It is functionally related to both the blood and the gastrointestinal tract. In many respects, liver and spleen are polar opposites. The liver is supplied primarily with venous blood, which flows from the intestine via the portal vein, but the spleen is completely oriented toward the arterial system. The spleen contains the body's only example of open circulation, meaning that blood leaves the vascular system. Within the spleen, the splenic artery branches into many arterioles that ultimately empty blindly into the spleen's reticular tissue (red pulp, Figure 90). Alongside this open system, however, the spleen also has a closed circulatory system in which

capillaries merge directly with veins. As a result, blood can either flow freely through the spleen (Figure 91) or leave the vascular system and enter the organ's reticular tissue. This dual circulation system offers several regulatory possibilities:

1. Blood cells that leave the vascular system can be inspected "from outside." In the spleen, aging or damaged erythrocytes (as well as other blood cells such as leukocytes and thrombocytes) are removed from the bloodstream and broken down. This process takes place primarily in the *red pulp*. Within the spleen, the arteries divide into the many fine penicillar arterioles, giving rise to a capillary network surrounded by macrophages and reticular cells (Figure 90). At the end of each arteriole is a contractile thickening of the arterial wall known as the sheathed capillary. The adjoining capillary empties directly into this reticular tissue. From there, the blood makes its way into the slightly widened terminal section (sinus) of a vein. The walls of this sinus, however, are netlike rather than completely closed (see Figure 90 for details). Because normal erythrocytes are very flexible (as they must be to squeeze through very narrow capillaries), they readily pass into the sinuses and then flow into the veins of the spleen. Toward the end of their roughly 100-day life span, however, erythrocytes become less and less flexible as the structure of their cell membranes changes. Older, inflexible erythrocytes can no longer pass through the net of the sinus wall. They remain trapped in the spleen's reticulum (red pulp), where they are consumed (phagocytized) and broken down by macrophages or sinus endothelial cells. The presence of blood in tissues outside of the spleen's vascular system makes it possible for aging or unusable blood cells to be "recognized" and then promptly eliminated from the bloodstream. This is the first of the major cleansing processes that take place in the spleen.

2. A second major complex of functions related to blood cleansing involves the spleen's *immune system*. Just below the point where the branches of the splenic artery subdivide into the penicillary arterioles, lymph follicles develop in the arterial walls. These nodules are collectively

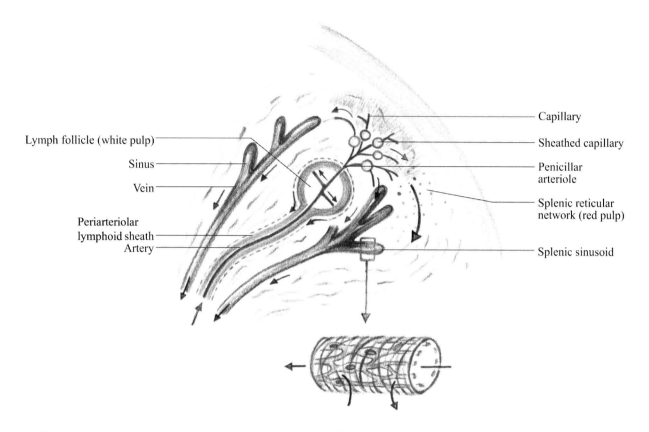

Labels on figure:
Lymph follicle (white pulp)
Sinus
Vein
Periarteriolar lymphoid sheath
Artery
Capillary
Sheathed capillary
Penicillar arteriole
Splenic reticular network (red pulp)
Splenic sinusoid

*Fig. 90. **Structure of the spleen. Open circulation.** Blood flows from the penicillary arterioles through the capillary network into the red pulp. To reenter the bloodstream, blood cells (especially erythrocytes)must first pass through a netlike splenic sinus (arrows in enlarged detail), where their age (flexibility and membrane structure) is monitored. In the **lymph follicles**, collectively known as the white pulp, blood is filtered. The resulting lymph flows first into the periarteriolar lymphoid sheath and is then carried in closed lymphatic vessels to the splenic hilum.*

called the **white pulp**, in contrast to the blood-filled reticulum and sinuses, which constitute the red pulp. The arrangement of vessels within each lymph follicle allows blood to be filtered and then conducted through the follicle's edge zone (where immune reactions occur) and finally into a lymph vessel. The spleen's lymph vessels lie in tissue gaps around the arteries (periarteriolar lymphoid sheaths). As a result, each artery is surrounded by a centripetal stream of lymph (Figures 90 and 91). The spleen has no afferent lymphatic vessels.

In summary, the spleen's arterial system presents a dual picture: on the one hand, the centrifugal flow of blood into the red pulp, which serves to break down blood cells, and on the other the centripetal flow of lymph, which defends against foreign antigens that have broken through the last of the body's major barriers and entered the bloodstream.

3. The spleen's third and final sphere of activity involves **regulatory** functions. By increasing or decreasing the amount of blood that flows out of it, the spleen can either withdraw blood or add to the amount in circulation, i.e., regulate the volume of circulating blood. Thus the spleen serves as a **blood reservoir**. The spleen is muscular throughout—even its capsule is muscular. As a result, it can contract and adapt to changing blood volumes. X-ray images reveal rhythmical contractions, and the spleen has thus been called the "heart" of the portal vein system. Because the

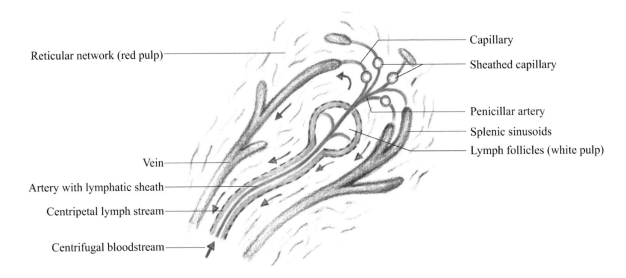

Reticular network (red pulp)

Capillary

Sheathed capillary

Penicillar artery

Splenic sinusoids

Lymph follicles (white pulp)

Vein

Artery with lymphatic sheath

Centripetal lymph stream

Centrifugal bloodstream

Fig. 91. **Structure of the spleen. Closed circulation.** *Here, the branches of the splenic artery, after passing through the lymph follicles, divide further into penicillary arterioles and form capillary networks that connect directly to the sinusoids of the splenic veins.*

splenic vein empties into the portal vein and not into the inferior vena cava, it belongs functionally to the portal vein system.

All of these features may allow the spleen to regulate blood circulation and perfusion in the upper abdominal area and perhaps also to serve a harmonizing function with regard to the rhythm of food intake. At our current level of civilization, we eat not only relatively informally but at very irregular times, which puts a strain on the metabolic system. It is true that the pylorus opens at regular intervals (independent of stomach fullness) to convey semiliquified food (chyme) to the duodenum in small batches. The peristaltic contractions that originate in the duodenum and run through the entire small intestine also occur in rhythmical waves in conjunction with secretion by digestive glands (the autonomic functions of the interdigestive or migrating motor complex). Nonetheless, these normal rhythms are repeatedly disrupted by the completely arhythmical timing of our food and fluid intake. In this context, the spleen may serve a rhymicizing and harmonizing function (cf. 65).

Liver, Biliary System, and Spleen: The Organ Trinity of the Upper Abdomen

The liver is the body's largest metabolic organ. In the liver, building blocks that flow in from the intestine via the portal vein are synthesized into endogenous compounds. The liver is also the source of blood. Although most blood cells develop in the bone marrow, blood fluid and most plasma components originate in the liver. The counterpart of this awesome regenerative process is the no less admirable breakdown of blood in the spleen. But the spleen does more than simply monitor blood cells, which it sorts out and breaks down if they are too old. In the white pulp, the plasma of inflowing blood is filtered and "cleansed" of antigens and foreign elements. In the spleen, therefore, the blood arrives at a boundary where its essential nature can be preserved or restored as needed. The alchemists of earlier centuries considered Saturn (the most distant planet of the then-known solar system) as

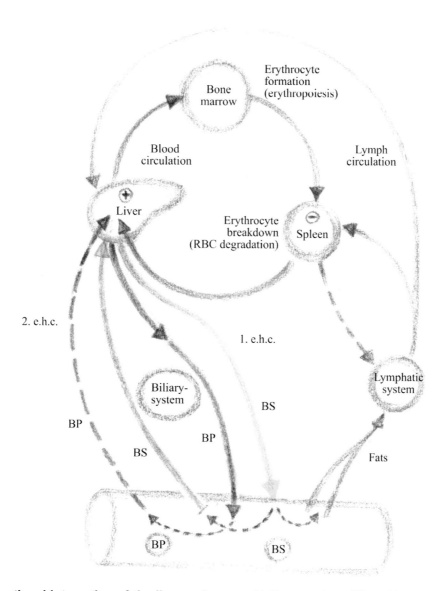

Fig. 92. **Functional interaction of the liver, spleen, and biliary system.** *Bile acids and bile pigments circulate between the liver and the intestines in the so-called enterohepatic circulation (e.h.c.). BP: bile pigments; BS: bile salts; RBC: red blood cells (for details, see text).*

the force that draws boundaries and preserves individual elements, and spoke of the spleen as a Saturnian organ. Unlike the spleen, the liver does not have the ability to ward off foreign elements immunologically, through antibodies. It can only render foreign substances or toxins harmless by metabolizing them. A third system comes into play when the liver accumulates antibodies produced elsewhere in the body, concentrating them in its

cells and excreting them along with bile. Thus the **biliary system** is inserted between the anabolic processes of the liver and the catabolic processes of the spleen. The biliary system, which is primarily excretory in character, is incorporated into the cycle of blood renewal in three ways. First, it serves an important immune function by excreting antibodies concentrated in the liver. In this role, it supports the spleen, which works in the immune system from the other side, the side of the blood. Second, by secreting bile salts, which circulate between the intestine and the liver (enterohepatic circulation), the biliary system relieves the liver of the task of digesting fat (Figure 92). Bile salts and the metabolic activities of the intestinal wall prevent fats from entering the blood. Instead, as we saw earlier, fats flow primarily into the body's lymphatic vascular system via the intestinal lymphatic vessels and lymph nodes. The third process has to do with the recycling of bile pigments, which are produced when hemoglobin is broken down in the spleen and are secreted into the intestine along with bile. In the large intestine, they are partially reabsorbed with the help of coli bacteria. This is a second form of enterohepatic circulation (Figure 92).

Ultimately, therefore, the liver's biliary system constitutes a third functional element that mediates between anabolic liver processes and catabolic spleen activity. Because it is related to secretory processes and is of central importance for blood regeneration, this system is an important foundation for the human experience of the "I". Wherever excretion processes occur, spiritual forces are released and made available either for new metabolic or structural processes or for conscious activities. The functions discussed here are probably especially related to the "I" experience, which explains why popular psychology has always associated bile secretion with the choleric temperament. (Think of expressions such as "The bile rose in his throat" or "What gall!") Temperamental individuals who are easily angered and "boil over" when their ebullient activity encounters resistance often have biliary systems that are out of balance.

Thus the specific forces of the upper abdomen's three organ systems are also reflected on the soul level. The alchemists of earlier times attributed the biliary system to Mars and the liver, with its sunlike, radiant power, to Jupiter. With the spleen as the Saturnian organ, all three of the planets beyond the sun are represented in the upper abdomen.

The Urogenital System:
The Organs of Excretion and Reproduction

In the liver-biliary system, anabolic processes related to the intestinal tract predominate. These processes make it possible for us to incarnate into space on the material level and to produce earthly substances. This complex of processes leads from the fluid to the solid (bones, cartilage) or semisolid (intracellular matrix, proteins, blood). The opposite occurs in the organs of excretion (kidneys, etc.). By removing salts and metabolic wastes (for example, urea as an end product of protein metabolism), the kidneys revitalize the fluid element. Elimination is simultaneously an excarnation process. All excretory functions release forces that are then available for new tasks. The greatest elimination process is death, which releases the soul-spiritual element from a body that has become unusable and is discarded. The less radical elimination processes that take place during our lifetime form the basis of our sense of life and self-awareness. Goethe once said that death is an artifice employed by nature to ensure abundant life (129). It is not surprising, therefore, that the organs of elimination are closely associated with the organs of reproduction. Reproduction is a special instance of elimination that serves to maintain the species, whereas urinary elimination serves to preserve the individual. In the animal kingdom, the same ductal system often transports germ cells (gametes) and urine. Consequently, the umbrella term "urogenital system" is used for the urinary tract and reproductive system.

The organs of reproduction serve the preservation of the species first and foremost. They play almost no role in the individual's own life processes. The purpose of "eliminating" germ cells and associated elements is not to free the body of metabolic wastes but to make space for a new being (embryo, fetus) to live. As in the kidneys, the primary process here is one of excretion, but instead of flowing back into the natural world, the excreted elements serve the incarnation of a new human being.

Morphology of the Urinary System (Kidneys)

The spleen, as the organ responsible for immunological monitoring of the blood, is the immune system's final guarantor of the organism's material independence from the outside world. In effect, the spleen draws a protective ring around the body, defining an interior space in which the body's independent material life can develop. The kidneys monitor the processes occurring in this interior space, especially fluid movements and electrolyte concentrations in the extracellular matrix. The spleen looks outward, as it were, but the kidneys look inward. Ten to fifteen times each day, all of the body's extracellular fluid is cycled

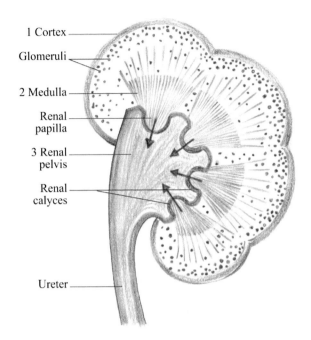

1 Cortex

Glomeruli

2 Medulla

Renal papilla

3 Renal pelvis

Renal calyces

Ureter

Fig. 93. ***Threefold functional division of the kidney.*** *The cortex (1) houses approximately 1.2 million renal corpuscles with their loops of blood vessels (glomeruli, red dots). The medulla (2) contains the renal tubules, the loops of Henle, and the collecting tubules. The renal pelvis (3) forms the calyces of the kidney, which surround the renal papillae, into which urine drips (arrows).*

through the kidneys, where its concentrations of salts, urea, etc. are tested. Without this tremendous movement of fluid, the life of the organism could not be maintained.

We can distinguish three major ***kidney functions*** that ultimately reflect the functional threefold division of the body as a whole (Figure 93). The renal cortex, which is extremely well supplied with blood vessels, monitors body fluids. Ultrafiltration occurs in the roughly 2.5 million renal corpuscles of the cortex. In the radially structured renal medulla, which has fewer blood vessels and is paler in color, primary urine is concentrated to form urine. This is a rhythmical process involving multiple exchanges between inside and outside. The third process, eliminating urine from the body,

begins in the renal papillae and continues via the calyces, renal pelvis, and efferent urinary ducts. Suction, absorption, and active movement are the processes involved here.

The ***renal cortex*** contains the renal corpuscles (approximately 1.2 million in each kidney) and the convoluted sections of the renal tubules. The ***corpuscles*** or Malpighian bodies develop out of cup-shaped depressions that form where the renal tubules dead-end. Each cup holds a dense tangle of capillary loops (glomerulus, Figures 94 and 95). The cell layer bordering the glomerulus becomes very thin; its closely spaced cell processes leave slits of not more than 4 x 14 nm, forming an extremely fine filter that traps blood cells and larger protein molecules. The capillary endothelial cells and the basal membrane of the glomerular capillaries also form a filter with a pore size of 50-100 nm (Figure 95). This differentiated filtration system allows blood plasma to pass through but holds back blood cells—a process known as ultrafiltration. This process is incredibly dynamic. Each day, 1,500 to 1,800 liters of blood (20 to 25 percent of total cardiac output) pass through the renal corpuscles. Of this amount, 150 to 180 liters per day of ultrafiltrate pass into the renal tubules, but only about 1.5 liters of urine are eliminated. The amount of fluid filtered daily by the corpuscles of the two kidneys has been calculated as four times the entire amount of water in the body, ten to fifteen times the amount of extracellular fluid, or sixty times the total volume of blood plasma. Almost all of the ultrafiltrate, however, is reabsorbed into the blood. Thus urine elimination is not a straightforward excretory process; it consists in selectively ***not reabsorbing*** fluid that has already been excreted. To help us visualize this process, let's imagine that a lecture room contains a hundred chairs, one of which is defective. Instead of having one person carry the chair out of the room to get rid of it, ***all*** of the chairs are carried out, checked for defects, and carried back into the room. Only the defective chair is left outside and discarded. This comparison clarifies two points: First, elimination and reabsorption constitute a sensory process

A

B

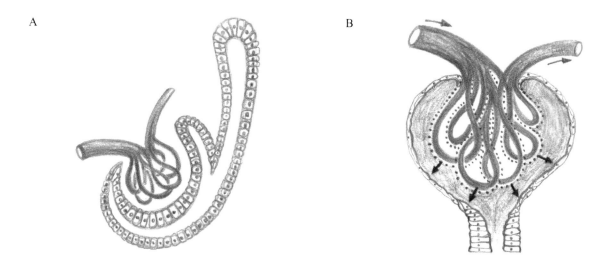

Fig. 94. **Development of a renal corpuscle.** *A tangle of capillaries (glomerulus) descends into a spoonlike depression in the blind end of an embryonic renal tubule (A). Together with the glomerulus, the resulting cup-shaped structure (Bowman's capsule) forms the renal corpuscle (Malpighian body, B). The inner layer of the Bowman's capsule (that is, the epithelial cells bordering the vessels) develops into a cellular filter (the podocyte filter), while the remaining cells form a cup to collect primary urine (blue), which is filtered out of the glomerular capillaries (ultrafiltrate, arrows). Upper arrows indicate direction of blood flow.*

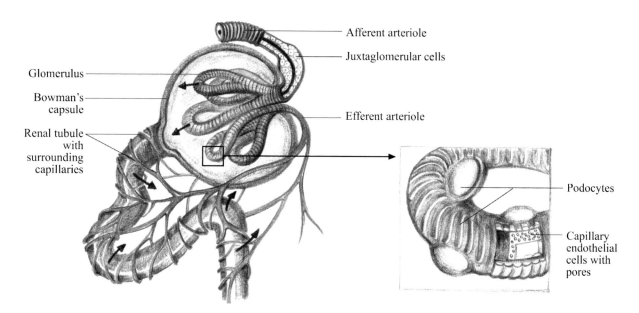

Afferent arteriole

Juxtaglomerular cells

Glomerulus

Bowman's capsule

Efferent arteriole

Renal tubule with surrounding capillaries

Podocytes

Capillary endothelial cells with pores

Fig. 95. **Structure of a renal corpuscle.** *The capillaries (glomerulus) of the renal corpuscle are surrounded by cells (podocytes) whose closely spaced processes constitute an essential part of the renal filter (see enlarged detail). The ultrafiltrate extracted from the glomerulus (arrows) is collected in the Bowman's capsule and flows into the adjacent renal tubule. The capillaries surrounding the tubule reabsorb fluid from the filtrate (arrows) so that the urine in the tubules becomes increasingly concentrated.*

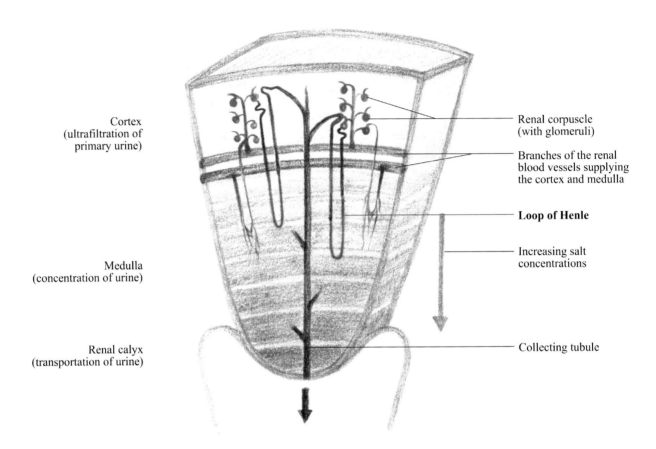

Cortex
(ultrafiltration of
primary urine)

Medulla
(concentration of urine)

Renal calyx
(transportation of urine)

Renal corpuscle
(with glomeruli)

Branches of the renal
blood vessels supplying
the cortex and medulla

Loop of Henle

Increasing salt
concentrations

Collecting tubule

Fig. 96. **Architecture of a kidney.** *The cortex contains the renal corpuscles with their glomeruli; the medulla contains the elongated sections of the renal tubules and the loops of Henle, which point downward (in the direction of the papilla) through zones of increasing salt concentration (represented by shades of gray)—an important prerequisite for urine concentration in the kidney.*

of sorts, which allows body fluids in the tubules to be "seen from outside" so that substances needing to be removed are "perceived" and not reabsorbed into the blood. Second, elimination of substances means that forces are set free. After the defective chairs are removed, the people involved in eliminating them have "nothing left to do" and are free to perform other tasks. In the kidneys, this type of elimination releases internal forces. Steiner calls this process "kidney radiation" (67).

The proximal tubules (the sections of the tubules closest to the renal corpuscles) are also able to eliminate substances directly. Toxins, foreign matter, metabolized medications, etc., can

move directly from the blood into the urine and be eliminated from the body in this way. Thus the kidneys, like the liver, also serve a detoxification function.

The renal medulla. The second major functional process involves the concentration of ultrafiltrate to form urine. This process takes place in the renal medulla (Figure 93). Each *renal tubule* forms a narrow loop (loop of Henle) pointing toward the renal papillae. In the medulla, the loop merges into the distal convoluted tubule and then into the collecting tubule (Figure 96). The many closely spaced loops of Henle and collecting tubules produce the medulla's characteristic radially striped pattern, which also extends into the cortex. Toward the papilla, concentrations of salt (NaCl) in the medulla's extracellular space increase, as if the loops of Henle were submerged in a pool of salt water (Figure 96). Consequently, the fluid in the tubules becomes more concentrated as it flows toward the papilla but is diluted again as it moves back toward the cortex. Final urine concentration takes place in the collecting tubules that run throughout the medulla and terminate in the renal papillae, where urine drips into the renal calyces. The repeated exchanges of Na, Cl, and K ions and urea between renal tubules and interstitial fluid within the medulla constitute a rhythmic process that makes it possible to fine tune the distribution of salts between body fluids and urine. This adjustment occurs primarily in the distal sections of the tubules and is regulated by adrenal cortical hormones (aldosterone), among other factors. Final urine concentrations, however, are achieved only in the collecting tubules (that is, in the renal papillae), where the posterior pituitary hormone vasopressin (antidiuretic hormone, ADH) is heavily involved. This middle, rhythmic function, which is comparable to a respiratory process, allows the kidney to perform adjustments and equilibrations made necessary by metabolic disturbances, environmental stress factors such as heat, or inappropriate fluid and salt intake.

Thus the kidney keeps a watchful, highly sensitive "eye" on the body's circulating fluids (blood and lymph) and extracellular matrix fluids, ensuring that they stay clean (i.e., not overly salty) and that concentrations of individual electrolytes necessary for organ functions (especially Na^+, Ca^{++}, K^+, and Cl^-) remain constant.

The urinary tract. Highly concentrated, slightly acidic urine is received by the renal calyces, collected in the renal pelvis, and transported via the ureter to the bladder. In the ureter, regular waves of contractions move small volumes of urine toward the bladder. As more fluid spurts in from the ureter, bladder muscle tone decreases. Together with the ureter's peristaltic motions, which produce a pumping effect of sorts, this decrease in muscle tone results in suction that helps move urine toward the outside. In a certain respect, the urinary tract consists of hollow spaces with inherent suctional effects that support kidney function as a whole. The ureter adds an active component to urine transport processes that function on the cellular level in the kidneys. At the transition from the renal pelvis to the ureter, a spontaneously rhythmical "pacemaker" system has been discovered. It induces peristaltic contractions at regular intervals. Each contraction "milks" only about three to five ml of urine out of the renal pelvis and moves it toward the bladder. This process is governed by the autonomic nervous system.

Elimination itself, which occurs via the urethra, is a partially involuntary (autonomically regulated) and partially voluntary act. The involuntary internal urethral sphincter lies at the neck of the bladder and is subject to the autonomic nervous system; the external urethral sphincter, located in the pelvic floor, is subject to voluntary control. Conscious control over emptying of the bladder, however, must be learned with considerable effort after birth and coincides approximately with the first awakening of the forces of the "I".

Ontogeny and Phylogeny of the Urinary System

The organs of elimination and reproduction are closely associated in both ontogeny and phylogeny. As habitats changed (from salt water to fresh water to dry land), the metabolism, body size, internal organization, and reproductive processes of evolving species also changed. According to Kipp, increasing individuation (that is, increasing separation from the outside world and increasing autonomy of the organism's life processes) can be observed in the vertebrate evolutionary series (54). This phenomenon is apparent even with regard to the limbs and their relationship to three-dimensional space (see p. 64). It is also evident in the intensification of metabolic processes and in warm-bloodedness (the ability to maintain a constant body

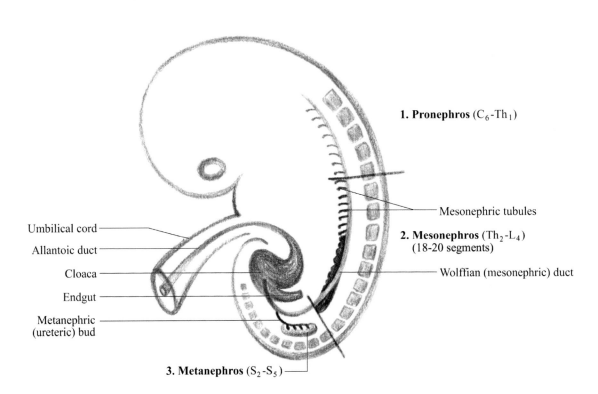

1. Pronephros (C_6-Th_1)

Mesonephric tubules

2. Mesonephros (Th_2-L_4)
(18-20 segments)

Wolffian (mesonephric) duct

Umbilical cord

Allantoic duct

Cloaca

Endgut

Metanephric
(ureteric) bud

3. Metanephros (S_2-S_5)

*Fig. 97. **Schematic representation and locations of the three kidney generations** in early human embryonic development. The Wolffian or mesonephric duct, which gives rise to the metanephric bud, still empties into the cloaca together with the hindgut.*

temperature independent of the environment), which is achieved for the first time by birds. And finally, it is apparent in reproductive behavior. Fishes and amphibians are still inseparable from their environments. They lay eggs in water, entrusting their further development to nature. The water, light, air, and warmth of the local milieu constitute the protective sheaths of the developing ova. Reptiles and birds achieve a degree of separation from the outside world by providing the amnion as a casing for their eggs. Each ovum is encased in a shell that also encloses its food supply (yolk, egg white, etc.). As a result, the developing organisms become less dependent on their surroundings and the embryonic period can be lengthened. These eggs, however, require incubation, which also influences their metabolism. Because fats are

the richest energy sources of all nutrients, fat metabolism comes to the fore. The main waste product is uric acid, which is insoluble and can therefore be allowed to accumulate and concentrate harmlessly in an extraembryonic bladder, the allantois, which serves that specific purpose.

Among mammals, the egg's dependence on the outside world is totally abandoned and the logical next step occurs: embryonic development relocates to the interior of the mother's body. A tendency toward more internalized development is found even in various bird species such as the weaver birds of Africa. Their closed nests, which have tubelike entrances accessible only from below, bear a striking resemblance to a uterus. In mammalian intrauterine development, all of the protective coverings originally found

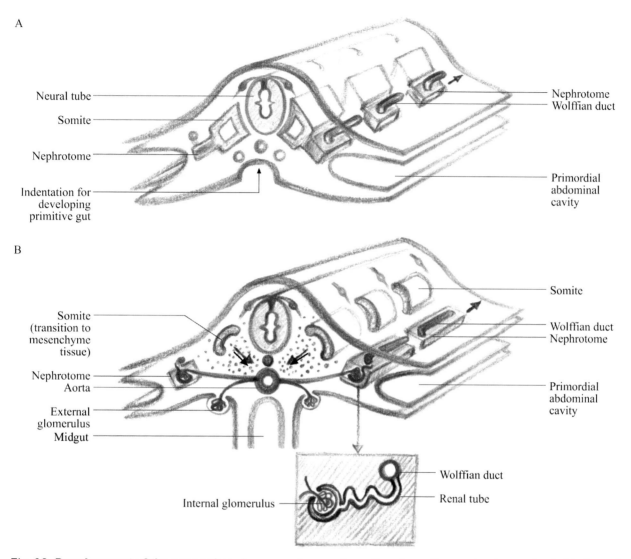

Fig. 98. **Development of the pronephros/mesonephros primordium from the nephrotomes** *(red). Each neph-rotome forms a duct (blue) that grows downward and connects with the corresponding duct of the next nephrotome segment. The result is the long Wolffian duct that empties into the cloaca. A: early stage; B: later stage (somites dissolving: arrows).*

in the outside world (water, warmth, air for respiration) shift to the interior of the body; together with the chorion (trophoblast, etc.), they create the new organism's initial habitat (see pages 56-57). This decisive step toward individuation presents two important challenges: Can metabolism be intensified and adapted to other substances that need to be eliminated (specifically, urea instead of uric acid)? And can the gestation period and hence the amount

of time available to develop important organ systems (brain, etc.) be significantly lengthened? As Portmann demonstrated, cerebralization (the increasing size and differentiation of the CNS) correlates with the length of both gestation and its "extension" in protracted infancy (56, 66). In humans, infancy provides an unusually long and intensive maturation period for the nervous system and sensory organs of an already highly individualized organism (54).

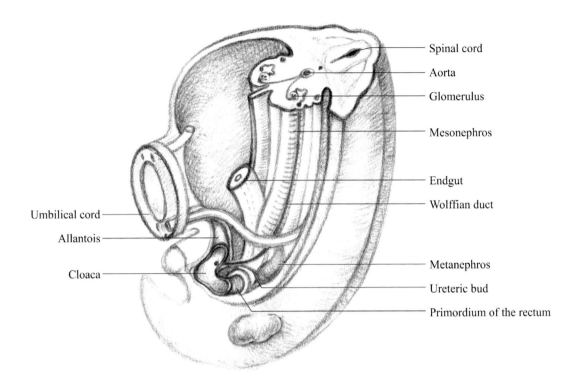

Spinal cord

Aorta

Glomerulus

Mesonephros

Endgut

Wolffian duct

Umbilical cord

Allantois

Metanephros

Cloaca

Ureteric bud

Primordium of the rectum

*Fig. 99. **Lower half of a five-week-old human embryo** (adapted from an illustration by Hamilton, Boyd, and Moss-man (122)). A longitudinal fold containing the mesonephros develops along the rear abdominal wall. The Wolffian duct (red) empties into the cloaca. The ureteric bud (green) sprouts from the Wolffian duct and unites with the nephrotome material of the sacral segments to form the primordium of the metanephros.*

This evolutionary individuation process—not to mention the increase in the size of the body itself—is also accompanied by a tremendous upgrading of the body's internal organization (that is, of various organ systems), which we will discuss in greater detail later with regard to the heart (see p.185ff).

Through a process of integrated concentration, the cardiovascular system evolved from a segmented, bilaterally symmetrical form of organization into a more highly differentiated and efficient structure. In the evolution of the kidneys, a similar process occurs. Through a tremendous process of concentration over the course of evolution, the segmented organization that first appeared in lower vertebrates was abandoned and an isolated, more efficient organ (the so-called metanephros) evolved. This stage is achieved only by amniotes (sauropsids and mammals).

In the ontogeny of the kidney, as with other organ systems, previous evolutionary stages are repeated. As a result, human embryonic development encompasses *three kidney "generations"*—the pronephros, the mesonephros, and the metanephros (Figure 97). The pronephros, which is the permanent kidney in lower vertebrates (cyclostomes, amphioxus, bony fishes), develops primarily in the area of the cervical segments (C_6-Th_1). In the human embryo, the mesonephros—which serves as the kidney in mature anamniotes (cartilaginous fishes, amphibians)—develops in the thoracic and lumbar segments (Th_2-L_4). The metanephros (S_2-S_5) develops only in amniotes (reptiles, birds, mammals) and becomes the permanent kidney after the two previous versions degenerate. At this level, segmental kidney structure is abandoned and a concentration process comes into play.

Originally, only one renal tubule is developed in each segment. Even in the mesonephros, however, several tubules develop in each segment, for a total of eighteen to twenty, and the number of renal tubules and renal corpuscles (Malpighian bodies) increases further as the metanephros develops (Table 14).

The **kidney primordia** develop out of the intermediate mesoderm—specifically, out of connections between the somites and the splanchnopleura (the lateral plates surrounding the body cavity) or nephrotomes (Figure 98). After freeing themselves from the somites and lateral plates, the nephrotomes develop tubelike canal segments that elongate until they join up with the next lower segments. In this way, a long duct develops. Ultimately, it connects the urinary tubules of all the segments and extends all the way to the cloaca at the lower end of the digestive canal (Figure 97). At the end of this primary ureter, also called the Wolffian duct, an offshoot called the ureteric bud develops. It grows toward the renal blastema of the sacral segments and unites with it to form the primordium of the metanephros (Figure 97). Metanephric tissue develops in the sacral segments (S_2-S_5) out of somite stalks, which rapidly lose their segmental organization and form a coherent mass of embryonic tissue, the metanephrogenic blastema. As the embryonic body grows, this kidney primodium is increasingly displaced (but does not actively move) from the pelvic region into the upper lumbar area (ascent of the kidneys). Unlike the pronephros, the mesonephros does not disintegrate completely. Its remnants, which develop a connection to the reproductive organs, shift downward as the primordial kidneys shift upward.

In the area of the primordial pronephros and mesonephros, segmented tubules develop out of nephrogenic tissue. These tubules develop into the Wolffian duct. They also develop an open connection to the body cavity (coelom) and an additional connection to the blood vessels that develop into glomeruli (Figures 98 and 99). The similar vascular bundles that occasionally develop in the wall of the body cavity, as well as the ductal connections to the abdominal cavity, are phylogenetic relics (Figure 98).

The Phylogenetic Development of the Kidneys

To better understand not only the kidneys' strangely circuitous ontogeny but also their structure and functioning, we must take a closer look at the dramatic restructuring of the different phases of kidney evolution. The simplest forms of kidney organization, as found in anamniotes (lower vertebrates such as fishes and amphibians, whose eggs have no amnion), consist entirely of segmentally arranged renal tubules whose contents empty into the cloaca of the endgut and usually have an open connection (nephrostome) to the body cavity. The tubules are somewhat convoluted and embedded in a dense network of veins, which are fed by an afferent vein and drained by an efferent vein. This is a **renal portal vein system**, which also exists in all other vertebrates except mammals (Figure 100 A). In this system, the arterial vascular bundles (glomeruli) are of secondary functional importance. They can appear anywhere in the walls of the body cavity and along the renal tubules or may even be completely absent (in so-called aglomerular kidneys). Elimination of metabolic wastes occurs primarily through absorption from the venous system into the upper sections of the renal tubules; the glomeruli merely serve to promote the flow of fluid—either from the blood or in the abdominal cavity, as the case may be. The ductal sections of the urinary tubules, which are connected to the abdominal cavity via a nephrostome, are often lined with ciliated cells that sweep fluid from the abdominal cavity toward the urinary tubules (Figure 100 A).

In the next higher group of vertebrates, the sauropsids (reptiles and birds, whose eggs are covered by the amnion and the allantois), connections to the abdominal cavity are

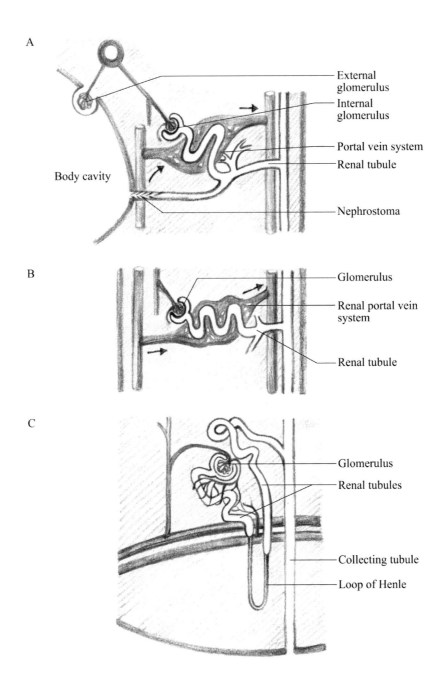

A
External glomerulus
Internal glomerulus
Portal vein system
Renal tubule
Body cavity
Nephrostoma

B
Glomerulus
Renal portal vein system
Renal tubule

C
Glomerulus
Renal tubules
Collecting tubule
Loop of Henle

Fig. 100. **Phylogenetic kidney series.** *In mammals and primates, the portal system of the kidney does not develop. In its place, the system of glomeruli and tubules (loop of Henle, collecting tubules) is further differentiated. A: fishes, amphibians; B: reptiles, birds; C: mammals, primates, humans.*

Species	Number of glomeruli per kidney
Acanthogobius (goby)	450-490
Frog (Rana)	~ 2,000
Pigeon	~ 50,000
Guinea pig	~ 30,000
Rabbit	~ 140,000
Human	1,200,000

Table 14. The process of concentration in kidney development in various vertebrates, as evidenced by the number of renal corpuscles (glomeruli) (134).

abandoned. The number of urinary tubules increases and the portal vein system becomes more elaborate (Figure 100B). The functional significance of the glomeruli also increases. Since the primary metabolic by-product is now uric acid, excretory processes are played out primarily between the venous portal vein system and the renal tubules. Although the abdominal cavity has been eliminated as a factor, body tissues and their interstitial fluid (that is, the actual interior of the body) do not yet play a larger role in kidney function.

In mammals and primates (which are also amniotes, of course), no portal vein system develops. Mammalian kidneys relate primarily to the arterial system, and the glomeruli and renal tubules now play major roles. Segmental organization is abandoned, the number of glomeruli and renal tubules increases enormously, and the tubules themselves become highly differentiated. Among other features, each tubule develops a loop of Henle, a long, narrow loop like the eye of a needle (Figure 100C). The kidney's new primary tasks relate to maintaining consistent conditions in the internal milieu, that is, monitoring water balance and maintaining constant ion concentrations in body fluids and blood. All blood plasma is filtered through the glomeruli several times a day to monitor its ion concentrations. The renal tubules gain the ability to reabsorb and concentrate metabolic wastes (especially salts and urea) that must be eliminated in the urine. Uric acid metabolism has been abandoned.

Here we see another example of the orthogenetic evolutionary principle. Evolution appears to be aiming deliberately for a higher functional state. On the first level, the body cavity (as a surface where exchanges occur) and the renal portal vein system still play a part. The total surface area, however, is very small, the pressure in the venous system is low, and the overall effectiveness of this elimination system is very limited. At the second level (sauropsids) the arterial system (glomeruli, etc.) plays a somewhat more important role. The urinary tubules become more convoluted (thus increasing their internal surface area), but because of the insolubility of uric acid and low pressure in the portal vein system, the capacity of such organs of elimination remains relatively low. The effective monitoring of water and mineral balances is not yet possible.

What has nature "learned" from these experiences? What had to happen to allow the emergence of an organism that could safeguard the function of highly differentiated internal organs through an effective monitoring of water and mineral balances, until ultimately "kidney radiation" and the development of consciousness became possible? In mammals and primates, the third and final group in this series, the portal vein system is totally deconstructed, the arterial system (glomeruli, etc.) is greatly elaborated, and consistent further differentiation of the renal tubule system (elongation of the loops of Henle, etc.) greatly enhances the concentration of kidney functions.

Thus a third basic evolutionary principle becomes apparent. Because it is based primarily on experience or information, we will call it the **empirical principle.**

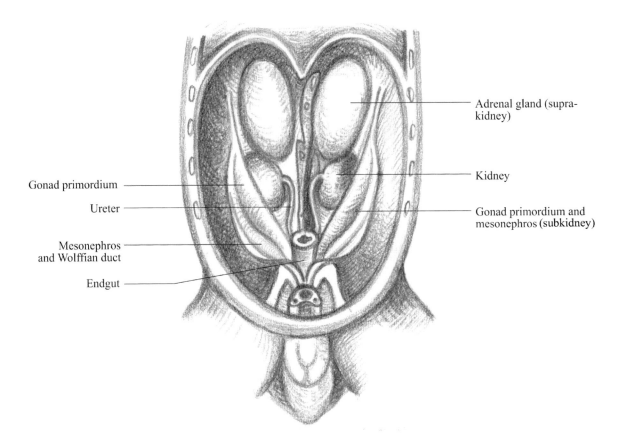

Adrenal gland (supra-kidney)

Kidney

Gonad primordium and mesonephros (subkidney)

Gonad primordium

Ureter

Mesonephros and Wolffian duct

Endgut

Fig. 101. **Development and basic threefold subdivision of the excretory system** *(view of the rear abdominal wall of a 36 mm-long human embryo at 8 weeks, adapted from an illustration by Hamilton, Boyd, and Mossman, 122). The three superimposed or adjacent ridges represent the primordia of the three major organ areas of the excretory system (suprakidney/adrenal glands, kidneys, and subkidney/gonads; for details, see text).*

Morphology and Development of the Reproductive Organs

The unique position of the reproductive organs is immediately apparent when we consider them in connection with the entire urogenital system. If we see the kidneys as its middle domain, then the adrenals (Latin *suprarenalis*, suprakidneys, or upper kidneys) constitute its upper and the reproductive organs (subkidneys or lower kidneys) its lower domain. The adrenals with their two parts (medulla and cortex) are the "head" of the whole system. They are informational in

character, assume regulatory functions within the system as a whole, and implement the connection to the nervous system through the medulla. The reproductive organs, as the lower domain, represent an area of "extra space" that can be safely occupied by foreign forces belonging to a new incarnating being.

This **threefold division of the urogenital system**, the system of excretion in its broadest sense, is already apparent at the back of the abdominal cavity during human embryonic development (Figure 101). The adrenals, which are much larger during the embryonic period, are located in the upper part of the system, directly under the diaphragm. The kidney primordia (metanephros) are located in the middle part,

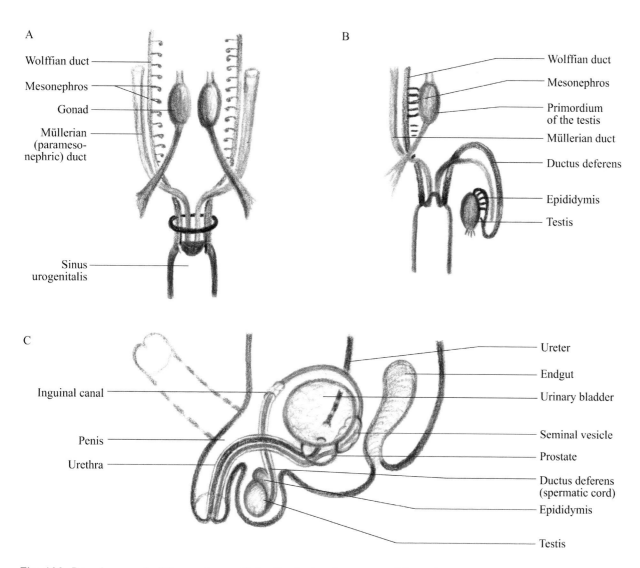

Fig. 102. **Development of the male genitals.** *Beginning from an undifferentiated state (A), the gonad primordium is transformed into the testis, which migrates through the inguinal canal into the scrotum on the outside of the body (testicular descent, B). The epididymis develops out of the primordium of the mesonephros. The Wolffian duct becomes the spermatic duct. It runs through the inguinal canal to the posterior aspect of the bladder (fundus) and through the prostate before emptying into the urethra (now located in the penis), which thus also serves as the ejaculatory duct (C).*

and the mesonephros and primordia of the reproductive organs are in the lowest part, extending into the lesser pelvis.

Initially, these primordial reproductive organs are the same in both sexes. Differentiation into male or female organs occurs later, beginning from a state that includes both possibilities (Figures 102 and 103). The common primordium consists

of the completely undifferentiated gonads, which emerge from the rear abdominal wall as elongated ridges and initially consist only of loose embryonic connective tissue (mesenchyme). These formations become more and more concentrated in the central parts of the longitudinal ridges as they develop into organs. Because they do not produce germ cells in the same way that salivary glands produce secretions, these organs are not true glands. They simply make it possible for these cells to develop within their tissues. The adjacent ductal systems (mesonephros, Müllerian ducts, etc.), which assume the function of transporting and/or further developing the germ cells, differentiate into the internal sex organs. Here again, contrasting formative principles are evident: The radial tendency dominates in the male and the more spherical formative principle in the female.

The male genitals. In male embryos, the pronephric tubules degenerate rapidly. Only the primary duct (Wolffian duct) persists for a while in the form of the mesonephric duct. In the male, the middle section of the mesonephros establishes a connection to the adjacent gonad primordium and undergoes a change in function as a result. The mesonephric tubules and duct become seminal tubules and then differentiate into the epididymis and the ductus deferens (Figure 102). The gonads (testes) migrate through the inguinal canal into the scrotum on the outside of the body. To reach the ureter, the ductus deferens of the adult male must run back through the inguinal canal to the fundus of the bladder (Figure 102C). Once the ductus deferens is linked to it, the urethra, which is enclosed in the penis, also serves as the ejaculatory duct. Through the swelling of its extensive spongy tissue, the penis becomes erectile and suitable for depositing sperm cells in the female's vagina during intercourse. The limblike, radial structural principle is clearly at work here.

The migration of the testes through the inguinal canal into the external scrotum is usually accomplished before birth and is an indicator of full-term gestation. It is a mysterious process. In some animal species, testicular descent occurs only during rutting season. In humans, undescended testes can lead to the development of malignant tumors (seminomas). This phenomenon gives the impression that sperm cell production sets in motion a prodigious cellular replication process (each ejaculation contains as many as three million sperm cells) that can degenerate into tumor growth if it cannot be expressed in insemination. Body warmth seems to play a role in this process. The external testis exists in a cooler milieu than a testis that remains in the abdominal cavity. The exact relationship, however, remains largely unexplained.

The female genitals. In female embryos, the pronephros and mesonephros are not involved in the development of the reproductive organs but degenerate completely, leaving only vestigial tubules behind. Instead, the two Müllerian ducts, which parallel the mesonephros and are connected to the abdominal cavity, develop into the Fallopian tubes and (through fusion of their lower sections) the uterus (Figure 103B). It is interesting to note that in the male, the same ducts are present but later degenerate, leaving behind only the prostatic utricle (a small channel enclosed in the prostate) and other small duct remnants.

At this point, therefore, we confront the remarkable fact that the point of departure for embryonic development of the reproductive organs is the same in both sexes. Specialization proceeds from an undifferentiated stage common to both. Neither the gonads nor the internal and external genitals exhibit any gender differentiation at this stage. Differentiation occurs only in the further course of embryonic development, which explains the numerous cases of intermediate forms (so-called intersexes) in which differentiation in one or the other direction is incomplete.

In the female embryo, the gonads also migrate downward, although only as far as the lesser pelvis, not to the outside of the body, as they do in the male (Figure 103B). The ovaries remain within the warm, protective enclosure of the abdominal cavity. As a result, the fallopian tubes, which loop around the ovaries in an expansive "hug," do not have so far to go to reach the uterus. The uterus becomes a hollow organ; at regular intervals (menstrual cycle), its mucous membranes prepare to receive a fertilized ovum. Over a relatively long period of time (approximately 280 days or ten lunar months), the "free space" thus created within the

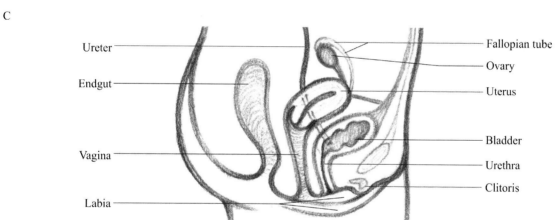

A

Wolffian duct

Mesonephros

Gonad

Müllerian
(parameso-
nephric) duct

Sinus
urogenitalis

B

Primordium of
the ovary

Wolffian duct

Müllerian duct

Fallopian tube

Ovary

Uterus

Vagina

C

Ureter

Endgut

Vagina

Labia

Fallopian tube

Ovary

Uterus

Bladder

Urethra

Clitoris

*Fig. 103. **Development of the female genitals.** Beginning from an undifferentiated state (A), the gonad primordium develops into the ovary, which migrates downward only as far as the lesser pelvis (B). The primordium of the mesonephros degenerates. The two Müllerian ducts form the fallopian tubes; their lower portions fuse to form the uterus. In the female, therefore, the urinary and genital tracts remain separate (C).*

mother's body supports a foreign organism's first steps into earthly existence. This process makes it strikingly clear that the genitals constitute an internal space whose life processes are determined not by the body's own needs but by a future-oriented principle that transcends the individual. Emptiness and receptivity to another being are the characteristic, determining qualities of this domain, especially of the gonads and the gametes that develop within them.

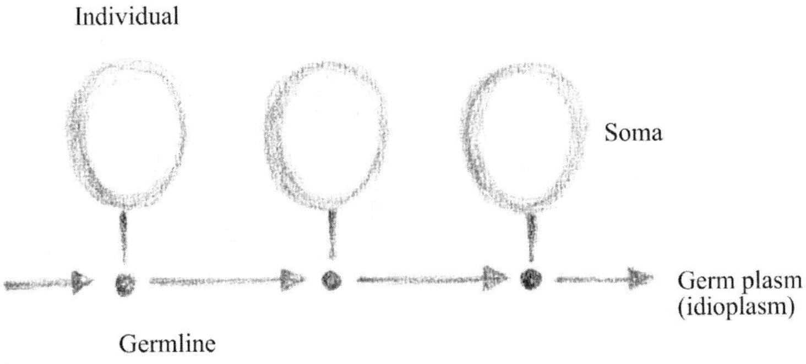

Individual

Soma

Germ plasm
(idioplasm)

Germline

Fig. 104. **Schematic representation of the germline.** *Germ plasm (idioplasm) is transmitted from generation to generation, although the body (soma) that results from it ends with death.*

Development of the Gonads

At this point, we encounter a basic mystery of reproductive biology: Undifferentiated primordial germ cells migrate *from outside* into the gonad blastema, where they later complete their development into male or female gametes (sperm, oocytes). The gonads merely provide the space where this differentiation occurs. The germ cells themselves are descended from cells produced in the earliest stages of embryonic development— specifically, from the cleavage cells of the early morula stage. As early as the first cleavage divisions (see Figure 20), some cells lag behind in their development and do not participate in subsequent steps leading to the embryo. These cells subsequently become the precursors of the primordial reproductive cells. Later, after the development of the embryonic body, they migrate via the body stalk (i.e., from outside) along the rear abdominal wall to the primordial gonads. This phenomenon is known as *germline development,* or migration of the primordial germ cells (Figure 104).

In the gonad, the primordial germ cells initially come to rest in the surface epithelium (modified peritoneal tissue) but later shift to the interior, where they are surrounded and metabolically supported by epithelial cells as they undergo further maturation (Figure 105). This maturation is a process of specialization in which the gametes increasingly lose their ability to survive

independently (Figure 17). The neighboring epithelial cells not only manage all necessary movements of the gametes within the gonad but also nourish and support them (described in Figures 15 and 17) as they undergo an increasingly extreme and one-sided differentiation that brings them close to death. In the process of becoming sperm cells, male gametes lose not only half of their original complement of chromosomes but also most of their cytoplasm and essential organelles. In contrast, female gametes nearly suffocate as a result of one-sided increases in cytoplasm. An earlier chapter described how this increasing one-sidedness and "devitalization" and the subsequent recombining of "fragments" creates the prerequisites for a new entity (that is, a new organism) to develop. This new organism, however, needs a space of its own that is as independent of the mother organism as possible.

In female embryos, the primordial germ cells migrate via the surface (germinal) epithelium into the embryonic connective tissue (stroma) of the gonad. Together with epithelial cells, they form globe-shaped cell clusters (primordial follicles), each with a primordial germ cell in its center (Figure 105 B). Here again we see the signature of the spherical formative principle. As the ovum continues to develop, its covering of epithelial cells persists. The follicle epithelial cells and corona radiata continue to form a protective and nourishing sphere around the ovum, which is on the verge of death (Figure 15).

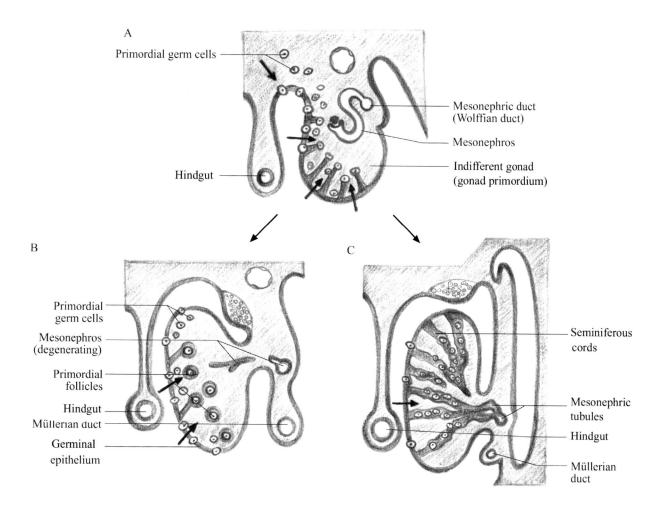

*Fig. 105. **Embryonic development of the gonads out of an undifferentiated primordium.***
A: Primordial germ cells migrate into the indifferent gonad (gonad primordium).
B: In the female gonad, the primordial germ cells, shown here translocating from the germinal epithelium into the interior of the primordium, initially come to rest in the cortex. They are accompanied by germinal epithelial cells, which develop into the follicle epithelial cells that support the egg cells. Note the spherical structural principle at work in the shape of the primordial follicles.
C: The male gonad develops strands of cells (radial structural principle) that then become the seminiferous cords that house the primordial germ cells. These strands connect to the mesonephric tubules, which then differentiate into the efferent ductules.

The picture is very different in the male gonad. Here, too, the primordial germ cells migrate via the germline to the gonad primordium, where they initially come to rest in the surface epithelium (germinal epithelium). This stage, however, is followed by the radial growth of tubes into the interior of the gland. These tubes, which carry the primordial germ cells with them, develop into the seminiferous tubules. In their walls, further differentiation of sperm cells occurs (Figure 105 C). Since the radial strands of sperm cells that grow into the stroma end blindly in the interior, they must gain access to an efferent system of tubules, which the body recruits from the mesonephric

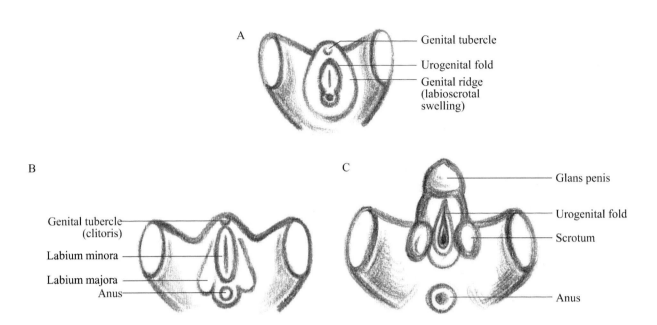

A   — Genital tubercle

— Urogenital fold

— Genital ridge
(labioscrotal
swelling)

B   C   — Glans penis

Genital tubercle   — Urogenital fold
(clitoris)
                                                                                  — Scrotum
Labium minora

Labium majora
Anus   — Anus

Fig. 106. **Development of the external genitals.**
A: Development of the external genitals from a common, undifferentiated primordium, which consists of a single genital tubercle, a pair of genital folds, and a pair of genital ridges.
B: The female genitals. The folds and ridges become the labia, the tubercle the clitoris.
C: The male genitals. The genital folds grow together; together with the tubercle, they form the penis, while the ridges become the scrotum.

system. The mesonephric tubules and the Wolffian duct become the epididymis and the ductus deferens, which allows the sperm cells to move outward through the ureter (now embedded in the penis, which is also radially structured).

The external genitals. The same polar structural principles—radial and spherical—are also evident in the development of the external genitals. Here again, the point of departure is the same for both sexes. Initially, two ridges, two folds, and one genital tubercle develop in the genital area (Figure 106). In the female, the genital folds and ridges develop into the labia minora and labia majora and the tubercle into the clitoris. In the male, the genital folds grow together. With the radially elongating tubercle, they form the penis, while the genital ridges form the scrotum and receive the testes as they migrate down through the inguinal canal. In the female, the radial thrust of growth that leads to phallus development in the male is restrained and the original stage persists longer. As a result, the female organs (together with the development of the corresponding hollow organ, the vagina) serve to receive sperm into the "holy space" of the mother's body and thus support the development of a new human being.

The Organs of the Rhythmic System

Blood and the Organs of Circulation

Functional Threefoldness of the Circulatory System

In the threefold human body, the rhythmic system is located in the middle domain, or "chest person," balancing and harmonizing functions that mediate between the upper (nervous) system and the lower (metabolic) system. This middle system is characterized by regular, rhythmic, repetitive activity, which is especially apparent in the beating of the heart and the rhythm of the breath. The rhythmic system is subdivided into two major groups of functions: the respiratory system (which tends to be oriented upward, toward the head) and the system of blood circulation (which is oriented downward, toward the metabolic system). The circulatory system itself is also threefold, consisting of:

1. The constantly moving blood, which exchanges vital substances with all organs of the body;

2. The vascular system, which serves to contain the flowing blood but is also adaptable and flexible;

3. The heart, which serves as the organizing center of the entire system (Table 15).

Heart	Upper	Form pole (structure, organization, sensory function)
Vessels (arteries, veins)	Middle	Rhythm (balance, compensation)
Blood	Lower	Substance pole (metabolism)

Table 15. The threefold circulatory system.

Blood vessels are constructed in three layers (tunics). The innermost lamella (tunica intima) is covered with a single cell layer (the endothelium), which is in contact with the flowing blood and regulates exchanges between blood and tissues (Figure 107). The middle layer (tunica media) consists of smooth muscles whose contraction determines the vessels' diameter and thus the degree of perfusion in the organs. This muscular wall transmits the pulse wave. Blood pressure is also largely dependent on the degree of contraction of the media in specific sections of the circulatory system such as the arterioles. The outermost layer (tunica adventitia), which consists primarily of connective tissue, is especially well developed in veins. It connects the vascular system with its surroundings (Figure 107).

The circulatory system. From the heart, blood flows through muscular vessels (arteries) toward the periphery and into a network of very fine vessels (capillaries) in the organs. This network's huge surface area permits an extensive exchange of substances. The heart, which develops out of a vascular tube during the embryonic period, regulates and redistributes the flow of blood, ultimately resulting in three major circulation areas (Figure 108). Systemic circulation supplies the organs and limbs—in other words, the metabolic system. This part of the circulatory system is accessed primarily from the left side of the heart (via the aorta), and blood returning to the heart empties into the right atrium via the inferior vena cava. Circulation to the head (the brain and sense organs) is served primarily by the carotid arteries and the vertebral artery. Blood returning from the head flows through the jugular vein to the superior vena cava and then into the right atrium. In contrast to the more-or-less

Heart

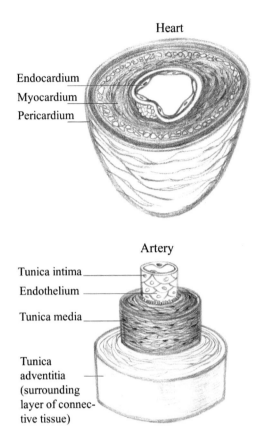

Endocardium
Myocardium
Pericardium

Artery

Tunica intima
Endothelium
Tunica media
Tunica adventitia (surrounding layer of connective tissue)

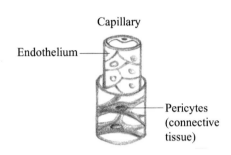

Capillary

Endothelium

Pericytes (connective tissue)

Fig. 107. **Layered structure of the blood vessels**. *The innermost layer (intima) is covered with a single layer of endothelial cells that is in contact with the flowing blood. The middle layer (media) consists primarily of smooth muscle cells (red), while the outer layer (adventitia) consists primarily of connective tissue, which anchors the vessel in its surroundings. In the heart, these three layers are further differentiated into the endocardium (intima), myocardium (media), and pericardium (adventitia).*

vertical circulation of blood through the head and body, pulmonary circulation is roughly horizontal. This part of the circulatory system involves the right side of the heart, where the pulmonary trunk originates. The pulmonary veins empty into the left atrium (Figure 108).

This functional subdivision of the circulatory system is a telling reflection of the threefoldness of the body as a whole. In the body's lower domain, circulation is influenced by metabolic processes in the organs. There, the capillaries are often fenestrated (permeable due to large gaps between endothelial cells) to permit extensive exchanges of substances between vessels and organ tissues (Figure 109B and C).

In contrast, brain capillaries are not at all permeable. They are completely sealed off from sensitive nerve tissue (Figure 109A). Exchange of substances between blood and nerve cells takes place via specialized non nerve cells called glia cells. Consequently, the brain, unlike the other organs, possesses practically no interstitial tissue. The brain can remain highly sensitive to neural stimulation only because it is protected against the direct effects of the blood and any possible breakthrough of metabolic processes. In order to serve our consciousness by "mirroring" all kinds of sensory and informational processes, the brain needs its "peace and quiet."

These two areas of circulation are separated by the pulmonary circulation, which serves gaseous exchange and supports metabolism through oxygen intake and carbon dioxide elimination. But inhalation and exhalation also have subtle effects on our consciousness: With inhalation we awake, and with exhalation we fall asleep. In a certain respect, breathing always entails a bit of waking up or falling asleep. Ultimately, death is the great exhalation—the body falls asleep and the spirit awakens.

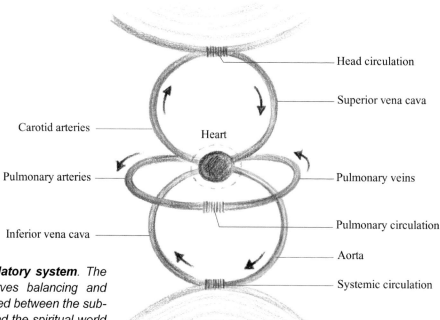

Carotid arteries

Heart

Pulmonary arteries

Inferior vena cava

Head circulation

Superior vena cava

Pulmonary veins

Pulmonary circulation

Aorta

Systemic circulation

*Fig. 108. **The threefold circulatory system**. The circulatory system, which serves balancing and harmonizing functions, is inserted between the substance world (lower domain) and the spiritual world (sensory-nervous system, upper domain). The heart is the central organ of the circulatory system.*

Thus a polarity exists between the upper (head) and lower (body) portions of the circulatory system, right down into the details of their vascular structure. These poles are harmonized and balanced by pulmonary circulation and respiration (Figure 108). In terms of their respective processes, the greatest possible contrasts exist between "upper" and "lower" circulation.

In earlier times, the human body was often seen as a microcosmic reflection of the universe, with each of its internal organs associated with a planet. When the outer world affects the sensory-nervous system, the blood "experiences" (as if from outside) the forces at work in the macrocosmic domain. And when the blood flows through the body's organs, it experiences the world of microcosmic forces as if from within. As Rudolf Steiner once formulated it, the blood is like a double-sided tablet that is written on from both the outside and the inside (65). The bloodstreams of head and systemic circulation come together in the heart, where their direction changes from

centripetal to centrifugal or vice versa. The heart is the point of reversal between upper and lower circulation, between outside and inside, and between the world and the "I". Thus the heart is the center of our circulation, the dynamic midpoint of the entire system, indeed the center of the individuality itself.

A similar view of the central importance of the heart was held by William Harvey (1578–1657), the discoverer of the circulation of the blood, which he described as follows:

It is possible to call this movement a circulation in the same sense that Aristotle compared the weather and rain with a circular movement in the upper regions. For the moist earth, warmed by the sun, develops vapors; the rising vapors again densify to rain and fall downward again, moistening the earth. Here we have the circulation of the sun. In this and in similar manner through the movement of the sun, through its approach and retreat, thunderstorms and other heavenly phenomena are brought about. So also it could

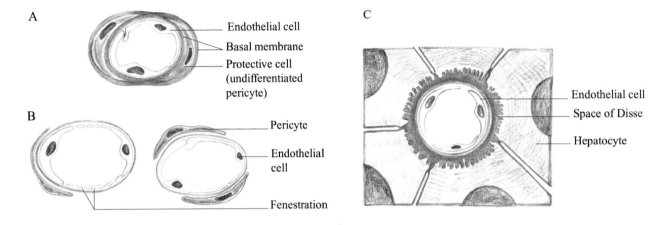

*Fig. 109. **Different types of capillaries**. A: Brain capillaries. The vascular wall is thoroughly sealed, not only by a multilayered basement membrane but also by the cells around it. The endothelial cells form the blood-brain barrier.*
B: Organ capillaries. The endothelial layer may be either permeable (fenestrated) or completely closed.
C: Liver capillaries (sinusoids). These vessels are fully permeable to allow blood plasma to pass through to the surrounding space of Dissé.

possibly happen in the body that all parts are nourished, warmed, and vitalized by way of a warmed, perfect, vaporlike, spiritual and (if I may so express myself) nourishing blood, whereas the blood, in the various parts of the body, is cooled down, densified, and weakened and therefore returns to its origin, to the heart, its source, to the altar of the body, in order to regain its perfection. There, through the naturally powerful fiery warmth, this treasure of life, liquefied anew, is impregnated with spirit and with balsam, as it were, and from here it is again distributed: and all that is dependent upon the beating movement of the heart. Thus is the heart the primal source of life and the sun of the small world, just as the sun in the same relationship deserves to be named the heart of the world. By virtue of this force and its beat, the blood is moved, brought to perfection, nourished, and preserved from decay and disintegration.... The heart is the root of the lives of living beings, the lord of them all, the sun of the small world upon which depends all life and from which radiates all freshness and all force (116).

The Lymphatic Vascular System and the Body's Fluid System

Bone marrow is the source of blood, but body tissues are the source of lymph fluid. Interstitial fluid accumulates in lymph vessels that originate either within organs or in connective tissue and then merge into larger vessels. Most of this lymph accumulates in the thoracic duct, which empties into the subclavian vein of the neck in the left jugular angle (Figure 89). Thus the lymphatic vascular system is connected to venous circulation. Ultimately, interstitial fluid originates in the blood or in the tissues themselves. Because this lymph is funneled back into the venous system, lymphatic circulation is incomplete in itself and is actually only a subset of blood circulation. The lymphatic vascular system belongs to the immune system. Lymph nodes, which are inserted into the lymphatic vessels at frequent intervals, monitor and "cleanse" the circulating lymph to protect the blood from contamination. In the lymphatic system, powerful life forces are at work. The lymphatic system is older than the circulatory system. Its forces, which hearken back to archaic times, protect the blood (the most important vessel for the human "I"-being) against invasion by "unclean" elements (Figure 89). Lymph is a preliminary stage of blood. It has not yet achieved the level of true blood, which is warmer and circulates more rapidly. Although lymphatic vessels do have a rhythmical pulse, their pulsations are slower and less regular than those of blood vessels and are often totally absent. Lymph circulation differs from organ to organ.

The lymphatic system's relationship to the immune system is only one aspect of this mysterious system. Its other aspect relates to the body's fluid system. All of the cells in the body are surrounded by fluid that ultimately drains into the lymphatic system. In children, this interstitial fluid accounts for 25 percent of body weight, as compared to 5 percent for blood plasma. In adults, intercellular fluid accounts for 15 to 20 percent of body weight. (Because adipose tissue stores little water, this figure is lower in obese individuals and higher in those who are thin.) The amount of fluid present inside cells (intracellular fluid) is relatively constant at approximately 40 percent of body weight, but the amount of intercellular fluid fluctuates, depending on physiological processes within the organs. In contrast to interstitial fluid, which is low in protein and high in sodium, cells are very high in protein and potassium. The first living things evolved in salty, protein-poor sea water. More highly evolved species abandoned the marine habitat but internalized this "seawater" milieu. As a result, the protein-rich cells must expend energy on transporting solutes against the concentration gradient to avoid becoming flooded with salt-rich fluid (especially sodium). When this "pumping" fails, cells swell up and die as they fill with sodium and water. Thus the survival of cells and organs is heavily dependent on constant levels of ions and salts in the interstitial fluid, through which all substances exchanged between the blood and the organs must pass. The kidneys prevent excess accumulation of salt in this life-giving, life-maintaining space. They keep

a "watchful eye" on all the substances moving within it and regulate its life-giving flows, primarily by increasing or decreasing the elimination of sodium.

Because the lymphatic vessels originate in fluid-filled interstitial tissues and end in the venous system, they represent a link between the body's organs and the blood. All exchanges of substances between blood and organs (with the exception of the organs of the nervous system) take place via interstitial tissues. We can imagine the currents of life forces flowing through this fluid-filled space. These currents manifest and become recognizable in the patterns of lymph flow. Because interstitial tissues are drained by the lymphatic system, organ processes that affect fluid movement in this space ultimately affect the entire body. The "fluid body" has its own dynamics.

Blood and Bone Marrow

We can see the blood as a liquefied organ system given shape by the blood vessels. The arrangement of these vessels allows the blood to come into contact with several experiences: impressions conveyed by the senses in the upper body, influences of the internal organs in the lower body, and consequences of respiration in the middle of the body. Though impacted by these extremely varied influences, the blood has an astonishing ability to maintain constant composition and structure and to restore equilibrium rapidly when imbalances occur. It is the harmonizing organ par excellence.

Bone marrow. Blood originates in the bone marrow. Hematopoesis takes place in the spongy marrow tissue of the long bones, vertebrae, ribs, sternum, etc. The fact that blood forms in the dark cavities of the bones is profoundly astonishing and an archetypal phenomenon of the greatest significance. On the functional level, compact bone is connected to muscles. Together with our joints, this allows our limbs to move in three-dimensional space. The structure and arrangement of our

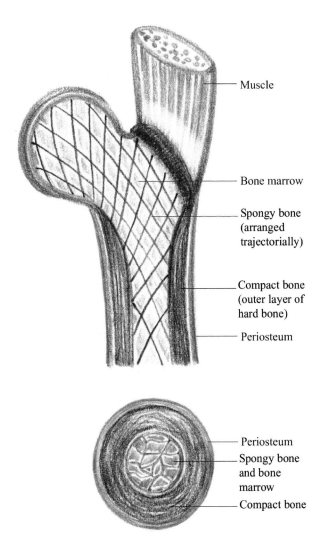

Fig. 110. **The head of the femur as an example of the location of bone marrow**. *Functional relationships between the spongy bone and the blood-producing marrow on the one hand and the compact bone and the muscles on the other.*

muscles brace the skeletal system, allowing our bones to remain relatively delicate in structure. Compact bone is deposited from outside—that is, directly from the surrounding periosteal connective tissue—onto the spongy bone at the core. Thus the compact bone's formative gesture can be described as circular, in spite of the bones' essentially radial, longitudinal structure. Bones interact with muscles, which constantly attempt to free themselves from the forces of the Earth's gravity and to overcome three-dimensional space through movements that are new, individual, and personal. In this process, compact bone, although forming radial bones, opens up to peripheral, cosmic forces within the earthly domain.

In contrast, the spongy bone within the long bones is endochondral (formed through ossification of cartilage) and develops from within. It is totally receptive to the radial forces proceeding from the center of the Earth. Here, bone formation occurs radially. The trabecular (archlike) network of the spongy bone is arranged along actual lines of force. Functionally, therefore, the structure of the spongy part of the bone is fully adapted to the demands of support (stasis) within the Earth's gravitational field. The spongy bone has no direct connection to muscles, which counteract the earthly force of gravity. The bone marrow that fills the interstices between the trabecular network develops out of embryonic mesenchyme and remains a juvenile tissue with high potential for growth. The same mesenchyme or reticulum cells that form bone tissue under the influence of earthly forces can also differentiate into blood cells, which collectively form the "organ" of blood. As such, they escape from earthly forces through movement, i.e., circulation (Figure 110).

Both of the fundamental formative processes active in shaping bones are also evident in the development of the head. In a process similar to the development of the compact bone in limb bones, the skullcap (calvarium) forms from outside and develops out of connective tissue. Here, the limbs' circular and columnar tendency becomes spherical. From a dynamic point of view, the strength and mobility of the limbs metamorphoses into the activity of thinking in the head. In contrast, the facial skull exhibits the beginnings of a radial formative tendency in the shape of the protruding chin and nose. The face, with its individual features, deviates from the spherical shape of the rest of the head. Like the spongy bone, it is a place where the individuality manifests, and as such it develops from the inside. Spongy bone, which is fully receptive to earthly forces, is the source of blood formation (hematopoiesis), providing the foundation for the human experience of the "I".

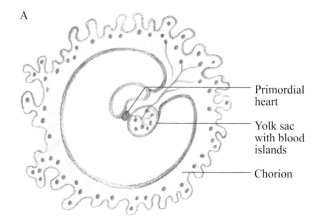

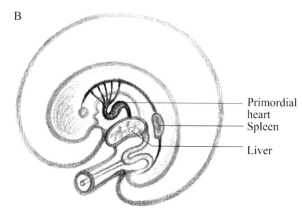

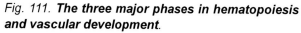

Primordial
heart

Yolk sac
with blood
islands

Chorion

Primordial
heart
Spleen

Liver

*Fig. 111. **The three major phases in hematopoiesis and vascular development**.*

A: Extra-embryonic phase. From week three onward, blood islands begin to appear on the yolk sac and in the chorion, along with vessels that merge into a primitive network.

B: Hepatosplenic phase (approximately months 3 to 8). Blood-cell production now occurs within the embryo, in the liver and spleen.

C: Myeloid phase. From the fifth month onward, the bone marrow of the long bones, pelvic and pectoral girdles, and skullcap assume the function of blood-cell production.

D: In the adult, centers of blood-cell production become limited to the torso (vertebrae, ribs, sternum) and joints.

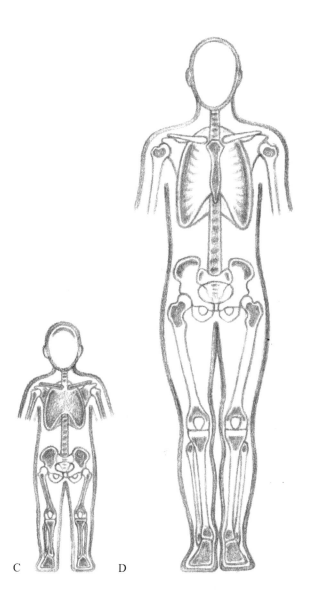

The head and the limbs are separated by the torso, where cosmic and earthly forces are in balance. This is where the heart, the center of the circulatory system, is located.

***The blood as an organ**. As early as the third week of gestation, blood-cell formation begins outside the embryo, in the "blood islands" of the yolk sac and chorion (megaloblastic phase). Blood-cell production first takes place in the embryonic body itself during the second month, when the liver assumes this function. During the third month, the spleen becomes active as another source of blood cells (Figure 111). Medullar (bone marrow) blood-cell production begins to dominate over hepatosplenic blood production only around the middle of pregnancy (month 5). After birth, the liver and spleen no longer produce blood cells.

	Cells	**Blood-plasma components**	**Functions**
Coagulation system	Thrombocytes, basophilic leukocytes	Fibrinogen	Formative processes
Transport system	Erythrocytes	Albumin	Respiratory and equilibration processes
Immune system	Leukocytes, lymphocytes	Gamma globulins	Substance processes

Table 16. Functional threefoldness of the blood.

In the growing child, blood production retreats from the limbs and becomes concentrated in the ribcage—that is, in the central torso (Figure 111), which also houses the heart and lungs, the organs of the "middle" system. In an impressive process of internalization, blood production shifts from peripheral organs surrounding the embryo to the interior of the skeletal system.

Bone is the hardest tissue in the body. It con-tains calcium salts (in the form of hydroxylapatite) and a dense, closely packed network of collagen fibers. In the bones, the body is completely subject to the Earth's gravitational force. Bone, however, is not dead tissue. Its dense network of branching bone cells (osteocytes) can release or redeposit calcium salts at any time. Because bone (unlike cartilage) is well supplied with blood vessels, minerals (Ca^{++} ions, phosphate ions, etc.) are readily mo-bilized from or redeposited in it. The bone is the body's largest repository of minerals. Blood is the opposite of bone. It frees itself from the telluric forces active in bone, repeatedly enlivening the mineral element and bringing it into circulation.

The body's total **bone marrow**, which weighs about 2,600 grams, contains approximately 400 grams of blood-producing cells. Since red blood cells (the blood's most important cellular component) number around 25×10^{12} and have a life span of only 100 to 120 days, they must be produced at a rate of approximately 150×10^6 per minute. This figure gives us an inkling of the tremendous scope of the cellular renewal taking place in the marrow's blood-producing centers, which are a constant and inexhaustible source of new life and therefore of circulation itself.

Because the blood, as a fluid organ or organ system, pervades all of the body's organs and comes into contact with all of their processes, it reflects everything going on in the body. This is why almost all pathological processes in the body can be identified through blood tests. Just as the nervous system mirrors the outside world, the blood mirrors the internal milieu. Like the nervous system, the blood represents the organism as a whole. This means that all of the basic processes of the threefold organism are also present in the blood, and the blood itself is functionally threefold (Table 16).

The blood's basic functions are to maintain homeostasis within the body (that is, to keep physiological conditions in the internal milieu relatively constant) and to **transport respiratory gases** (oxygen and carbon dioxide). These arche-typal rhythmic functions are served by two of the blood's most important components, namely, red blood cells (erythrocytes) and low molecular weight plasma proteins (albumins). The surface area of these protein molecules is large, with many hydrophilic and lipophilic receptors that allow them to bind and transport both water-soluble and fatty compounds. As a result, these proteins serve a very important function in maintaining constant oncotic pressure. The anucleate red blood cells, which develop from nucleated cells in the bone marrow, are shaped like little discs with indented centers. They contain hemoglobin, and their iron content makes it possible for them to transport oxygen.

The apatite crystals in bones serve as points of focus for physical, earthly forces. Similarly, the iron in blood cells provides a vehicle for the "I". There is something archetypal in the fact that the cells facilitating the human spiritual entity's entry into the physical body dispense with the genetic material of the cell nucleus, which links all other cells to their hereditary past. Furthermore, when erythrocytes are broken down in the spleen and heme is released, this iron-containing pigment is transported in a protein molecule (ferritin) with the shape of a pentagonal dodecahedron. (This structure is significant. The pentagon has always been seen in relationship with the human form; the twelve pentagonal sides of the dodecahedron can be seen to relate the human form to the twelve aspects of the cosmos.) With the first breath we draw, we become citizens of the Earth. Oxygen helps us incarnate into our physical bodies and fulfill our earthly karma. Iron is the tool that enables the "I" to be active in the physical world, because all life processes are ultimately based on the release of energy through the molecular "combustion" of sugars and other compounds, which is supported by the blood's oxygen supply. Thus oxygen is the substance most characteristic of life on Earth (cf. Wolff, 62). Internal (tissue) respiration is the central process in the life of the human body. Life ends when respiration ceases. At death, the purely physical and chemical processes of the outside world reassert control over the matter in the body, and it begins to disintegrate.

Two support functions—preserving the structure of the vascular system and warding off damaging influences—are essential to the blood's primary task, the uninterrupted transport of respiratory gases, etc. The coagulation system guarantees the vascular system's structural integrity; the immune system serves the defensive function. Like the blood itself, these two systems have both cellular and humoral components.

The *coagulation system* prevents loss of blood from a leaking or damaged vessel. The breakdown of specialized cells (thrombocytes) triggers the transformation of fibrinogen (a high molecular weight plasma protein) into fibrin, producing a clot (thrombus) that plugs the hole in the vessel wall. If the injury is extensive, tissue proliferation is also triggered. Ultimately, the thrombus dissolves and circulation is restored. Of course this complex sequence of events involves many factors. In the blood, equilibrium is maintained between thrombocytes, which promote coagulation, and basophils, which inhibit coagulation through the release of inflammatory mediators. The same is true of the corresponding plasma factors. Coagulation guarantees the structure of the circulatory system as a whole and preserves its subdivision and differentiation in individual organs. As such, coagulation serves the informational function within the circulatory system, as the sensory-nervous system does for the organism as a whole.

In contrast, the *immune system* is dominated by metabolic functions. Although the processes that trigger immune responses are certainly comparable to informational processes, the end result is always a breakdown of compounds—in other words, a digestive process. As discussed earlier, modern science distinguishes between cellular and humoral immune defenses. In the cellular defense system, specialized cells in the blood (leukocytes or white blood cells) ingest and digest (phagocytize) noxious and foreign substances. In contrast, the specialized cells (lymphocytes) of the humoral defense system produce antibodies that circulate in the blood and deactivate foreign compounds. Antibodies are high molecular weight proteins (gamma globulins, immunoglobulins) that bind with antigens to produce complexes that can then be ingested and digested by macrophages.

Within the blood, therefore, the immune system serves as a highly differentiated metabolic system whose function is to keep the circulating blood free of contaminants. Wherever inflammation appears in the body, it is always underlain by an immune response in which the circulatory system is heavily involved. Inflammation indicates an excess of metabolic functions. Its opposite is sclerosis, which indicates an excess of formative processes.

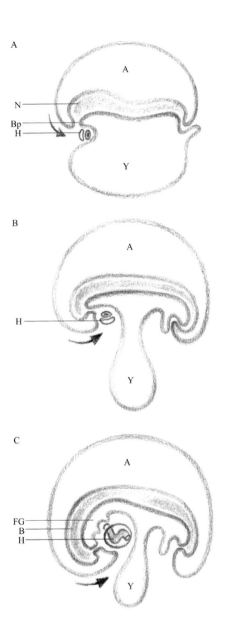

Fig. 112. *Early embryonic stages and descent of the heart.*
A: Around day 21, the earliest heart primordium (H) becomes visible in front of the buccopharyngeal membrane (Bp) and neural plate (N).
B: On day 26, the cardiac tube (H) begins to rotate (arrow).
C: Day 28. The heart primordium shifts to a location under the brain primordium (B) and foregut (FG) (arrow).

A: amniotic cavity
Y: yolk sac
H: heart primordium

The Heart

The heart is one of the most mysterious organs in the human body. The widely held view of the heart as a mechanical pump that drives circulation seriously underestimates its importance in human existence. Idioms such as "speaking from the heart," "to love someone with all one's heart," or "a good-hearted person" retain hints of more exalted connections and suggest that the heart is more than just a pump. The heart has always been experienced as an organ that is uniquely connected to a person's soul-spiritual nature. Let's attempt a phenomenological approach to the mystery of this organ. We will begin by considering its developmental history.

The Ontogenetic Development of the Heart and the Dimensions of Space

Early embryonic development of the human heart. The primitive heart is the first organ primordium to develop in human beings. Toward the end of the third week of gestation (days 19 to 21), the pericardial cavity appears as a little gap between the endoderm and the ectoderm. The mesenchymal vascular islands that develop here merge into networks and later form a thin-walled endocardial tube. These vascular islands and the early heart primordium appear outside of the future embryo, near the yolk sac. The pericardial cavity, initially located near the front of the future head, is increasingly displaced downward, along with the endocardial tube. As the head (especially the neural tube) becomes distinguishable from the embryonic disc and the foregut shifts to a more caudal location, the heart primordium also shifts and comes to rest under the brain primordium (Figure 112). Later, the heart descends further, "sinking" into the ribcage and ultimately (after birth) all the way to the diaphragm. (The cardiac apex is aligned with the third or fourth intercostal space in newborns and the fifth in adults.)

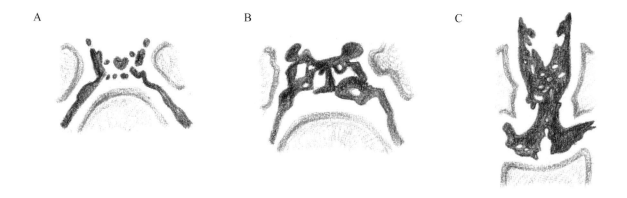

*Fig. 113. **Early heart primordium in the Stage-10 embryo** (approximately day 21). Lumina are shown in black. The vessels, initially paired, later merge to form the endocardial tube (adapted from Hinrichsen, 38).*

These displacements add up to a significant inward and downward shift in the location of the heart primordium, from the periphery of the embryonic disc to the center of the embryo. The early vascular system, which also includes the entire ring of chorionic villi (the future placenta)—that is, a major peripheral functional domain (Figure 111A)—gradually pervades the embryonic body. The centrally located heart, which soon begins to beat, forms the only bridge between the functions of peripheral organs (chorion, placenta, etc.) and the developing embryonic body. The shifting location of the heart mirrors the progressive incarnation of the human spiritual being, beginning in the peripheral embryonic sheaths (chorion, placenta) where all organ functions initially take place, and then moving into the interior of the embryonic body via the bridge of the umbilical cord, with the help of the blood and blood vessels (cf. Figure 31). Thus the primitive heart, which supports circulation from the periphery (embryonic sheaths) to the center (embryo) and vice versa and undergoes extensive differentiation as early as week 8, becomes the portal through which the individuality incarnates into the body, the threshold that the human spirit must cross on its journey from the "other world" of the protective embryonic membranes into the world of the developing body.

Cardiac Development and the Dimensions of Space

Within the spherical sheath of the embryonic membranes (chorion, etc.), the laws of space do not yet apply. The human individual becomes "earthly" only after taking hold of the embryonic body and developing it. The new (spatial) dimensionality of the body is reflected in cardiac development in very surprising ways. Let's explore this development step by step.

It was formerly believed that an endocardial tube developed on each side of the primitive gut after mesoderm and somite development, and that these tubes then merged along the median line. And in fact, this is what happens in lower vertebrates. In humans, however, early vascular development produces an irregular network of vesicles and strands in the vicinity of the future heart. This network then develops into a single cardiac tube in the embryo with two to four somites (Stages 9 and 10). When only isolated individual vesicles or islands are present, the yolk sac veins have already formed and the embryonic disc with its somites, lateral plates, etc., is bilaterally symmetrical. At this stage, the heart primordium can be described as paired (Figure 113). As soon as a single, unpaired cardiac tube develops, it begins to divide again by forming septa. Thus the

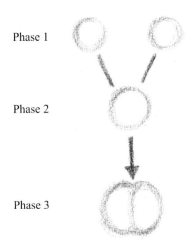

Phase 1

Phase 2

Phase 3

Fig. 114. **Three phases of cardiac development.**
Paired endocardial tubes (Phase 1) unite into a single cardiac tube (Phase 2). Phase 3: Right and left halves of the heart develop through septation of the cardiac tube.

transitory paired structure of the heart primordium gives way first to an unpaired arrangement and then to a double structure that is part of a new, combined entity, which becomes fully functional only after birth (Figure 114).

We can therefore identify three stages of cardiac development:

1. An approximately symmetrical initial stage;

2. A single cardiac tube, which is inserted in front of the pharyngeal arches and is part of a bilaterally symmetrical circulatory system;

3. The stage of cardiac septation, which transforms embryonic circulation into an asymmetrical system.

Development of the Cardiac Tube

As soon as the cardiac tube is formed, bends and distortions begin to develop. Many attempts have been made to attribute these changes in shape to the somewhat confining space of the pericardial cavity. But the characteristic loop shape must be intrinsic to the organ, because it is evident even in pathologies where the heart primordium develops outside of the embryo. The changes most essential to the metamorphosis of the cardiac tube are the downward shift of its upper section and the upward shift of the lower section (Figure 115). The initially slightly S-shaped tube consists of a sequence of four cavities. From bottom to top, they are:

1. The venous sinus, into which the yolk sac veins, body veins, and umbilical veins empty;

2. The primitive atrium;

3. The primitive ventricle; and finally

4. The bulbus cordis, from which the arterial trunk emerges.

The aortas and the trunks of the pharyngeal arteries emerge in pairs from the arterial trunk. At first, therefore, the entire system is bilaterally symmetrical in structure.

Initially, blood flows into the cardiac tube from below—that is, from its "venous" end. Next, the tube widens; horizontal bulges that later develop into the cardiac auricles surround the "arterial" end of the tube on both sides. This arterial or exit portion, initially located at the very top of the primitive heart, shifts downward, forming the cardiac apex and the ventricle area (Figures 115 and 116). Simultaneously, the "venous" or entrance portion shifts upward. What was below is now on top and vice versa.

In other words, *a reversal has occurred in the up-down dimension*. Is this reversal qualitative as well as spatial? The portion of the tube that has shifted upward (venous sinus and atrium) later develops into the atria, which receive blood flowing in from the body and the lungs and channel it into the ventricles. The blood that collects in the atria comes from all different parts of the body and reflects the full variety of peripheral processes. For example, nutrient-rich blood from the liver mingles with blood from the brain, which contains cerebrospinal fluid, and so forth. From the perspective of the blood, "substance" processes predominate in the atrial area, although not in the form of the true metabolism characteristic of the lower domain of the threefold body.

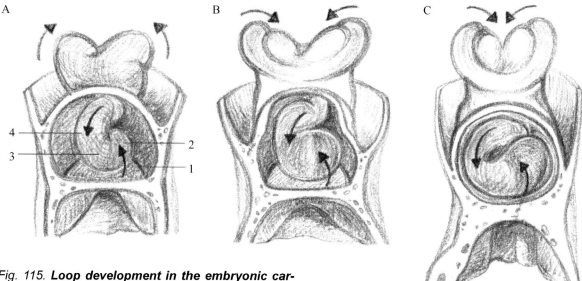

Fig. 115. **Loop development in the embryonic cardiac tube**. *The upper section of the tube shifts downward as the lower section moves upward (view from in front; the pericardium has been opened). (Adapted from Hinrichsen, 38.)*
A: 9-somite stage (approximately day 22).
B: 11-somite stage (day 22/23).
C: 11-12-somite stage (approximately day 23).
Sequence of blood flow through the cardiac spaces:
1: Venous sinus; 2: Primitive atrium; 3: Primitive ventricle; 4: Bulbus cordis. Arrows indicate directions of growth.

The processes taking place in the ventricular area are qualitatively very different. The downward shift of the initially uppermost, "arterial" portion of the cardiac tube produces a sharp bend (the future cardiac apex). As a result, the heart's pattern of contraction changes from a peristaltic wave to the saccadic rhythm of systole and diastole. The flow of blood, initially constant, is interrupted and ceases for a fraction of a second before its direction is reversed. Muscle contraction puts pressure on the blood in the ventricles and discharges it to the periphery. At this stage, therefore, the ventricular portion of the heart creates a rhythmical pulse wave that interrupts the previously constant flow and briefly compresses the blood. Rhythmicization, heart rate, blood pressure, etc., all conform to conditions on the periphery. Ventricular activity

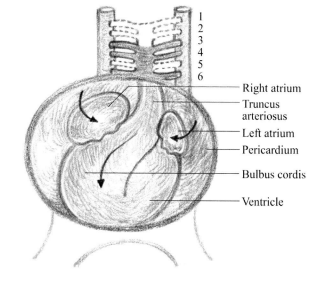

Fig. 116. **Embryonic heart primordium** *(approximately day 35, view from in front through the opened pericardium). 1-6: Schematic representation of the pharyngeal arteries. Arteries 1, 2, and 5 already show atrophy. The atria develop horizontally, from back to front (arrows) around the bulbus cordis, which is shifting downward. (Later, continuation of this development results in the cardiac auricles.) Septation produces the right and left sides of the heart.*

mirrors circulatory conditions on the periphery. Thus the heart becomes the organ that reflects circulation as a whole, both "perceiving" the body's circulatory status and regulating it through meaningful responses. Ordinarily, however, perception and regulation are functions of the "upper" human being or informational system. In a certain respect, therefore, the heart is a sense organ; it serves sensory as well as motor functions in the adult organism. We will revisit this phenomenon later. For the moment, let's simply note that the qualitative aspects of up and down as they apply to the upright human being are reversed in the heart. Figuratively speaking, the human heart is "standing on its head." It is also worth noting that this reversal, which occurs during embryonic development, is the very first step in the development of the heart as an organ.

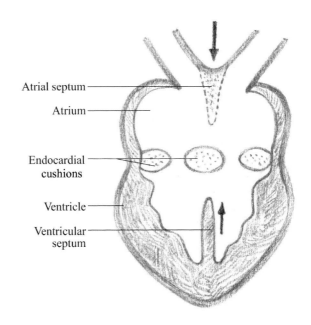

Fig. 117. **Septation of the embryonic cardiac tube.** *In the ventricular area, the ventricular septa form in the direction of the flow of blood, but in the atrial area, the atrial septum grows toward the endocardial cushions (i.e., against the bloodstream; arrows).*

Septation of the Cardiac Tube and the Right-Left Dimension

Immediately after the above-mentioned reversal, the initially unitary cardiac tube begins to divide into left and right halves as the septa develop. Cardiac septation is a complex process. It takes place **with** the flow of blood in the ventricular area but **against** it in the atrial area and bulbus. The septa grow from both ends of the cardiac tube toward the center, where they unite with the endocardial cushions, which later give rise to the atrioventricular valves (Figure 117).

As the septa grow, the veins emptying into the atrial area become asymmetrical. The left branch of the sinus venosus atrophies while the right widens, forming the vertical superior and inferior venae cavae. Simultaneously, the pulmonary veins enlarge on the left in preparation for the future separation of pulmonary and systemic circulations (Figure 118).

In the bulbus, four ridges grow together to form a septum that divides the stream of blood exiting the heart. The plane in which they meet shifts from a peripheral to a central location, separating the bulbus into two major vessels (aorta and pulmonary trunk). Because the plane of separation spirals to the right, rotating almost 300°, the aorta is connected to the left ventricle and the pulmonary artery to the right (Figure 119). In this way, the right side of the heart is linked to pulmonary circulation, the left side to systemic circulation, and their respective bloodstreams cross in the heart in the form of a lemniscate. This septation process, which is completed only after birth, separates venous from arterial blood. During the fetal period, however, the blood remains mixed for the most part, in spite of septation, because arterialization (oxygenation) of blood cannot occur in the lungs but only in the placenta (that is, outside of the embryonic body). Within the embryo itself, anastomoses (foramen ovale, ductus arteriosus) allow blood to bypass pulmonary circulation. Consequently, right-left differentiation is completed only after birth.

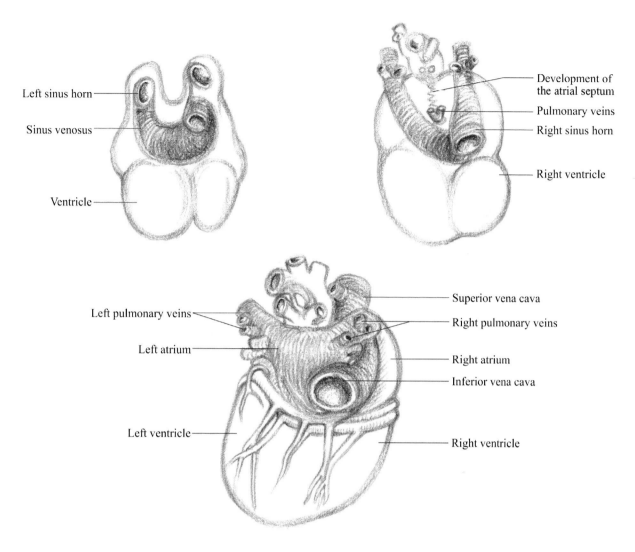

Left sinus horn

Sinus venosus

Ventricle

Development of the atrial septum

Pulmonary veins

Right sinus horn

Right ventricle

Left pulmonary veins

Left atrium

Left ventricle

Superior vena cava

Right pulmonary veins

Right atrium

Inferior vena cava

Right ventricle

*Fig. 118. **Embryonic heart primordium** (rear view). Development of asymmetry in the ventricles in conjunction with septation. The initially symmetrical (U-shaped) venous sinus atrophies. In its place, the pulmonary veins widen on the left and are incorporated into the left ventricle (adapted from Clara, 124).*

If we apply the qualitative concepts of dimensionality that we worked out in an earlier chapter, what is the significance of this phenomenon? The right side of the body, at least in right-handed people, is the more active side. The right hand is used to complete all-important work related to life on Earth. Our right side is more earth-oriented, active, and giving; the left is more reserved, supportive, and passive. With regard to metabolic functions, it is important to note that most of the liver lies on the right side of the body. The liver, as the organ that synthesizes substances for the body, makes it possible for the individuality to incarnate into physical existence. In the metabolic system, asymmetries appear as early as the embryonic period, when the liver shifts to the right and the stomach rotates to the left. The stomach is more involved in breaking

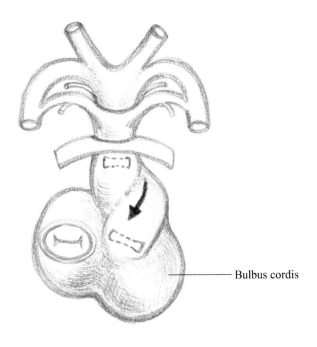

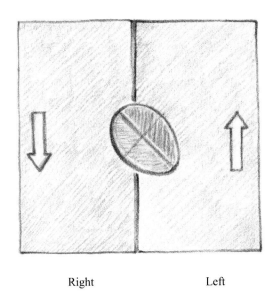

Right   Left

*Fig. 120. **The chambers of the heart in relationship to the right/left dimension**. This diagram illustrates the reversal of the qualities of right and left in the differentiation of the right and left sides of the heart.*

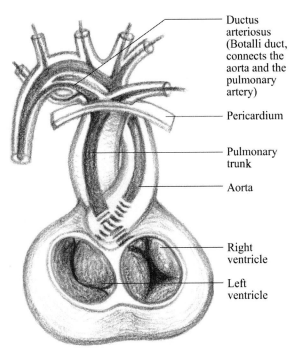

Ductus arteriosus (Botalli duct, connects the aorta and the pulmonary artery)

Pericardium

Pulmonary trunk

Aorta

Right ventricle

Left ventricle

Bulbus cordis

*Fig. 119. **Embryonic heart primordium and blood vessels** (atria removed; view from behind and above). Division of the outgoing flow of blood is accomplished as the bulbus ridges grow together to form the aorto-pulmonary septum, which grows in a spiral from the periphery toward the center (arrow). At the same time, the ventricle divides into right and left chambers.*

down matter, although this function prepares the way for synthesis on the far side of the intestinal wall.

From the qualitative perspective, arterial and venous blood tend to relate to different sides of the body. Oxygen absorption in the lungs (i.e., arterialization of the blood) makes cellular activity possible through the accumulation of small amounts of energy in the tissues (for example, in the form of ATP). All bodily or cellular activities require adequate supplies of oxygen. Our activity in earthly space is based on oxygen consumption in the body's tissues. Since the right side is the more active side of the body, we would expect arterial blood to flow through the right side of the heart and venous blood through the left, but in fact **another reversal occurs here**. As a result of the septation described above, oxygen-enriched blood from the pulmonary veins enters the left atrium from the outside (lungs) and leaves the heart through the aorta (which is connected to the left ventricle) for distribution throughout the interior of the body. Conversely, the direction of flow on the right side

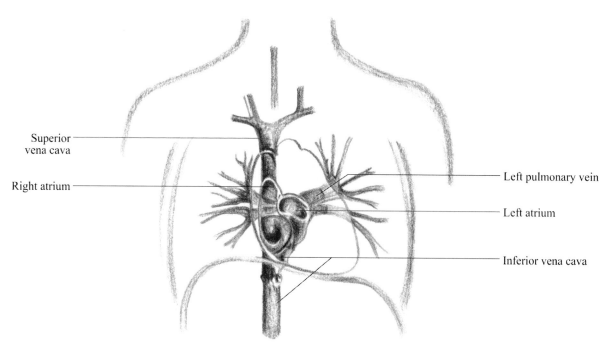

*Fig. 121. **Crossing of veins in the heart** (view with ventricles and atria removed; adapted from Benninghoff, 70).*

of the heart is from the interior toward the outside. The right atrium fills with venous blood from body tissues; the pulmonary artery exits the right side of the heart, linking it to pulmonary circulation. Venous blood, however, always tends to come to rest, to become inactive, and to release the spirit (interestingly, the ancient Greek word *pneuma* meant both "breath" and "spirit") bound in arterial blood—tendencies characteristic of the left side of the body. In functional terms, therefore, the heart reverses the situation in the body: The left half of the heart is more closely related to the right side of the body and vice versa (Figure 120). At this stage in our discussion, we will disregard the reversal of dimensionality that occurs in the head (lateralization of the brain, etc.).

The Heart and the Front-Back Dimension

The separation of the originally unitary cardiac tube into two functionally distinct sides of the heart becomes effective only after birth. After birth, venous and arterial blood no longer mingle, and the baby becomes a true Earth dweller with a functioning pulmonary circulation and two completely separated kinds of blood. This separation is achieved with the closing of the foramen ovale in the atrial septum and the atrophy of the ductus arteriosus linking the pulmonary artery and the aorta (Figures 119 and 141). Only at this stage can the blood flow separately through the two halves of the heart in the front-back dimension. Let's take a closer look at these flows.

The major vessels leading to the heart lie behind it—the superior and inferior venae cavae on the vertical axis and the pulmonary veins

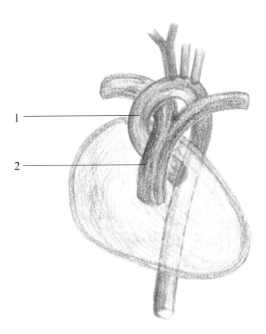

Fig. 122. ***Intertwining of major vessels leaving the*** ***ventricles****. The aorta (1) emerges from the left ventri-* *cle and spirals around to the back of the heart in a great* *arch (red). The pulmonary arterial trunk (2) emerges* *from the right ventricle and wraps around the aorta.*

(which carry arterial blood) on the horizontal axis. Together ***these veins form a cross*** (Figure 121). These veins with their relatively elastic walls are firmly embedded in their surroundings and thus hold the heart in place. The apex of the heart, however, is not secured. In rhythm with the heart's contractions (systole/diastole), it moves away from the crossed veins and snaps back into place elastically. The heart organ as a whole, therefore, is bound to the cross of veins and moves back and forth rhythmically in front of it. Contemplating this remarkable image can fill us with awe and wonder.

The flow of blood away from the heart carries a very different signature. When the "shortcut" of the ductus arteriosus closes with the newborn's first breath, venous flow is channeled from the right side of the heart to the lungs through the horizontal pulmonary arteries, which wrap around the ascending aorta (Figure 122). This blood

flows first through the almost sagitally oriented arch of the aorta and then through the vertically aligned (unpaired) descending aorta. During the embryonic period, two aortas were present, but the right aorta atrophies, leaving only the one on the left. With the septation of the embryonic heart and the degeneration of the branchial circulation (pharyngeal arches), bilateral symmetry is abandoned in favor of an asymmetry in the right-left dimension. In the front-back dimension, a contrast emerges between the crossing of the veins in the back and the intertwined vessels in front (Figures 121 and 122). It's as if the blood "experiences" something while passing through the heart's inner chambers from back to front. Since we typically move in a forward direction, the front-to-back motion of blood exiting the heart through the major arteries does not correspond to the direction of our bodily activity. Thus the heart also reverses the dimensions of front and back.

In summary, we can conclude that the development of the heart qualitatively reverses all three of the spatial dimensions in which the human body moves. Thus the heart is a place where spatial tendencies are reversed or "turned inside out." This archetypal phenomenon will become even more apparent when we consider the heart's phylogenetic development.

The Function of the Heart

Blood enters the heart "under the sign of the cross," i.e., through the crossing veins. Blood from all parts of the body mingles in the atria and then enters the sacred temple of the ventricles, the "holy of holies," through the atrioventricular valves. This space, with its columnar papillary muscles and arching chordae tendineae, is truly reminiscent of a cathedral (Figure 123). When the muscles contract (systole), the atrioventricular valves close, "sectioning off" a specific volume of blood from the continual flow. As the ventricle contracts, this quantum of blood is pressurized until the semilunar valves spring open, sending the blood

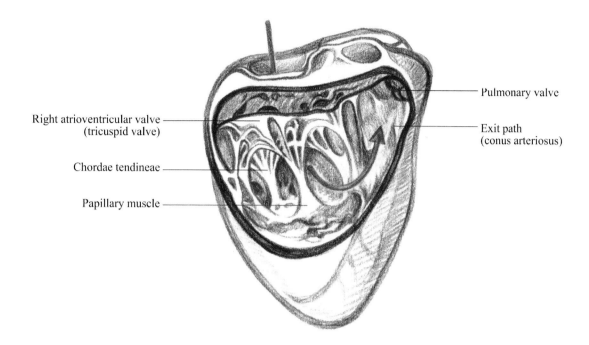

Fig. 123. **Right ventricle** *(view through front opening with atrium removed). The structure of the papillary muscles with their arching chordae tendinae is reminiscent of the interior of a cathedral. Exiting blood flows toward the pulmonary valve. The arrow indicates the reversal in the direction of flow.*

out into the major vessels. Its exit path, however, does not fall in a straight line with its entrance; a reversal occurs in its direction of flow (Figure 123). In the heart, therefore, the bloodstream is quantized (rhythmically isolated and interrupted) and then redirected (from outside to inside, from inside to outside, etc.). But the entire quantum of blood is not ejected. Part of it always remains behind and mixes with the next quantum. Keeping this in mind, we can see the whole process as comparable to homeopathic potentization. This comparison, however, will only prove valuable if there is some functional significance to this mixing of the blood as well.

Let's take another look at the relationships between the shape of the heart and the dimensions of space. If the heart qualitatively reverses the dimensions of space, as described above, this can only mean that the forces of life and soul that are carried by the blood are released from the confines of space. And in fact we can observe that the heart's rhythmic contractions and the quantization of the bloodstream (pulse) insert a rhythmic (i.e., temporal) element into this elemental flow of life. In the organs on the periphery, blood is "used up" as it comes into contact with earthly or material (i.e., spatial) processes. The flow itself is constant, almost "timeless." In the heart, the blood is released from space, so to speak, and enters time. In other words, it takes on temporal structures that serve as healing elements in the body as a whole. The blood's rhythms are not dictated by the heart; they adapt to whatever we are doing at the moment. The heart is simply the place where this adaptation occurs.

Time structures, however, are also the structures of life forces. According to Rudolf Steiner (67), when we are awake, supersensible etheric (life) forces flow constantly from the heart to the head, forming the basis for conceptualization and perception. Steiner called this process the "etherization of the blood." Because these forces are spatial forces by origin, it makes sense that they enable us to "recreate" space as we perceive (in seeing, for example) or when we form mental images of spatial elements.

These thoughts also shed new light on familiar physiological facts. The heart's muscle contractions increase blood pressure from near zero to 80 to 120 mm Hg. Because of this fact, the heart has always been described as a mechanical pump, a view that does not do full justice to its function (cf. reference 68). What is the real significance of blood pressure? Isn't it an indicator of our soul's activity, our desire to be active in space, and our confrontation with the earthly world? Ultimately, the will activity that arises in the heart and radiates into the entire body originates in the human individuality itself. On the periphery, this will activity triggers metabolic processes that in turn (through the blood's respiratory capacity) support very subtle "combustion" processes, that is, warmth processes and life processes. Warmth makes the transition between bodily and soul processes possible.

A brief detour is called for at this point. Under normal circumstances, core temperature remains constant in the torso, which houses the heart in its center. In contrast, body temperatures fluctuate widely in the skin and limbs. Thus streams of warmth, generally following the pathways traveled by the blood, are present in the body. If we consider the qualities of the four "elements"—earth, water, air, and warmth—we can say that cells and organs (especially bones) are the most solidified and "earthly." At the boundary with interstitial or extracellular space (which has a total volume of approximately ten to twelve liters), these (relatively) solid features give way to fluid. Because the circulating blood (about four to six liters) transports respiratory gases (O_2, CO_2, etc.), the entire body is also pervaded with the element of air. Blood, however, is also the organ of warmth transportation.

In metabolic processes in the organs (and especially in the muscles), energy transfers take place constantly. To a certain extent, these transfers are temperature-dependent. Metabolic intensity can be increased by warmth and reduced by cold. (Fevers and hypothermia are impressive examples.) It is conceivable that the will (the actual driving force in metabolic processes) makes use of the warmth in order to manifest its intentions in the form of physical movement. If this is so, the warmth transported by the blood is the actual bridge between bodily and soul processes. Conversely, it is also conceivable that the warmth energy released through metabolism is taken up by the soul and "radiated" into our surroundings in the form of love, empathy, compassion, or devotion. In this case, the blood and circulation serve not only the regulation of (physical) warmth but also the actual transformation of physical forces into soul-spiritual forces, which is how Rudolf Steiner describes the true task of our earthly existence (65). The heart organ, which lies in the center of the circulatory system, is then the place where physical warmth is transformed into soul warmth and vice versa. After all, our language is full of expressions such as "warmth of heart" or "a warm-hearted person." Perhaps what the blood carries into the interior of the organism is more than simply gaseous components (oxygen, etc.) that serve the "combustion" of energy-rich compounds in the tissues. Perhaps the blood also carries forces of intentionality, mediated by warmth. Ultimately, this view could lead to an understanding of psychosomatic processes that originate in the soul but cause bodily health or illness.

Phylogenetic Development of the Heart and Circulatory System

The heart's ontogenetic development, described above, becomes understandable only when we see it against the backdrop of phylogeny (cf. 69, 70).

Centralization

Among **fish** species, the heart still takes the form of a unitary, non septated vascular tube. This S-shaped cardiac tube is located very close to the cranium and directly behind the gills. In the absence of lungs, only venous blood flows through it. As is also the case with the human primordial heart, the cardiac tube in fishes consists of a sequence of four compartments (venous sinus, atrium, ventricle, bulbus cordis) that are separated by constrictions and, in some cases, valvelike structures. There is no "motor" driving systemic circulation. In fishes, circulation is truly "circular" in that the heart is inserted into the venous branch, directly preceding the gills (Figure 124). The heart does not yet occupy a central position in the circulatory system. Capillary surface area, total blood volume, speed of flow, and blood pressure are all still very low in fishes. The pericardium still has an open connection to the abdominal cavity; in effect, the heart is located in a bulge in the abdominal wall. Constant waves of peristaltic contractions run through the cardiac tube from the venous sinus to the bulbus cordis. When valves are present at all, their function is simply to regulate the flow.

Fundamental changes occur in these structures only when branchial respiration is replaced by **pulmonary respiration**. Blood from the lungs, unlike blood from any other organ, has to flow back to the heart instead of simply continuing into systemic circulation. This fact places the lungs in opposition to the other organs, and pulmonary circulation comes to occupy a unique position within the system as a whole. The emergence of pulmonary respiration supplies the heart with two different types of blood, arterialized blood from the lungs and venous blood from the body. The necessary consequences of this development are cardiac septation and the transition from circular to lemniscatic circulation (Figure 125). The division of the heart into chambers is a dramatic process that is achieved only through multiple interim steps and "detours" in phylogeny. We will call this process **centralization** because the fully septated heart abandons its original peripheral location and descends into the ribcage to lie in the center of the circulatory system as a whole.

Centralization of circulation begins with the **Dipnoi** or lungfish (Figures 125 and 126). These animals live in mud, or sometimes in water-free habitats in the transition zone between water and land. Lungfish have gills, but they also have a metamorphosed swim bladder or related organ that also serves respiration. As a result, arterialized blood flows into the heart at least some of the time. The veins coming from the air-breathing organ are still branches of the portal vein, so venous and arterial blood mingle in the circulatory vessels as well as in the heart. Septa begin to develop, however, as the heart makes a first attempt to live up to its new task of separating the two types of blood. It is important to emphasize that the transformation of the heart is peripherally triggered; the heart simply reacts to what comes toward it from outside. Mirroring of peripheral processes, in fact, is one of the fundamental attributes of this miraculous organ, which always "selflessly" attempts to optimize the functioning of the entire system.

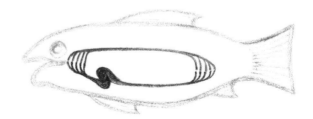

*Fig. 124: **Circulatory system in fish** (adapted from Portmann, 48). The S-shaped cardiac tube is located in the venous branch of circulation and directly precedes the branchial (pharyngeal) arches.*

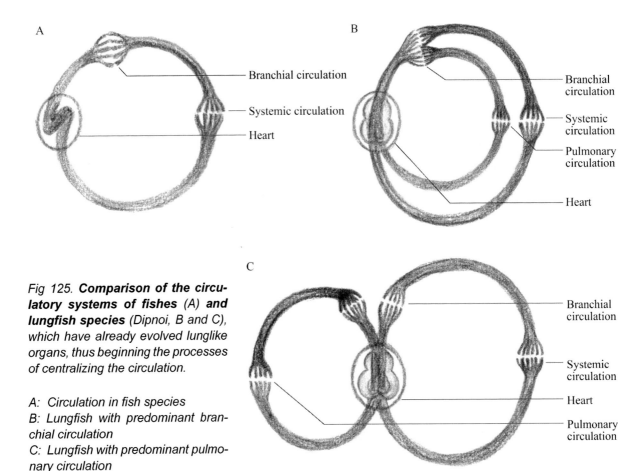

A

B

— Branchial circulation

— Systemic circulation

— Heart

— Branchial circulation

— Systemic circulation

— Pulmonary circulation

— Heart

C

— Branchial circulation

— Systemic circulation

— Heart

— Pulmonary circulation

Fig 125. **Comparison of the circulatory systems of fishes** (A) **and lungfish species** *(Dipnoi, B and C), which have already evolved lunglike organs, thus beginning the processes of centralizing the circulation.*

A: Circulation in fish species
B: Lungfish with predominant branchial circulation
C: Lungfish with predominant pulmonary circulation

Distinct progress in the direction of centralization occurs in **amphibians**, who are clearly "dual citizens" of land and water. Their larvae are "fish" with tails, branchial respiration, and completely venous hearts. As adults, they abandon the tail and develop limbs. This decisive step toward mastering terrestrial life is possible only because amphibians also develop lungs. Amphibians' lungs, however, are not their only organ of respiration. They must compete with the skin, which serves as a powerful respiratory organ and can completely substitute for the lungs under certain conditions (Figure 127). Clearly, the "internalization" of respiration is not completed in amphibians. However, the development of lungs is not the only milestone in this process. The pulmonary vessels connect to the heart, laying the foundation for independent pulmonary circulation; the pulmonary veins already empty into the atrium. (In salamander embryos, this junction still occurs lower down, near the spot where the inferior vena cava enters the heart.) In contrast, the vessels of cutaneous circulation remain on the periphery throughout the animal's life. In a certain sense, cutaneous circulation and pulmonary circulation form a polarity (Figure 127). In species in which the heart takes precedence, septation is more advanced; where cutaneous circulation predominates, cardiac septation is minimal. The lungs send arterialized blood into the left atrium, the skin sends it into the right atrium (via the subclavian vein). In evolutionary terms, cutaneous circulation has little influence on the shape of the heart and must be seen as a retarding element.

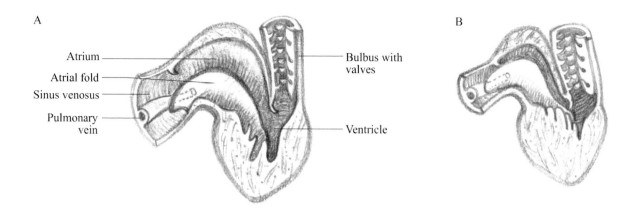

Fig. 126. **Structure of the heart in a lungfish,** Neoceratodus *(adapted from Portmann, 48). A: dilated atrium. Branchial circulation predominates, and the blood flowing through the heart is primarily venous. B: contracted atrium. Pulmonary circulation predominates. The atrial fold permits a certain degree of separation of venous and arterial blood. The blood flowing into the heart is more mixed.*

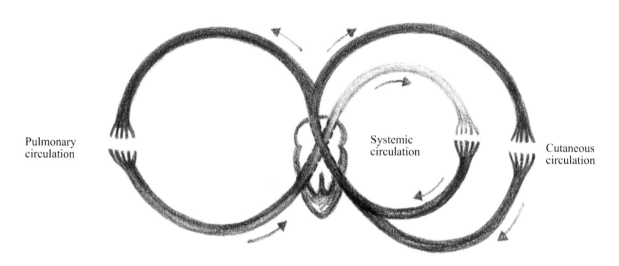

Fig. 127. **Structure of the circulatory system in amphibians.** *A septum begins to divide the atrium into two sections, partially separating venous and arterial blood. Cutaneous respiration is a retarding factor.*

Organisms become increasingly independent of the outer world through the evolutionary concentration of respiratory processes in an internal organ (lung), beginning with amphibians, and the later development of warm-bloodedness (the ability to maintain a constant body temperature independent of external temperatures). Upgrading the body's internal organization, which is asso-ciated with an increase in capillary surface area, initiates a process of separation from the environment that achieves its zenith in humans, ultimately providing the bodily basis for the development of the "I". This evolutionary process, which is especially evident in the development of the circulatory system, can also be called ***individuation***—in other words, evolution in the

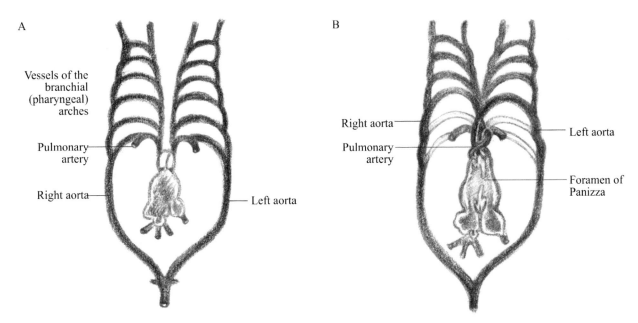

A

Vessels of the branchial (pharyngeal) arches

Pulmonary artery

Right aorta

Left aorta

B

Right aorta

Pulmonary artery

Left aorta

Foramen of Panizza

*Fig. 128. **Comparison of circulatory organization in amphibians** (A) **and primitive reptiles**, e.g. lizards (B). The structure of the circulatory system is still bilaterally symmetrical. Separation of venous and arterial blood in the heart increases in reptiles as a result of improved septation, but since the left aorta originates in the right ventricle and the right aorta in the left, this separation must be partially reversed by the foramen of Panizza.*

direction of an entity independent of its environment, as typified by the human being as an "I"-being (cf. 54).

The earliest beginnings of individuation occur in amphibians, through the development of a still-imperfect **centralized circulation** and the first steps toward independent pulmonary circulation.

Reptiles. It is interesting to note that cutaneous respiration generally disappears in reptiles (crocodiles, tortoises, snakes, lizards), whose skins become scaly. This represents a major step in the centralization of circulation. Cardiac septation would be almost complete in reptiles were it not for a few new "errors" or imperfections that creep in. Reptilian species are still heavily dependent on their environment because they cannot maintain constant body temperatures. In reptiles, the major vascular trunks close to the heart (such as the right and left aortas) are still bilaterally symmetrical. In amphibians, the atria are separated by a septum but the ventricles remain united. In reptiles, an interventricular septum develops for the first time. In

lower reptilian species such as lizards, ventricular separation remains incomplete, while in higher forms such as crocodiles the separation extends as far as the roots of the aortas. Were it not for the bilateral symmetry of the major vessels, complete separation of pulmonary and systemic circulation would now be possible. As things stand, however, complete ventricular septation would shut the left aorta off from the right (venous) side of the heart and the right aorta off from the left (arterial side). Since this arrangement is functionally untenable, a secondary hole develops in the septum (the so-called foramen of Panizza, see Figures 128 and 129) to allow arterial blood from the left ventricle to pass into the right ventricle and thus also into the left aorta.

Because they are not yet able to regulate their body temperature, reptiles remain heavily dependent on their environment. They live partly in water and partly on land, and their circulation adjusts accordingly. On land, pulmonary circulation predominates. Blood pressure in

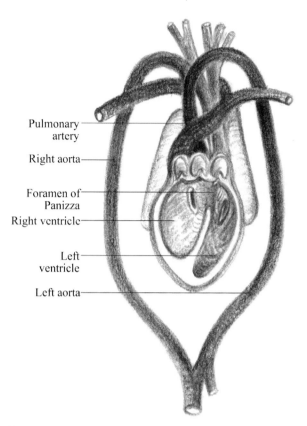

Pulmonary artery

Right aorta

Foramen of Panizza

Right ventricle

Left ventricle

Left aorta

*Fig. 129. **Structure of the heart in more highly evolved reptiles**, e.g. crocodiles (Benninghoff, 70). The ventricular septum is almost complete but must remain partially open (foramen of Panizza) so that the left aorta, which emerges from the right ventricle, does not receive only venous blood.*

the left ventricle (the more muscular of the two ventricles) and the right aorta increases, so that more arterialized blood passes through the foramen of Panizza and into the left aorta. As a result, the body (especially the brain and sensory organs) is pervaded with more **oxygen-enriched** blood. Body temperature increases, and the animals become more alert and active. Before submerging in water, a reptile such as a crocodile usually breathes deeply to expand its lungs. Once underwater, it often remains relatively motionless for long periods. Due to the resulting congestion in the lungs, blood pressure increases in the pulmonary circulation and the right ventricle begins to work harder. Blood pressure then also increases in the left aorta

(which originates in the right ventricle), and more **venous** blood reaches the systemic circulation. The animal becomes less active and less alert and begins to doze off. By abandoning cutaneous respiration and relying exclusively on pulmonary respiration, reptiles take a major evolutionary step toward lemniscatic reconfiguration of the circulatory system. But they still do not achieve complete separation of pulmonary and systemic circulation, and circulating blood always remains more or less mixed, depending on activity levels and ambient temperatures.

Birds are the first group to develop complete cardiac septation. It is interesting to note that they do so by simply abandoning the "offending" left aorta, which creates the need for secondary perforation of the intraventricular septum in reptiles. Birds retain only the right aorta, which emerges from the left ventricle. As a result, both branchial circulation and the bilateral symmetry of the major vessels near the heart are abandoned for the first time in the history of evolution. Also for the first time, the structural principle of asymmetry is realized. The absence of the second aorta in birds is not the result of secondary regression but occurs directly and seemingly deliberately, as if bird species "learn" from the example of reptiles. In birds, development of the interaortic septum is suppressed, and only a **single** aorta develops from the very beginning. Thus the "proximal aorta of birds corresponds to the undivided aorta in the trunk and bulbus cordis of lower vertebrates" (Benninghoff, 70). In birds, the lungs become the exclusive organ of respiration. They are highly differentiated and capable of completely arterializing the circulating blood. Pulmonary and systemic circulation are completely separated; the mingling of venous and arterial blood no longer occurs in the heart.

Nonetheless, the avian circulatory system does not achieve the degree of perfection evident in mammals and primates. Asymmetry develops in the wrong direction, so to speak (Figure 130). As discussed above (cf. Figure 120), the right side of the heart, which is pervaded with venous blood, belongs qualitatively to the left side of the body, while the left (arterial) side of the heart

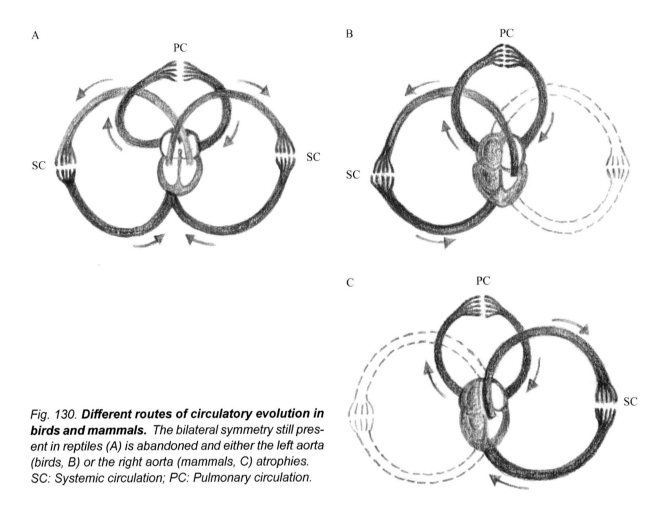

*Fig. 130. **Different routes of circulatory evolution in birds and mammals.** The bilateral symmetry still present in reptiles (A) is abandoned and either the left aorta (birds, B) or the right aorta (mammals, C) atrophies. SC: Systemic circulation; PC: Pulmonary circulation.*

belongs more to the body's right side. In birds, development of the ***right*** aorta, which comes from the left side of the heart and is filled with arterial blood, results in an incomplete reversal of right and left. Asymmetry is accomplished "inappropriately." In contrast, mammals "correctly" accomplish the reversal of laterality in the heart by suppressing the development of the right aorta while retaining the left (Figure 130).

From the functional perspective, the structure of the avian heart is the most advanced among vertebrates. Birds' rapid metabolism corresponds to high body temperature, rapid pulse, relatively high blood pressure, and the relatively great weight of the heart in comparison to the rest of the body. Birds are alert, highly active animals that have freed themselves from the Earth and

conquered the atmosphere to a large extent. They could be described as "head animals," beings dominated by processes that take place in the head in humans. Birds are most active in the sensory domain; metabolism as such takes a back seat. Therefore, metabolically inefficient use of blood in bird tissues places greater demands on the heart. The chambers of the heart are enlarged, smooth-walled, and largely lacking in netlike (trabecular) internal structures. The heart muscles are powerful, and the heart's relative weight is 1.4 times greater than in mammals of similar size. In birds, life processes are not yet "internalized" by the heart as they are in humans. Birds live as if in a fever, fully active in and interacting with their environment. Consequently, the heart (as the inner, resting pole of centralized circulation

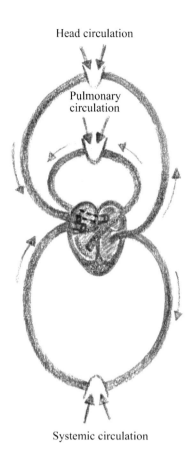

Fig. 131. **Organization of the circulatory system in mammals and humans.** *Paired aortas disappear; the system has become asymmetrical. Functional three-foldness first appears in mammals and is perfected in humans.*

Concentration

To understand the final evolutionary stage of the cardiovascular system as achieved by humans, we must still consider a second major evolutionary trend, namely, the process of **concentration**. Centralization leads to cardiac septation and the vertical separation of the heart into right and left halves; concentration leads to a restructuring of the chambers and the formation of valves in the horizontal plane, i.e., to the development of two functionally different types of chambers, the atria and the ventricles.

In **fish** species, the heart is a simple tube consisting of a linear sequence of spaces (venous sinus, atrium, ventricle, bulbus). The ventricle compartment is nothing more that a loose-meshed spongy mass (Figure 132).

In **amphibians**, leaflike septa develop in the ventricle area. This is the first evidence of the evolutionary tendency to concentrate the four types of interior cardiac spaces into two by incorporating the venous sinus into the atrium and the bulbus cordis into the ventricle (Figure 133). This process occurs simultaneously with centralization and is finalized only in mammals. In the mammalian heart, the atrium still has two visibly different sections, a smooth-walled portion (the

and thus as the place where the dimensions are reversed) cannot develop completely. Birds "overshoot the mark." Although they do achieve complete cardiac septation (i.e., centralization), warm-bloodedness, and asymmetry of the vessels near the heart, they do not achieve complete dimensional reversal or (more importantly) the final stages in the development of the heart's internal structure.

Mammals and humans. The last stage in the transition from a bilaterally symmetrical vascular system with paired aortas to a completely asymmetrical system appears for the first time in mammals, which retain only the left aorta, thus completing the reversal of dimensions in the heart (Figures 130 and 131).

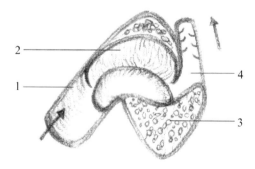

Fig. 132. **Structure of a fish heart** *(Benninghoff, 70). The heart consists of loose-meshed spongy muscle tissue and takes the form of an S-shaped tube with four successive compartments: 1: venous sinus, 2: atrium, 3: ventricle, 4: bulbus cordis.*

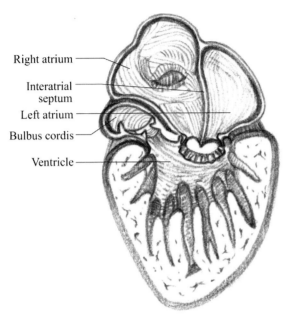

Fig. 133. **Structure of an amphibian heart** *(frog, from Portman, 48). The leaflike ventricular septa are clearly visible.*

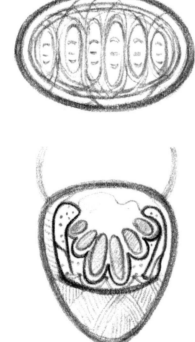

Fig. 134. **Muscle structure of the amphibian heart** *(frog, from Benninghoff, 70). Leaflike septa separate the ventricle into many little fissurelike spaces. Muscle fibers are arranged in perpendicular circular and longitudinal bundles.*

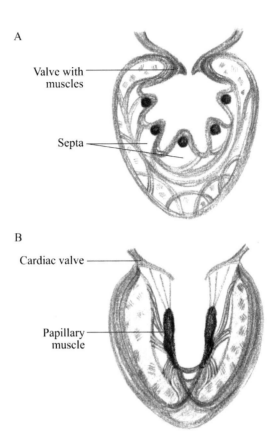

Fig. 135. **Comparison of ventricular muscle structure in amphibians and mammals**. *A: In amphibians (cold-blooded), the ventricle is subdivided by septa and the muscles are arranged three-dimensionally. The valves are still muscular. B: In mammals, this arrangement is transformed into a lemniscatic system of compact heart muscles, papillary muscles, and tendinous valves.*

former venous sinus) and the netlike (trabecular) auricle (the former atrium). In the ventricle, the smooth-walled outflow channel corresponds to the former bulbus, the trabecular influx channel with its papillary muscles to the former ventricle compartment.

As concentration progresses, the **heart muscles** are also transformed. In **amphibians and reptiles**, the spongy, undivided ventricle muscles become a system of hollow spaces separated by leaflike septa. The walls of these spaces consist of strands of muscles that run at right angles to each other in all three dimensions of space (Figure 134).

A

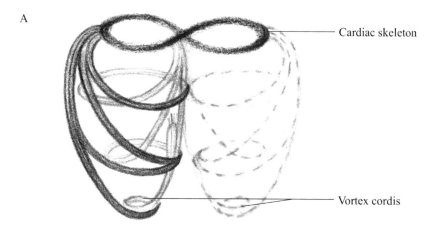

Cardiac skeleton

Vortex cordis

B

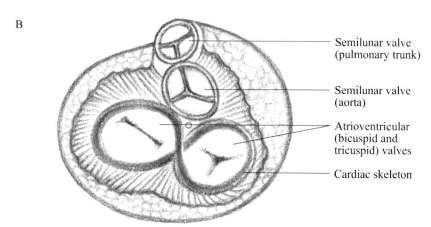

Semilunar valve
(pulmonary trunk)

Semilunar valve
(aorta)

Atrioventricular
(bicuspid and
tricuspid) valves

Cardiac skeleton

*Fig. 136. **Spiral arrangement of ventricular musculature and the structure of the cardiac skeleton in the human being** (adapted from Benninghoff, 70). The muscles spiral to the left in the right ventricle and to the right in the left ventricle. The tricuspid and bicuspid valves are anchored in a lemniscate of tendons (the cardiac skeleton), which also provides attachment points for the atrial and ventricular muscles.
A: Arrangement of muscle fibers in the left and right ventricles;
B: View of the geometric plane of the valves of the human heart, showing the cardiac skeleton in red.*

The outer and inner longitudinal muscle bundles are separated by a central layer of perpendicular bundles. Along with the system of septa, therefore, the original spongy chamber has developed differentiated musculature consisting of a compact outer layer and inner, leaflike septa. Through concentration of the cardiac compartments, the originally sequentially arranged valves shift to a single plane (the valve plane) for the first time in **birds and mammals**. Muscles that formerly ran in all three directions are linked into lemniscates and spirals, and the original muscular bulges at the transitions between the compartments of the cardiac tube are transformed into the tricuspid, bicuspid, and semilunar valves. The ventricular musculature now consists of right and left muscle spirals, which together form a large lemniscate (Figure 135).The papillary muscles are fibers left

over from the many little ventricular septa, some of which remain in place instead of shifting to the ventricle wall. Through the disappearance of these septa, the interior volume of the ventricles increases and their muscular walls become more compact (Figures 135 and 136).

Upgrading of the body's internal organization in the course of evolution greatly increases the capillary surface area of organs, with a corresponding increase in peripheral vascular resistance. In response, the heart muscle becomes thicker, the heart's internal space enlarges to increase its capacity, and the heart begins to work more efficiently. In a related phenomenon, the valves of the heart become mechanized, i.e., muscle folds are replaced by the plates of tendon and connective tissue that form the tricuspid, bicuspid, and semilunar valves.

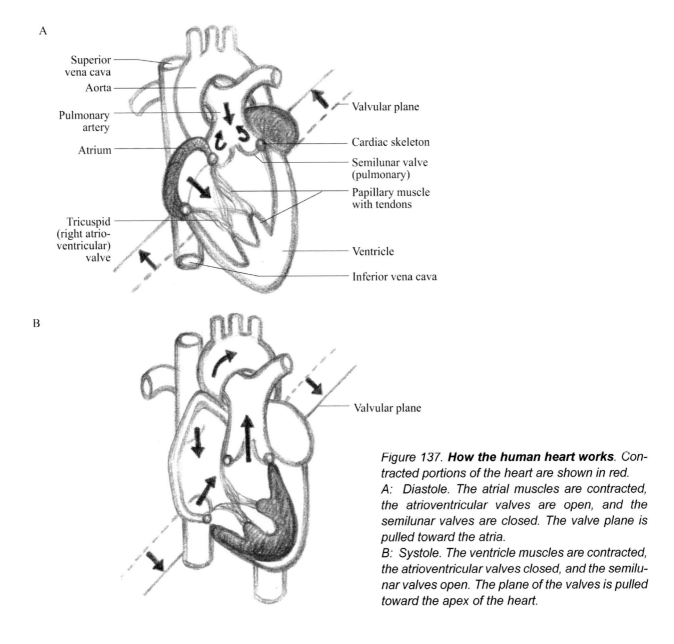

A

Superior vena cava
Aorta
Pulmonary artery
Atrium
Tricuspid (right atrio-ventricular) valve

Valvular plane
Cardiac skeleton
Semilunar valve (pulmonary)
Papillary muscle with tendons
Ventricle
Inferior vena cava

B

Valvular plane

Figure 137. **How the human heart works**. *Contracted portions of the heart are shown in red.*
A: Diastole. The atrial muscles are contracted, the atrioventricular valves are open, and the semilunar valves are closed. The valve plane is pulled toward the atria.
B: Systole. The ventricle muscles are contracted, the atrioventricular valves closed, and the semilunar valves open. The plane of the valves is pulled toward the apex of the heart.

In lower vertebrates, **cardiac action** still takes the form of a peristaltic wave running from one end of the S-shaped cardiac tube to the other. In the course of the concentration process, as the heart's interior spaces enlarge and its muscles are transformed from perpendicular, crossing bands (septa) to spirally arranged strands (Figure 136), the heart's contraction pattern also changes from a peristaltic wave to rhythmic, saccadic contractions (systole and diastole). This change, however, is predicated on the development of the **cardiac skeleton**. Between the atrial and ventricular muscles, a lemniscate of tendons develops around the bicuspid and tricuspid valves (Figure 136) and serves as a tendon attachment for the muscles. In many mammals, this tendinous structure incorporates bits of cartilage or even bone. The cardiac skeleton with its valves defines

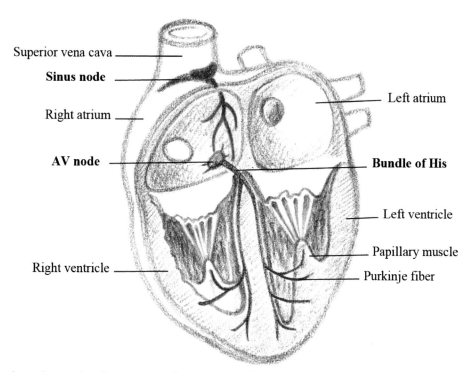

Superior vena cava

Sinus node

Right atrium

AV node

Right ventricle

Left atrium

Bundle of His

Left ventricle

Papillary muscle

Purkinje fiber

*Fig. 138. **The heart's conduction system**. Spontaneous rhythmical impulses emanate from the sinus node ("pacemaker") in the right atrium. These impulses spread through the atrial muscles and finally reach the atrioventricular node (AV node), which directly determines ventricular rhythm. The bundle of His enters the ventricle through a hole in the cardiac skeleton and divides into two branches that run along the cardiac septum to the ventricular muscles, where they subdivide into the Purkinje fibers carrying the electrical impulse to the papillary muscles.*

the valve plane, which shifts either toward the apex of the heart (at systole) or toward the atria (at diastole) as the heart contracts rhythmically (Figure 137). But development of the cardiac skeleton and valves, which is a prerequisite for the functioning of the human heart, breaks the connection between the atrial and ventricular muscles. To maintain a functional connection between atria and ventricles, a small portion of the original muscle connection is maintained and differentiates into the **conducting system** of the heart, which does not exist in lower vertebrates. This system consists of specialized muscle fibers with the ability to send out spontaneous stimuli in rhythmic succession (70 to 80 per minute). These stimuli originate in the sinus node (Keith-Flack), which serves as the heart's natural pacemaker. They cause the atrial or ventricular muscles to contract (Figure 138). The stimuli spread through the atrial muscles until they reach the atrioventricular node (Aschoff-Tawara), which lies at

the base of the right atrium (Figure 138). The waves of impulses (40 to 50 per minute) that determine the rhythm of ventricular contractions originate in the AV node and spread via the Bundle of His and its two branches, which follow the ventricular septum, into the ventricular and papillary muscles.

Restructuring the heart's muscles and shifting the location of the valves splits the heart into two functional domains, and the conduction system, which is both autonomic and independent, reunites it. Concentration of the cardiac spaces and rhythmical movement necessitate this heart-specific automatism. Interruption of blood flow in the ventricles and the action of related valve mechanisms rhythmicize the formerly more-or-less constant flow of blood on the periphery. *The pulse originates in the heart.* Through the heart's rhythmical activity, a temporal element enters the (spatial) vascular system. In mammals and humans, metabolism is more of a factor than it is in

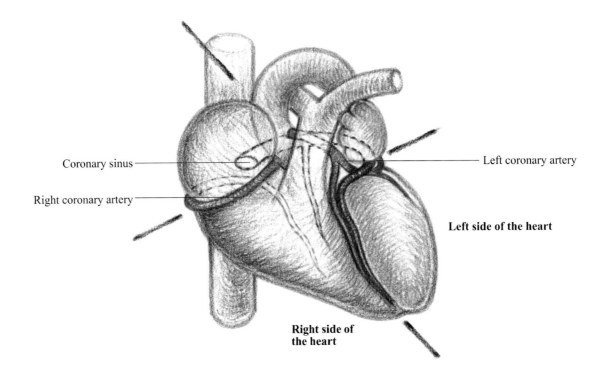

Coronary sinus

Right coronary artery

Left coronary artery

Left side of the heart

Right side of the heart

Fig. 139. **Architecture of the coronary vessels**. *The arteries and veins of the right and left halves of the heart have different characteristic signatures (for details, see text).*

birds, and the rhythmicization of the bloodstream is correspondingly more harmonious. Blood pressure, blood flow, and respiratory intensity are all more moderate. In higher mammals, and especially in humans, time and space interact harmoniously in the heart, the center of the rhythmic system. In humans, this interaction supplies the basis for the development of individuality, i.e., the incarnation of the "I"—a step that also depends on an appropriate integration of the body into the dimensions of space (in other words, on uprightness). Only in the upright human body can the heart assume its "correct" position within the three dimensions and ultimately also achieve the reversal of the front-back dimension as described above. In humans, the smooth-walled interior spaces of the avian heart are replaced by cathedrallike ventricular structures where the direction of the bloodstream is reversed and blood flow is rhythmicized and redirected (Figures 123 and 137).

The evolutionary process of concentration explains still another phenomenon, namely, the development of the **coronary vessels**. Like the musculature of the conduction system, these vessels are not present in lower vertebrates. The spongy muscle of a fish heart (Figure 132) can still be supplied by the general flow of blood. A dedicated system of vessels to supply the heart becomes necessary in higher vertebrates due to increasing thickness of the chamber wall musculature. Two coronary arteries emerge from the root of the aorta. The right artery runs relatively horizontally, following the atrioventricular groove, while the main branch of the left artery is nearly vertical and follows the groove between the right and left ventricles (Figure 139). At the back of the heart, the veins empty into a fairly large venous sinus (coronary sinus, see Figure 139) in the atrioventricular groove. The signature of this vascular architecture is indeed surprising. The right side of the heart is venous, the left side arterial—a reversal of the bilateral symmetry of the body as a whole (cf. Figure 120). In the coronary arteries, which connect the two ventricles, the gesture is again reversed. The great cardiac *vein* and coronary sinus wrap around the *arterial* left side of the heart, while the major vessel on the right, the right coronary artery, which wraps around the *venous* side of the heart, carries *arterial* blood. On the left side of the heart, the venous system is horizontally oriented and the arterial vertically, while on the right side the arterial system is horizontal and the venous vertical (Figure 139). It is as if the heart's own supply system, which wraps the ventricles in a loving embrace, is attempting to functionally harmonize the whole by balancing out the reversed dimensionality that the heart has acquired in the course of evolution. The coronary vessels occupy a unique position within the vascular system as a whole, which may help to explain why they are often the first to develop pathologies (heart attack, etc.) as a result of psychological stress and rhythmical disharmonies (dysrhythmias, arrythmias).

Fetal Circulation

In the adult body, the functional domain of circulation lies in the polarity between the upper and lower body (the nerve-sense system on the one hand and the metabolic-limb system on the other) and in the center (pulmonary circulation, etc.; see Figure 108) that balances these opposing systems. In the fetal stage, however, polarities have not yet developed. Everything the fetus needs comes from the placenta—in other words, from the outside, from the protective surrounding sphere. The umbilical vessels permit a circulation of sorts between placenta and fetus, but this circulation still lacks any polar differentiation since the major organ systems (especially the lungs as the organ of respiration) are not yet functional. As in lower vertebrates, the heart still receives mixed venous and arterial blood (Figures 140 and 141). The venous and arterial bloodstreams are separated

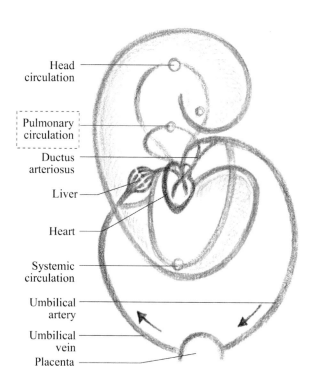

Head circulation

Pulmonary circulation

Ductus arteriosus

Liver

Heart

Systemic circulation

Umbilical artery

Umbilical vein

Placenta

Fig. 140. ***Diagram of fetal circulation.*** *Circulation within the embryo is still "dormant" and not yet structured as a threefold system. Gaseous exchange takes place exclusively in the placenta, outside of the embryonic body. Arterialized (oxygenated) blood flows through the umbilical vein to the liver and then to the right atrium, where it mingles with venous blood from systemic circulation. Bypassing the right ventricle, the blood passes through the foramen ovale into the left atrium and out through the aorta into the body. Most of the venous blood in the right ventricle does not flow through the pulmonary artery to the lungs, which are not yet functional, but instead flows into the aorta via a second shortcut, the ductus arteriosus. As a result, the aorta carries mixed blood. Complete separation of venous and arterial blood occurs only after birth.*

in the heart only after birth, when the foramen ovale and ductus arteriosus close. With the baby's first breath, circulatory threefoldness, with all of its inherent tensions, suddenly becomes functional (Figures 140 and 141) as the all-encompassing security of the womb is abandoned. From now on, the human individuality must proceed, step

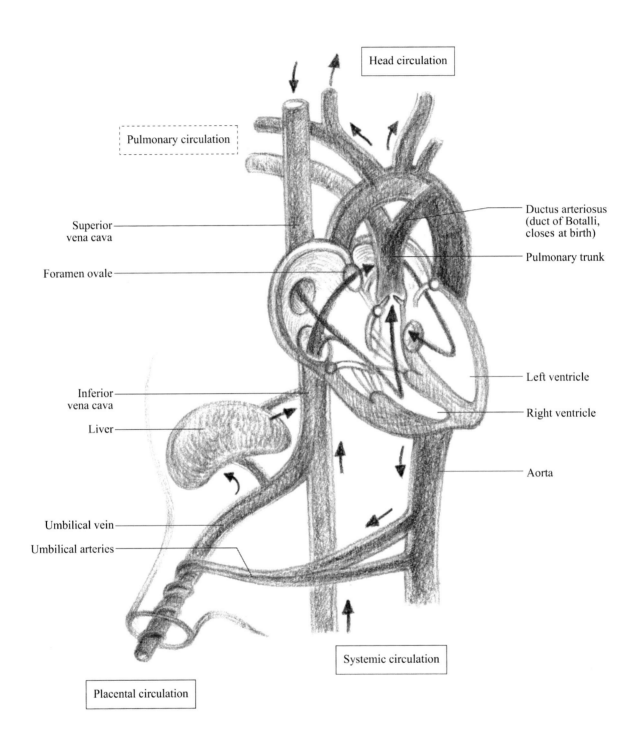

Head circulation

Pulmonary circulation

Ductus arteriosus
(duct of Botalli,
closes at birth)

Superior
vena cava

Pulmonary trunk

Foramen ovale

Inferior
vena cava

Left ventricle

Liver

Right ventricle

Aorta

Umbilical vein
Umbilical arteries

Systemic circulation

Placental circulation

Fig. 141. **The heart in fetal circulation**. *The blood that flows to the brain and sense organs contains more oxygen than the blood supplied to the lungs and the organs of the lower body. Thus an oxygen gradient exists between the upper and lower halves of the body. From the pulmonary trunk, venous blood from the right ventricle (ultimately, primarily from the brain) flows through the ductus arteriosus into the aorta below the point where the arteries supplying the head branch off. The aorta then carries mixed, oxygen-poor blood to the rest of the body.*

Age	Relative weight of heart (g/kg body weight)
Newborn 1 month 2 months 3 months	7.6 5.1 4.8 3.8
4-15 months	5.0

Table 17. Postnatal changes in relative heart weight.

by step, to assume control of the functional tensions that result from the activities of various organs. Pulmonary respiration is the first step. Next, the nerve-sense system comes into play as the vital reflexes of sucking and grasping are activated. Gradually, the metabolic system adapts to "earthly" food. Thermoregulation, in which the circulatory system plays a central role, is initially very weak; in the first few weeks of life, infants cannot perspire. The heart also gradually begins to adapt to its new functional circumstances. The relative weight of the heart, quite large in the embryo, decreases rapidly after birth and gradually increases again only after the third month (Table 17). This phenomenon demonstrates the dramatic scope of the functional changes in the heart and circulatory organs in the transition from embryonic to "earthly" life. It takes about twenty years for this system to mature completely and become a secure foundation for the individuality.

The Empirical Principle In the Evolution of the Circulatory System

To an unbiased view, the consistent, logical "improvements" to the circulatory system from one evolutionary level to the next—cardiac septation, for example—are quite striking. But the goal-oriented (orthogenetic) thrust of this development

becomes fully apparent only in view of the final stage, the human heart and circulatory system. As the human heart takes its place in three-dimensional space, it "reverses" the dimensions, qualitatively speaking. The heart is a place where space gives way to time, where spatial forces intermingle with temporal structures (rhythm, pulse). This function of the human heart, which is incisive for the incarnation of the human "I" and its existence in earthly space, can proceed smoothly only once the heart becomes the actual center of the body; that is, when circulation is fully centralized and the dimensions (right/left, up/down, etc.) have been reversed—or better, turned inside out—in the heart. In the entire vertebrate series, the heart only achieves this unique position in the human body because only we humans walk completely upright, with our heads oriented toward the heavens and the Earth at our feet (cephalocaudal orientation). Thus the phylogenetic development of the cardiovascular system is also intimately related to the development of the individuality, or *individuation*. A completely upright organism inserts itself into the dimensions of space in "functionally appropriate" ways, and a heart that reverses the body's relationships to these dimensions makes it possible for the organism to step outside of space. Ultimately, only such a body can receive an "I"-being for whom individual freedom is a reality.

This, then, is the *goal of evolution*. Animal species are preliminary stages in this development, and the ultimate goal is not achieved in the first attempt. The structural plan of each level represents an additional step toward the goal. Here we are not comparing individual animal species or groups of species, which always adapt to specific environments, but only the structural plans of the major vertebrate classes (fishes, amphibians, reptiles, etc.). There are no transitional stages between these classes—a fact that no theory of evolution can avoid. It has often been said that nature learns only from its successes, not from its mistakes (49). While indubitably true of the processes of adaptation and selection, this statement is not true of antiadaptation, which we discussed in an earlier chapter (cf. Figure 48), nor is it true of the empirical principle we will describe now. In the end, there is no getting around the fact that progress occurs from one structural level to the next and that this progress is cumulative in a way that suggests nature does indeed "learn" from the mistakes or imperfections of each previous level.

With the transition to life on dry land ("setting foot on the Earth") in amphibians, an initially very imperfect pulmonary circulation began to develop, and with it the centralization of circulation into a lemniscate with the heart at its center. The crossing point of a lemniscate is clearly a point of reversal. In amphibians, this lemniscatic pattern of circulation lays the foundation for later dimensional reversals, but centralization is limited by cutaneous respiration, which is still possible in amphibians and plays a substantial role in some species.

On the next structural level, reptiles—as if having "learned" from amphibians—do away with cutaneous respiration and associated circulatory features. The reptile body becomes covered with protective scales. Cardiac septation (and thus also the reversal of the right-left dimension) can now be completed, but once again "mistakes" are introduced. The bilateral symmetry of the vessels near the heart (right and left aortic arches, etc.) is still preserved, necessitating a secondary perforation of the ventricular septum in the foramen of Panizza.

The next level once again seems to learn from the previous structural stage. From the very beginning, birds abandon the bilateral structure of the vessels close to the heart, introducing an asymmetry of the major vessels (aorta, etc.) and atrial veins. Concentration of the heart's compartments continues but is not quite completed. Complete septation is achieved for the first time, and pulmonary and systemic circulations are completely separated. Warm-bloodedness is also achieved on this level. Once again, however, "mistakes" are introduced. Birds become one-sided sensory beings; their metabolic organs are underdeveloped and they give up contact with the Earth and its spatial

dimensions to the greatest extent possible. In the avian heart, reversal of the dimensions occurs in the "wrong" way—the right aorta (instead of the left) is preserved, the transformation of the heart (concentration of its interior spaces, etc.) is not completed, and the right atrioventricular valve is still muscular. In effect, birds "overshoot the mark" and become one-sidedly "antidimensional," shunning the Earth.

Again, this experience seems to have consequences on the next structural level. Mammal species master metabolism and develop a "system-appropriate" cardiac asymmetry: the left aorta becomes the primary vessel. In mammals, the process of concentration is completed, and warm-bloodedness leads to a harmonious balance between sensory and metabolic processes. The full scope of this harmonization, which is accompanied by a considerable degree of independence from environmental conditions and represents the final stage in the individuation process, becomes evident only on the human level.

This does not mean that the ancestors of humans were mammals, birds, or reptiles. Instead, we must imagine a central stream in evolution that always remained flexible and capable of further development; its very flexibility meant that it left few or no traces in the paleontological record. This stream is where we must look for the unfinished, still flexible, perhaps "primitive" organisms that allowed evolution to continue in the physical world (cf. 52). This stream is the fertile ground that repeatedly produced new organizational forms, each with a structural plan more perfect than the last. Organizational forms that remained plastic and flexible allowed the "experience" gained from adaptive processes to influence each level's new structural model (the empirical principle). This new model then formed the basis for the great variety of new species and individual organisms that appeared on that level. As newly emerged species gradually adapted to specific habitats, the principles of adaptation and selection took effect as a matter of course.

The Respiratory System

Along with the heart and its major blood vessels, the chest cavity also houses the lungs, the other major organ of the rhythmic system. The lungs are the center of the respiratory system just as the heart is the center of the circulatory system. If we are not content to view the subject of gaseous exchange superficially, we will find that the rhythmic activity of respiration conceals many secrets that are intimately bound up with the essential nature of the human being and with human life on Earth. These secrets are not easy to fathom.

We have already seen that pulmonary respiration begins to play a significant role in vertebrate phylogeny only with the transition from aquatic to terrestrial life. In the evolution of the respiratory organs, three unique features or "archetypal phenomena" become apparent:

1. The lungs and respiratory passages do not develop independently but originate as part of the digestive tract (specifically, as a ventrally located glandlike offshoot).

2. Because the lungs develop only one ductal system, the same air passages must be used for both inhalation and exhalation. This illuminates the need for rhythmic respiration.

3. Surprisingly, the entrance to the respiratory passages is not located at the beginning of the respiratory organs themselves. Instead, it lies above the oral cavity, in the area of the (future) nostrils. As a result, the respiratory and digestive tracts cross. Although this arrangement possesses certain inherent complications (the possibility of choking or of food entering the air passages, etc.), it ultimately provides the basis for the development of speech.

The Connection between the Respiratory and Digestive Systems
(First Archetypal Phenomenon)

Because the respiratory system separates from the digestive tract in the course of development, it is often seen as belonging exclusively to the metabolic system. In fact, however, it can be divided into three functionally distinct sections:

1. The lungs, where gaseous exchange occurs and air encounters the "inner world" in the form of the blood;

2. The airways, which transport air and link the system to the outer world;

3. The organs of speech (larynx, etc.), which serve speech and sound production.

The first archetypal phenomenon (the respiratory system's connection to the digestive tract) makes sense when we take a closer look at the processes of gaseous exchange. Although the lungs are the primary organ of gaseous exchange (oxygen absorption and carbon dioxide elimination), in a much more comprehensive sense this function is incorporated into the entire organism and pervades all of its life processes. Each individual cell "breathes"; in other words, it needs oxygen to do its job, and it gives off carbon dioxide as a waste product. Just as the pulse wave moves from the heart to the body's periphery, respiration also pervades the entire organism. As a result, we must distinguish between "internal"

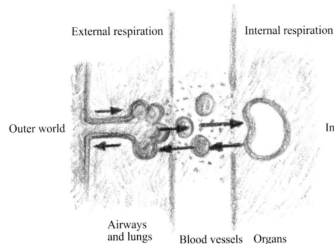

External respiration

Internal respiration

Outer world

Inner world

Airways
and lungs

Blood vessels   Organs

*Fig. 142. **Basic respiratory processes**. External respiration (via the airways and lungs) is complemented by internal respiration, i.e., gaseous exchange between the blood and tissues (organs, cells, etc.). The blood vessels link and balance these two processes.*

respiration (in cells and tissues) and "external" respiration (ventilation and gaseous exchange in the lungs). The vascular system links these two types of respiration (Figure 142).

Together, external and internal respiration ensure that we are able to survive on Earth. Death sets in when respiration ceases, and earthly life begins at birth with an infant's first breath, which is soon followed by the ingestion of food, energy transfers, and internal tissue respiration. Oxygen absorbed from the air is the body's very stuff of life.

But what does ***internal respiration*** really involve? Within the body's cells, three basic types of energy-consuming processes take place:

1. "Imbalances" that support *life* are maintained by combating the physical tendencies of pure matter (e.g., ion exchange to maintain cell compartments).

2. Cell and tissue ***structures*** are continually being renewed.

3. Energy is expended on tissue-specific cellular ***functions*** such as muscle contraction, secretion, etc.

These three basic functions require energy, which cells acquire by breaking down the three basic types of nutrients (proteins, carbohydrates, and fats). As discussed in an earlier chapter, the body does not simply "burn" these compounds with the help of oxygen (cf. Figs. 73 and 74) in order to produce energy. It is astonishing to discover that the breakdown of these different basic nutrients always results in the same substance, acetyl-CoA, which then supplies H_2 ions via the citric acid cycle. With the help of respiratory enzymes (cytochromes) in the cells, these ions combine with the oxygen supplied by respiration to form water: $2 H^+ + 1 O_2 = 2 H_2O$. This multistep process, known as biological oxidation, releases energy and makes it available to cells (Figure 143).

Thus the primary purpose of the oxygen we inhale is not to oxidize ingested nutrients ("combustion") but rather to drive the cytochrome cycle in the cells and to ensure that the transport of H_2 ions (protons) in cellular respiration does not come to a halt. The energy produced when water is formed is not released immediately but is stored in the form of ATP, to be released later when ATP is split into ADP. This energy is utilized not only for intracellular functions but also to reconstruct proteins, fats, etc., for use throughout the body. In the body's cells, therefore, a cycle of breakdown

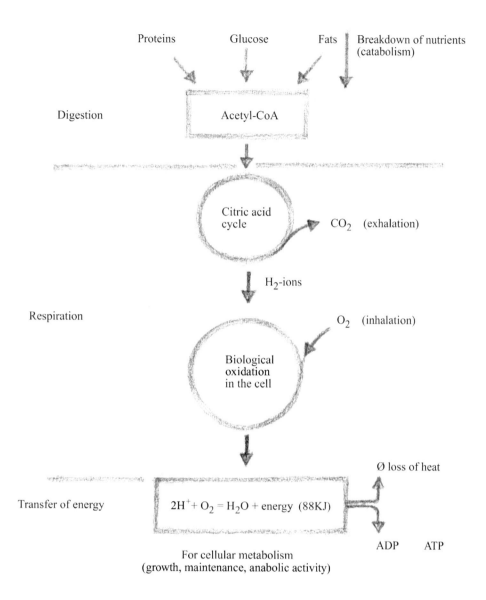

*Fig. 143. **Basic processes in the production of energy in tissues and in cellular respiration.***

and synthesis develops in which substances are recycled and energy transfers occur. This cycle would persist in a balanced state ("perpetual motion") were it not for the fact that a certain amount of energy is always lost in the form of heat. Nutrients must be ingested to compensate for this loss. Ultimately, therefore, the purpose of the oxygen that reaches the tissues via the blood is to ensure that hydrogen can be bound up in the form of water, thus making energy available to the cells. All cellular activity is powered by oxygen, which is supplied by respiration. Ultimately, not only specific organ functions but also the maintenance of the body's structures depend on respiration. But for oxygen to enter the body, we need an organ that is open to the air, namely, the lungs.

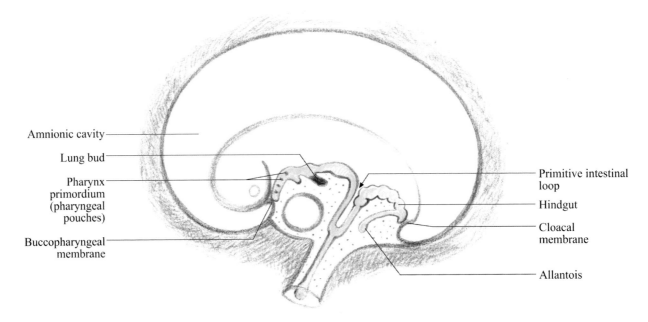

Amnionic cavity

Lung bud

Pharynx primordium (pharyngeal pouches)

Buccopharyngeal membrane

Primitive intestinal loop

Hindgut

Cloacal membrane

Allantois

Fig. 144. **Lung primordium in the 28-day-old embryo**. *The lung bud (red) originates in the foregut and grows into the surrounding mesenchyme. It divides rapidly into two and then (dichotomously) into additional buds (cf. Figure 145).*

Lung Development and Respiration

As early as the end of the third week of gestation, the initial lung primordium appears in the form of a little ventral offshoot of the embryonic intestinal tube near the foregut, i.e., in the neck (Figure 144). Through constant dichotomous divisions, this bud sprouts branches, rapidly forming a "tree" whose bulbous terminal buds (the future pulmonary alveoli) continue to grow on the periphery while the "stalks" become the bronchi (Figure 145). In the lungs, as in a plant, growth occurs in the terminal organs while the branching structure (the future bronchial tree) is preserved at each stage. In this respect, lung development is very similar to gland development. The parotid and pancreas, the major glands of the digestive tract, also develop actively growing, dichotomously dividing terminal portions while the "stalks" remain behind, forming the future ductal system. The lung primordium displays the same contrast in growth dynamics between its active buds (which grow from the inside outward) and its differentiating structures, where division is imposed from the outside (Figure 145). In contrast to the digestive glands, however, which display purely dichotomous growth, the pulmonary lobes develop asymmetrically from the very beginning through the sympodial-dichotomous growth pattern that is familiar to us from plants. After the first division, the right pulmonary bud grows somewhat more rapidly and divides again while the left bud is still increasing in volume. The resulting three and then five buds are the primordia of the future pulmonary lobes (three on the right and two on the left). This asymmetry is retained in later development, resulting in differences in structure and size between the left and right sides of the lungs (Figure 145).

A   B   C

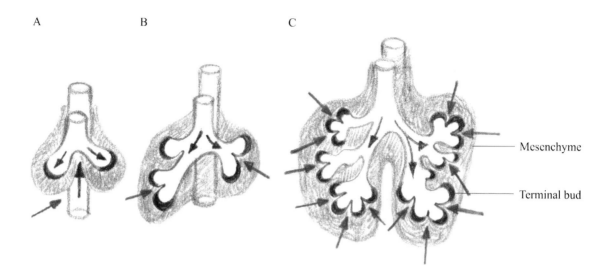

Mesenchyme

Terminal bud

Fig. 145. **Three successive stages in embryonic lung development**. *A: 4 weeks; B: 5 weeks; C: 6 weeks. The asymmetry of the right and left lobes is evident at an early stage. The lung primordium grows like a gland (i.e., through constant dichotomous divisions of its terminal portions) into the surrounding embryonic connective tissue (mesenchyme, red shading). Growth of the terminal buds (black) from within is counteracted by a differentiation process working from the outside in (red arrows). Inhibition of cellular replication in the terminal buds causes these buds to divide and leads to the development of the lung's ductal system.*

What is actually going on here? Let's take another brief look at the major digestive glands and their important contributions to digestion. To prepare for the absorption of basic building blocks, these glands secrete enzymes that dissolve and break down complex nutrients (proteins, fats, carbohydrates) and eliminate their source-specific attributes. The secretions from these glands flow into the intestines; together with the activity of the intestines themselves, they liquefy foods, releasing them from the spatial context of their origins and preparing them to cross the "threshold" of the intestinal wall to be incorporated into a new spatial entity, the human body.

To implement the reentry of digested substances into space, however, respiration is required. In this context, it is interesting to note that the chief organ of respiration is a "negative gland"—it develops like a gland but becomes hollow. The lungs and the bronchial tree can

be compared to a hollow digestive gland that eliminates space-filling matter in its interior in order to admit air from the outside world. Normally, the human body scrupulously avoids air bubbles or gases in its tissues, but in the chest it generates an organ that consists largely of hollow spaces. This organ empties itself of space-filling matter in order to take in the outside world's gaseous element. Through tissue respiration and with the help of blood circulation, the "negative space" of the lungs makes possible the synthesis of space-filling compounds.

As a result of a prenatal growth spurt, the walls of the alveoli become thinner and adapted to respiration, which sets in at birth. The amniotic fluid that fills the lungs during the embryonic stage is absorbed immediately after birth. Through secretion of a surfactant, the alveoli develop to the point where gaseous exchange with the blood is possible. Red blood cells take in oxygen and transport it via the bloodstream to the cells and organs where anabolic activity occurs. Carbon dioxide, released when substances are broken down, is then transported back to the lungs and eliminated.

Ultimately, the oxygen-dependent activities initiated and supported by respiration include not only space-filling anabolic functions but also the body's movement in space (cellular activity, limb movements, etc.). The organism is pervaded by respiratory gases, whose concentrations in different organs and tissues reflect their overall concentrations in the body, regardless of the chemical makeup of specific tissues. Inside each of us, therefore, is an "air body" that obeys laws of its own and is enlivened and regulated by the negative space of the lungs as a hollow organ.

Respiratory Rhythm
(Second Archetypal Phenomenon)

Unlike food, which enters the digestive tract at one end and exits at the other, the air we breathe does not follow a unidirectional route through the body. Inhalation and exhalation are channeled through a single conduit system, namely the airways (nasal cavity, trachea, bronchial tree; see Figure 146), resulting in **rhythmic respiration**. Through its rhythmic functions, the respiratory system breaks out of its metabolic context and becomes part of the middle or rhythmic system.

Respiratory rhythm is an astonishing archetypal phenomenon. Just as the heart spontaneously contracts and relaxes at regular intervals, so too the lungs are ventilated through regular, rhythmic movements of the ribcage and diaphragm. The ribcage rises and expands during inhalation and sinks during exhalation. Contraction of the diaphragm increases the volume of the chest cavity, sucking air through the airways (trachea, bronchi) into the lungs (inhalation); relaxation of the diaphragm reduces the volume of the chest cavity, causing exhalation (Figure 146). But contractions of the diaphragm are able

to ventilate the lungs only because the lungs are highly elastic and secured to the ribcage in a way that allows them to move. The lungs owe their elasticity to the development of an extensive elastic network and their mobility to the structure of the two pleura: the visceral and costal pleura. These features make it possible for suction (negative pressure) to develop in the chest cavity, resulting in inhalation.

If we look at the three major body cavities from the perspective of their relationship to the Earth's gravitational field, we discover characteristic differences among them. In the abdominal cavity, pressure corresponds to outer conditions, i.e., the pressure on the pelvic floor corresponds to the weight of the column of water above it. In the chest cavity, pressure values alternate rhythmically between positive and negative. And in the cranial cavity, the brain is subject to the buoyant force of the cerebrospinal fluid, which reduces its weight from an average of 1,500 grams to 20 to 40 grams, according to Archimedes' principle. As a result, our head always feels light; we never consciously experience its weight (64). But this inner buoyancy and freedom from the Earth's gravitational field begins already in the chest and its respiratory processes. A short poem by Goethe (113) is a wonderful expression of this unique aspect of the breathing experience:

> In breathing we two blessings know:
> Drawing air in, and letting it go;
> One winds us tight, the other relieves;
> How wonderfully breathing in all life weaves!
> So thank we god when we are pressed
> And thank him again when he grants us rest.

The rhythm of respiration is regulated and coordinated by specific centers in the brainstem (inspiration and expiration centers, the pneumotactic center, etc.). These centers contain neurons whose spontaneous action corresponds to the rhythm of respiration (normally eighteen breaths per minute). Cardiac rhythm is faster (72 beats per minute) and more oriented toward the lower body (metabolism, etc.). In contrast, the significantly slower rhythm of respiration is

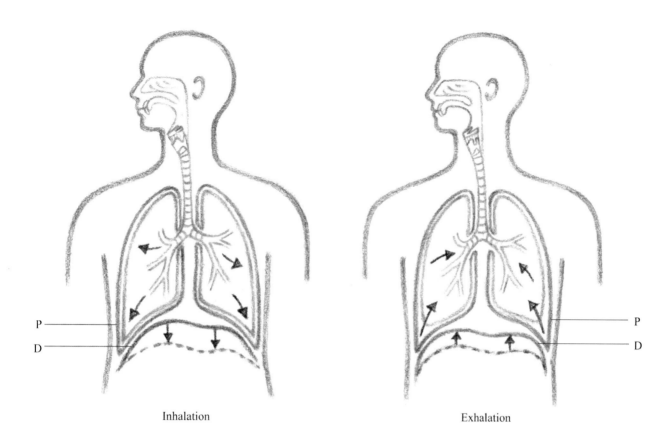

Inhalation   Exhalation

*Fig. 146. **Interaction of the diaphragm and lungs in respiration**. When the ribcage is lifted, the lungs expand and air is sucked into them (inhalation, left picture). When the ribcage sinks, the lungs contract, causing exhalation (right picture). However, breathing can also be initiated by the diaphragm. Through contraction of the diaphragm (D), the chest cavity expands, sucking air through the airways (nasal cavity, trachea, and bronchial tree) into the lungs (inhalation). When the diaphragm muscle relaxes, the ribcage presses the air out of the lungs again (exhalation). P: pleura, D: diaphragm.*

oriented more toward the upper human being, i.e., toward perception and cognition.

Respiration links us to cosmic rhythms. At a normal rate of approximately eighteen breaths per minute, we breathe 1,080 times per hour and 25,920 times in twenty-four hours. Surprisingly, this number corresponds to the macrocosmic cycle of the Platonic cosmic year. Each year, the point in the zodiac where the sun rises on the vernal equinox (March 21) slightly precedes the previous year's location. (In astronomy, this is called "precession of the equinoxes.") As a result,

the point where the sun's path (ecliptic) crosses the heavenly equator moves through the entire Zodiac approximately once every 25,920 years. This period has been called a Great Year or cosmic year.

As we see, the solar rhythm of the cosmic year corresponds to the human respiratory rhythm. But the number 25,920 also conceals other mysteries. If we consider a year to have 360 days, as the ancient Babylonian calendar did, then a typical human lifespan (72 years) encompasses 25,920 days. Normally, each day consists of one

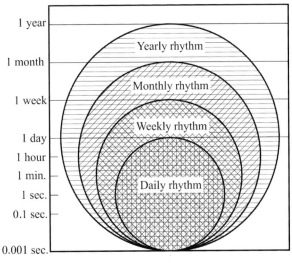

Period duration (log)

Fig. 147. **Schematic representation of the interaction of cosmically determined longer frequencies in the human being.** *In the frequency range shorter than the daily rhythm, all functions are influenced by all four rhythms (from Hildebrandt, 73. See also 114).*

alternation between waking and sleeping. Thus the number of these alternations in a lifetime is roughly the same as the number of breaths in a day and as the number of years in the great sun rhythm of the cosmic year (71). A human life, therefore, corresponds to one 360th of a Platonic cosmic year, i.e., one Platonic cosmic day.

Thus the Earth's relationship to the sun is the source not only of our world's time structure but also of the rhythmical structure of space, which pervades the human body through the respiratory and circulatory systems and even becomes consciously perceptible through our sensory organs (eye/light; ear/sound; Figure 147).

Human Chronobiological Rhythms

In addition to the above-mentioned rhythms of the cardiovascular and respiratory systems, there is a broad spectrum of other rhythmical functions in the body, ranging from the high-frequency rhythmical processes of the nervous system, which serve information exchange, to the slow rhythms of the autonomous metabolic system. In total, these rhythmical functions cover a range of 2 x 12 octaves.

"While informational rhythms are strictly bound to highly differentiated spatial structures in the nervous system, metabolic rhythms affect all tissues and organs, more or less, and are therefore less specific. These contrasting poles are linked by the central domain of the autonomic rhythmic system, principally the rhythms of circulation and respiration" (Hildebrandt, 73). The result is a functional threefoldness that is also reflected in individual rhythmic processes (Figure 148).

"Thus the activities of the informational system are expressed in frequency modulations in the rhythms of neural action, with each frequency mirroring a corresponding degree of excitation of neural elements and therefore (essentially) the influences of the outer world. In contrast, the frequencies of metabolic rhythms do not modulate significantly. Instead, each functional domain has at its disposal a series of different, predetermined frequency bands; it jumps between them as performance intensity changes. All of these frequency bands, however, relate to each other in simple, whole-number proportions as the expression of a harmonious, "musical" arrangement. For example, the ratio of the stomach's digestive movement (stomach peristalsis) to the basic one-minute rhythm of the fundus muscles is 3:1; the ratio of the duodenum's rhythm to stomach peristalsis is 4:1. Even an isolated bit of smooth intestinal muscle displays spontaneous rhythmical contractions whose period duration constantly changes, jumping between frequencies related by whole-number ratios" (Hildebrandt, 73).

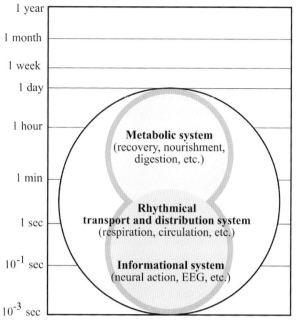

Period duration (log)

Sleeping/waking
Deposition/excretion (bowel, bladder), metabolic activities

Smooth muscle tone
Secretion
Peristalsis-circulation

Respiration
Movement

Heartbeat
Ciliated epithelium
Brain activity

Neural activity

Fig. 148. **Threefoldness of autonomic rhythmical functions**, *with period durations of less than one day; for details, see text (from Hildebrandt, 73).*

Table 18. Typical frequencies of cardiac rhythm, respiratory rhythm, blood-pressure rhythm, and minute rhythm of peripheral circulation in healthy subjects during sleep (adapted from Rauschke et al. in Hildebrandt, 73).

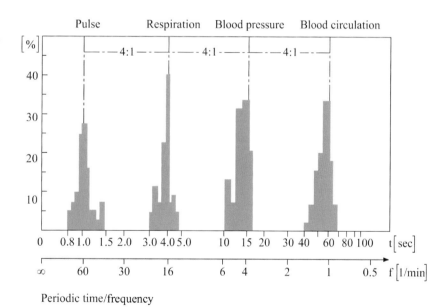

Thus the center of the rhythmic system—the organs of circulation and respiration—must produce harmony and balance between the poles of the sensory-nervous system, which is oriented toward and randomly influenced by the environment, and the metabolic system, which is will-dependent and works autonomously. The rhythmic system must mediate "between one time structure whose frequencies are constantly being modulated by incoming information and another whose frequencies are firmly anchored in a predetermined and ultimately cosmic, harmonious musical order. The rhythmical functions of the middle system that connect these inherently polar

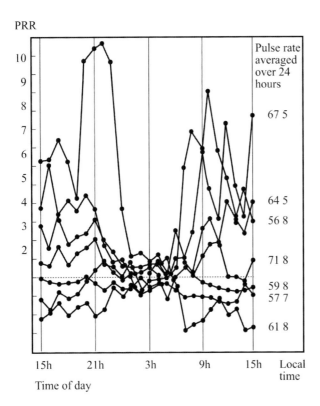

PRR

Pulse rate averaged over 24 hours

67 5
64 5
56 8
71 8
59 8
57 7
61 8

15h 21h 3h 9h 15h Local time

Time of day

Fig. 149. **Daily changes in pulse-respiration ratio** *(PRR) in healthy subjects with similar sleeping habits. The right column, which shows each subject's average pulse rate for the 24-hour period, demonstrates that nocturnal stabilization is largely independent of day-time rates (from Hildebrandt, 73).*

ordering principles are able to do so because they display relatively large variations in frequency and respond to the need for increased performance with frequency modulations (e.g., increases in heart and respiratory rates when working), yet tend to revert to preferred or normal frequencies (especially when at rest) that relate to each other in whole-number ratios" (Hildebrand, 73).

For example, the ratio of pulse rate to respiration during sleep is 4:1, which is also the ratio of respiratory rhythm to blood-pressure rhythm and of blood-pressure rhythm to the minute rhythm of peripheral circulation (Table 18).

Pulse-respiration ratio. Cardiac and respiratory rhythms relate to each other in ratios of 4:1

in the resting state (pulse-respiration ratio). They undoubtedly play a central role in the ordering of rhythmical functions. Respiratory rate and heart rate often vary considerably during the day, but in healthy adults the pulse-respiration ratio stabilizes at around 4:1 at night, between midnight and 3 a.m. (Figure 149). It is interesting to note that this stabilization does not occur in children until about age twelve (74). It is also absent in patients with circulatory disorders or heart disease, even in the preclinical stage, but may be restored after physical recovery or a lengthy stay at a health resort.

To summarize, we have ascertained that two (polar) domains meet in the body's middle or rhythmic system. The lower domain is not subject to our voluntary, conscious control. Cardiovascular rhythms belong to this domain, since we cannot directly influence our heart rate. The respiratory system relates more closely to the upper domain, which is open to the outer world and can be experienced consciously. We can directly and consciously alter our respiratory rate but not our heart rate. Within limits, we can hold our breath, breath deeply or shallowly, and consciously alter the timing of inhalation and exhalation. Psychological stimulation usually affects respiration directly and unconsciously. Conversely, voluntary changes in respiratory rhythm can also affect our consciousness—a phenomenon that plays a significant role in yoga.

The Organs of Speech and The Faculty of Speech
(Third Archetypal Phenomenon)

The essential character of the respiratory process becomes fully revealed when we consider its connection to the production of the sounds of speech. The Word (Logos) was held sacred by the ancient Greeks, who saw our human ability to produce words and sounds as evidence of our spiritual nature and kinship with the divine.

Evolution of the Speech Organs

The faculty of speech is truly a uniquely human attribute. Only humans are able to use the oral cavity to produce speech sounds. Using their larynx or other organs, animals may produce sounds and signals but not meaningful, highly differentiated, content-rich, and thought-filled speech.

The bodily foundations of the faculty of speech began to evolve only with the shift to terrestrial life and pulmonary respiration. In *fishes*, respiration (through the gills) and food intake still run parallel (Figures 45 and 150). In *amphibians*, the ventrally located lung primordium develops out of the intestinal tube, while the primary nasal cavity develops on the opposite side of the head. This is the first evolutionary appearance of the crossing of the airways and the digestive tract in the pharynx. In *reptiles*, elongation of the palate restricts this crossing to a smaller area; the entrance to the airways is safeguarded by sphincter muscles and protective reflex mechanisms. In *mammals* and nonhuman *primates*, an articulated larynx appears for the first time but is not yet used to produce the differentiated sounds necessary for speech. The anatomical prerequisites for speech and song appear only in human beings, as a result of laryngeal descent, which is related

to uprightness. In higher apes, the anatomy of the larynx is humanlike, but prognathism of the jaw develops so quickly after birth that the larynx retains its higher, fetal location. Consequently, the epiglottis extends all the way to the palate, and the oral cavity cannot be used for speech.

When a *human being* begins to stand upright approximately one year after birth, the larynx begins to descend. As a result, the distance between the epiglottis and the soft palate increases until speech sounds can be produced when small quantities of air are forced from the lungs and airways into the oral cavity. Now the crossing of the airway and the alimentary canal, which initially seemed so problematic in amphibians, begins to make sense because speech requires an open section of pharynx so that exhaled air can flow out through the mouth (Figure 150).

This is another impressive example of the *goal-oriented orthogenetic trend in evolution*, which was described in an earlier chapter in relationship to heart development. Once again, the human being is the goal, the zenith of the phylogenetic stream of evolution, and once again the goal is not achieved at the first attempt but only step-by-step. The "weighing" of specific experiences whose results are always incorporated into the structural model of the next level demonstrates that an empirical principle is at work here.

The Human Speech Organs

In the development of speech, we must distinguish between two different and independent components: *articulation* and *phonation*. Phonation, or voice formation, is based on oscillation of the vocal cords, whose frequency determines the pitch of the sound. As exhaled, pressurized air is forced against the more or less closed glottis, the previously continuous stream of air is interrupted and begins to vibrate (Figure 151). The vibrating air is then blown into the oral cavity, which shapes it in various ways that determine what type of sound is produced (articulation). For example, the oral cavity is wide open and undivided when the vowel sound "ah" is pronounced but divided by the

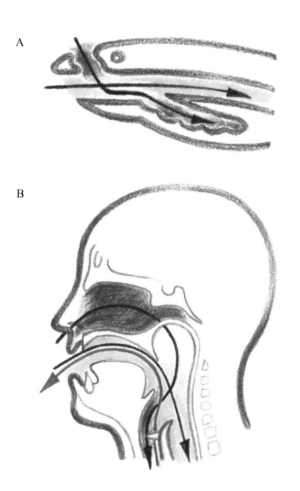

A

B

Fig. 150. **The crossing of the airways and the alimentary canal is important for the formation of speech sounds.**
A: In phylogeny, crossing of the airway and alimentary canal appears for the first time in amphibians.
B: In the upright human being, the crossing of airways and alimentary canal makes possible the development of speech. Air from the larynx (red line) can be forced through the pharynx into the oral cavity, which then serves as the "nozzle" for speech.

raised tongue when "ee" is pronounced (Figure 152). Through changes in the position and/or movements of the lips, teeth, tongue, soft palate, and other structures of the oral cavity, different consonants (labial or guttural sounds, etc.) can be produced. In some cases the nasopharynx also serves as a resonating cavity.

What is actually going on here? Breathing is an inherently rhythmical activity that takes place in the element of air rather than in the fluid element that provides the medium for the rhythms of blood circulation. In the organs of speech, however, the rhythmic aspect of breathing is enhanced, raised to a higher level, and individually (i.e., deliberately) shaped. The stream of exhaled air is interrupted (as the bloodstream is in the heart) and shaped into speech sounds by being forced into the "nozzle" of the oral cavity in quantized form. But at the same time a spiritual content, the meaning of a word, is imprinted on the air, and the word takes on a life of its own. The word is "born" out of the oral cavity like a baby out of the uterus. Imbuing newly created word elements with spiritual content requires the participation of the nervous system—in other words, of our consciousness. In the organs described above, the conscious activity of our spirit, supported by brain functions, transforms the sounds that are produced into speech.

Speech is not automatically organized and guided by the brain's "speech centers," as materialistic theories would have it. We can easily recognize the involvement of a superordinate "I"-being in the fact that the brain's different types of speech centers are located in different places and connected only by complicated, still hypothetical associative networks (Figure 153). The unity of meaningful speech, therefore, originates in the human "I" with its intentions to learn, adapt, and creatively shape speech and imbue it with content. Neural and organic processes merely serve as the physical basis.

For example, a "motor speech center" (Broca's center) has been identified in the left frontal lobe, a sensory speech center (Wernicke's area) in the upper temporal lobe next to the auditory centers, and finally an "optical speech center"

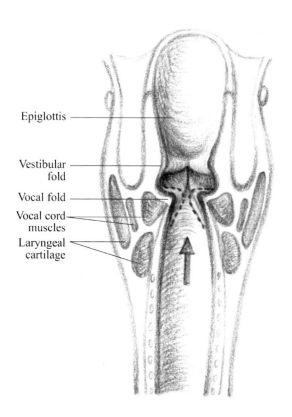

Epiglottis

Vestibular
fold

Vocal fold

Vocal cord
muscles

Laryngeal
cartilage

*Fig. 151. **Cross section through the human larynx**. The vocal folds block the airway except for a slit (the glottis). When air strikes them from below (arrow), the vocal folds begin to vibrate horizontally. The frequency of these oscillations determines the pitch of the voice (phonation).*

(also called the "reading center") in the parietal lobe of the cerebral cortex near the higher visual centers (Figure 153). The "motor" speech center is involved in coordinating movement processes that play a role in producing speech. In right-handed individuals, the motor speech center develops in the left hemisphere—specifically, in the inferior frontal gyrus (triangularis). Its development coincides with the emergence of right-hand dominance. (Because of the crossing of the nerve tracts, the left cortex is the dominant side of the brain in right-handed people and is responsible for limb movement on the right side of the body.) The "motor" speech center develops only on one side of the brain, on the left in right-handed individuals and usually (but not always) on the right in left-handed people. This phenomenon suggests that the development of limb activity, upright walking, and hand dominance in the first few years of life provides incisive impulses for the differentiation of both the cortex and the faculty of speech, not the other way around. In other words, the brain is not the primary initiator of speech motor mechanisms.

The several different levels of the sensory speech center make it possible for us to understand speech. The visual "speech center" allows us

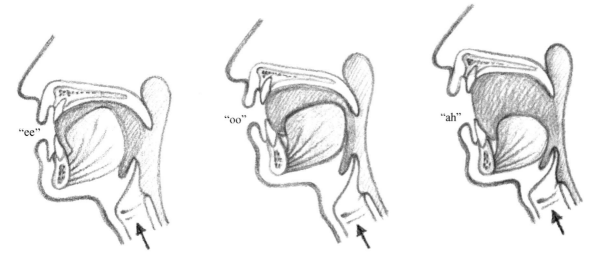

"ee"   "oo"   "ah"

*Fig. 152. **The oral cavity as the resonating cavity for speech**. In the articulation process, the oral cavity functions as a "nozzle" for the larynx. The positions of the tongue, palate, teeth, lips, etc., alter the shape of the resonating chamber and thus the sound that is produced. The illustrations show tongue positions when speaking the vowel sounds ee, oo, and ah.*

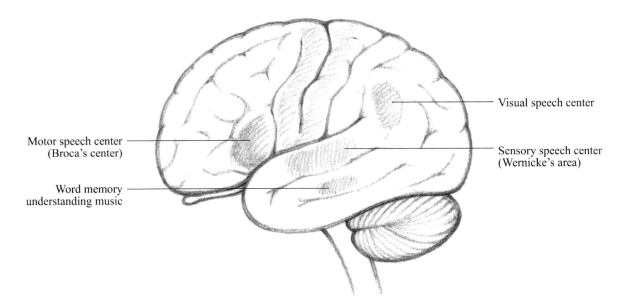

Fig. 153. **Location of the three major speech centers**. *The visual speech center in the parietal lobe is also called the "reading center" because it is involved in recognizing visual shapes (letters, symbols). Wernicke's area in the temporal lobe is connected to cortical fields responsible for language understanding, musicality, and auditory memory. The motor speech center (Broca's center) in the frontal lobe is located on only one side of the brain (usually on the left in right-handed individuals and in many left-handed people as well).*

to recognize signs (letters, lip movements, etc.) relevant to speech. Every artist knows that producing words or tones is not simply a function of the brain. Everything "born" out of the oral cavity ultimately comes from the entire body; the brain merely provides the basis for the spiritual, upper element to incarnate/incorporate into the substance coming from below (the "sacrificed" aspects of air) so that the Word can appear.

In physical terms, the Word (Logos) consists of rhythmicized air imbued with warmth and droplets of fluid. But more than that, it always contains something of the individual's soul-spiritual aspect, which is often evident even in the quality of the voice. On the spiritual level, the Word houses an idea that the speaking person understands and shapes creatively—an idea that may encompass the entire universe. After all, cultural history tells us

that ultimately the characteristic speech of an era— that is, how people shaped their words—reflects all of its ideas and even the level of development of human consciousness at that time.

Human beings become creative on three different levels: in conceiving offspring, in producing words and sounds, and in bringing forth thoughts and ideas ("conceiving" in a higher sense). As Schiller so convincingly argued in his letters on esthetic education, we are truly free only in the middle domain, where we creatively shape speech and song (75).

The Nervous System
and the
Sense Organs

A

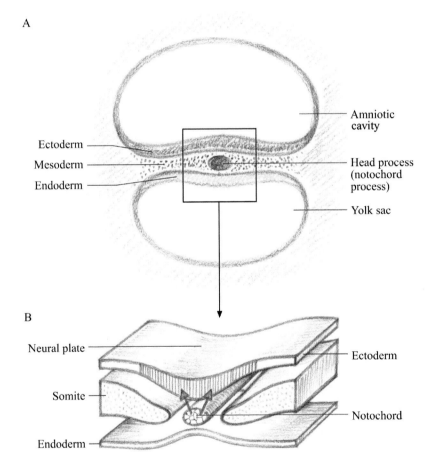

Ectoderm

Mesoderm

Endoderm

Amniotic cavity

Head process (notochord process)

Yolk sac

B

Neural plate

Somite

Endoderm

Ectoderm

Notochord

*Fig. 154. **Embryonic development of the nervous system.***

A: In a 17-day-old embryo, the embryonic disc consists of three germ layers (ectoderm, mesoderm, and endoderm). The axis of the body is determined by the notochord process of the mesoderm, which gives rise to the notochord.

B: The notochord sends out induction stimuli (red arrows) that initiate development of the nervous system, which consists initially of a flat neural plate within the ectoderm.

The Functional Threefoldness of the Nervous System

In many respects, the nervous system occupies a unique position among organ systems. For example, it is made up almost entirely of cells, whereas the tissue-specific (parenchyma) cells of all other organs are surrounded by fluid-rich, highly vascularized connective tissue. All metabolic exchanges take place in this connective tissue where swelling or shrinkage may develop and inflammation or immune responses occur. Here, blood cells or connective tissue cells can move from the vascular system to organ tissues or vice versa, and gases and other substances are exchanged between organ tissues and the blood. In adults, the volume of fluid in the body's extracellular space is approximately ten to twelve liters, in comparison to only four or five liters of blood. This extracellular space, the true interior of the body, is also very important for generative and regenerative processes. In plants, there is no extracellular space as such; it appears for the first time in animals. Plants grow through replication and incorporation of new cells at the growing point. Individual plant organs (leaves, flowers, etc.) do not regenerate and are eventually discarded.

Although the cells of the nervous system are more complex than those of a plant, the nervous system also consists of similarly densely packed cells. Between these cells are very narrow gaps (Ø 100-200 nm) but no larger spaces for connective tissue. Instead, the necessary movement of fluids and solids occurs through helper cells (neuroglia) that specialize in various transport and exchange processes. Of course the nervous system also includes blood vessels, but they are a secondary development and are separated from nerve tissue by a close-fitting membrane of glial cells. The vessel walls themselves form the blood-brain barrier, which many substances cannot breach.

Development of the Nervous System

The purely cellular character of the nervous system is most evident in its developmental history. In human embryonic development, the nervous system is one of the first organ systems to appear. It develops out of an invagination in the outer germ layer (ectoderm, see Figure 154). As a result of this invagination, the notochord process inserts itself between the epiblast and the hypoblast (the future ectoderm and endoderm) and then induces another invagination process in the ectoderm. Two longitudinal neural ridges appear, grow toward each other, and fuse to form the neural tube, located below the ectoderm (Figure 155 B). Because neural-ridge fusion begins in the middle, the neural tube is initially open on both ends (anterior and posterior neuropores). But these openings soon close, creating a sealed tube that initially consists only of epitheloid cells. This tube is the primordium of the entire nervous system. Its cellular character, otherwise found only in the epithelia covering internal or external surfaces, is a permanent feature in the nervous system, persisting even after the cells develop complex processes and synapses and become extremely

A

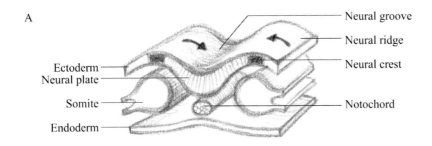

Neural groove
Neural ridge
Neural crest

Ectoderm
Neural plate
Somite
Endoderm

Notochord

*Fig. 155. **Development of the spinal cord.***

A: The neural plate develops in the middle of the neural groove, the neural ridges on either side. The ridges move toward each other to form a tube (neural tube, see B).

B

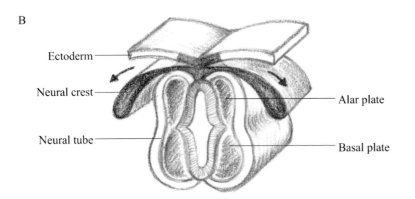

Ectoderm

Neural crest

Neural tube

Alar plate

Basal plate

B: The fusion zone of the neural ridges is an area of especially active growth. This is where the neural crest (black) develops. It produces cells that grow toward the periphery of the body (arrows) to form the peripheral ganglia and plexuses. The neural tube is divided into a dorsal plate (alar plate, blue) with primarily afferent (sensing) functions and a ventral plate (basal plate, red) with primarily efferent (motor) functions (arrows in illustration C).

C

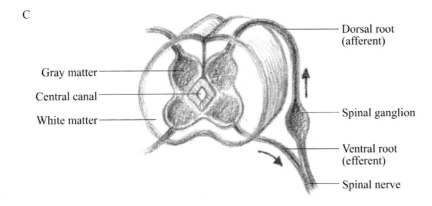

Dorsal root (afferent)

Gray matter
Central canal
White matter

Spinal ganglion

Ventral root (efferent)

Spinal nerve

C: Embryonic spinal cord with ventral and dorsal roots, which come together in the spinal nerve. The spinal ganglion is located in the dorsal root. The spinal cord's gray matter consists primarily of nerve cells, its white matter of nerve fibers.

varied in shape. Neurons develop out of initially undifferentiated embryonic cells, the neuroblasts, and are the only cells that serve neural functions. The second major cell group, the neuroglia, are strictly supportive (facilitating functions such as the transportation of fluids and solids) and are necessary to nourish the neurons and maintain their functioning. Blood vessels migrate into neural tissue only secondarily; for the most part, they remain spatially and functionally separated from it, as noted above.

During embryonic development, nerve tissue pervades the entire body, growing outward from the **neural crest**, which develops out of the neural tube (Figure 155B). Cells from the neural crest migrate toward the periphery and settle in various parts of the body, often producing large clusters of cells (ganglia, Figures 156A and B). One such migration produces the solar plexus, which is located in front of the abdominal aorta. (Editor's note: The solar plexus is the largest major autonomic plexus in the body and includes the mesenteric plexus, the

A

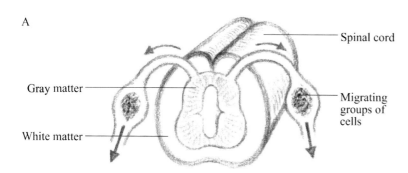

Spinal cord

Gray matter

White matter

Migrating groups of cells

*Fig. 156. **Reversal of cellular migration processes in the peripheral and central areas of the nervous system**. In both cases the migration begins in the neural tube.*

B

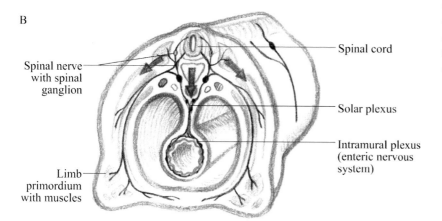

Spinal nerve with spinal ganglion

Spinal cord

Solar plexus

Intramural plexus (enteric nervous system)

Limb primordium with muscles

A and B: Cells migrate from the embryonic spinal cord (A) to the periphery (B) and colonize the torso and limbs with nerve cells (ganglia) and nerve fibers (plexuses, arrows). In the spinal cord, gray matter is on the inside and white matter on the exterior.

C

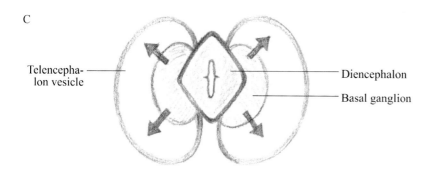

Telencephalon vesicle

Diencephalon

Basal ganglion

D

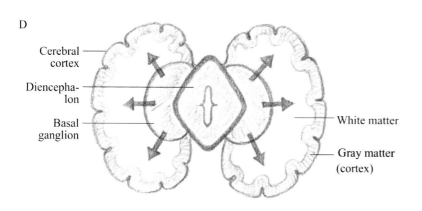

Cerebral cortex

Diencephalon

Basal ganglion

White matter

Gray matter (cortex)

C and D: Embryonic brain. From a basally located cell mass (basal ganglion), cells migrate outward to form the cerebral cortex (arrows indicate direction of migration). In the brain, most of the gray matter lies on the outer surface (cortex), and the white matter inside, reversing the situation in the spinal cord.

A

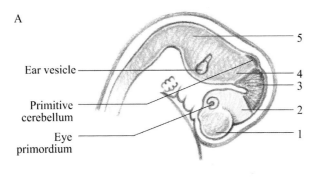

Ear vesicle

Primitive
cerebellum

Eye
primordium

5
4
3
2
1

B

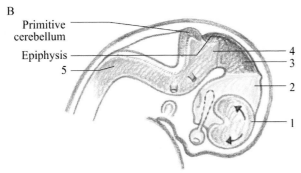

Primitive
cerebellum

Epiphysis

5

4
3
2
1

C

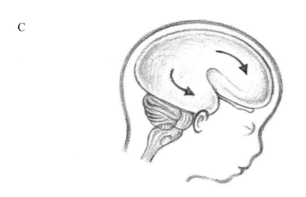

D

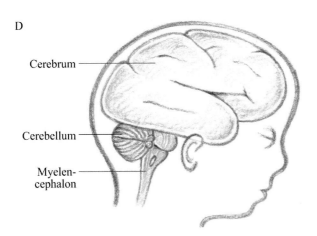

Cerebrum

Cerebellum

Myelen-
cephalon

Fig. 157. **Neural tube development in the head** *(from Rohen, 16). Side views of four stages in the development of the human brain.*
Age of fetus:
A: 35 days; B: 44 days; C: 5 months; D: 6 months.
Development of the five brain vesicles (1-5) varies greatly. The endbrain, which becomes the cerebrum, overwhelms all subsequent sections of the brain and develops more and more convolutions (gyri and sulci).

1: Endbrain (telencephalon)
2: Interbrain (diencephalon)
3: Midbrain (mesencephalon)
4: Metencephalon
5: Medulla oblongata (myelencephalon)
4+5: Hindbrain (rhombencephalon) and cerebellum

celiac ganglion, and the renal plexus. While they are often described in their individual detail, this is overshadowed by their inherent connectivity with each other.) Neurons also settle inside organs such as the lungs, kidneys, etc. In the intestinal wall, they form extensive multicellular networks (intramural plexuses), which constitute the enteric nervous system. Ultimately, as a result of these massive migrations, the entire body is pervaded with nerve tissue and the nervous system comes into contact with every cell system. The sum total of nerve tissue that migrates into the organs is called the vegetative or **autonomic nervous system** because it is not subject to voluntary control and its functioning is largely autonomous or independent of our consciousness.

In the **head**, the development of the nervous system is completely different. Although a migration of cells also occurs here, the cells move only from the brain's interior to its surface (Figures 156C and D). The five brain vesicles that form in the developing head later become the different sections of the brain (Figure 157). The largest vesicle, the telencephelon, develops into the cerebrum (cerebral hemispheres—cerebral cortex with the ventricles). It increases dramatically in size during the embryonic period, gradually overwhelming all other sections of the brain as it grows in a semispiral (Figure 157). The wall of the telencephalon is initially very thin and smooth, but

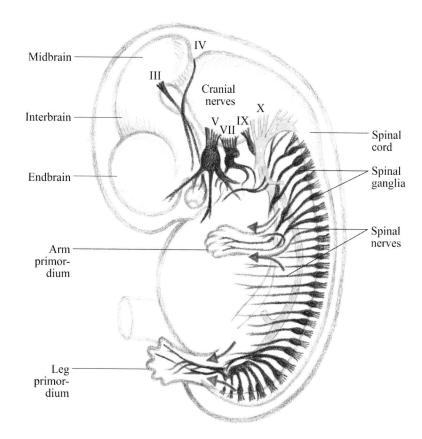

Midbrain

IV

III

Cranial
nerves

X

V IX
VII

Interbrain

Spinal
cord

Endbrain

Spinal
ganglia

Spinal
nerves

Arm
primor-
dium

Leg
primor-
dium

*Fig. 158. **Human embryo** at 2 months. Nerve cells migrating from the neural tube (the future spinal cord) colonize the body, forming the segmentally arranged spinal nerves. The spinal nerves extend into the primordia of the limbs, where they abandon their segmental character and form large plexuses (the brachial plexus, which serves the arm, and the lumbosacral plexus, which serves the leg). The primordia of the cranial nerves (III, IV, V, VII, IX, and X) develop in the head.*

it thickens and develops ridges (gyri) and furrows (sulci) as a result of the large numbers of cells that migrate from the interior to the surface (gyrification of the brain, see Figure 156D). The cells that accumulate in each gyrus are functionally related and later develop into a specific brain center. The number of cells migrating to the surface of the brain is no smaller than the number migrating to the organs on the periphery. Similar increases in numbers of cells occur in the other brain vesicles, and in some cases substantial nuclei develop. Cell migration also plays a role in the development of the cerebellum.

The movement of embryonic nerve cells toward the surface of the brain reverses the relationship of gray matter to white matter relative to the spinal cord. In the spinal cord, white matter lies on the outside and gray matter on the inside; in the cerebrum, specifically the cerebral cortex, the mass of nerve cells (gray matter) is outside and the white matter inside (Figure 156).

Basic Morphological Divisions of the Nervous System

In the head, a massive concentration of nerve tissue develops in a very limited space. In contrast, dispersion and decentralization characterize the periphery. Brain centers in the head (cerebral cortex, etc.), which additionally develop connections to the major sense organs, form the basis of our conscious experience, but the nerve centers of the peripheral, autonomic nervous system elude consciousness.

Between these two extremes lies a third domain that functions partly unconsciously ("reflexively") but in some cases is also subject to conscious influence. This "middle section" of the nervous system, which encompasses the *spinal cord* and its connections to the muscles and the body's surface, is functionally related to the torso and extremities. As with the torso in

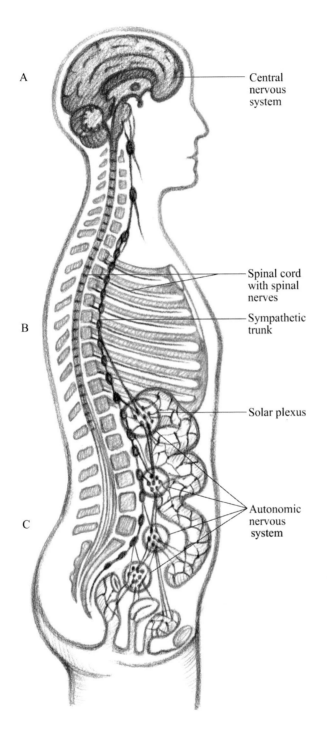

Central
nervous
system

Spinal cord
with spinal
nerves

Sympathetic
trunk

Solar plexus

Autonomic
nervous
system

A

B

C

*Fig. 159. **The threefold nervous system**. A: Head (dense concentration of nerve tissue in the brain and major sense organs); B: Spinal cord (segmental structure, spinal nerves serving the limbs and the body's surface; C: Intestines (autonomic nervous system, decentralization of nerve tissue, formation of plexuses and ganglia).*

general, the nervous system in this part of the body is morphologically segmented, revealing its rhythmic character (Figure 158). Each pair of ribs is associated with a pair of nerves that innervate the intercostal muscles and related areas of skin (dermatomes). Thus the number of spinal nerves emerging from the spinal cord corresponds to the number of torso segments or vertebrae. Because the limbs begin their development as protrusions emerging from the torso's ventral side, spinal nerves (specifically, their ventral branches) also innervate the limbs in the adult body. (Editor's note: As Dr. Rohen so succinctly describes in the unpublished translation of his text *Functional Neuroanatomy*, "As the limbs grow in length... the muscles pull their innervating nerves along with them.") The segmental arrangement of these nerves becomes more radial as the limbs grow and the nerves intertwine to form the plexuses of the extremities (brachial plexus, lumbosacral plexus, etc.). Yet the nerves never completely abandon their relationships to their respective segments.

Thus the morphology of ***the nervous system is visibly threefold*** (Figure 159). In the head, nerve tissue is concentrated in a limited space. The cerebral cortex with its roughly sixteen billion neurons is the seat of our most conscious mental activity. It is divided into many functional areas which are primarily involved with the major sense organs (the sensorium). In contrast, nerve tissue in the visceral organs is spread out over a huge surface area. Here, in the autonomic nervous system, decentralization and dispersion, not concentration, are the rule. Neural processes here run their course unconsciously and automatically, regulating and directing vital processes in the organs. This is why L. R. Müller calls them the "life nerves" (cf. 16 and 140). The spinal nervous system (spinal cord, etc.) lies between these poles—it is the middle portion of the nervous system. It is structured in segments, and the nerves from the spinal cord extend into the torso wall and extremities. These spinal nerves also innervate the skin, transmitting sensations (of pressure, touch, temperature, etc.) from sense organs in the skin. First and foremost, however, the spinal system is responsible for the skeletal muscles (which are subject to voluntary control) and thus for the body's entire system of voluntary movement. The brain is oriented toward the outer world, the autonomic nervous system toward the body's interior, and the spinal cord's segmental system toward both. For example, if we pay attention to what is going on inside the body, we can perceive the tension in our muscles (so-called deep sensibility or bathyesthesia) or use our respiratory muscles to change the rhythm of our breathing. But our organs of movement and the sensorimotor portion of the nervous system also allow us to interact with the outside world.

Throughout the body, therefore, the nervous system plays a decisive role in organ processes, limb movements, the rhythmic functions of the cardiovascular and respiratory systems, and of course also in sensory processes. But it never performs these functions itself. It stands on the sidelines, so to speak. This separation is evident even in the morphology of nervous tissue: Wherever it is found in organs, glial tissue separates it from organ tissue. Nerve tissue obeys its own laws, which are significantly different from those of other organ systems. This distinction will become especially apparent when we consider the structural idiosyncrasies of nerve tissue, which exists only to serve information exchange. In other words, nerves "reflect" organic processes but do not produce them.

Basic Nerve Tissue Functions

The nerve tissue of the brain consists of densely packed neurons whose cell bodies lie primarily within the gray matter of the cerebral cortex or in nuclei in the brain; for the most part, their axons end in white matter. Each nerve cell consists of a cell body (soma or perikaryon), usually with numerous processes called dendrites, and a single longer process, the axon, which conducts impulses away from the cell body. A nerve cell with all of its processes is called a neuron (Figure 160A). It is connected to other neurons through synapses (contact points at the membrane), which take a variety of different forms and can be located on dendrites, cell bodies, or axons (Figure 160C). An axon may end in a synapse on a dendrite or cell body of another neuron, or it may connect to a structure of a different sort, such as a muscle cell (Figure 160A).

Three **fundamental functions** are evident in all neurons, regardless of variations in size and shape. The cell body (soma) is the neuron's metabolic organ and maintains the life of the cell as a whole. The cell's processes (nerve fibers) represent the conduction or transportation function. The synapses, which transmit stimuli, serve the functions of information exchange and neural regulation.

Nerve fibers. In contrast to the physiological processes of other cells, which take place primarily within the cytoplasm, neural stimulation takes place on the outer surfaces (membranes) of neurons. As a result of the unequal distribution of Na^+ and K^+ ions (Na^+ ions on the outside, K^+ on the inside), neuronal membranes at rest are negatively charged, with a negative membrane potential of -80 to -90 mV. When an impulse is transmitted, Na^+ ions flow into the cytoplasm while K^+ ions flow out, and the membrane is depolarized (Figure 161). This change in potential moves along the cell membrane until it reaches a synapse, where either a new action potential develops or the transmission is extinguished. To restore negative membrane potential so that new impulses are

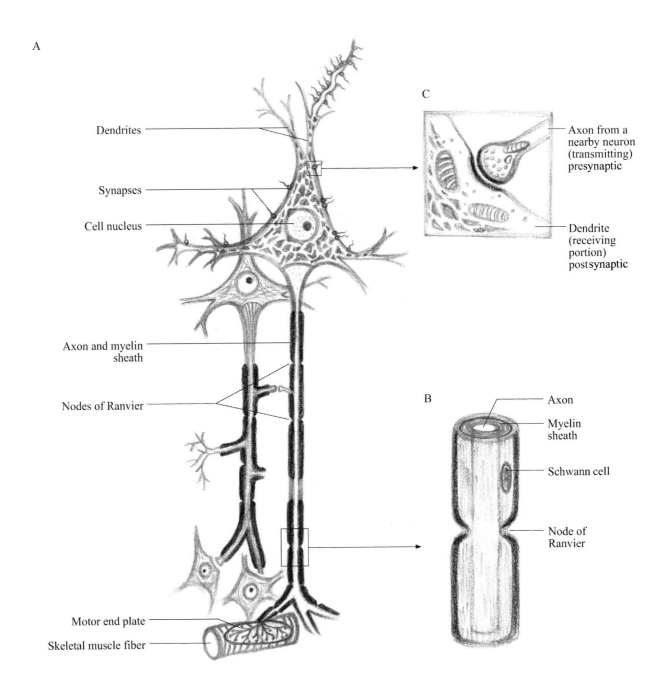

A

C

Dendrites

Synapses

Cell nucleus

Axon from a
nearby neuron
(transmitting)
presynaptic

Dendrite
(receiving
portion)
postsynaptic

Axon and myelin
sheath

Nodes of Ranvier

B

Axon

Myelin
sheath

Schwann cell

Node of
Ranvier

Motor end plate

Skeletal muscle fiber

Fig. 160. Structure of a neuron (pyramidal cell) with all of its processes and specialized structures.
A: *Diagram of a neuron with its processes (motor neurons);*
B: *Detail: section of an axon showing the myelin sheath and node of Ranvier;*
C: *Detail: a synapse on the cell body (axo-somatic synapse).*

A

Na⁺ channels

Open   Closed

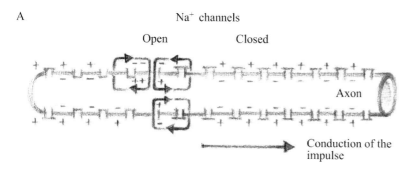

Axon

Conduction of the impulse

B   Na⁺ influx

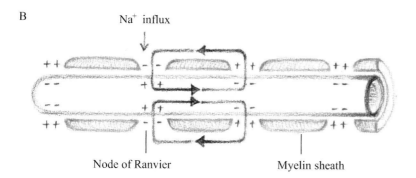

Node of Ranvier   Myelin sheath

*Fig. 161. **Membrane processes in neural stimulation of nonmyelinated (A) and myelinated (B) nerve fibers**. Nerve impulses traveling along a myelinated axon must jump the gaps formed by the nodes of Ranvier. In an unmyelinated axon (A), the movement of the impulse (here, from left to right) is continuous and uninterrupted, but in myelinated fibers impulses "jump" from one node to the next (B). When the sodium channels open and Na⁺ ions flow into the axon, the negative ion potential at that point on the cell is reduced (depolarization). The membrane can be recharged by actively pumping out Na⁺ ions.*

possible, the cell must expend energy to actively pump Na⁺ ions out of the cytoplasm.

Impulses are transmitted much faster along nerve fibers that have lipoprotein (myelin) sheaths because ion displacements occur only at the ring-shaped interruptions (nodes of Ranvier) in the sheaths. As a result, impulses hop from node to node (saltatory conduction, see Figure 161). The thicker the myelin sheath and the longer the distances between nodes, the faster impulse transmission occurs. In the brain, white matter (such as that underlying the cerebral cortex) is made up of myelinated nerve fibers. The cortex itself, also called gray matter, is more grayish in color because it consists primarily of the cell bodies of neurons.

Now let's consider **neural impulse transmission** from a more qualitative perspective. To remain excitable, each neuron must repeatedly restore its negative membrane potential (Figure 161). This takes energy, which is supplied by the

cell body and reaches the membrane via the cytoplasm. At death, when these energy-transport processes cease, Na⁺ ions flow into the cytoplasm, eliminating differences in concentration, and the cell fills with fluid and dies. Wherever concentration differences and ion gradients break down—in other words, wherever and whenever the purely physical and chemical laws of the outer natural world gain the upper hand—cells die off. The largest manifestation of this process is the death of the body. Death, however, also involves the freeing of an individual's soul-spiritual aspect from the body.

If neural impulse transmission begins with Na⁺ ions flowing into the neuron, this means essentially that a catabolic, dying-off process is taking place, if only for a fraction of a second. Neural stimulation always incurs a tiny death. The consequences are not catastrophic simply because the neuron always summons up the energy to recharge its membranes, to reenliven

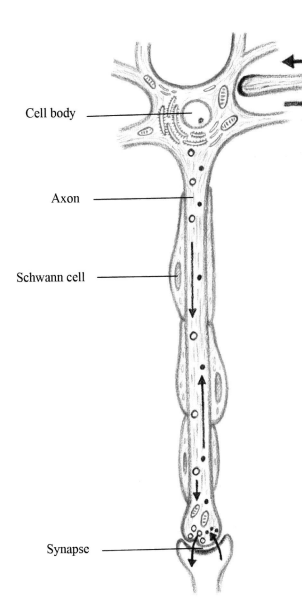

Cell body

Axon

Schwann cell

Synapse

Blood vessel

Astrocyte
(fluid transport)

*Fig. 162. **Neuron with Schwann cells and a glia cell for metabolic support**. Inside axons, plasma flow in both directions (so-called axoplasmatic transport, arrows) maintains metabolic connections between the cell body and terminal organs such as synapses.*

itself. In little death processes of this sort in nerve fibers and synapses (white matter), soul-spiritual forces are also released. In the nervous system, therefore, death processes are the prerequisites for the development of consciousness. These instances of localized, controlled "deaths" unleash informational processes that become conscious in the soul, which consciously mirrors the events that trigger neural impulses.

Neuron cell bodies. Conversely, the energy-consuming, regenerative, and enlivening metabolic activity proceeding from the cell body or soma is consciousness-deadening or "sleep-inducing." In comparison to other cells, the soma of a neuron is extremely large (Figure 160). Within each axon plasma is constantly flowing. In humans, the proteins in this flow reach speeds of 25 to 40 cm per day, while cell organelles (e.g., parts of the cytoskeleton) move at 1 mm per day. In the nervous system as a whole, this flow of substances is monumental. Not only recycled membrane proteins (for maintenance) but also new organelles, neurotransmitters, etc., are transported in a centrifugal direction toward the neurons' terminal formations and synapses (ante-grade ***axoplasmatic transport***, Figure 162). Neurotransmitters are broken down in the termi-nal structures and are largely reabsorbed, but some of the catabolic products are returned to the cell body via retrograde (centripetal) axoplas-matic flow in the axon and are resynthesized. In other words, transmitters are recirculated in the nerve fibers and are repeatedly recycled. As usual, a small amount of matter falls out of this cycle and must be replaced. Thus centrifugal and centripetal plasma flows run parallel in the axon (Figure 162). These intracellular processes of renewal and reenlivening are the only thing that allows neurons as such to retain their outer form for the life of the body and to maintain information exchange in their axons and synapses in the long term.

A cell that constantly changes shape would not be able to function as an information-transmitting organ, just as the surface of a body of water produces recognizable reflections only when it is not moving. The relatively constant structure of nerve tissue (the principle of rest) is thus an important component of the nervous system's "reflective" function, which develops consciousness and produces images of the external or internal world.

The third fundamental function in neurons involves their contact points (synapses). In *Synapses* (Figure 160C) neurons are (reversibly) linked into functional groups (reflex loops, neuron chains, or conduction pathways). Ultimately, the number of synaptic connections determines the nervous system's level of functional differentiation. A more highly developed nervous system is more adaptable because it has more potential connections that can be established and then dissolved again.

These three fundamental functions of nerve cells also reflect the threefoldness of the body as a whole. In a certain sense, the cell body and plasma represent the neuron's "metabolic" system, which handles regeneration, substance recycling, and energy transfers. Metabolic processes dominate in the gray matter of the cerebral cortex and spinal cord, which consists primarily of neuron cell bodies. Metabolic processes, as we know, are related to will processes in our soul life; in the nervous system, the will element affects mental activity through neuronal metabolism. This is especially true of the activity of remembering. Modern methods such as PET imaging show that metabolic activity increases in specific brain centers during strenuous thinking or intense concentration.

Unlike the metabolic processes inside the cytoplasm, impulse transmission occurs on the surface, on the membranes of axons and neurons (Figure 161). The partial death (catabolic) and reenlivenment (anabolic) processes that generate signal conduction make up the neural and informational activity typical of nerves as such. In the cerebral cortex, this activity brings about the "reflective process" that allows us to become conscious of events in the outer world.

The third distinct functional element is the system of interneuronal connections through *synaptic membrane contacts*. These connections are where impulses are transmitted or inhibited. Plus/minus, yes/no, or excitation/inhibition is the basic principle underlying neural circuitry. Ultimately, synapses that connect or separate different neurons or neuron groups are responsible for the nervous system's great variety of functional possibilities. Collectively, the synapses constitute the "middle" or rhythmic element of nerve tissue. Their primary task is to dissolve and reestablish connections. This alternation (like inspiration and expiration in the rhythmic system) serves harmonizing, balancing, and transforming functions. It is the centralized activity in the nervous system.

On the soul level, "connecting" and "dissolving" signify feelings of sympathy and antipathy. An emotional component is always involved in any conceptual activity that truly relates to reality. Goethe wrote, "If you do not feel it, you will never get it" (*Faust*, line 534). Upon careful consideration, one notes that real understanding and learning require empathy and adaptability. Mastering new skills requires making new neural connections and abandoning old ones. The human brain is distinguished by the fact that it remains flexible, plastic (i.e., capable of producing new synaptic connections) into old age. In animals, these connections become largely fixed and nonadaptable after the initial imprinting phase. Inherent mobility of periodicity and a capacity for transformation, however, are characteristic of the rhythmic system, which plays a central role in all evolutionary processes.

General Structure of Reflex Arcs in the Three Functional Domains of the Nervous System

For events in the outer world or inside the body to be reproduced or "mirrored" in the nervous system, circuitlike connections must exist. These connections are made up of neurons linked into shorter or longer pathways via their synapses. Ultimately, therefore, the nervous system consists of an abundance of cellular units. The position of neurons within each pathway determines the direction of impulse conduction along it. If the function of a group of neurons is to convey information from the sense organs to the brain, the direction of conduction is centripetal and the pathway is called an **afferent** system. Centrifugal pathways leading from the center toward the periphery (to muscles, for instance) are made up of **efferent** neurons. The interrelationship of these two nerve types is clearest in the spinal cord, where afferent and efferent neurons are combined in functional sensorimotor systems.

To better understand this fundamental phenomenon, let's take another brief look at the **embryonic development of the spinal cord**. Neurons from the dorsal half of the primitive spinal cord (alar plate) migrate toward the periphery along the nerves of the dorsal spinal root, while the cells of the ventral half (basal plate) remain in the gray matter of the spinal cord (Figure 163). Initially, the dorsally migrating neurons remain in the dorsal spinal root, forming the spinal ganglion. The cells of the basal plate develop large cell bodies with multiple dendrites, which connect with other spinal neurons, and a single long neurite (group of axons) that extends into the periphery and connects with muscle fibers in the torso or primitive extremities. Neurons that connect with muscle fibers are called motor neurons. Because they conduct impulses centrifugally, from the spinal cord to the muscles, they are also called efferent neurons. The neurons in the spinal ganglia become bipolar; in other words, each one sends one process out toward the periphery and another back toward the spinal cord. Because these cells conduct impulses from the periphery to the spinal cord, they are called sensory or afferent neurons. Even in the embryonic stage, therefore, functional neural pathways develop to link the muscles and the spinal cord. In the simplest instance, such a system consists of two neurons, one afferent neuron that reaches the spinal cord via the dorsal root and one efferent neuron whose neurites (or axons) run from the ventral spinal root to the muscles (Figure 164). This pair of neurons constitutes a reflex arc or conduction circuit.

Functional threefoldness of conduction systems in the nervous system. Reflex arcs of afferent and efferent neurons are found not only in the spinal cord but elsewhere in the nervous system as well, where they assume very different forms in each of the three major functional domains of the nervous system (Figure 165). The differences in these three domains are tellingly revealed in the makeup of their respective reflex arcs and are the key to understanding the threefoldness of the nervous system itself.

In the **head** (brain), sensory systems are functionally dominant. The major sense organs (eye, ear, organs of smell, etc.) supply the central nervous system with the information we need to orient ourselves in our surroundings. Here, the afferent function comes to the fore, although this does not mean that efferent neurons (represented by dashes in Figure 165A) are not present. Sensory systems are based on the general model of the reflex arc, but the two branches of the arc are not given equal emphasis. The efferent neurons play a supporting role, regulating the stimulus threshold of sensory cells. Thus they contribute to optimizing the (afferent) sensory process but do not directly influence it.

The opposite is true in the **autonomic nervous system**, where the efferent branches of reflex arcs predominate. Here, in contrast to

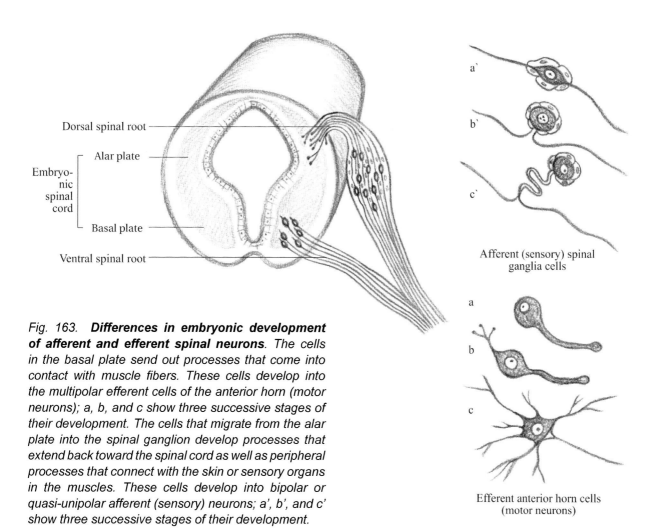

Fig. 163. **Differences in embryonic development of afferent and efferent spinal neurons.** *The cells in the basal plate send out processes that come into contact with muscle fibers. These cells develop into the multipolar efferent cells of the anterior horn (motor neurons); a, b, and c show three successive stages of their development. The cells that migrate from the alar plate into the spinal ganglion develop processes that extend back toward the spinal cord as well as peripheral processes that connect with the skin or sensory organs in the muscles. These cells develop into bipolar or quasi-unipolar afferent (sensory) neurons; a', b', and c' show three successive stages of their development.*

the spinal system, each efferent branch consists of two neurons (the pre- and postganglionic neurons), which usually synapse in an enteric ganglion of the intestinal wall. The efferent neurons of the autonomic nervous system are divided into two major functional groups (the sympathetic and parasympathetic systems) with different and usually opposing functions. An afferent branch is of course also present, but its role is only to optimize functioning rather than to determine it, so it is indicated by dashes in Figure 165C.

Thus afferent and efferent neurons are relatively harmoniously balanced only in the middle portion of the nervous system—the **spinal cord**, the domain of the so-called sensorimotor systems (Figure 165B). This domain, which has to do primarily with bodily movement, is not limited to the spinal cord. It extends far into the brain where the afferent branches of sensorimotor systems ultimately reach the cerebral cortex and synapse with the corresponding efferent branches, which originate there. Thus the brain also includes a "middle" domain within the threefold organization of the nervous system where the architecture typical of sensorimotor reflex arcs is located.

In contrast to this "middle" domain, the sensory (upper) and autonomic (lower) systems are structural opposites. We become conscious of the activity of the higher sensory systems, which

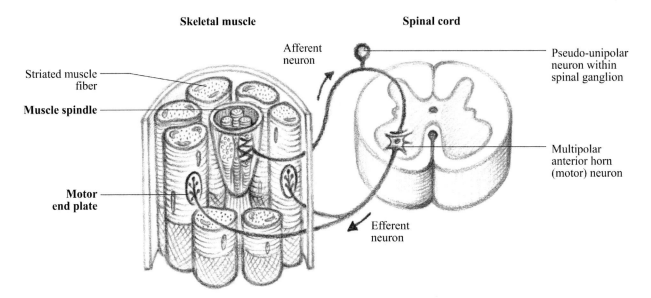

Skeletal muscle   **Spinal cord**

Afferent neuron

Pseudo-unipolar neuron within spinal ganglion

Striated muscle fiber

Muscle spindle

Multipolar anterior horn (motor) neuron

Motor end plate

Efferent neuron

Fig. 164. **Connection between the spinal cord and a muscle**. *The simplest form of a reflex arc between the spinal cord and a skeletal muscle. It consists of one afferent (sensory) neuron, which enters the spinal cord through the dorsal spinal root, and one efferent (motor) neuron, whose axon leaves the spinal cord through the ventral root and connects with a striated muscle fiber in the motor end plate (sensory-motor system). Impulses that originate in tiny sensory organs (muscle spindles) in the muscles are transmitted to the motor neuron by the afferent neuron, thus closing the circle.*

are functionally associated with the cerebrum, but remain unconscious of the activity of autonomic systems. Any sensory process that leads to perception begins in sensory cells, where specific compounds (for example, visual pigments such as rhodopsin) often play a role. Conversely, the unconscious process of impulse conduction in the autonomic nervous system ends with the release of specific neurotransmitters that regulate the activity of organs such as glands, blood vessels, or intestinal muscles. This does not mean, however, that the autonomic nervous system causes the activity of internal organs. Blood circulation, glandular secretion, intestinal activity, and many other such functions run their course largely independently. The primary task of the autonomic nervous system is to enable the exchange of information *among* organs so that their functions can be coordinated and fine tuned.

In other words, the autonomic system allows organs to "know about each other" so that their cellular activities can be harmonized or adapted to current needs such as changing environmental conditions (heat, cold, exertion, stress, etc.).

In principle, the situation is no different in the "middle" (spinal) system (Figure 165B), except that the efferent (motor) neurons are in direct contact with their effector organs (striated muscle fibers) and can be influenced deliberately. Even here, activity is not directly guided by consciousness. In the case of the striated or skeletal muscles, movement may be initiated by consciousness, but actual muscle contraction depends primarily on metabolic processes and energy transfers (Table 19). Energy is stored in the cell in the form of adenosine triphosphate (ATP), released when ATP is converted to ADP (adenosine diphosphate), and expended when myofibrils contract. Contraction depends on a sudden increase—more than a hundred-fold—in the concentration of Ca^+ ions in the cytoplasm (Figure 72). This increase is triggered by the influx of Na^+ ions into the cell. Like stimulus conduction in nerves, this process, which ultimately leads to a contraction (i.e., hardening) of the muscle, can be compared to a tiny, reversible "dying off" process. To overcome this hardening and become soft again, the muscle needs energy, supplied either from glycogen reserves in its cells or by the vascular system. Energy is expended to move Ca^+ ions back into their "containers" in the endoplasmic reticulum, eliminate sodium from the cell, and build up energy-rich phosphate molecules (ATP) anew.

The muscle hardening that sets in at death, when these energy transfers cease, is called rigor mortis. The muscles soften again only later, when the body's cells begin to break down. In the living body, however, muscle relaxation indicates not disintegration but successful energy expenditures that have made the muscle soft again.

Muscles must be well vascularized because oxygen and the compounds (especially glucose) that supply energy "travel" in the bloodstream. Blood vessels also carry away metabolic wastes (lactic acid, carbon dioxide, etc.). Thus circulation is the third important function involved in muscle movement.

Efferent nerves (motor neurons), whose motor end plates link directly to muscle membranes, release transmitters such as acetylcholine, which trigger sodium influx, and with it the intracellular "flood" of Ca^+ ions and subsequent muscle fiber contraction. This does not mean, however, that efferent nerves "cause" movement. The actual movement depends on independent muscle-cell activity, which in turn depends on intracellular metabolic processes. The nervous system simply regulates this activity and reconciles it with the activity of the motor system as a whole. For example, when one group of muscles contracts, cramping or movement disorders will occur unless the opposing group relaxes. In this context, the

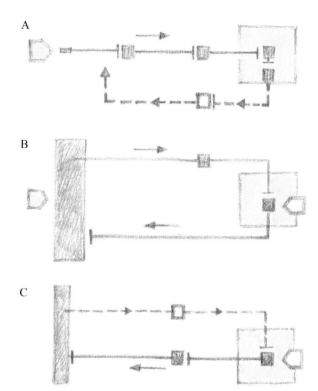

Fig. 165. **Neural structure of the nervous system** *(16). The three basic forms of neural circuits in the nervous system reflect the functional threefoldness of the nervous system as a whole.*
A: Head (sensorium, central nervous system). Afferent neuron chains dominate.
B: Spinal cord (spinal, segmented domain of the nervous system). Afferent and efferent connections are balanced.
C: Visceral domain (autonomic nervous system, peripheral nervous system). Efferent neurons are functionally dominant.

job of the nervous system is to "direct traffic," to organize and harmonize the flow of movement forces, just as traffic lights activate but do not cause the movement of vehicles in traffic. The actual causes of moving traffic are the drivers' intentions to reach specific destinations; traffic lights and regulations simply serve to organize and coordinate the activities as a whole.

In line with the aforementioned observations, it becomes clear that the metabolic activity

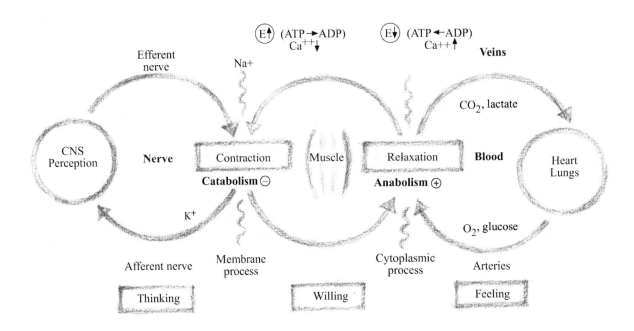

Table 19. **Basic processes involved in muscle contraction** and their relationships to cellular and psychological processes (for details, see text).

underlying movement is a process in the domain of the will, whereas events triggered by the so-called "motor" (efferent) nerves are essentially neurological (i.e., informational) in character. Efferent nerves, in their direct link to muscles, allow us to **implement the movements we have in mind**, but they do not produce the movements themselves. Of course a muscle can become paralyzed when the relevant nerve is severed or damaged, but it may also be paralyzed or its movement disturbed when its cellular metabolic processes are disrupted.

Between the "will aspect" and the neurological or mental aspect of movement lies the balancing and harmonizing effect of the vascular (rhythmic) system, in which the element of feeling comes into play. Thus each movement includes not only an informational or mental component (i.e., the movement we have in mind) and a will element (the application of strength and energy) but also a

feeling (e.g., enthusiasm, depression) that humanizes the movement (Table 19).

These perspectives may help us understand why Rudolf Steiner repeatedly and emphatically rejected the notion of motor nerves as "will organs" (27, 65). He pointed out that the metabolic system is the physical basis for will activity, with the nervous system serving only to coordinate and regulate functions as well as convey movement-related sensory experiences and mental images (see reference 60 in particular).

Thus the sensorimotor system, which we will discuss in the next chapter, is not primarily involved in human will activity but rather in informational processes. With regard to voluntary movements, it also has to do with the mental images we have of intended movements. Implementing these movements, however, requires not only neurological coordination and regulation but also functioning metabolic and circulatory systems.

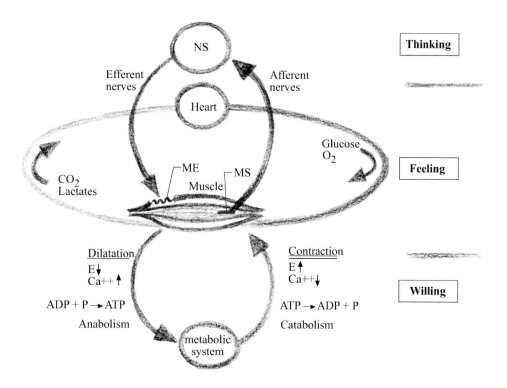

Fig. 166. **Functional threefolding of the musculoskeletal system.** *Striated muscles are functionally placed between the nervous system (sensorimotor systems), metabolic system (energy transfer in the cytoplasm of the muscle cell), and circulatory system (blood vessels for the delivery and removal of energy-bearing O_2, CO_2, etc.). (Arteries: red, veins: blue.)*
Willing acts upon the muscles primarily by way of the metabolism, feeling by way of the blood circulation, and thinking (picturing movement) by way of the nervous system.

ADP: adenosine diphosphate
ATP: adenosine triphosphate
ME: motor end plate
MS: muscle spindle
NS: nervous system (sensorimotor systems)

The Major Sensorimotor Systems

The sensorimotor systems represent the nervous system's middle functional domain, which lies between the sensory systems (sensorium) in the brain on the one hand and the autonomic (vegetative) nervous system in the body on the other. The sensorimotor systems are located primarily in the spinal cord (Figure 159). For the most part, they are involved with the motor apparatus and voluntary movements.

The human body has an infinite variety of possible movements at its command. As we have seen (pp. 112-114 ff.), these movements originate first and foremost in our will or intentionality, not in the nervous system. The nerves that innervate the motor system are initiating factors only in that they provide vital informational processes related to movement that are necessary to coordinate the activities of the will, which works within the metabolic processes of the muscles. From the informational perspective, the great variety of possible movements can be reduced to five major divisions (referred to as "systems" here), each regulated by a specific sensorimotor system of the nervous system.

Sensorimotor Systems Within the Nervous System			
	Type of Motor Activity	**Superordinate CNS Organ**	**Functional Systems**
1.	Controlling muscle length and tension	Spinal cord (individual segments)	Monosynaptic, myostatic stretch reflexes
2.	Isolated, purposeful individual movements (defense, fight or flight reactions); primitive, rhythmical locomotion	Spinal cord (multiple segments)	Complex polysynaptic (flexor) reflexes
3.	Regulating equilibrium; muscle tone in relation to maintaining equilibrium (stand and stance reflex); temporal coordination of movements	Hindbrain, cerebellum, midbrain	Vestibulocerebellar system, brain stem reflexes
4.	Subcortical motor activity, learned movements, posture control, mimicry, habits (instinctive, unconscious movements)	Brain stem, basal ganglia (lentiform nucleus, corpus striatum, globus pallidus), thalamus	Subcortical motor systems
5.	Conscious, creative, voluntary movement; aiming, skilled movements	Cerebral cortex	Cortical motor system (pyramidal system)

Table 20. Overview of the five great human sensorimotor systems.

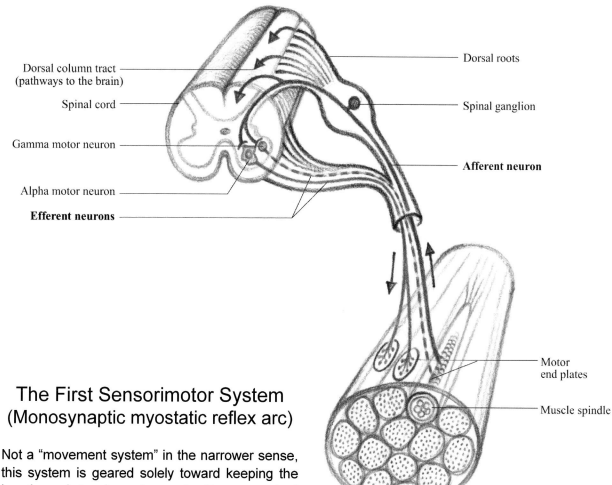

Dorsal column tract
(pathways to the brain)

Spinal cord

Gamma motor neuron

Alpha motor neuron

Efferent neurons

Dorsal roots

Spinal ganglion

Afferent neuron

Motor
end plates

Muscle spindle

The First Sensorimotor System
(Monosynaptic myostatic reflex arc)

Not a "movement system" in the narrower sense, this system is geared solely toward keeping the length and tension of muscle fibers constant —providing muscle tone (Figure 167). In the simplest example of such proprioceptive (stretch) reflexes, one afferent and one efferent (motor) neuron linked to a muscle form a reflex arc in which neural impulses circulate constantly to maintain consistent muscle length. The afferent sensory fibers that spiral around intrafusal muscle fibers in the muscle spindles are actually tiny sensory organs that register changes in the length of muscle fibers (Figure 167). How does this system function? For example, if the knee joints threaten to collapse (perhaps because of a heavy weight carried on the head), muscle tension is automatically increased. This system keeps the muscle tone adapted to the Earth's gravitational pull in order to maintain uprightness (an antigravity feedback loop). Thus this first sensorimotor system is "hostile" to movement, so to speak, and can be thought of as a myostatic system.

*Fig. 167. **Neural structure of the first functional sensorimotor system**: Simple monosynaptic reflex. Arrows indicate direction of impulse conduction to (afferent) and from (efferent) the spinal cord. (For details, see text.)*

The Second Functional System of the Sensorimotor Systems
(Complex polysynaptic reflexes)

The first system always provides the foundation for the more complex neural circuits required by specific movements. For example, when you shoo away a biting insect or pull your hand away from it in a reflexlike gesture, complex impulse patterns run back and forth between your spinal cord and

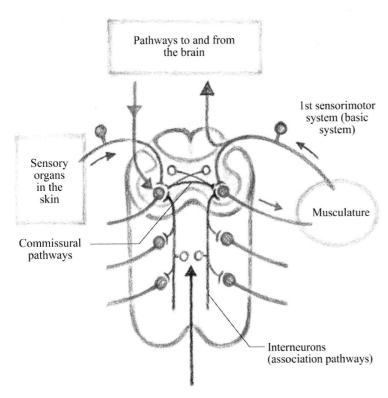

Pathways to and from the brain

1st sensorimotor system (basic system)

Sensory organs in the skin

Musculature

Commissural pathways

Interneurons (association pathways)

Fig. 168. **Structure of the second-order sensorimotor system** *(polysynaptic reflex system). Impulses flow from sense organs in the skin to the spinal cord, where they are processed by commissural and associational pathways in such a way that coordinated, directed individual movements become possible. Ascending and descending projection pathways provide connections to higher centers in the brain.*

force of gravity and maintaining muscle tone, while the movements of individual flexors must be repeated for each step forward to keep the motion of walking going.

From the neurological perspective, higher centers in the brain stem (supraspinal systems) play important roles in the simple motions of walking or running. The descending reticular pathways, the medial and lateral reticulospinal tracts, affect the flexors and extensors through inhibition or facilitation. Because these pathways end in spinal motor neurons, they also influence underlying proprioceptive reflex pathways, which are directly connected to the muscles (Figure 168).

Here we encounter a general structural principle: Higher sensorimotor systems are never directly connected to muscles but always use the first and second sensorimotor divisions as their common endpoint or starting point. All higher neurological regulation ultimately influences muscles only through the first system, which is in direct contact with them. The higher supraspinal systems are hierarchically arranged inasmuch as their nuclei are located one above the other in the hindbrain, midbrain, interbrain, and endbrain and are connected by feedback loops. First of all, let's consider the systems having to do with the endbrain (cerebral cortex, etc.).

the muscle groups needed to implement a single, directed, reflexive movement. As individual flexor muscles contract, the length of the corresponding extensors must be increased by the same amount. We are usually barely conscious of such "*heteroceptive*" circuits, which originate not in sense organs of the muscles themselves but in other locations (skin, mucous membrane, etc.). In this second sensorimotor system, internuncial neurons in the spinal cord play a role in switching impulses between left and right (commissural pathways) or up and down (associative pathways); (see Figure 168).

When we walk or run, the first and second sensorimotor systems work together. The extensors preserve uprightness by counteracting the

Cortical Motor Systems (Pyramidal system—the 5ᵗʰ sensorimotor system)

The most highly evolved form of movement — directed, consciously intended, voluntary movement—always requires a functioning cerebral cortex. The pyramidal tract (lateral corticospinal tract) is a long efferent pathway that begins in the precentral gyrus (the somatomotor cortical region in front of the central sulcus), crosses to the other side of the midline in the medulla oblongata (pyramidal decussation), and then runs directly to the motor neurons of the spinal cord (Figure 169). Afferent nerve fibers coming from the sense organs of the muscles run in the opposite direction.

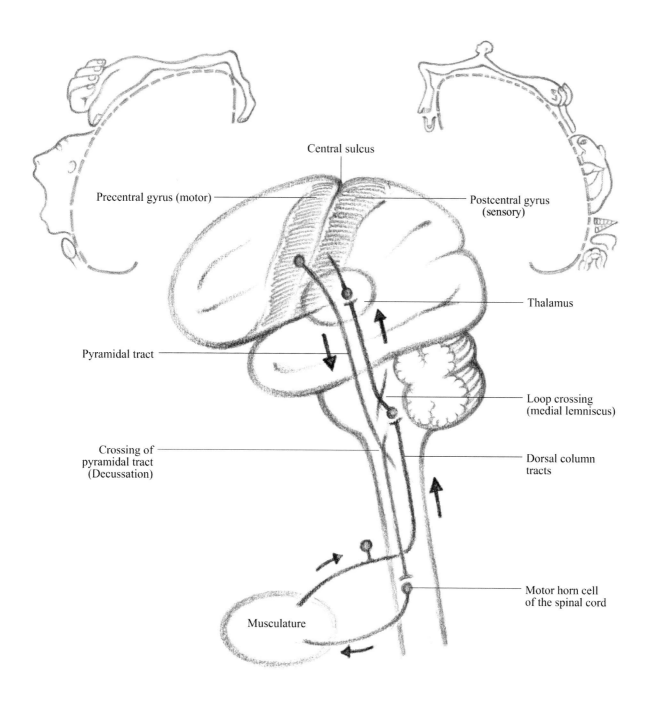

*Fig. 169. **Neuronal structure of the 5th sensorimotor (pyramidal) system. The efferent (pyramidal) pathway** runs without interruption from the so-called somatomotor cortex (precentral gyrus) to the anterior horn cells of the spinal cord, crossing the midline in the medulla oblongata. After crossing in the brain stem at the medial lemniscus, the associated **afferent dorsal column pathway** ends in the somatosensory cortex (postcentral gyrus). Each of these cortex areas contains a projected "map" of the body, standing on its head and distorted according to the functional importance of its parts (important areas are larger, less important ones smaller). These reflected maps are the so-called sensory and motor homunculi.*

Central sulcus

Precentral gyrus (motor)

Postcentral gyrus
(sensory)

Thalamus

Pyramidal tract

Loop crossing
(medial lemniscus)

Crossing of
pyramidal tract
(Decussation)

Dorsal column
tracts

Motor horn cell
of the spinal cord

Musculature

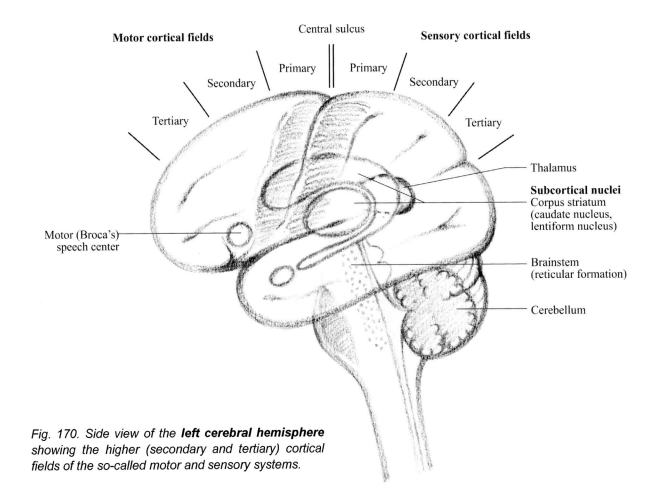

Motor cortical fields

Central sulcus

Sensory cortical fields

Primary

Secondary

Primary

Secondary

Tertiary

Tertiary

Thalamus

Subcortical nuclei
Corpus striatum
(caudate nucleus,
lentiform nucleus)

Motor (Broca's)
speech center

Brainstem
(reticular formation)

Cerebellum

*Fig. 170. Side view of the **left cerebral hemisphere** showing the higher (secondary and tertiary) cortical fields of the so-called motor and sensory systems.*

Their cell bodies are located within the spinal ganglion. The afferent fiber tracts run in the dorsal (posterior) column of the spinal cord towards the brain stem where they cross to the opposite side (dorsal column/medial lemniscal pathway), finally ending in the postcentral gyrus of the brain (somatosensory region of the cortex). Together with the pyramidal tract, they form a reflex loop that passes through the cerebral cortex. This loop is of a higher order than the first sensorimotor system and reflects all of the muscles in the body, as well as the functional importance of individual muscle groups or corresponding areas of skin (sensory and motor homunculi; Figure 169).

The job of the pyramidal sensorimotor system is to regulate and organize the skilled gestures and voluntary movements that are so characteristically human. Our artistic and technological achievements would be impossible without this system's precise informational "programs." Along with our deliberate, "will-filled" intentions, the pyramidal system makes possible the many impressive, exclusively human accomplishments in art, technology, and sports.

Subcortical Motor System
(4th sensorimotor system)

Differentiated, consciously intended, voluntary motor activity would still be impossible, however, without the involvement of major subcortical nuclei. The putamen, caudate nucleus, and globus pallidus all belong to the telencephalon (endbrain). The caudate nucleus and the putamen make up the corpus striatum; the globus pallidus and putamen together form the lentiform or lenticular (lens-shaped) nucleus. The thalamus, which belongs to the interbrain, and the red nucleus (ruber) of the midbrain and substantia nigra also

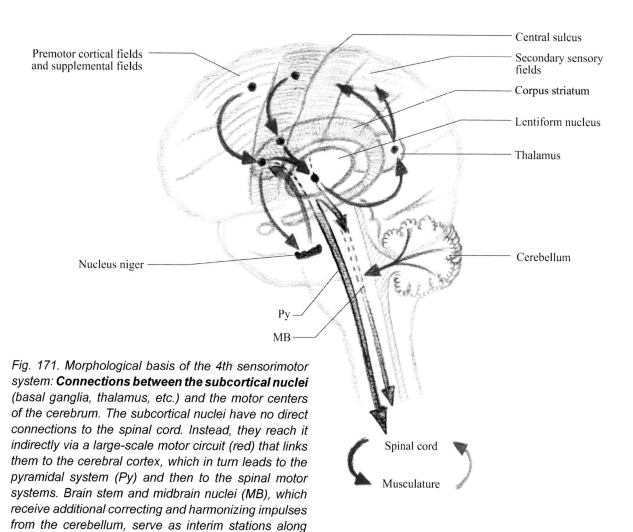

Premotor cortical fields and supplemental fields

Central sulcus

Secondary sensory fields

Corpus striatum

Lentiform nucleus

Thalamus

Nucleus niger

Cerebellum

Py

MB

Spinal cord

Musculature

Fig. 171. Morphological basis of the 4th sensorimotor system: **Connections between the subcortical nuclei** *(basal ganglia, thalamus, etc.) and the motor centers of the cerebrum. The subcortical nuclei have no direct connections to the spinal cord. Instead, they reach it indirectly via a large-scale motor circuit (red) that links them to the cerebral cortex, which in turn leads to the pyramidal system (Py) and then to the spinal motor systems. Brain stem and midbrain nuclei (MB), which receive additional correcting and harmonizing impulses from the cerebellum, serve as interim stations along this route.*

belong to the subcortical motor system (Figures 170 and 171). Feedback loops among major subcortical nuclei are connected to the cerebral cortex and use the pyramidal tract system as their common exit (Figure 171).

The subcortical nuclei are especially important for organizing and mastering new forms of movement. Every new movement pattern must be learned, often with great effort over a long period of time, as it is planned and practiced—clumsily and slowly, at first—with the help of the cortical motor and premotor centers. Think about learning to play a piece of music, for example. Once you've finally learned the specific movements, they happen automatically and semiconsciously,

as if by themselves. When you master the piece, the system of subcortical nuclei, which form large feedback loops ("motor circuits") with the cerebral cortex, takes over the program.

The human ability to acquire motor skills is immense. From the neurological perspective, this ability is based on motor and premotor cortical systems, which are highly evolved and differentiated in humans. Substantial evolutionary advances in other parts of the cerebrum also make it possible for other systems (sensory systems, etc.) to contribute to this kind of learning. For example, the part of the cortex called the motor speech center of Broca (Figure 170), located in front of the precentral gyrus, influences the larynx muscles in ways that make speech movements possible. If this center, which is normally present only in the left half of the brain, is damaged, speech becomes impossible even though the laryngeal muscles are not paralyzed. This is known as motor aphasia. Thus higher (secondary and tertiary) motor centers of the frontal lobe are involved in specialized functions (speaking, writing, etc.) that coordinate the movements of individual muscle groups into complex movement in the service of a superordinate overall function.

A similar functional arrangement of higher (secondary and tertiary) centers exists on the sensory side, i.e., in the parietal lobe of the cerebrum (Figure 170). These centers, however, are involved in the sensory evaluation of afferent impulses from the motor system—in other words, in experiencing the body's orientation and location in space. Here we become conscious of muscle tension and the location of muscles in space (proprioception). These centers are important for body awareness and kinesthesia. Visual spatial orientation and recognition of symbols and letters are also located here, in the so-called optical reading center.

The sensory organs for cortical sensorimotor functions are located in muscle and tendon spindles and joints. Afferent impulses that originate in these sensory organs are processed like reflexes in the spinal cord in the first and second sensorimotor systems; they are also conducted to the cerebrum, primarily via the dorsal column pathways, where they constitute the most important source of information for cortical and subcortical motor systems. But as a result of the activity of the higher sensory cortex fields of the parietal lobe, which border on the postcentral gyrus, these impulses can also become conscious—a fact of central importance for our ability to experience space, our own bodies, and our orientation in three-dimensional space.

The current state of knowledge allows us to *summarize* the neural foundations of voluntary motor activity as follows: The pyramidal tract, which runs directly from the motor cortex (precentral gyrus) to the spinal cord, is the common efferent tract (output) for all of the brain's

motor systems. Precise functional representations of individual muscle groups (the so-called motor homunculus) are found in the cortex. Planning and "programming" complex movement sequences, however, require the involvement of higher brain centers, especially those located in front of the primary motor cortex. These areas, the so-called premotor and supplementary motor area (secondary motor centers, Figures 170 and 171), increased radically in size as the human brain evolved. Together with the brain's associative systems, they occupy six times more space in humans than in apes. Experiments have shown that these centers become active even before a consciously intended voluntary movement is carried out and are therefore involved in planning the program for such movements. Now that accurate measurement of activity in specific brain areas has become possible—even in humans— through imaging techniques (PET) based on changes in circulation, it has been determined that premotor brain areas really do become active before a voluntary movement is performed. It is interesting to note, however, that such activity also increases during "mental rehearsal," that is, when the movement in question (for example, opening and closing a hand) is simply imagined. This demonstrates that secondary and tertiary motor cortex areas (Figure 170) are involved in planning and producing specific movement programs for voluntary motor activities. Ultimately, the motor feedback loop that involves the major subcortical groups of nuclei (Figure 171) allows long-term stabilization of these programs, which in turn makes it possible for us to learn movement sequences, to monitor and adjust the details of complex movements involving aim and skill, and to produce "involuntary," automatic accompanying movements (mimicry, gestures, etc.). Ultimately, however, learning voluntary motor "programs" also requires the harmonizing and balancing activity of an intermediary system—specifically, the system of equilibrium and the cerebellum.

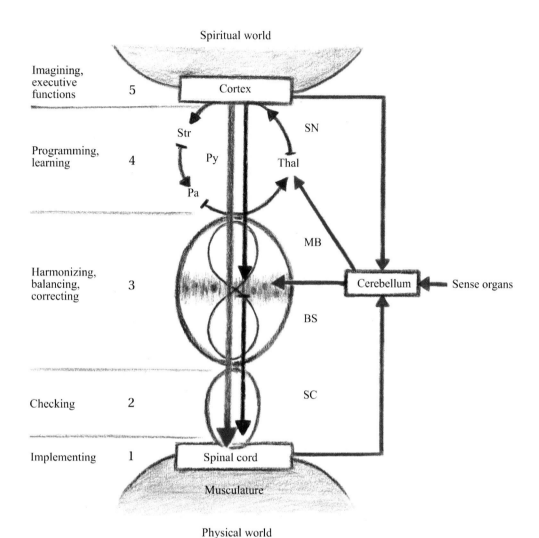

Fig. 172. **Functional interaction of the five major sensorimotor systems** *(1-5)* **in connection with the cerebellum**. *The cerebellum receives input (blue) from the cerebral cortex, spinal cord (SC), and from the major sense organs (eye, ear, labyrinth) and exerts corrective and harmonizing effects on the motor system via efferent tracts (red) to the thalamus (Thal), midbrain (MB, e.g., red nucleus), and brain stem (BS, e.g., reticular formation and vestibular nuclei). Consequently, the third sensorimotor system becomes a mediating, balancing element between the two upper (cortical, 5 and 4) and the two lower (spinal, 2 and 1) systems. Implementing conceived movements takes place in multiple stages (planning, programming, monitoring or correcting, and implementing). In this multistep process, only the base system (1) of the spinal cord is in actual contact with the muscles, i.e., with the will aspect of the movement process. The pyramidal system (Py), however, can skip these steps and intervene directly in the motor systems of the spinal cord, which is what makes fine motor activity possible (e.g., the finger movements of writing or the vocal cord movements of speech). Pa: globus pallidus; Str: Corpus striatum; SN: subcortical nuclei.*

The Vestibular System and the Cerebellum
(3rd sensorimotor system)

The two upper (higher) sensorimotor systems of the brain (system 4 and 5) and the two lower, more reflexively working systems of the spinal cord (system 1 and 2) are linked by the vestibular system and cerebellum. Voluntary motor activity and reflexes could not occur in parallel without the mediation and harmonization of the system of equilibrium. This system does much more than merely maintain the body's balance in three-dimensional space. It also has balancing and harmonizing effects on the other four sensorimotor systems.

The central organ of this activity is the *cerebellum*. Afferent pathways supply it with the necessary information from all other parts of the brain:

1. From the cerebrum via the pons (corticopontocerebellar pathways);

2. From the spinal cord (and thus ultimately from the muscles and joints) via the lateral column tracts (spinocerebellar tracts);

3. From the dedicated organ of balance, the labyrinth in the petrous portion of the temporal bone, via the vestibulocochlear nerve (CNVIII).

The *organ of balance* consists of three semicircular canals that stand perpendicular to one another, forming three planes like the corner of a room. The canals emerge from the two little sacs (the utricle and the saccule) that together make up the vestibule (hence the name "vestibular apparatus"). The sense organs lining the fluid-filled canals make us conscious of the body's (or more precisely, the head's) position in space and inform the cerebellum about bodily movements so that it can work out the appropriate reflex "programs" necessary for maintaining balance.

In the cerebellum, information that originates in the labyrinth is compared to information coming from the cerebral cortex and from the motor apparatus itself, which is conveyed toward the center by the spinal cord. Our consciousness is not involved in the cerebellum's responses to this information. The efferent pathways leading out of the cerebellum connect with the cortical and subcortical motor systems via the thalamus and the red nucleus and with the spinal cord via the vestibular nuclei of the brain stem and the reticular formation of the midbrain (Figure 171). Here too, the first sensorimotor system serves as the common final section of the route for all of these regulatory pathways (Figure 172).

The *cerebellum* functions like an extremely fast computer that monitors and corrects all of the movement "programs" originating in the brain. The cerebellum's activity harmonizes the movements of the motor organs, ensures balance, and refines and smoothes out individual movements. Without the system of equilibrium, even relatively simple directed motions—such as grasping an object, throwing (aiming) a ball, or producing different notes on an instrument—would be impossible.

Thus this "layered" sensorimotor system, the middle functional domain of the nervous system, consists of five major neural systems that are associated with specific forms of movement and differ significantly among themselves with regard to both the complexity of their neuronal circuits and the degree to which we become conscious of their activity (Table 20).

Greek gymnastics. Ancient Greek mystery-wisdom may have already been aware of these five major sensorimotor systems (16). To a considerable extent, the five disciplines of the classical Olympic pentathlon (running, jumping, wrestling, discus, and javelin) correspond to these five sensorimotor systems. Running and jumping primarily involve the spinal cord (first and second sensorimotor systems) in which reflexes predominate. In the third discipline, wrestling, maintaining balance (especially in the horizontal dimension) plays a decisive role; from the neurological perspective, the vestibular system is heavily involved. In the discus throw, which involves mastering a complex voluntary movement that becomes largely automatic with practice, the subcortical system comes to the fore. In the fifth and final exercise (javelin), learned gestures again play a role, but the essential elements in this voluntary motor activity are a good aim and a high degree of consciousness—characteristics of the pyramidal motor system.

The Sensory Systems

Functional Subdivision and Action of the Sensory Systems

The sensorium constitutes the upper domain of the nervous system (Figure 165A). Within it, each sense has its own characteristic level of consciousness. For the most part, we become fully conscious only of the functions of the higher senses (seeing, hearing, etc.). In contrast, we are normally totally unaware of the activity of visceral sensory receptors and become conscious— usually painfully so—of the functioning of our internal organs only when they are diseased. Although there are many different sense receptors in the internal organs, they typically convey only a dull sensation of well-being when the organs are healthy or discomfort when they are not.

Thus our sense organs can be categorized according to the scope of their specific activity and the degree of consciousness they achieve. At the top of this list are the organs of sight and hearing. The organs of smell and taste are somewhat less differentiated, as are the organs of the various skin senses, which collectively convey not only sensations of touch, pressure, and vibration but also temperature differences and sensations of pain. At the lower end of the scale are the sensory receptors in the body's interior, which function completely unconsciously and are responsible only for basic regulatory processes such as osmoregulation, chemoregulation, or blood pressure regulation (Figure 173). The upper group of sense organs conveys perceptions from the outer world, while the lower group (the visceral senses) conveys perceptions from inside the body.

Between the upper and lower groups lie the senses of balance, with its organs located in the inner ear, and of deep sensitivity, with receptors located in muscles and tendons (muscle and tendon spindles) and near joints. These senses mediate between the upper and lower senses. Receptors in muscles are essential for movement in three-dimensional space because they register not only the tension and length of the muscles as such but also (indirectly) the effect of gravity on the organs of movement (sense of position). In contrast, the body's movements in three-dimensional space are directly registered by the organ of balance, which therefore mediates between events in the outside world and factors related to the body itself, such as its static or changing location in space or its voluntary movements.

Thus each of the many senses can be assigned to one of three major groups, with the upper group being oriented toward the outside world, the lower group toward the body's interior, and the middle group toward both, so that it serves a mediating function between the other two groups (Table 21).

For human beings, however, all of these sensory apparatuses form a functional whole. The "I"-being, the essential core of the personality, always compiles a unitary image of the world from sensory inputs from various organs. Thus it is more useful to arrange the senses in a circle centered on the sense of pain, which is relatively undifferentiated but is an "archetypal" sense with the potential to be transformed into any of the other senses

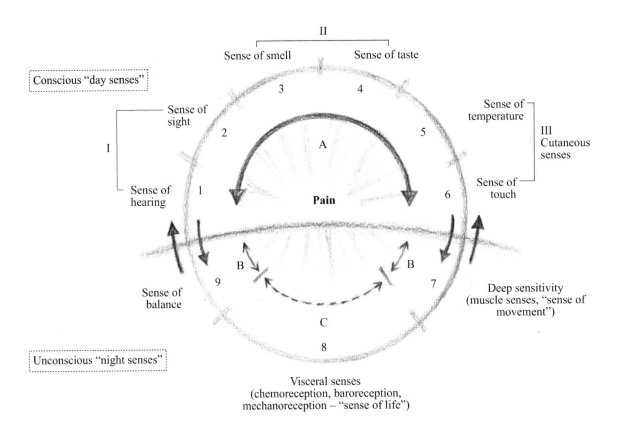

Fig. 173. **Human sensory systems.** *In this array, pain appears in the center as an undifferentiated "archetypal sense." The "day senses" (A), which belong to the world of conscious perception, can be subdivided into three groups with varying degrees of differentiation and consciousness (I, II, and III). Each group consists of two contrasting senses (e.g., sight/hearing). The "night senses" (B and C), which work more unconsciously, have to do with life and movement functions inside the body (for details, see text).*

This circular arrangement clarifies still another phenomenon. If one sense is eliminated, other sense organs fill the gap, becoming more important and enhancing their performance, sometimes to an unbelievable extent. For the individual, the sensory world remains a coherent whole even if sight, hearing, or other senses fail. Although the specific character of the missing sensory input cannot be replaced, the system remains intact as other sensory domains expand to fill the void. The "I" then uses other sensations to compensate (often extensively) for the ones that are missing. The extent of this compensation is evident in accounts by Jacques Lusseyran or Helen Keller, for example (77, 78).

General Functioning of the Senses

Whether morphologically simple or complex, all the senses function quite similarly. To understand the reality of movement as a whole, we found that we had to consider not only neurological but also metabolic and rhythmic processes involved in muscle activity. Similarly, with regard to sensory activity, we cannot consider neural processes in isolation. To gain a completely valid picture of sensory processes, we must also take into account the rhythmic foundations (circulation, respiration) of sensations and emotions and the

	Sensory system	Sensory modality	Related nerves and brain areas	Level of consciousness	
Higher senses (oriented toward the outer world)	Auditory system	Hearing (perception of sounds and pitches)	CN VIII, temporal lobe (Heschel's gyrus, Wernicke's area)	Fully conscious	Hearing
	Visual system	Seeing (forms, colors, space)	CN II, occipital lobe (striate cortex, etc.)	Fully conscious	Sight
	Olfactory system	Smelling	CN I, rhinencephalon and temporal lobe (piriform lobe)	Conscious	Smell
	Gustatory system	Tasting	CN IX (also CN X), temporal lobe	Conscious	Taste
	Cutaneous senses	Surface sensitivity (temperature, pressure, touch, vibration, pain)	Spinal nerves, CN V, temporal lobe (postcentral gyrus)	Wide range in degrees of consciousness	Warmth, Touch
Middle senses (oriented toward the outer and inner worlds)	Vestibular system	Equilibrium, experiencing space	CN VIII, cerebellum	Unconscious, semiconscious	Balance
	Muscle senses	Deep sensitivity	Nerves in the spinal cord and brain; cerebellum, temporal lobe	Partly conscious, partly unconscious	"Sense of movement" (kinesthesia and proprioception)
Lower senses (oriented toward the inner world)	Visceral senses	Osmoreception, baroreception, chemoreception, mechanoreception	Autonomic nervous system	Unconscious	"Sense of life"

Table 21. Overview of sensory systems, related nerves and brain centers, and levels of consciousness. "Sense of movement" and "sense of life" are terms coined by Rudolf Steiner (76).

metabolic foundations of our will (Figure 174). As with muscle activity, what the soul experiences through sensory perception cannot be traced back exclusively to neural processes. Neural processes enable us to become **conscious** of external or internal events but in no way represent the entire scope of the activity. Sensory experience involves many elements other than nerve activity. Our sense organs are like channels or "ports of entry" that provide the outer world with access to the

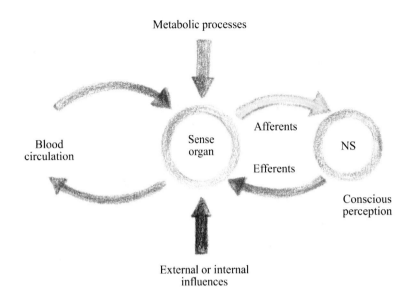

Metabolic processes

Blood
circulation

Sense
organ

Afferents

Efferents

NS

Conscious
perception

External or internal
influences

*Fig. 174. **Basic life processes in sensory systems**. Neural processes are complemented by circulatory and metabolic processes, which are as essential to perception as sensory cells and neuronal circuits. NS: nervous system.*

body (79). In many cases, elements characteristic of the outer world must even be present inside the body for perception to occur. For example, the otolith organs (see Figure 189C, p. 263), which are directly affected by gravity, help us sense the vertical up-down dimension.

But our senses do more than simply impart consciousness of the forces at work outside or inside the body. They also open up a world of experience that is as varied as the possibilities for movement in our limbs. Each sense is ***specific***, as Johannes Müller formulated it in the mid-nineteenth century in his "law of specific sense energies." It shows us only part of the world. The eye perceives only light, the ear only sound, and the organ of smell only odors. Thus each sensory system specializes in one particular ***modality***. Sensory experiences are not based exclusively on neurological processes, however, but are also related to rhythmical and metabolic processes within the sensory apparatus. In other words, sensory events are associated with correspondingly differentiated experiences of feeling and will. As a result, understanding a sensory system as a totality is usually possible only if we also take supposedly auxiliary functions such as respiration and metabolism into account (Figure

174). If we do so, the problem of correlating psychological experience with sensory processes also disappears. In the modern view of the sensory process, the world is a dark, silent box filled with "quivering particles of matter" that contact our sense organs and then call forth subjective experiences in the brain. We can describe neurological pathways to the cortex in detail, but the subsequent development of qualitative sensory experiences (color, sound, etc.) remains an insoluble mystery. Here, as with the question of the origin of movement, overcoming our customary epistemological reductionism requires a fundamental shift in our thinking. We will return to this issue when we discuss individual sensory systems.

But first, let's look at the ***neurological aspect of these systems***. As mentioned above, the level of consciousness achieved by individual sensory systems varies greatly, and the connections of individual sensors to the nervous system are equally varied. The highly differentiated sensory systems (seeing and hearing) that dominate our consciousness are projected onto the cerebral cortex, where they occupy extensive areas. In contrast, the sensory systems of the internal organs and of the body itself (our third or "lower"

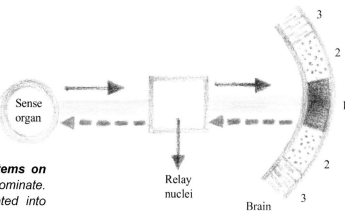

Fig. 175. **Basic structure of sensory systems on the neuronal level**. *In general, afferents dominate. Subcortical synapses are always incorporated into neural pathways. The cerebral cortex includes (primary) projection fields (1), higher processing centers (2), and often also still-higher areas (3) for "understanding" and remembering perceptions.*

group; see Table 21) have almost no connection to the cerebral cortex; their relay nuclei are located in the brain stem or in the medulla oblongata. Most of their activity relates to reflexes and does not become conscious except as a generalized "sense of life" (76).

The sensory systems belonging to the musculature and to the vestibular apparatus (Table 21, middle group) occupy an intermediary position. In most cases, they have connections to the spinal cord, which is segmentally (i.e., rhythmically) structured. The cerebellum is associated with the organ of balance, whose activity remains totally unconscious. In some cases, the muscle senses (proprioception) are also projected onto the cerebral cortex. This activity becomes conscious, but reflexes, which are played out in the spinal cord and brain stem, do not.

At least with regard to the higher senses, we can now recognize a characteristic **threefold functional division** in the neurological domain (Figure 175). At the first level are the sense organs themselves, where receptors (usually highly specialized) and related auxiliary organs (lens, middle ear, etc.) are located. The second level consists of relay nuclei in the interbrain and midbrain, whose activity occurs unconsciously and

usually reflexively. The third level encompasses cortex functions, of which we become conscious. As a rule, we can identify a hierarchy of three functional cortex fields. The sense organs themselves project onto primary cortex fields. The adjacent secondary cortex fields have to do with "processing" sense impressions that contribute to higher individual functions such as understanding images or words. Tertiary fields are located even farther from the primary projection fields. According to neurophysiologists, their primary function is to store perceptions in short- or long-term memory—a function that must not be interpreted one-sidedly (i.e., in strictly neurological terms), as we shall see in a subsequent section.

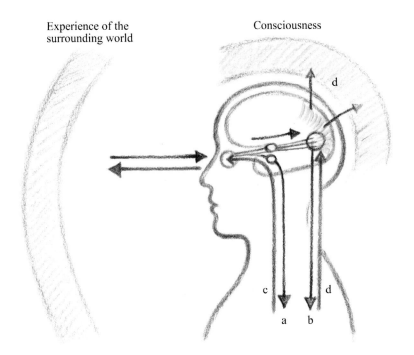

Experience of the surrounding world

Consciousness

*Fig. 176. **The sensory process involves the entire human being**. The process of perception does not consist simply in projecting afferent stimuli onto the associated brain centers. It also requires the cooperation of the entire body, i.e., of metabolic, circulatory, and respiratory processes (a-d), which must also be taken into account. (For details, see text.)*

Asymmetry of Sensory Reflex Loops

Every sensory system, like every sensorimotor system, includes a reflex loop consisting of an afferent branch and an efferent branch (Figures 165 and 175). In sensory systems, however, the reflex loop is always highly asymmetrical and one-sided in structure, dominated by the afferent branch. The efferent branch becomes much less visible and has nothing to do with projecting perceptions but simply serves to optimize the reception of stimuli—by influencing the stimulus threshold, for example. As we will see later, the opposite asymmetry is characteristic of the autonomic nervous system (Figure 165C).

As mentioned above, the process of sensing is in no way limited to neurological processes in the sense organs and nervous system (Figure 176). For example, instead of experiencing images of the outer world on the brain's outer surface, as if they were pictures on a television screen, we perceive them as outside our bodies, as the surroundings we see or hear. This phenomenon presents profound problems that still remain largely unsolved.

Every sensory experience involves not just the nervous system but the ***entire human being***. What we take in with each sense impression is not merely a dead image of nature but also includes life and soul forces that are active in the natural world. These forces, however, are "filtered out" before reaching the cerebrum. They act only on the human subconscious, i.e., on our own subconscious life and soul forces (*a* in Figure 176). But what we perceive consciously—the abstracted image of the outer world—also sinks down into the subconscious domain of the body (*b* in Figure 176), where its effects can vitalize or damage the body or even make it ill. Retrieving this image from within also involves forces of life and soul or (in other words) metabolic, respiratory, and circulatory processes (*c* in Figure 176). Once this happens, the higher cortical centers (secondary and tertiary cortex fields) can ***reenliven*** "stored" images of the past and recall them as memories (*d* in Figure 176).

But the entire organism is involved even in transient perceptions. At least with regard to the higher senses, we "project" sense impressions back into our surroundings and experience the world as being around us, not inside us. The life and soul forces necessary for this projection also originate in the organism as a whole, reaching the sense organs via the blood (*c* in Figure 176). Plato is an example of someone who was still able to perceive this stream of life emerging from the body (from the eyes, for example). In modern times, Jacques Lusseyran, blinded at the age of eight, clearly and convincingly describes this aspect of the perceptual process (77).

Thus sensory activity is clearly asymmetrical not only in the neurological part of the system but also in associated processes of life and soul, which are based on rhythmical and metabolic organ activity. The result is not only our characteristic modern form of sense perception but also the way we think and conceptualize. In the Old Testament, the first appearance of asymmetry in the perceptual domain (the so-called Fall) is described in the words, "Their eyes were opened." This and the sentence "You will be like God" may indeed refer to subsequent shifts in sensory brain centers, which led to the development of mental images and memories and thus to our enhanced experience of personality.

The Organs of Hearing and Balance

The organ of hearing is subdivided into three functionally distinct sections: the outer ear, which funnels sounds into the hearing system; the middle ear with its sound-conducting apparatus; and the inner ear, where the receptors are located. In the visual system, the head's longitudinal direction (front/back) dominates, but the auditory system lies predominantly in the right/left dimension, and a spiral tendency is clearly evident in its structure, beginning with the gently spiraling external auditory meatus. Although the inner ear is ultimately located deep inside the petrous bone (the hardest bone in the body), the labyrinth vesicle develops out of an invagination in the outer germ layer (ectoderm) during the embryonic period. In other words, the ear develops from the outside

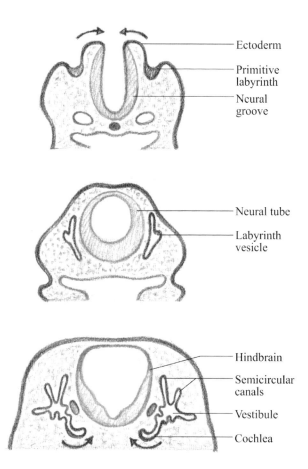

Fig. 177. **The labyrinth separates from the ectoderm through strangulation** *(adapted from Clara, 124). These illustrations show three successive stages in the development of the labyrinth (through cross sections of the embryonic head at the level of the hindbrain, to which the labyrinth later develops neuronal connections).*

in, unlike the eye vesicle, which originates in the interbrain and then moves to the outer surface of the body. Thus these two major sense organs are polar opposites, even in their developmental gestures.

Embryonic development of the inner ear. The labyrinth vesicle separates from the ectoderm through strangulation and elongates toward the interior (Figure 177). Distinct upper and lower sections soon become evident, along with two little sacs (the utricle and the saccule), which connect them. The upper section develops into

A
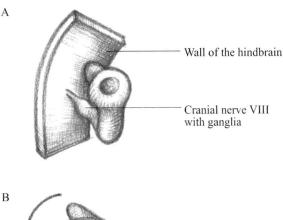

Wall of the hindbrain

Cranial nerve VIII
with ganglia

Fig. 178. **Three-dimensional model of the embryonic labyrinth vesicle in three successive developmental stages.** *Arrows indicate contrasting gestures in the development of the semicircular canals and cochlea. The eighth cranial (vestibulocochlear) nerve also grows outward from the labyrinth and connects with the hindbrain, forming the spiral ganglion, which serves the cochlea, and the vestibular ganglion, which serves the semicircular canals and vestibule (utricle and saccule).*
A: Approximately day 31
B: Approximately day 40
C: Approximately day 56

B
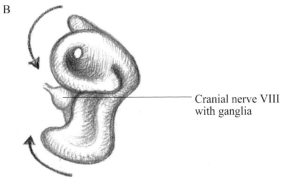

Cranial nerve VIII
with ganglia

C
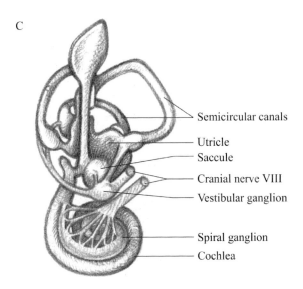

Semicircular canals

Utricle
Saccule
Cranial nerve VIII
Vestibular ganglion

Spiral ganglion
Cochlea

a spiraling plate whose central portions fuse and atrophy, leaving only little tubes along the edges. These tubules remain connected with the utricle as they develop into the three semicircular canals of the organ of balance.

In a contrasting developmental gesture, the cochlea, as the organ that serves hearing, emerges from the saccule in the form of a tubelike bud, which then elongates into a spiral canal (Figure 178). It is astonishing to realize how well this early developmental gesture reflects the organ's ultimate function. Hearing makes it possible for us to consciously perceive the inner world of another being. Through the word, we experience other people's ideas, and the character of other beings or objects is always revealed by their sounds. The ear is not as easily deceived as the eye. A gold-painted pottery jar looks like gold but sounds like clay. We experience the essential character of a substance through its vibrations.

The organ of balance is very different. It "looks" at the external aspect, at matter itself. What we experience (unconsciously) through this organ is not the inner aspect of a being or object but simply its mass, its relationship to space. The three semicircular canals that make up the outer portion of the labyrinth vesicle reflect the three planes of space. These formations "see" the spatial world from outside, while the cochlea exposes its inner aspect or the essential nature of its forces, as Goethe so beautifully expressed in the line "The Sun intones, in ancient tourney" (see p. 208).

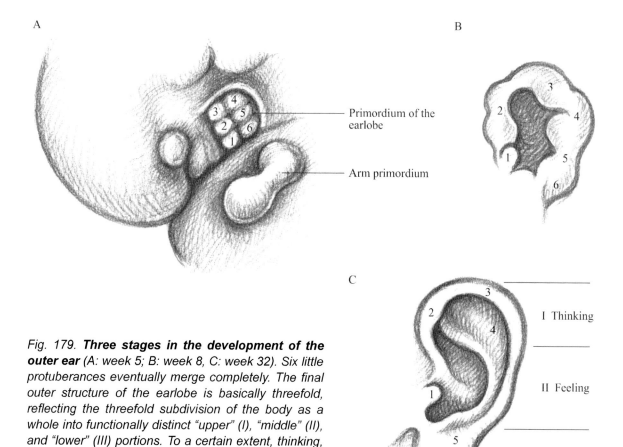

Fig. 179. **Three stages in the development of the outer ear** (A: week 5; B: week 8, C: week 32). Six little protuberances eventually merge completely. The final outer structure of the earlobe is basically threefold, reflecting the threefold subdivision of the body as a whole into functionally distinct "upper" (I), "middle" (II), and "lower" (III) portions. To a certain extent, thinking, feeling, and willing (metabolism) are evident even in the shape of the ear.

The Outer Ear

The polarity between outward and inward orientation, between spherical and linear/spiral form, or—in more general terms—between "form" and "matter" is already evident in the outer ear. The temporal bone, which houses the inner ear, displays the same polarity of form.

Embryonic development of the outer ear. As early as the fifth week of gestation, the outer ear begins to develop out of six little protuberances, which are initially all the same size (Figure 179). They later merge, forming the earlobe. The large, flat arch of the earlobe (pinna) corresponds to the upper part of the embryonic labyrinth vesicle (which gives rise to the semicircular canals), while

the lobule of the auricle, which has no cartilage to stiffen it, corresponds more to the cochlea. Especially in the art of ancient Greece, which dates from a time when such forms were instinctively seen in their true context, artistic representations often depicted the lobule as a circle or spiral and the upper earlobe as a winged or radiant curve (Figure 180).

Such symbolic representations also offer new perspectives on the *physiognomy of the ear*. The curved shape of the upper earlobe primarily reflects an individual's capacity for thought, while the lobule reflects strength of will and the midsection the capacity for emotional experience (Figure 179). The shapes and relative sizes of these parts of the ear vary widely among individuals and often correspond surprisingly well

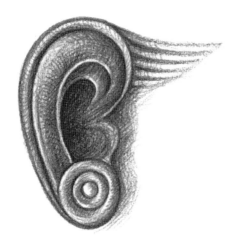

Fig. 180. **The ear of the Sounion Kouros,** *Greece (National Museum, Athens, no. 2720, ca. 600 BC).*

to fundamental personality traits. The shape of the lobule says a lot about a person's connection to the material world (strength of purpose, avarice, tendency toward action or weakness, etc.), while the shape of the upper earlobe tells us about his or her ability to develop abstract concepts or creative ideas. In this sense, the physiognomy of the ear is as revealing as the face.

The Temporal Bone, the Middle Ear, and Pneumatization

A structural polarity is also found in the **temporal bone**. Although the temporal bone is a composite of several elements with different developmental histories, on a phenomenological level its overall form is very telling. The squamous portion, which is part of the skullcap, is flat and scalelike and appears to radiate outward and upward. Like the large, curving upper portion of the earlobe, it represents the "form pole." In contrast, the plump, drop-shaped mastoid process is comparable to the lobule and represents the "matter pole" (Figure 181). The zygomatic process, which looks like the horizontal beam of a balance, connects

the upward-directed forces of the squama and the downward weight of the mastoid process and mediates between them. It is interesting to note that the zygomatic process includes the jaw joint as well as the outer opening of the ear, which is partially enclosed by a ring of bone (the tympanic annulus, Figure 182). The mastoid process is part of the pyramid-shaped petrous bone, which extends inward all the way to the sella turcica of the sphenoid bone. A fourth structural element of the temporal bone is the styloid process, which originates in the branchial apparatus (the remnant of the second branchial arch) and attaches to the petrous bone only secondarily. The branchial apparatus (gills), which serves respiration in fishes, is still present in human embryos but undergoes a radical change in function; its structural elements are transformed into the organs of chewing and speech. In this context it is interesting to note that the organs of hearing and speaking develop at the same time.

The ability to perceive sounds depends heavily on the development of a **sound-conduction mechanism** consisting of the eardrum, the three ossicles (malleus, incus, stapes) and the tympanic cavity (middle ear space). Unlike cavities elsewhere in the body, which are filled with vascular or connective tissue, the sound-conduction channel must be filled with air. Toward the end of the gestation period, the tympanic cavity is emptied of tissue and filled with air from the pharynx. This process is called pneumatization. The tympanic cavity connects to the upper throat (pharynx) via the Eustachian tube. In the process of pneumatization, an epithelial bud grows from the Eustachian tube into the middle ear cavity, forcing the loose network of embryonic connective tissue back against the cavity's bony walls. This allows air from the throat to penetrate the middle ear so that the ossicles and eardrum can begin to vibrate.

It is interesting to note, however, that **pneumatization** does not stop at the walls of the middle ear but continues into the inner ear, where ultimately the mastoid process also develops. The **mastoid process** is almost totally absent in newborns. It becomes clearly apparent only when a child is two or three years old and achieves

A

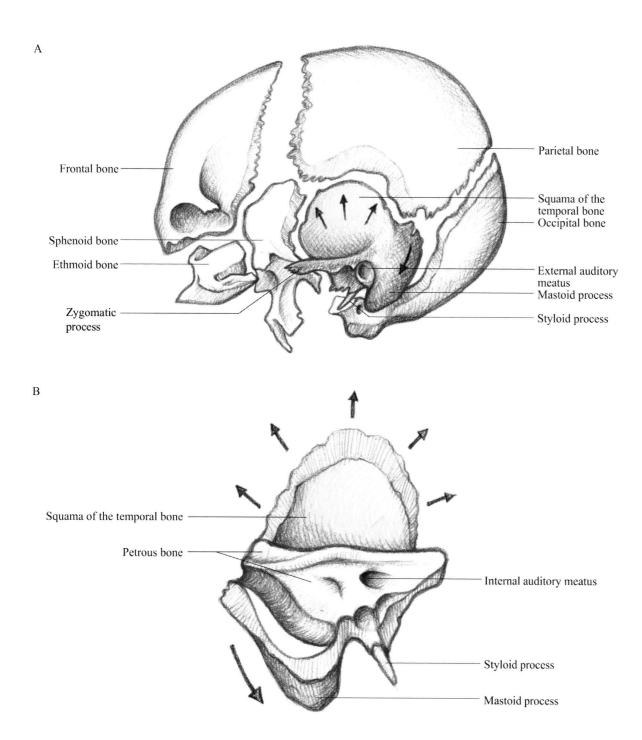

Frontal bone

Parietal bone

Squama of the
temporal bone

Occipital bone

Sphenoid bone

Ethmoid bone

External auditory
meatus

Mastoid process

Zygomatic
process

Styloid process

B

Squama of the temporal bone

Petrous bone

Internal auditory meatus

Styloid process

Mastoid process

*Fig. 181. **The signature shape of the temporal bone**. On one side, the temporal bone develops a radially structured squama (yellow, arrows) that completes the mosaic of the skullcap. On the other, the heavy, downward directed mastoid process develops (red, arrow). The horizontal zygomatic process (blue, A) lies between them like the crossbar of a balance.*

A: Left temporal bone in the mosaic of the skullcap bones (view from outside);

B: Left temporal bone (view from inside). Like the beam of a balance, the petrous bone lies between the temporal bone's structurally contrasting parts (squama and mastoid process). The petrous bone houses the organs of hearing and equilibrium, whose nerves exit through the internal auditory meatus.

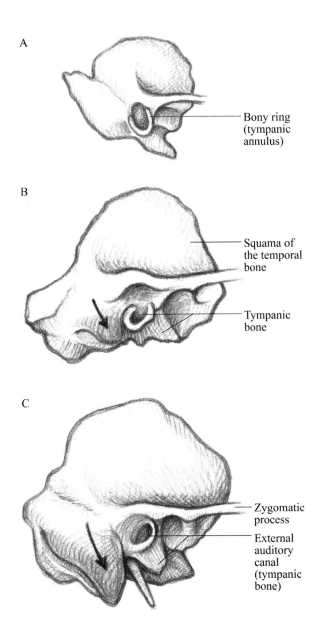

A

Bony ring
(tympanic
annulus)

B

Squama of
the temporal
bone

Tympanic
bone

C

Zygomatic
process

External
auditory
canal
(tympanic
bone)

Fig. 182. **Development of the mastoid process** (red)
of the temporal bone as a result of increasing pneumatization during the first five years after birth.
A: newborn; B: three-year-old; C: five-year-old.

its final form only around the age of five (Figure
182). Its growth is the result of increasing inner
ear pneumatization, which ultimately replaces
the marrow-filled cavities of the spongy bone
with air spaces (mastoid cells, Figure 183A).
Here, pneumatization takes place in a way that is
completely different from analogous developments

in the middle ear. Characteristically, the mucosa of
the middle ear begins to grow into the spaces in
the spongy bone of the mastoid process only after
preliminary transformation of the marrow through a
process that resembles the development of a tumor
(Figure 183B). Shortly before birth, embryonic
connective tissue in the marrow spaces of the bone
suddenly begins to proliferate, eating away all the
structures around it, including the trabeculae, just
as an infiltrating proliferative tumor would do. This
condensed, actively growing connective tissue is
then invaded and displaced by epithelium-covered
mucous membranes expanding out of the middle-
ear cavity, ultimately resulting in air-filled hollow
spaces in the mastoid process.

In the middle ear, we see a conflict between
growth processes, so to speak. The epithelium
"fights" with highly vascularized connective tissue,
which is finally forced back to the bony walls of
the cavities. If the connective tissue "wins," a thick
layer of well-vascularized mucous membrane
remains in the middle ear. In children, this
condition can cause a predisposition to middle-
ear infections.

In the inner ear, in the pneumatization of the
mastoid process (and ultimately of the entire
temporal bone), these developments "***cooperate***"
instead of "***fighting***" each other. Only when the
connective tissue in the middle ear has been
completely pushed back is this development
reversed at the threshold of the inner ear, where
connective tissue begins to proliferate to prepare
the way for subsequent pneumatization. If this
dynamic transformation of connective tissue into a
proliferative growth does not occur, the epithelium
does not advance and the mastoid process is not
effectively pneumatized. We see that in this case
these two types of tissues work together instead
of against each other.

Such cooperation or interaction is also characteristic of the auditory process as a whole.
In hearing, we make ourselves inwardly empty
and allow something to enter us, which we then
immediately recreate (using similar forces) in
order to experience sound. When a process of
this sort descends to the physical level, the result
is pathological growth, or even tumors in extreme

A

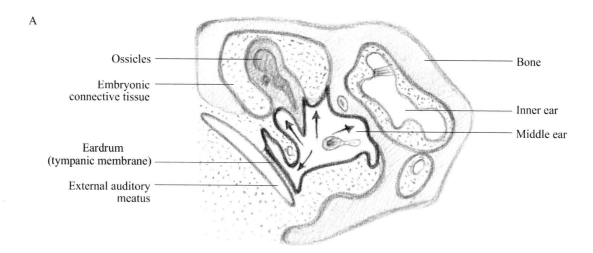

Ossicles

Embryonic
connective tissue

Eardrum
(tympanic membrane)

External auditory
meatus

Bone

Inner ear

Middle ear

*Fig. 183. **Pneumatization of the middle ear and
mastoid process** (adapted from Wittmaack, 125).*
*A: Diagram (7x magnification) of a histological section
through the middle and inner ear of the fetus at eight to
nine months. Mucous membrane growing in from the
pharynx displaces embryonic connective tissue in the
middle ear (arrows).*
*B: Diagram (7x magnification) of a histological section
through the mastoid process of a newborn. "Tumorlike"
proliferation of connective tissue (red arrows), which
moves in from the middle ear, paves the way for
transformation of the bone marrow.*
*C: Diagram (5x magnification) of a histological section
through the mastoid process of a two-year-old child.
Large parts of the mastoid process (x's) have already
been pneumatized, but the tip of the process has not.
Red: remnants of proliferated connective tissue.*

B

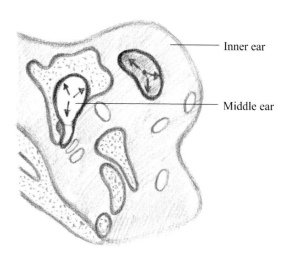

Inner ear

Middle ear

C

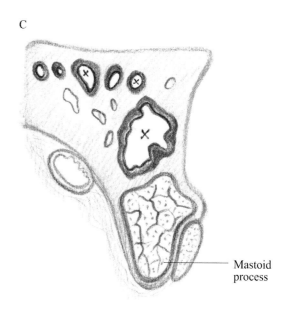

Mastoid
process

cases (80). In a certain sense, preliminary marrow
transformation is comparable to a tumor process,
but in this instance growth does not become
destructive because the middle-ear mucosa
immediately eliminates the proliferating tissue
and creates air-filled spaces in its place. Of
course true tumors (such as cholesteatomas) can
also develop in this area, but they originate in the
epithelium of the external auditory meatus, not
in the connective tissue of the mastoid process.
These carcinomas grow from the middle ear into
the inner ear, as if attempting to recapitulate the
process of pneumatization, but what they really
do is destroy tissue.

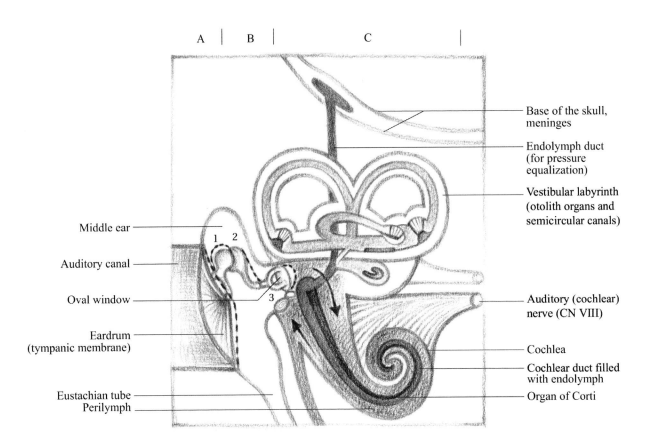

A | B | C

Base of the skull, meninges

Endolymph duct (for pressure equalization)

Vestibular labyrinth (otolith organs and semicircular canals)

Middle ear

1 2

Auditory canal

Oval window

3

Auditory (cochlear) nerve (CN VIII)

Eardrum (tympanic membrane)

Cochlea

Cochlear duct filled with endolymph

Eustachian tube
Perilymph

Organ of Corti

*Fig. 184. **Threefold subdivision of the organ of hearing in the outer ear** (A, sound reception), **middle ear** (B, sound conduction), **and inner ear** (C, sound perception). The middle ear contains the bridge formed by the auditory ossicles—hammer (malleus, 1), anvil (incus, 2) and stirrup (stapes, 3)—which transmit vibrations of the eardrum (tympanic membrane) to the perilymph of the inner ear via the oval window (arrows). The cochlea is filled with endolymph (red) and houses the sensory organ for sound perception (organ of Corti).*

The Organ of Hearing

Hidden away deep within the petrous bone lies the inner ear, whose sensory terminals make both hearing and spatial orientation possible. The inner ear consists of a membranous labyrinth that encompasses the three semicircular canals, the vestibule with the utricle and the saccule, and the cochlea. This membranous labyrinth is filled with endolymph, bathed in perilymph, and enclosed in a bony labyrinth of similar shape (Figure 184). Growth and development of the petrous bone are essentially complete at birth; it does not undergo any of the postnatal modifications typical of other bones in the body. Bone marrow tissue, present throughout the skeletal system as an organ of blood formation, is absent in the petrous bone, where pneumatization has replaced the marrow with hollow air spaces. As a result, the petrous bone consists of bone that is unusually "dead," highly calcified, and perhaps the hardest bone in the body, hence its name ("petrous" = stony).

Within this extremely mineralized "grave" lies the most sensitive sense organ in the human body, namely, the ***organ of hearing***. It includes three distinct sections:

1.   The outer ear, which includes the auditory canal and tympanic membrane (eardrum);

2.   The middle ear with its auditory ossicles (malleus/hammer, incus/anvil, stapes/stirrup);

3.   The inner ear, which includes the spiral-shaped cochlea housing the organ of Corti with its receptors (Figure 184).

Regardless of which stage in the transformation of stimuli we may be considering, two elements are always essential for understanding how *hearing* works: the soul-spiritual content of the complex of sounds and the material basis of "stimulus transduction" (vibrations in air, waves in fluid, changes in potential in receptors and nerves). Modern physiology explores only the material process, relegating the soul-spiritual component to the subjective sphere of psychology. These two elements, however, are inextricably linked, and we must not fail to consider how they interact.

The spoken word produces sound waves in the air. The frequencies of these vibrations are transmitted to the eardrum and then, in the *middle ear*, through the auditory ossicles to the oval window, which is attached to the stapes (Figure 184). The vibrating plate of the stirrup creates pressure waves in the perilymph in the scala vestibuli of the inner ear. In turn, these waves produce vibrations in the endolymph in the cochlear duct. These vibrations are transduced into neural stimuli by receptors in the organ of Corti and then transmitted to the brain via the auditory nerves.

The *inner ear* has a remarkable ability to sort and "take apart" the complex frequency patterns of speech or music. The stirrup's vibrations produce traveling waves that move through the perilymph of the scala vestibuli at different speeds. Vibrations produced by these pressure waves are transmitted through the endolymph of the cochlear duct to the organ of Corti, located on the basilar membrane (Figure 185A). Basilar membrane fibers vary in length (shorter in the outer spiral and longer toward the center), with corresponding differences in amplitude. Lower frequencies (low tones) are perceived toward the center, higher frequencies (high tones) closer to the entrance to the spiral. The spectrum of perceptible frequencies ranges from 20,000 Hz at the base to 100 Hz at the center (Figure 186).

We know that any sound consists of a number of tones with different frequencies. In the inner ear, these frequencies produce pressure waves that move at different speeds. As a result, a sound's unique pattern of frequencies is taken apart ("traveling wave dispersion") and distributed over individual areas of the basilar membrane that have "strings" of different lengths. Surprisingly, the *organ of Corti* (Figure 185A) has two different groups of receptors (hair cells). The outer hair cells (approximately 12,000 of them) form two rows near the base of the spiral and up to five rows near its central point, where the basilar membrane fibers become longer. Regardless of where they are located in the cochlea, the inner hair cells form only a single row and thus total only around 3,500. Strangely enough, each inner hair cell is always in contact with multiple afferent nerve fibers (up to twenty fibers each), whereas ten or more outer hair cells are innervated by a single neuron. It is now assumed that these differences in innervation have to do with frequency selectivity in the perception of sound. Without outer hair cells, hearing is still possible but words don't make sense because individual frequency ranges cannot be distinguished.

Inner-ear *receptors* are called hair cells because each one has a small bundle of hair on its surface (Figure 185B). These hairs are in contact with the tectorial membrane, which lies directly above them. Traveling waves trigger vibrations in the organ of Corti, causing tiny distortions in the sensory hairs of the hair cells. The difference in potential (+155mV) between hair cells (-70mV) and the endolymph of the cochlear duct (+85 mV) is unusually high, in fact unique in the organism. Distortions of the sensory hairs produce frequency-synchronous changes in cell-membrane resistance, resulting in tiny ion flows that depolarize the hair cell. The distribution of transmitters at the base of the cell produces specific stimulus patterns in the afferent auditory nerves.

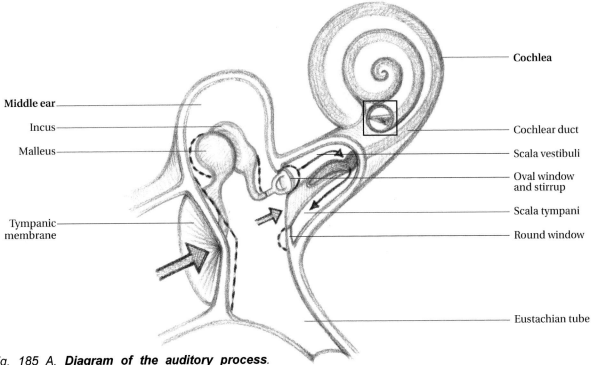

Cochlea

Middle ear

Incus

Malleus

Tympanic membrane

Cochlear duct

Scala vestibuli

Oval window and stirrup

Scala tympani

Round window

Eustachian tube

*Fig. 185 A. **Diagram of the auditory process**. Sound waves produce vibrations in the eardrum, which are transmitted via the auditory ossicles and oval window to the perilymph of the scala vestibuli (blue). The perilymph waves produce vibrations in the endolymph of the cochlear duct (red), which move both the basilar membrane, where the organ of Corti and its receptors (hair cells) are located, and the tectorial membrane, which is connected to the hairs of the receptors. These minute movements trigger stimuli in the auditory nerves leading to the brain. The lower illustration is an enlargement of the cross section shown in the square in the upper illustration.*

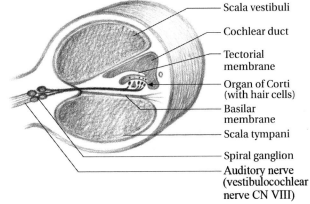

Scala vestibuli

Cochlear duct

Tectorial membrane

Organ of Corti (with hair cells)

Basilar membrane

Scala tympani

Spiral ganglion

Auditory nerve (vestibulocochlear nerve CN VIII)

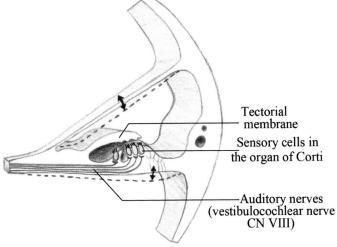

Tectorial membrane

Sensory cells in the organ of Corti

Auditory nerves (vestibulocochlear nerve CN VIII)

Fig. 185 B. The vibrations in the membranes of the cochlea are indicated by the arrows. In the process of hearing the hairs of the hair cells are stimulated by the vibrations of the tectorial membrane.

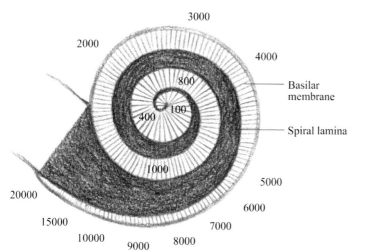

3000
2000
4000
800
Basilar
membrane
100
400
100
Spiral lamina
1000
5000
20000
6000
15000
7000
10000
9000 8000

*Fig. 186. **The cochlea** (view from above), showing only the spiral lamina, to which the basilar membrane is attached. The length of the fibers in the basilar membrane (light) increases toward the center of the spiral while the spiral lamina narrows. High tones with frequencies up to 20,000 Hz are perceived near the base of the spiral, low tones (100-1000 Hz) toward the center (tip).*

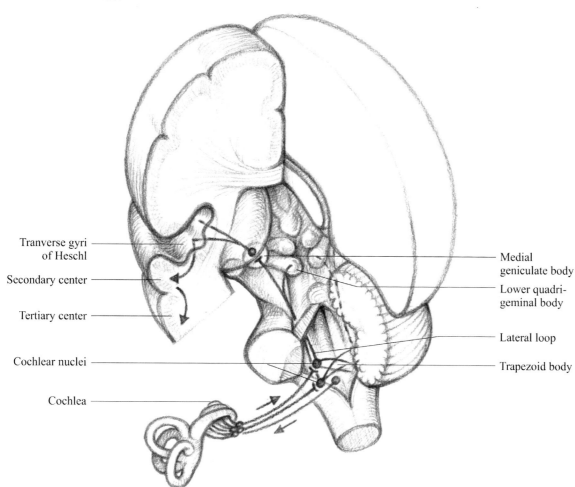

Tranverse gyri
of Heschl

Secondary center

Tertiary center

Cochlear nuclei

Cochlea

Medial
geniculate body

Lower quadri-
geminal body

Lateral loop

Trapezoid body

*Fig. 187. **Diagram of the auditory pathway** (auditory radiation). In the trapezoid body of the rhombencephalon, the auditory nerve (cranial nerve VIII) connects with the two auditory nuclei at the beginning of the auditory pathway. The auditory pathway runs via the lateral loop to the medial geniculate body and lower quadrigeminal bodies to Heschl's gyri (auditory centers) in the area of the insular cortex and upper temporal gyrus. The adjacent cortical regions of the temporal lobe house the higher secondary and tertiary cortical centers of the auditory system.*

Neurophysiological studies suggest that some type of frequency dispersion is probably also at work in the conduction of neural stimuli to the brain's auditory centers. (This principle has been applied extensively in telecommunications technology.) If receptors and the adjacent nerves conduct a sound's *different constituent frequencies* to the brain at different speeds, this means that the ear is a *temporal organ* or, in other words, a sense organ capable of converting spatial proportions into patterns in time (81, 82). It is well known that musical intervals are based on specific numerical proportions that can also be found in the material world and even in architecture. Spatial proportions appear to the ear as music.

The auditory neural tract and the process of hearing. Conscious perception of sound requires not only an intact inner ear but also a functioning nervous system. We become conscious of sounds through the activity of the auditory centers in the temporal lobe (Figure 187). The auditory nerve (N. cochlearis, cranial nerve VIII) connects the cochlea with the hindbrain, where stimuli are rerouted into the auditory pathway via the auditory nuclei at the base of the rhomboid fossa (floor of the fourth ventricle). The auditory tract passes through the brain stem via the lateral lemniscus, synapses in the medial geniculate body, then travels by way of the auditory radiations in the internal capsule to the primary auditory cortex (transverse gyri of Heschl) in the temporal lobe (Figure 187). Here, tonotopic projection breaks the sound apart into separate frequencies. High tones and low tones are "reproduced" in different places. The adjacent secondary and tertiary auditory centers of the cortex no longer have anything to do with perceiving individual tones or frequency ranges. The secondary centers play a role in understanding the sounds of speech or music, the tertiary centers in remembering auditory perceptions. When these centers malfunction, words are still heard but their content is not understood (acoustic aphasia) and it becomes impossible to develop relevant related concepts.

Stimuli streaming into the brain via the auditory nerves reach not only the cerebral cortex (the site of our highest waking consciousness) but also various centers in the hindbrain, midbrain, and interbrain. We do not become conscious of the activity of these centers directly because they are primarily involved in reflexes that serve as functional links between the auditory system and other systems within the nervous system (sensorimotor systems, for example). These links may result in reflexive head movements in response to noises, unconscious accompanying movements of the limbs or eyes, or even vegetative (ANS) reflexes in the intestines, genitals, or glands.

Thus the nervous system does not supply a comprehensive image of a sound but distributes incoming stimuli to different centers and nuclei in the brain. Therefore, the emergence of a unified experience of a word or sound depends on the collaboration of the entire human body and the soul-spiritual entity that inhabits it (83).

In conclusion, let's review the complicated *process of hearing as a whole*. Air vibrations produced by a word or sound are first received by the eardrum (tympanic membrane, Figure 185). In a certain sense, the auditory ossicles represent a little limb. The handle of the malleus, which is attached to the eardrum, is like a little hand that "touches" it and "feels" its vibrations. The stapes converts these tiny "limb movements" into fluid movements in the cochlea, which in turn cause minute distortions (that is, physical, mechanical changes) in the sensory hairs and subsequent changes in the potential in the associated nerves.

The cochlea is a spiral, a shape that is also found in the intestines of many species (Figure 188). The cochlea can be compared to a spiraling intestinal tract that dead-ends in the helicotrema, which lies between the scala vestibuli and the scala tympani. If we consider the hearing process from a qualitative perspective, the comparison to the digestive process is very apt. The double spiral is a universal symbol of a process that begins with breakdown (in the movement from outside to inside) but then reverses direction and is transformed into a building-up process as it leads from the center back to the periphery (Figure 188). Destruction and reconstruction take place in the intestinal system in a "spiral of substance" that leads from the breakdown of foods to the building up of body-specific compounds, making the spiral an apt image of functional processes of this sort (Figure 188C). And in fact breaking down and reconstructing the "substance" of a word—that is, its spiritual content—happen when we perceive sound, at least inasmuch as the human soul-spiritual aspect is involved. The word "incarnates" in the element of air, in a specific pattern of vibrations that is then taken apart or broken down step by step in the three successive sections of the organ of hearing. The listening individual's spirit pours into these hollow spaces, which have been emptied of organic activity, and recreates the word within. Instead of passively hearing another person's word, we replace it with a newly created word of our own that allows us to perceive the other person's spoken word and its content. All this happens on the basis of the highly differentiated impression the original word makes on our nervous system. Ultimately, this impression consists only of very subtle differences in neural potential in *various parts* of the brain.

Watch how subtly a deaf person observes a speaking person's intentions and understands the content of the words even though the breakdown process described above cannot take place. The astonishing accomplishments of someone like Helen Keller demonstrate that the sense for words remains intact in spite of deafness (78).

When we listen, we become inwardly empty and allow another being to occupy that space. In the physical, living world, however, the same thing happens in every process of growth and regeneration: the old is broken down and replaced with the new. In this instance, however, the new structure is determined by the body's own life forces, not by a foreign element such as a word or sound coming from outside. But when, in organic growth, a foreign "program"—or none at all—is implemented instead of the body's own architectural program, a tumor develops. (See above, pp. 252–55 for the unique cooperation of processes involved in the pneumatization of the

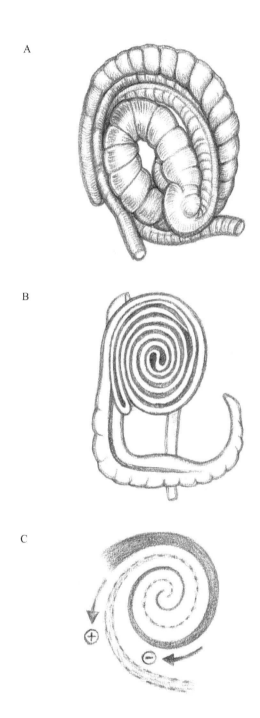

A

B

C

*Fig. 188. **The spiral principle in the biological realm**. A: Spiral of the large intestine in an Old World wild rabbit (Oryctolagus), adapted from Muthmann; B: Spiral rectum in a lemurlike prosimian (Propithecus); C: Symbolic spiral of forces. Breakdown (the inward spiral) and rebuilding (the outward spiral) follow the same pathway.*

inner ear.) From this perspective, Rudolf Steiner's initially fantastic-sounding statement that ear formation is "based on a process that becomes normal simply because a tumor-forming force has been halted at the right point" also begins to make sense (80).

The Vestibular Organ

In its development and structure, the other part of the inner ear, the organ of balance, is the complete opposite of the organ of hearing. Its receptors are stimulated directly by fluid movements *in the endolymph* rather than indirectly through perilymphatic vibrations (Figures 184 and 189). The organ formed by the semicircular canals is spatially oriented, while the organ of hearing relates to time. In phylogenetic terms, the organ of equilibrium is very old. It is already present in the most primitive vertebrates, whereas the organ of hearing is fully developed only in mammals. (Birds have only a lagena, not yet a true cochlea.)

The three *semicircular canals* stand at right angles to each other in an image of the three dimensions of space (Figure 189A). The planes of the canals, however, are not aligned with the planes bisecting the body but are rotated approximately 45°. As a result, the left superior and right posterior semicircular canals lie in the same plane. In other words, the three semicircular canals do not align themselves directly with the body's spatial axes but create with them a dynamic relationship through coordinated planar movements. Each of the three semicircular canals includes a dilated portion (ampulla) that contains a sensory organ consisting of sensory and supporting cells and covered with a brushlike cap (cupula). When the head moves in one of the three planes of space, the fluid in the corresponding semicircular canal moves in the opposite direction due to inertia, bending the cupula slightly (Figure 189B). The sensory cells whose hairs extend into the cupula register the cupula's mechanical movement and transform it into neural stimuli that are then conducted to the central nervous system, specifically to the vestibular system in the brain stem and cerebellum, which is responsible for maintaining balance.

Two other sensory organs, the *maculae staticae*, are also located in the vestibule, between the semicircular canals and the cochlea (Figure 189C). Here neural stimuli are triggered not by fluid movement but by the force of gravity itself. A membrane in which tiny aragonite crystals (otoliths) are embedded covers the receptors of the maculae staticae. As the body moves in space, the otoliths press on the hairs of the receptors, triggering neural impulses that set balance-regulating processes in motion. Move-ment of the body (or more precisely, of the head) in the vertical dimension activates the horizontally oriented utricular macula, whereas movement in the horizontal dimension activates the more vertically oriented saccular macula. In both cases, linear acceleration in the appropriate dimension constitutes an adequate stimulus for these sense organs, whereas the sense organs of the semicircular canals register rotational acceleration in their respective planes.

Stimuli generated by the organs of equilibrium normally remain unconscious, unlike those of the organs of hearing. We usually enjoy a general sense of feeling secure in space but know nothing about the activity of the sense organs involved. Pathologically extreme stimuli are required to produce the vertigo, nausea, and vomiting of seasickness, for example.

If we compare the *sensory activity* in the organs of balance and hearing, a clear polarity emerges. The ear breaks the spatial qualities present in a sound or a word down into temporal structures, thus allowing us access to the spiritual element at work in the spatial world. Through the organ of balance, however, the static spatial field within which the body moves is transformed into minute movements in a fluid medium; a dynamic image of space is produced, but it does not become sound. Hearing exposes us to the inner, spiritual aspect of space, the experience of balance only to its outer, physical aspect.

A

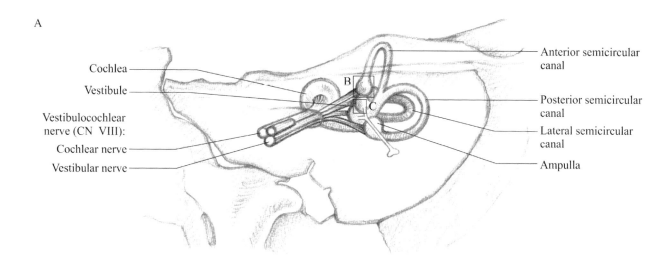

Cochlea

Vestibule

Vestibulocochlear
nerve (CN VIII):

Cochlear nerve

Vestibular nerve

Anterior semicircular
canal

Posterior semicircular
canal

Lateral semicircular
canal

Ampulla

Fig.189. **Structure of the labyrinth, which regulates equilibrium.**

A: Location of the labyrinth in the petrous bone (right side, view from behind). This system consists of tubes filled with endolymph—the three semicircular canals, each with its ampulla, and the vestibule with the two maculae staticae;

B: Ampulla of the superior semicircular canal. The "hairs" of the receptors extend into the cupula. Movement of the fluid in the semicircular canal (arrows) causes these hairs to move back and forth, stimulating the receptors and nerve fibers;

C: Static (gravity) sense organ (macula statica) showing the layer of otoliths capping the receptors. As the body moves in space, the otoliths press or pull on the sensory hairs, thus producing neural stimuli.

B

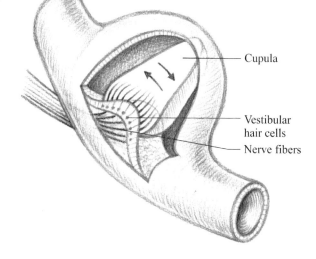

Cupula

Vestibular
hair cells

Nerve fibers

C

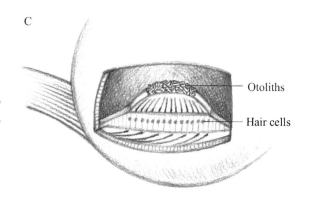

Otoliths

Hair cells

The Organs of Speech And the Functional Cycle of Hearing and Speaking

As with other sensory activities, hearing is by no means limited to the hearing apparatus but is subsumed into the body as a whole. Perception involves the whole body; the nervous system serves only to make us conscious of what we hear. As described earlier (pp. 260-61), the structure of the auditory system "filters out" the soul-spiritual content of another person's spoken word, leaving only its neural impression. But the sound of the word causes the soul's inherent capacity to experience sound to "resonate," so we are then able to use our own forces to recreate the spiritual content of what we hear. In every act of hearing, the entire body resonates or "vibrates" in sympathy. This is why we are able to dance to music and why everything we hear—especially as children—has such a profound impact on the body's life forces. We learn to speak only because we hear speech.

The process of producing words or musical sounds is the exact opposite of hearing. A specific content originating in an individual soul-spirit is imprinted on the exiting stream of air and sent out into the world. Each word is "born" out of the interaction of the larynx with the sound-sculpting capacities of the oral cavity. This activity involves the whole body. Although the respiratory system ("air body") plays a primary role, warmth and the fluid element are also involved. Blowing on the vocal cords in the larynx produces a sound (phonation), which is then shaped into vowels or consonants in the oral cavity (articulation). The oral cavity is the "mold" that shapes each quantum of expelled air into something that can house an incarnating idea. Different positions of the lips, tongue, and palate shape the hollow space of the mouth in many different ways (Figure 152)—a prerequisite for producing different speech sounds and different languages. Hearing is an inward catabolic process, speaking a creative, outward-directed one, but the two are functionally linked. Hearing and speaking form a functional cycle that will eventually allow human beings to play an active and creative part in the world's formative forces through faculties that we have yet to discover.

As we saw earlier, the faculty of speech evolved only as a result of achieving uprightness, laryngeal descent, and a persistently spherical skull, which allowed the oral cavity to serve as a "nozzle" for the larynx. When we view these evolutionary steps as a unity, it becomes obvious that a progressive evolutionary tendency is inherent in the organs of speech. If human beings of the future grasp the potential of these organs, they may be able to tap new, creative sources of life and influence their surroundings directly through speech and song, as Orpheus is reported to have done with his lyre.

The Eye and the Visual System

As evolution proceeded, the visual system became increasingly significant. Most mammals are nocturnal, and the sense of smell is still their dominant sense. The sense of sight becomes dominant only in diurnal primates, whose noses and snout are less prominent. To compensate for an underdeveloped sense of smell, the sense of sight becomes the dominant sensory system in humans, and vision also plays a leading role in our thinking and imagination. People who are blind lose significant, sometimes vital, aspects of the experiences that sighted individuals take for granted.

Morphology and Embryonic Development of the Eye

The formative gesture of the auditory system is the spiral, which, on the soul level, is a gesture of sympathy; the gesture of the visual system, however, is the cup, an expression of antipathy. The contrast between hearing and seeing is evident even in the characteristic gestures of the earliest stages of organ development. The development of the embryonic eye, like that of the embryonic organs of hearing and equilibrium, displays dis-tinctive formative processes that later become functional. The labyrinth primordium emerges from the ectoderm (i.e., it develops from the outside in), whereas the primitive eye develops out of the nervous system itself (from the inside out). At a very early stage, the eye primordium appears as a little vesicle emerging from the part of the endbrain that will later become the interbrain. This vesicle grows toward the skin, and its elongated stalk later develops into the visual nerve (Figure 190A). After reaching the skin, the optic vesicle develops a cuplike indentation (optic cup) and simultaneously induces development of the lens primordium in the adjacent skin (ectoderm). As the optic cup forms, the ***lens***

A

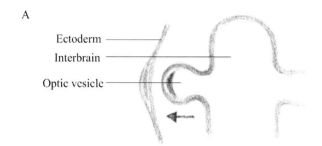

Ectoderm
Interbrain
Optic vesicle

primordium invaginates, ultimately separating from the ectoderm to form a closed lens vesicle within the optic cup. Both the vesicle and the cup continue to grow. The anterior (epithelial) lens cells divide and spread rapidly, crossing the lens equator and moving around to the back, where they are transformed into fibers that fill more and more of the vesicle's hollow space. The result is a compact body consisting of closely packed, roughly hexagonal cells that later become transparent (Figure 190D). Lens epithelial cells never completely lose their ability to divide, so the lens never stops increasing in size—a significant factor in the development of presbyopia.

The development of the ***optic cup*** is diametrically opposed to that of the lens vesicle (Figure 190C and D). The optic cup's inner layer

B

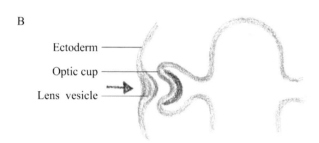

Ectoderm
Optic cup
Lens vesicle

C

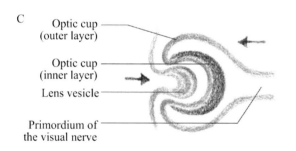

Optic cup (outer layer)
Optic cup (inner layer)
Lens vesicle
Primordium of the visual nerve

Fig. 190. ***Embryonic development of the human eye.***
A: The optic vesicle develops as a protuberance on the interbrain (diencephalon);
B: The optic cup begins to form; invagination of the lens primordium (Day 30);
C: Development of the optic cup and lens vesicle (Day 32);
D: The lens primordium has moved to the interior of the optic cup and is completely enclosed by a capsule of blood vessels (hyaloid artery). The inner layer of the optic cup becomes the retina, the outer layer the pigmented epithelium (PE). The photoreceptors develop in the direction of the pigmented epithelium, on the side of the retina that is not exposed to light (Day 40).
Red: blood vessels.

D

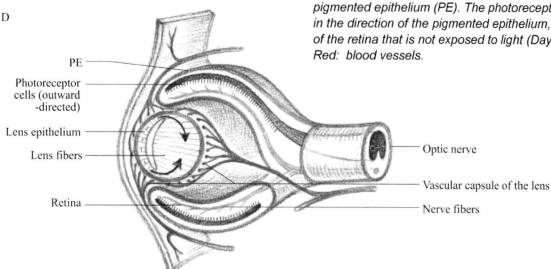

PE
Photoreceptor cells (outward-directed)
Lens epithelium
Lens fibers
Retina
Optic nerve
Vascular capsule of the lens
Nerve fibers

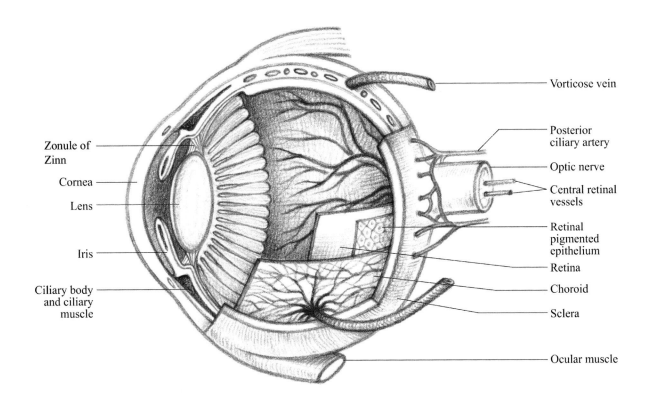

Vorticose vein

Posterior ciliary artery

Optic nerve

Central retinal vessels

Retinal pigmented epithelium

Retina

Choroid

Sclera

Ocular muscle

Zonule of Zinn

Cornea

Lens

Iris

Ciliary body and ciliary muscle

*Fig. 191. **Layered structure of the eye.** The inner layers are partially exposed to show their relative locations. The posterior ciliary arteries enter the eye at the back with the visual nerve, whereas the choroid veins (vortex veins) exit the eye at its equator. The retina is served from within by the central vessels, which enter the eye encased in the visual nerve. Note also the structural contrast between the anterior portion of the eye (lens, accommodation apparatus, iris, cornea, etc.) and the posterior portion (visual nerve, retina, choroid, and sclera).*

of cells exhibits the most active growth. Multiple growth spurts produce additional layers of nerve cells behind the first, forming the retina. This cellular "migration" is similar to what happens in the development of the cerebral cortex, so the retina can be imagined as a protruding bit of cortex that forms a flower-shaped cup to receive light from the outside world. The lens "sucks" light into the body's interior, so to speak, and focuses it on the retina. The optic cup receives light stimuli and responds by producing images, which we then experience as being "projected" back into the outside world. The lens develops through a cuplike invagination from the outside in. In contrast, the gesture of the optic cup's development is one

of actively reaching out. Like an opened hand (Figure 190), it extends peripherally toward the lens vesicle, which it incorporates into itself.

The primordial retinal cells that later become photoreceptors undergo a remarkable shift in location as a result of the indentation that ***transforms the optic vesicle into the optic cup***. Originally located on the optic cup's inner surface, these primordial retinal cells now lie on the outside. In other words, they are turned ***away from the light*** and face the optic cup's outer layer (Figure 190D). This outer layer differentiates and develops into the pigmented epithelium, which is very metabolically active and closely connected to the sensory cells. But the light-sensitive portions of

Incidence of light

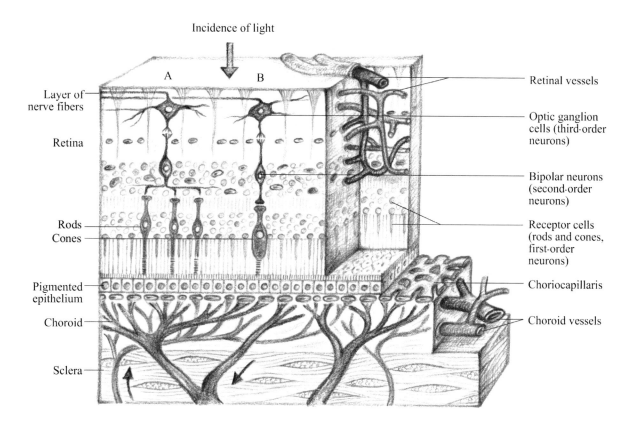

Layer of nerve fibers

Retina

Rods
Cones

Pigmented epithelium

Choroid

Sclera

Retinal vessels

Optic ganglion cells (third-order neurons)

Bipolar neurons (second-order neurons)

Receptor cells (rods and cones, first-order neurons)

Choriocapillaris

Choroid vessels

*Fig. 192. **Diagram of the structure of the retina.** The photoreceptors (first neuronal system) are turned away from the light and are in close contact with the retinal pigmented epithelium and the underlying vascular network (choriocapillaris). The relay neurons (second-order neurons) are primarily bipolar neurons. In contrast, the cells of the optic ganglia, which make up the retina's third neuronal system, are multipolar. Their axons make up the optic nerve. A: Rod circuitry; black/white perception; B: Cone circuitry; color perception.*

the sensory cells, instead of being turned toward the light (i.e., toward the lens) as we might expect, are turned away from it, toward the pigmented epithelium. In addition, the migrating nerve cells that make up the other retinal layers lie on top of the receptor cells, deflecting light so a clear image cannot develop at all. This reversal of location, which seems highly impractical at first glance, is an archetypal phenomenon of the vertebrate eye. Like the development of other organs described earlier, it begins to make sense only when we view evolution as a purposeful, orthogenetic development toward the human body. From a superficial perspective, this inversion could be

seen as a "bad design" on nature's part were it not for the immense enhancement of function that it ultimately produces in the human being.

At an early stage, an extensive vascular network called the **choroid** develops around the optic cup. This network is adjacent to the pigmented epithelium and provides the foundation for its exceptionally active metabolism (Figures 191 and 192). Being oriented outward (toward the pigmented epithelium) instead of inward allows the receptors to participate in this intense metabolic activity. Research has confirmed that ocular sensory cells actively regenerate. This means that the close functional relationships among the

	Anterior portion of the eye	**Posterior section of the eye**
Outer layer	Cornea	Sclera
Middle layer (uvea)	Iris, ciliary body	Choroid
Inner layer	Epithelial layers of the iris and ciliary body	Pigmented epithelium, retina

Table 22. The layered construction of the eye (see also Figures 191 and 192).

receptors, the retinal pigmented epithelium, and the choroid is crucially important to the visual system. To overcome the disadvantage of "intervening" retinal layers, humans (and also higher primates, to some extent) have evolved an area of sharpest vision, the so-called *fovea centralis*, in the center of the retina. Here in the fovea, the retinal layers are displaced to the side so that light strikes the receptors directly (Figure 194). Away from the fovea, visual acuity decreases rapidly. We will revisit the fovea's fundamental importance for human vision in a subsequent section.

The choroid is the posterior portion of the eye's middle layer, the uvea, which surrounds the lens and optic cup and consists of connective tissue, blood vessels, and muscles—in other words, of systems that support the work of the actual optical apparatus. The iris and the ciliary body make up the uvea's anterior portion (Figure 191). The uvea's sensitive structures of nerves and vessels would not be able to function without a solid covering, so the eye also has an outer layer (cornea and sclera) that serves as an outer skeleton of sorts to which the external eye muscles are attached (Figure 191).

Thus the fully formed eye consists of three spherical *layers*, which reflect in some respects the functional threefoldness of the body as a whole:

1. The inner layer, which consists of the retina and pigmented epithelium (the eye's informational system),

2. The outer layer, which consists of the sclera, eye muscles, and eyelids (the limb or motor system), and

3. The middle layer, which consists of the choroid, ciliary body, iris, and blood vessels (the eye's circulatory system). Together with the pigmented epithelium, this middle layer also serves metabolic functions (Figure 191).

The transparent, gel-filled vitreous body in the interior of the sphere and the anterior chamber in front of the lens filled with circulating aqueous humor ensure the internal stability of the eyeball. In contrast to the vitreous body, the anterior chamber contains constantly circulating fluid.

The eye is spherical in shape, as if it were an image of the cosmos, but there is a clear polarity in the architecture of its anterior and posterior sections (Figure 191 and Table 22). Neurological processes are concentrated in back and transmitted to the brain via the optic nerve. The front is the site of additional functional systems (centered on the lens) essential for vision. Within the eye as a whole, we can distinguish *five functional systems* that contribute to the perfection of vision in humans:

1. The eye's neurological apparatus (retina, optical tract, and brain centers);

2. The accommodation apparatus;

3. The iris, which serves as an aperture;

4. The motor apparatus, which consists of the outer eye muscles and sclera;

5. The cornea, connective tissue and eyelids, which protect the eye.

To clarify the contributions of the eye's "support systems" to the perfected human visual process, we must first understand the qualitative value of optical neurological functions.

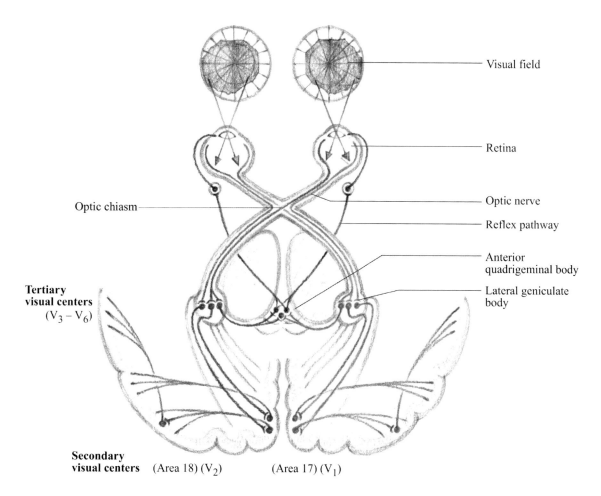

Visual field

Retina

Optic nerve

Reflex pathway

Anterior quadrigeminal body

Lateral geniculate body

Optic chiasm

Tertiary visual centers $(V_3 - V_6)$

Secondary visual centers   (Area 18) (V_2) (Area 17) (V_1)

Fig. 193 A. **Diagram of the optic tract**. *Images from the two eyes are transmitted separately to the primary projection fields in the calcarine cortex (area 17). From this "distribution center" visual stimuli are passed on to higher secondary and tertiary specialized centers (V_2, V_3-V_6).*

The Visual Process and the Optic Tract

Although the neuronal connections in the optical system are relatively easy to understand, central processing of visual stimuli is extremely complex.

In the retina, we find three sequentially switched neuron systems that are linked horizontally by specialized cells in each of the two synapse zones (Figure 192). The receptors can be considered the neurons of the first system. There are two types of receptors—rods (for scotopic vision in dim light) and cones (for photopic or color vision in bright light). The second neuron system consists of bipolar retinal switching cells of the retina, and the third of optic ganglia cells whose axons make up the optic nerve and run

all the way to the lateral geniculate body of the interbrain before connecting with a fourth neuron. The axons of the fourth neuron system end in the visual cortex of the occipital lobe, in the calcarine area (area 17, V_1), which is considered to be the visual projection center or primary visual cortex (Figure 193A). The calcarine cortex is connected to neighboring cortical areas of the parietal and temporal lobes (areas 18 and 19, as well as 20 and 21), which are involved in secondary and tertiary processing of visual "information." We now know that the nervous system transmits and

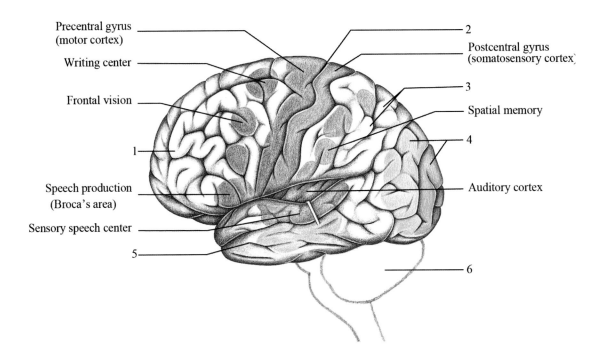

Precentral gyrus (motor cortex)

Writing center

Frontal vision

Speech production (Broca's area)

Sensory speech center

2

Postcentral gyrus (somatosensory cortex)

3

Spatial memory

4

Auditory cortex

Fig. 193 B. **Left brain hemisphere with its cortical fields** *(in color).*
1 *Frontal lobe*
2 *Central sulcus*
3 *Parietal lobe*
4 *Occipital lobe with its secondary and tertiary optical fields 18 and 19 (as well as primary area 17).*
5 *Temporal lobe (including areas 20 and 21)*
6 *Cerebellum*

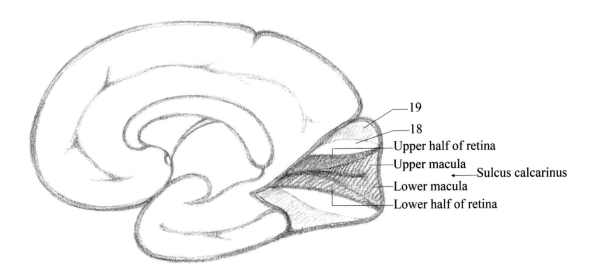

19
18
Upper half of retina
Upper macula
Sulcus calcarinus
Lower macula
Lower half of retina

Fig. 193 C. **Primary optical fields in the occipital lobe** *(medial surface of the right brain hemisphere).*

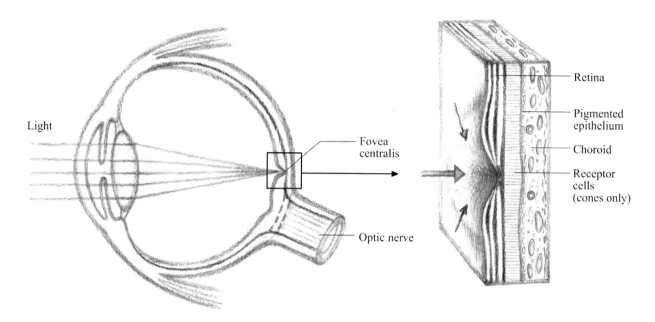

Fig. 194. **The retina's central fovea**. Rays of light are focused on the fovea. The fovea's switching neurons have shifted into the parafoveal zone (arrows) so that light can fall directly on the receptors (cones only; see enlarged detail).

processes different elements of an image (color, shape, orientation, depth perception) *separately*.

Here we confront the archetypal phenomenon of the visual system. We will now attempt to understand its essence. Let's consider the eye and the optic tract from the perspective of naïve image perception. We experience our surroundings as a colorful, organized, three-dimensional whole, but this whole never becomes visible anywhere in the neurological portion of the optic system. Our two eyes generate two images, which do not fit together, as a little self-experimentation readily reveals. Nonetheless, we experience these images as a unity. Each image is reversed by the lens, and this reversal is maintained throughout the optic tract, but we do not experience the perception as reversed. Finally, images from the two eyes are "projected" onto separate, columnlike zones of the brain's visual cortex. A third factor is the above-mentioned centralization of the retina with its more significant central region (*fovea*), along with constantly decreasing visual acuity toward the periphery (Figure 194). If a camera took double, reversed images that were fuzzy

everywhere except in the middle, we would hardly consider it a useable optical device! Moreover, the areas of the human visual cortex associated with the fovea are much larger than the areas that receive "projections" from the retina's periphery. Even in the primary cortex, therefore, no "true image" of our surroundings is present.

If we investigate the details of what happens to our image, its dissolution into individual elements becomes even more dramatic. In the last few decades, a great deal of scientific work has been done on this subject, so we now know fairly precisely which cells react to which types of stimulus and which areas of the cerebral cortex ultimately receive these stimuli. The primary visual cortex (area 17, or V_1), serves as a **distribution center** for stimuli coming from both eyes. This is where stimuli are sorted into colors, shapes, and movements. Color perception stimulates groups of cells in the parietal and temporal lobes (V_2 - V_4). Movements in space are registered in the upper occipital area (area 19), and details of form and pattern in the anterior and lower temporal area (areas 20 and 21, see Figure 193B).

Level	Human	Animal	Degree of consciousness
1.	Form concepts ("thinking in seeing") such as optical illusions	Signaling effects Primary information	"unconscious," automatic
2.	Learned visual concepts, e.g., written characters	Imprinting phase Learned behavior	Initially conscious, then unconscious (Threshold of consciousness)
3.	Creative concepts in optical perception (e.g. art, esthetics)	Absent	Conscious, proceeding from the (normal) "I"
4.	Supersensible perceptions (ideas become images), imaginations, etc.	Absent	Organ-free (brain-free) higher consciousness, proceeding from the "higher I"

Table 23. Conceptual elements in seeing and their respective levels of consciousness.

The coherent images of our de facto experience are nowhere to be found in the brain. On the contrary, our neurological apparatus picks each image to pieces, breaking it down into details such as color, shape, movement, and position in space. Optical images leave deep impressions on us, and we can pinpoint their spatial locations and movement. But where do these images arise? The typical modern response is that image formation occurs on the psychological level and that the pattern of neuronal stimulation is the "objective" element in this process, while our experience of optical images is unreal and subjective.

As we have already discussed, however, this argument is epistemologically untenable. We must take our experience of optical images seriously and acknowledge its reality. But there are multiple levels of reality. As we know, we cannot perceive a visual impression as such in isolation, without involving our capacity for thought. In other words, we must form concepts in order to see (2). Without the addition of concepts, perceptual images appear chaotic. Steiner (2) calls this "pure perception." For example, on awakening from anesthesia or a drunken stupor, we may perceive our surroundings as a chaotic confusion of colored blobs that do not immediately resolve into distinct objects. As a rule, this perception causes great anxiety, but inner calm is restored as soon as we

grasp the first few "organizing" concepts—this is a bed, that's a chair. Our thinking assigns individual perceptions to specific concepts, thus creating the mental images necessary for orienting ourselves in space. Like the actual perceptions, however, these concepts originate on very different levels that must then be taken into account in analyzing the visual process.

The lowest level of this process involves simple concepts of shape or structure. Whether we see two straight lines as parallel or curved is decided by the visual system itself, so to speak. Many familiar optical illusions prove that shapes we see appear as the result of inherent "conceptual" contexts that we can do little to change. Although we can deliberately correct optical illusions, doing so requires a certain amount of conscious effort. Normally, the processes involved in perceiving shapes are almost automatic and unconscious. We might say that there is an "unconscious thinking" at work in the activity of seeing. This simple type of perception is also found in animals, for whom optical impressions serve as signals for reflexive responses to stimuli.

A second and somewhat higher level involves learned concepts that influence our visual per-ception, as in the interpretation of writing. Although we must initially learn the meaning of these specific visual shapes, recognizing them ultimately becomes largely automatic. Animals achieve this level in the imprinting phase but unlike humans, they later lose the ability to incorporate new, complex signals into their behavior patterns.

The next two levels are achieved only by humans. The first involves creative concepts that flow into perception from the sphere of the "I". Such concepts make it possible for humans to interpret the artistic, esthetic, or moral elements of the perceived image and raise them to consciousness. The final and highest level is the level of supersensible perception, which is no longer bound to physical instruments (eye, brain, etc.) but allows us to become conscious of the spiritual intentionality inherent in a perceived image.

Regardless of the level of visual perception, the basic process is always the same: The sensory system registers the details of an optical image, breaking it down into its separate elements (shape, direction, color, space, etc.). The occipital brain center (area 17, V_1) distributes these elements to widely separated regions of the brain. In other words, the image as a whole is broken apart by the sensory system and cannot be put back together again within the nervous system. As a result, the rebuilding that necessarily follows this breakdown must originate in the domain of forces of a different type. We have already seen that thinking plays a decisive role here. But for thinking to create the relevant perceptual image in each case, the entire body's soul and life forces must be involved. Consequently, we must again distinguish between several different domains.

First, let's consider the **perception of space**. Unlike color perception, it has no actual anatomical corollary in the retina. Normally, both eyes are needed for spatial perception. When the visual axes of both eyes (which run through the fovea) cross in a point on the periphery (fixation point), "horizontal disparity"—the distance between the image of that point and that of a second point on the retina—allows us to determine whether the second point lies behind or in front of the fixation plane (Figure 195). As such, therefore, space is not "reproduced" either on the retina or in the

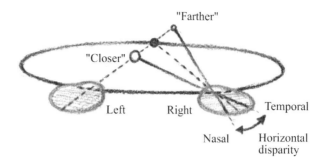

Fig. 195. **Perceiving distance by "measuring" horizontal disparity on the retina** (for details, see text).

brain but is "calculated" in the nervous system on the basis of incoming data. These "data" alone, however, cannot tell us what happens on the psychological level.

Let's take another look at the evolution of the head and eyes. The skull's evolution into a generally spherical shape is very closely related to acquiring uprightness and the resulting change in the center of gravity in the upright human body. In higher mammals with tube-shaped heads, the eyes are usually located well back on the sides of the head. Even in lower primates or insectivores such as tree shrews (*Tupaia* spp.), the eyes are still located quite far to the side (Figure 196A). Initially, the eyes of human embryos are also laterally located, but they later move to the front as part of the development of the face, which also involves the alignment of the forehead, mouth, and nose in the frontal plane. Laterally located eyes are relatively poorly suited to distance perception. In humans, the shifting of the eyes to the front and the development of the fovea centralis means that the visual axes of **both** eyes can be directed toward a single fixation point. The capacity for spatial perception is the result (Figure 196B). As a further consequence, human beings can distance themselves from objects in space and become conscious of the separation. The visual axes of both eyes "touch" each other so to speak in the object focused upon. This optical touching

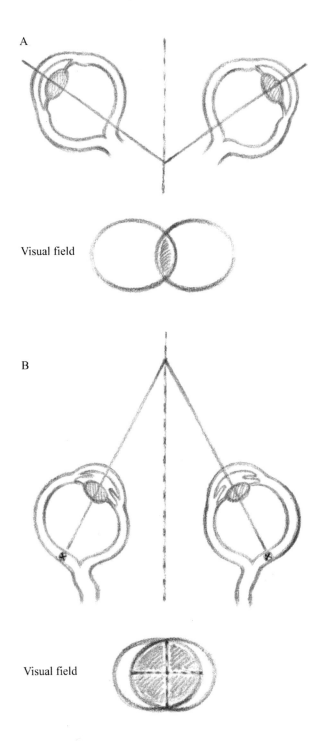

A

Visual field

B

Visual field

*Fig. 196. **Orientation of the visual axes** (red lines) **in tree shrews** (Tupaia, A) **and humans** (B). In humans, the field of binocular vision (red) is greatly increased because the eyes have shifted toward the center, simultaneous with the development of the fovea centralis (x) in the center of the retina.*

leads to consciousness. It is repeated within the visual system itself when the optic fibers from the right sides of both retinas (which lead to the right cerebral cortex) contact the fibers from the left halves (which lead to the left cortex) in the optic chiasm (Figure 193A; see also Figure 3, p. 5). Accurate spatial perception develops only when the fibers from the two eyes remain precisely separated in the visual tract.

On the psychological level, this distancing, confronting, or touching is ultimately a **will experience**. Thus, as Rudolf Steiner often emphasized, our perception of space is based on a will experience that is centrally important to the experience of our individual "I" (84).

Color vision leads us to a different level of visual perception. The retina contains three different types of cones ("blue," "green," and "red" receptors). Experiments have shown that we can distinguish approximately 200 hues, 26 levels of saturation, and approximately 500 levels of brightness, for a total of over one million perceived variations in color. This huge variety is a psychological phenomenon that cannot be entirely explained by the linear scale of wavelengths and the neuronal switching in the brain and retina. Goethe discovered the color circle and its soul-spiritual dimension. He demonstrated that the experience of color is always a whole (i.e., a circle) in which the individual elements produce infinitely many psychologically expressive possibilities through contrasts, similarities, modifications, etc. With the help of colors, the human "I" is thus able to manifest and become conscious of a great wealth of soul experiences.

In the perception of pure **form**, feeling plays less of a role. Here, the essential element is the dynamic of lines and shapes, such as we find primarily in the world of living things and which we sense through our own life forces. The fact that adding a radiating array of straight lines suddenly makes two parallel lines appear curved (Figure 197) demonstrates that we do not perceive abstract, geometrical laws but rather the dynamic of the elements in each image. The expansive

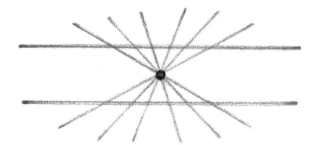

*Fig. 197. **Example of an optical illusion**. The two horizontal lines are parallel.*

thrust of the radiating lines affects the parallel lines, making them appear curved. The visual system, rather than evaluating images abstractly, always grasps them as wholes, i.e., in terms of their structural dynamics.

Table 24 below distinguishes the processes involved in the visual experience.

If, however (as explained above), the nervous system cannot possibly be the physiological vehicle of will and sensation processes, what are the anatomical and physiological foundations of the nonneural aspects of visual perception? Neurological processes are informational in character. They break down the image but do not reconstruct it. They can reflect or reproduce the outer world and allow it to become conscious, but the perceptual experience as a whole requires other, additional processes that science has barely touched on to date (see especially Zajonc, 85).

As discussed earlier, willing finds its basis in metabolic functions, feeling in rhythmical (circulatory and respiratory) functions. And in fact such activities play very significant roles in the eye.

The retina is closely underlain by the **retinal pigmented epithelium**, a layer only one cell thick, which is one of the most metabolically active

tissues in the body (Figure 198). Directly under the pigmented epithelium lies the inner layer of the choroid, a layer of closelyknit capillaries called the choriocapillaris (Figures 191 and 192). Unusually large quantities of blood circulate through this layer. Because only approximately five percent of the oxygen in the blood is removed from the choriocapillaris, its exceptional degree of vascularization cannot be entirely explained by the oxygen demands of the pigmented epithelium and retina. Hence it is assumed that this capillary system with its unusually large volume of circulating blood also serves as a cooling system removing excess heat generated when the retina is impacted by light. The recently discovered nerve-cell plexus within the human choroid (consisting of nearly 2,000 ganglion cells) might have an important function in this respect (regulation of blood volume and blood circulation in the choroids) (136). But when we consider the human being as a soul-spiritual entity, heat (warmth) can be seen as a link between physical and soul-spiritual functions (see p. 184) and possibly also as a connection between the different levels of thinking discussed above.

In this context, another significant function is the **regeneration** (so-called disk shedding) of the **photoreceptors**. In addition to their inner segments, which contain numerous cell organelles, both the rods (which number around 120 million) and the cones (approximately 6.5 million) have membranous outer discs that are in contact with the pigmented epithelium (Figure 198). These outer discs contain visual pigments (such as rhodopsin, a vitamin A derivative), whose stereoisomeric structures are changed by light. The bottoms of the photoreceptors constantly shed discs, which are phagocytized by the cells of the pigmented epithelium. The breakdown products

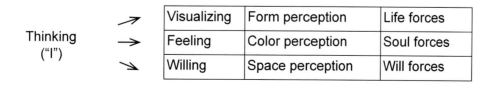

Thinking ("I")		Visualizing	Form perception	Life forces
		Feeling	Color perception	Soul forces
		Willing	Space perception	Will forces

Table 24. The fundamental processes involved in seeing.

Fig. 198. **Renewal of photoreceptors in the retina** *(disk shedding). Visual pigments (red) form in the receptors' inner segments and are then transported to the outer segments, where they are denatured by the effects of light. The altered disks slowly make their way to the tips of the outer segments, where they are phagocytized by the pigmented epithelium. Breakdown products of visual pigments are carried by the blood to the liver, where they are resynthesized. The new pigments are transported back to the blood vessels of the choroid, where they are absorbed into the pigmented epithelium and funneled back into the sensory cells (arrows). Radioactively tagged amino acids make it possible to trace the migration of visual pigments from the inner segment to the outer segment and then into the pigmented epithelium (arrows).*
1: 90 to 120 minutes
2: 180 minutes
3: 72 hours
4: 65 days
5: 82 days after injection of the radioactive marker.

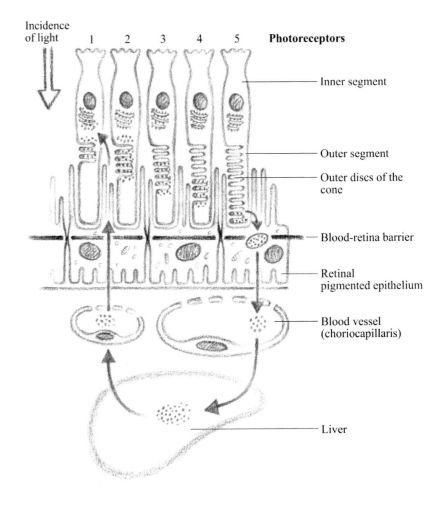

are channeled into the circulatory system via the choroid capillaries and ultimately regenerated in the liver. Carried back to the eye by the bloodstream, they are absorbed into the pigmented epithelium, transferred to the inner parts of the sensory cells with the help of small cytoplasmic processes (microvilli), and fed back into the external discs to regenerate them in a circadian rhythm. Within the receptors, therefore, discs are constantly streaming toward the inside (Figure 198). Thus a monumental cycle of building up and breaking down takes place in the eye. This cycle is triggered by light and ultimately involves the whole body.

Is it really so difficult to imagine that these unbelievably intensive and comprehensive metabolic processes in the eye have roles to play in

functions other than our experience of visual perceptions? Plato described the eye as having an "arm" of energy emerging from it to "touch" objects and make us conscious of them. Awareness of these connections was lost to humanity after Plato's time.

The Eye's Auxiliary Functional Systems

Up to this point, we have been considering the eye in general terms as the organ that perceives light. Perceiving a sharp image, however, also involves four auxiliary systems:

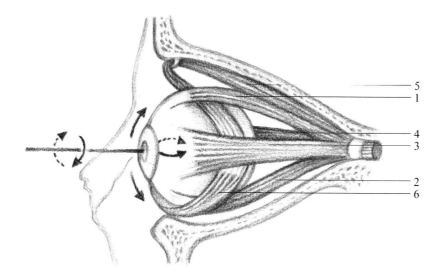

Fig. 199. **The eye muscles** *(illustration shows the left eye in its socket). With very little motion, the six (extraocular) eye muscles can shift the line of sight in every direction (arrows). There is one muscle for each direction of movement: up/down (1, 2), left/right (3, 4), inward/outward rotation (5, 6).*

1: *superior rectus muscle*
2: *inferior rectus muscle*
3: *lateral rectus muscle*
4: *medial rectus muscle*
5: *superior oblique muscle*
6: *inferior oblique muscle*

1. The iris;
2. The accommodation apparatus;
3. The movement apparatus;
4. The eyelids and lacrimal apparatus.

Each of these systems serves a specific function with regard to image quality.

The **aperture of the iris** ensures a relatively constant level of illumination. Reflex-controlled variations in pupil dilation increase depth of field by preventing excessive illumination of the retina. In this first step in seeing, the visual system itself actively "organizes" light-filled space.

Out of this initially undefined space, the **accommodation system** then "selects" a specific focal plane in which objects are seen clearly. Contraction of the ciliary muscles changes the curvature of the lens, thus shifting the focal point. This too is clearly an active process. This type of accommodation occurs only in higher primates and humans, and its evolution is closely associated with retinal centralization and the development of the fovea. Our capacity for accommodation allows us to "wander around" in light-filled space, focusing on objects at will, regardless of whether they are close or far away (see also Figures 194 and 195). Because accommodation involves muscles, it is largely a will process.

Conscious perception of three-dimensional space, however, requires yet a third active aux-

iliary system, the eye's **movement apparatus** (sclera, extraocular muscles, etc.), which adds the third dimension to the two-dimensional space we experience through accommodation. For three-dimensional vision, both eyes must work together. Each eye is equipped with three pairs of muscles, each of which moves the eye back and forth in one of the three planes of space (Figure 199). The two horizontal muscles (the medial and lateral rectus muscles) turn the eye inward and outward in the horizontal plane, the two vertical muscles (the superior and inferior rectus muscles) move it up and down, and the two rotator muscles (superior and inferior oblique muscles) rotate the eye. As a result, the human eye has a greater range of motion than any animal eye. Without any movement of the head, the human eye can extend its imaginary visual arm into space in all directions. But we are able to see in three dimensions only when our two "visual arms" or lines of sight cross in the focal plane or plane of accommodation. Then a truly three-dimensional perceptual image comes about (Figures 195 and 196).

The minute and extremely precise muscle movements needed to explore the visual field are possible because the eyeball moves back and forth almost weightlessly in the eye socket, as if in a joint, and because the **eye muscles** are among the most highly developed and richly innervated muscles

Horizontal motion (important for accommodation and space perception	Abduction (outward motion) Lateral rectus muscle	Abducent nerve (CN VI)
	Adduction (inward motion)	Oculomotor nerve (CN III)
Rotation (leaving space —REM phenomena)	Outward rotation Inferior oblique muscle	Oculomotor nerve (CN III)
	Inward rotation Superior oblique muscle	Trochlear nerve (CN IV)

Table 25. Antagonistic innervation of the eye muscles related to the two most important basic functions of the visual system.

in the body. The human eye has an antagonistic pair of muscles for each plane of space (up/down, right/left, etc.)—an ideal movement system for the optical perception of space.

A significant phenomenon is the rich and strangely complex *innervation of the extraocular muscles*, which involves three very densely fibrous cranial nerves (CN III, IV, and VI). Given the high functional value of the eye movements, however, this arrangement certainly makes sense. The two movements (horizontal and rotational) most important for exploring the field of vision each involve two antagonistic cranial nerves. The abducent nerve (CN VI) and the oculomotor nerve (CN III) are involved in horizontal eye movements, the trochlear nerve (CN IV) and the oculomotor nerve (CN III) in rotation (see Table 25). Because of horizontal disparity, horizontal eye motion is especially important for space perception.

In contrast, rotation plays a role in "leaving space" when we are self-absorbed and not involved with visual space. Normally, rotational eye movements are a way of achieving emotional release. We know, for example, that eye rolling (which involves the rotator muscles in particular) is an indicator of dream phases in sleep (so-called REM sleep). These phases are associated with psychological excitement and may serve to dissipate inner conflicts. In rotational eye movements, the human visual system "leaves space," as it were, similarly to the way closing our eyelids extinguishes the world of images and provides a respite from confronting our surroundings. This phenomenon may also shed light on the strange fact that the fourth cranial (trochlear) nerve is the only cranial nerve that emerges from the dorsal side of the brain stem. In a certain respect, this nerve sets itself apart from the other ocular nerves in its relation to counterspace. These connections can also lead to a new understanding of pathological eye movements such as strabismus convergens and divergence or rolling of the eyes under extreme psychological duress, etc.

The last auxiliary system consists of the *eyelids* and *lacrimal apparatus*, which are usually considered protective mechanisms. Unlike the organs of hearing, the organs of sight are capable of shutting themselves off from the outer world of light. But the fourth auxiliary system also points to a more profound aspect of the visual system. During the embryonic period, this system develops from the inside out, growing from the interbrain to the surface of the skin (Figure 190). The result is a permanent "wound" in the body's covering of skin. The conjunctiva of the eye is the only place in the body where a mucous membrane lies exposed on the surface. Like an open wound, it "oozes" constantly, as indeed it must, because lacrimal fluid is needed to keep the cornea transparent. The open eye is a gash in the body's protective covering. On the physical level, this opening allows light into the interior; on the soul level, it also facilitates the release of emotional tension, as in crying.

The Visual System as a Whole

In terms of its dynamics, the visual process is fundamentally different from the auditory process. In hearing, we make ourselves empty, so to speak, in order to take in a foreign element. The image of the double spiral illustrates this phenomenon. On the psychological level, the attitude of hearing is one of devoted cooperation or sympathy.

Seeing, however, involves a more active **confrontation** or contrasting of outer and inner processes. The optic cup receives light from outside but responds with a countergesture in that we "project" the resulting image into the outer world and perceive it there. Moving toward the outer world, confronting and taking hold of it, is an active process that creates consciousness through the meeting of forces (antithesis, antipathy).

Rudolf Steiner characterized this confrontation of life processes as a "latent inflammation" (80). Inflammation, regardless of where it occurs in the body, is always a nascent "eye development" in the wrong place: something foreign penetrating the body is met with an immune reaction in the blood or connective tissue. In this process, life forces are released. In a tumor, the opposite occurs: life forces remain *in* the tissue in question, where they cause pathological growth. We have seen how a tumorlike process plays an important role in the development of the auditory system (p. 254).

On the highest and purest level, therefore, the two most important sensory systems (eye and ear) reflect two major (and polar opposite) fundamental biological processes, which appear as inflammation and tumor growth, respectively, when they manifest pathologically.

In this connection, the recent discovery that the eye occupies an exceptional position in the immune system is almost archetypally characteristic. The eye is one of the "immune-exempt" organs in which immunological (inflammatory) reactions are normally suppressed. The eye overcomes its inherent, latent inflammatory potential and transforms it into a sensory process. Sensory processes can lead to accurate perceptions only when fundamental biological processes are "purified"—that is, when they operate completely selflessly, on a higher level.

The Chemical Senses (Taste and Smell)

Like the senses of sight and hearing, whose activities are polar opposites in many respects, the senses of taste and smell also reflect a polarity, although on a somewhat lower level. To an ingested substance, tasting is an antagonistic process that continues into the digestive organs. To be perceived, the substance must first be dissolved in fluid. The serous glands of the organs of taste, which produce this fluid, are an active and decisive component of the perceptual process. Tasting "tests" a foreign substance to determine its quality and suitability for digestion and absorption—is it toxic or nourishing? The organs of taste, which are located mainly on the tongue (with a few on the palate and in the back of the throat), have many little cup-shaped depressions that receive substances for assessment. In this respect, they are similar to the optic cup, which develops in the embryonic eye to "catch" light and react to it. In both cases, the process is "confrontational" in character.

The olfactory process is very different. As with hearing, it involves cooperation or inter-penetration, and the image of the double spiral is again applicable. Olfactory substances, along with air, directly contact the olfactory mucosa of the nose, where they trigger a perceptual process that reaches deep into the interior of the body. Ultimately, they provoke direct responses in the autonomic nervous system as well as emotional responses with physical consequences. In many vertebrates, the olfactory system (which is usually highly developed) is directly connected to reproductive processes via the brain's limbic system and the hypothalamus, and it directly influences reproductive behaviors. Even in humans, whose olfactory system has been severely impacted by more highly developed senses (especially sight), olfactory stimuli are still capable of triggering deep-seated emotions that extend into the sexual domain. Just think of perfumes, incense, etc. Figurative references

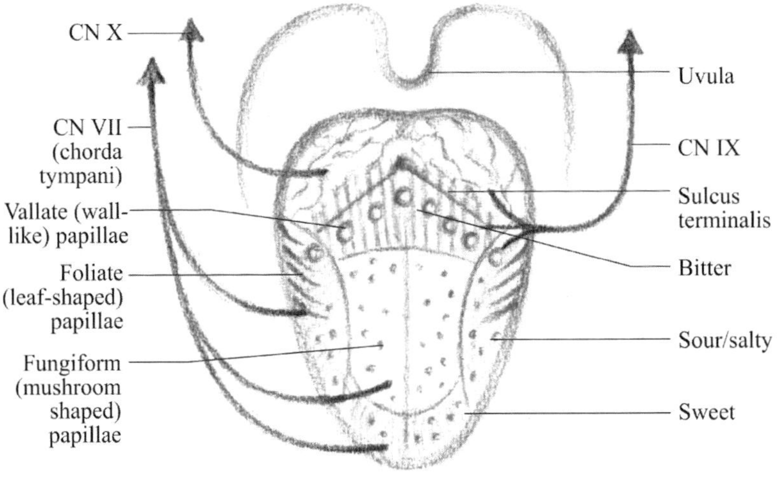

*Fig. 200. **Distribution of papillae and taste buds**. The vallate or circumvallate papillae (of which there are 10-12) lie in front of the V-shaped sulcus terminalis and house approximately 1,000 taste buds each. The foliate and fungiform papillae have significantly fewer taste receptors. Three cranial nerves (CN VII,IX, and X) serve the sense of taste.*

to smell (such as "it stinks to high heaven") in colloquial speech convey a deeply emotional response. Figurative references to the sense of taste ("tasteful," "tasteless," etc.) are completely different in character, dominated by the antithetical, objectifying, or appraising element.

The Sense of Taste (Gustatory System)

The organs of taste (taste buds) are irregularly distributed in the epithelium of the oral mucosa. They are most numerous on the tongue and palate. Taste buds are much more numerous in infants than in adults; their number decreases radically with age, which explains why older people need stronger stimuli in order to taste anything. With regard to the sense of taste, it is especially true that newborns are still "all sense organ" and perceive everything very intensely. Because the digestive system only gradually becomes accustomed to earthly food, the monitoring function of the sense of taste is vitally important in infancy. The sense of taste is one of the factors that help infants and toddlers make the challenging transition between intrauterine life and earthly life until speech

develops and offers them another means of self-defense.

The **organs of taste** and their receptors are located primarily on the tongue in the epithelium of the vallate, foliate, and fungiform papillae. The fungiform papillae are distributed irregularly over the top of the tongue, the foliate papillae lie along its edge, and the vallate papillae (of which there are usually ten or twelve) form a V-shaped line at the back of the tongue (Figure 200). Each vallate papilla is ringed by a trench housing up to one thousand onion-shaped taste buds (Figure 201), each of which consists of densely packed, elongated cells of two types—receptors and supporting cells. On their outer surfaces, the receptors develop little processes that protrude into cup-shaped depressions (taste pores). These processes are sensitive to substances that can be tasted (Figure 201). The basal portions of the taste buds have synapselike connections (ganglia) to nerve fibers that are branches of the three major cranial nerves innervating the tongue (CN VII, IX, and X, Figure 200). These nerves conduct taste impulses first to the "taste center" (nucleus tractus solitarius) in the brain stem and then via the thalamus to the postcentral gyrus in the cerebral cortex, where perceptions of taste become conscious.

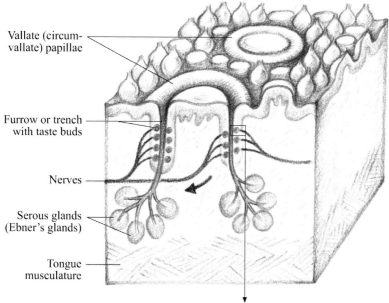

Vallate (circum-
vallate) papillae

Furrow or trench
with taste buds

Nerves

Serous glands
(Ebner's glands)

Tongue
musculature

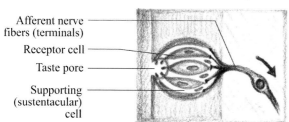

Afferent nerve
fibers (terminals)

Receptor cell

Taste pore

Supporting
(sustentacular)
cell

Fig. 201. **Cross section of the back of the tongue, showing vallate papillae**. *The taste buds, located in the trenches surrounding these papillae, consist of receptors and supporting (sustentacular) cells, which are actually immature taste cells (see enlarged detail). The receptors (red) have microvilli that extend into the taste pore. The bases of the receptors are in contact with nerve fibers.*

In the gustatory system, we rediscover a principle that is already familiar to us from the visual and auditory systems: incoming stimuli are distributed to different regions of the brain and are never reintegrated into a whole in any way that would adequately explain what we actually experience.

The adult oral cavity contains between five and ten thousand taste buds. To date, there is no evidence of any specialization of taste receptors. The sense of taste registers only four basic modalities, which are localized on different parts of the tongue's upper surface: sweet is perceived primarily at the tip of the tongue, bitter at the back, and sour and salty along the edges (Figure 200). Apparently, each receptor registers multiple modalities. In the brain, however, the modalities seem to be kept separate from each other and are separately connected to other sensory systems,

especially the olfactory system, and to parts of the autonomic nervous system (as indicated by increased secretion of gastric juices following taste stimuli).

Thus the gustatory system is broadly integrated into more general sensory activity. On their own, the organs of taste would play only a very modest role in how we experience our surroundings. We all know that a common cold can severely reduce our experience of taste, while seeing nicely presented foods may enhance it.

As with the eye and the ear, experiences of taste remain incomprehensible unless we also take emotional and will activity into account. Here again, we must ask, what are the morphological foundations of this activity? This question remains largely unanswered. One thing we must keep in mind, however, is that tasting dissolved substances would be impossible without the activity of the serous glands, which secrete a thin fluid into the base of the trench of each vallate papilla. This secretion flushes taste substances out of the openings (pores) of the taste buds and helps dissolve new substances. The tongue muscles aid in this process by "massaging" the glands to stimulate secretion. For this purpose, professional wine or water tasters always put bits of bread in their mouths between samples.

A second, equally important process is ***receptor regeneration***. Every ten to fifteen days, new taste receptors (complete with new surface processes and new nerve contacts at their bases) develop out of undifferentiated cells in the taste buds. This remarkably intense regenerative process is predicated on a high degree of metabolic activity and good circulation. The process itself is similar to the renewal of photoreceptors in the eye, which also takes place approximately every ten days. The connection between this metabolic regenerative activity and sensory experience has not yet been explained. It is conceivable, however, that the regeneration of receptors engages will elements in the perceptual process. As we have already mentioned several times, the will has no place in the purely neurological aspects of our perceptual experience.

The Organ of Smell And the Olfactory System

Unlike the process of tasting, which usually passes directly over into digestion, the olfactory process initially remains on the surface. The sense of smell fulfills the vital function of "guarding the gates" of respiration. In many mammals, the sense of smell is very highly developed, but in humans it is outweighed by sight and hearing. Nonetheless, our sense of smell is extremely sensitive. For example, we can smell ethyl mercaptan at concentrations as low as 10^{-13} g/ml of air, which is approximately 10^9 molecules (1). To be smelled, inhaled olfactory substances must be dissolved in fluid and must contact the receptors (in humans, approximately 10^7 cells) in the olfactory mucosa of the upper parts of the nasal concha and nasal septum, an area of approximately 300 mm^2 (Figure 202).

Olfactory receptors are unique in that they are actually nerve cells that have been transformed into sensory cells (Figure 203). On their upper surfaces, they have little bulbous swellings from which long processes (olfactory cilia) emerge, spreading out to cover a huge surface. Olfactory receptor cells are also unique in that they are constantly being regenerated, unlike any other neurons in the brain. In a sixty-day rhythm, new receptors develop out of the basal cells of the olfactory mucosa (Figure 203). This means that the ciliary membranes, which house the receptor proteins, also undergo constant restructuring. The cilia are embedded in a thin fluid (olfactory mucus) secreted by specialized glands (Bowman's glands) in the olfactory mucosa. This mucus not only traps olfactory substances but also dissolves them so that they can come into contact with the cilia's receptor molecules. This contact triggers neuronal impulses. In some animal species, a single molecule of olfactory substance is enough to trigger a stimulus in a receptor cell.

Olfactory receptor cells are unspecialized. In contrast to colors perceived in the eye, for example, there are no "primary smells" that

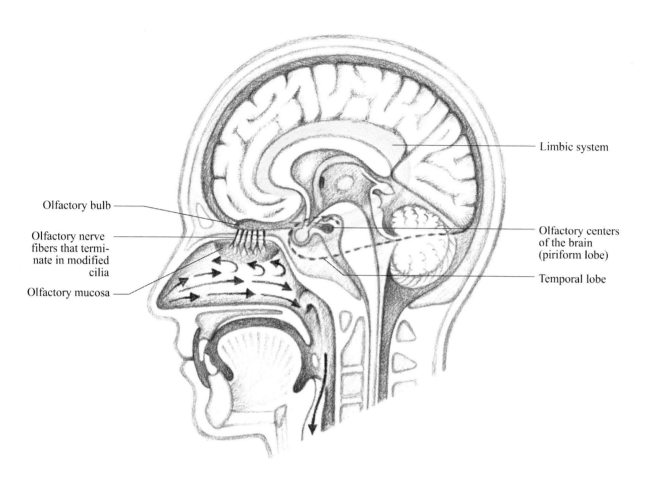

Olfactory bulb

Olfactory nerve fibers that termi-nate in modified cilia

Olfactory mucosa

Limbic system

Olfactory centers of the brain (piriform lobe)

Temporal lobe

*Fig. 202. **Overview of the olfactory system**. Inhaled air swirls against the roof of the nasal cavity, striking the olfactory mucosa (red). Stimuli from the olfactory receptors are transmitted first to the brain's olfactory bulb and then to the olfactory centers (red) of the temporal lobe, which are also connected to the limbic system (yellow).*

make up complex smells. Why some of the great variety of available substances trigger olfactory stimuli while others do not is a riddle that remains unanswered, even though the fundamental molecular processes underlying the sense of smell have been explained. The world of smell is mysterious and intimately related to the essential character of the beings and objects whose odors we perceive.

Although smelling involves only superficial contact with various olfactory substances, its psychological effects are often profound. The penetrating power of olfactory stimuli may be related to several surprising neurological features. **Stimuli from receptors in the nasal mucosa** are transmitted directly to the olfactory bulb (part of the brain!) and then via the olfactory tract to the higher olfactory centers in the piriform lobe in the anterior temporal lobe, where they become conscious (Figure 202). All other incoming sensory stimuli pass first through the thalamus (a huge collection of nuclei in the interbrain), but the nerve fibers of the olfactory receptors lead directly to the brain, specifically to the olfactory bulb, which makes up most of the brain in lower mammals such as opossums (Figure 204). The **thalamus** serves as an antechamber to the cerebral cortex, as an inhibition and filtration station that catches and suppresses most incoming sensory impulses. But the olfactory

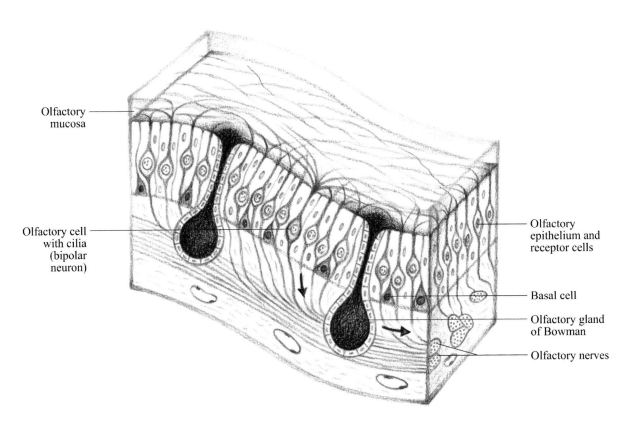

Olfactory mucosa

Olfactory cell with cilia (bipolar neuron)

Olfactory epithelium and receptor cells

Basal cell

Olfactory gland of Bowman

Olfactory nerves

*Fig. 203. **Structure of the olfactory mucosa**. The receptors are specialized nerve cells whose basal processes lead to the brain (olfactory bulb). On the surface of the mucosa, these cells develop long cilia that are embedded in olfactory mucus secreted by the Bowman's glands. Neural impulses are triggered when olfactory substances stick to the cilia. Basal cells constantly develop into new receptor cells.*

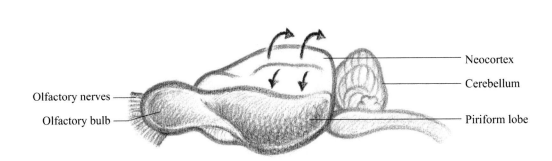

Neocortex

Cerebellum

Olfactory nerves

Olfactory bulb

Piriform lobe

*Fig. 204. **Brain of an opossum**. The olfactory system (gray) occupies most of the brain. The neocortex (white) is still relatively small. In higher mammals, it has become significantly larger (as indicated by arrows), forcing the rhinencephalon (olfactory brain) downward and inward.*

A

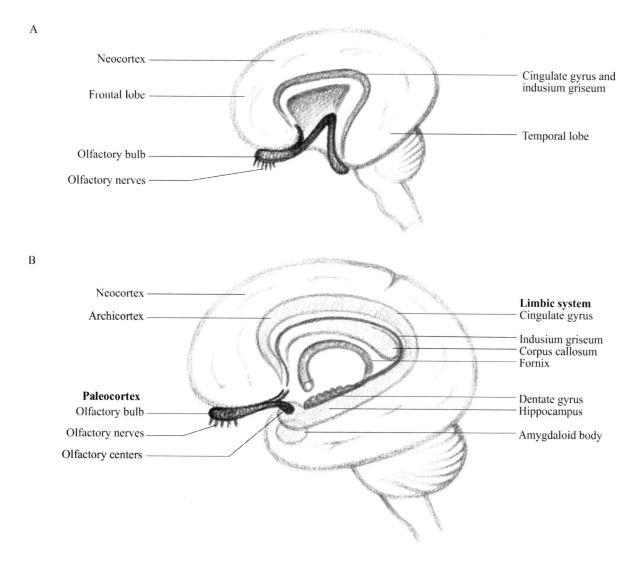

Neocortex

Frontal lobe

Olfactory bulb

Olfactory nerves

Cingulate gyrus and
indusium griseum

Temporal lobe

B

Neocortex

Archicortex

Paleocortex
Olfactory bulb

Olfactory nerves

Olfactory centers

Limbic system
Cingulate gyrus

Indusium griseum
Corpus callosum
Fornix

Dentate gyrus
Hippocampus

Amygdaloid body

Fig. 205. **Development of the olfactory** *(dark)* **and limbic** *(red)* **systems in humans**. *The olfactory system is forced toward the base of the brain as the cerebral cortex (neocortex) increases greatly in size. The cere-bral commissures bundled together in the corpus callosum separate the medially located limbic system (archicortex, red) into the indusium griseum (and its continuation, the dentate gyrus), which runs above the corpus callosum, and the fornix, which runs below. These areas, which are rolled up against the inside of the cerebral hemispheres, form the hippocampus in the area of the temporal lobe. The amygdaloid nucleus, also considered part of the limbic system, is in front of and connected to the hippocampus.*
A: Embryonic brain (5 months)
B: Adult brain (side view, with the frontal lobe on the left).

system has no such intermediate station. This is why olfactory stimuli often elicit actual organic effects (for example, in nausea, sexual behavior, and fight-or-flight reactions).

In humans, the cerebral cortex (neocortex) has undergone tremendous development and is therefore able to suppress the "archaic" brain regions associated with the olfactory system, including the rhinencephalon or olfactory cortex itself. In the course of evolution, the parts of the brain we now call the paleocortex and archicortex have been forced to the interior, where they lie rolled up at the base of the cerebral hemispheres. Also known as the limbic system, they now occupy little space in the adult brain (Figure 205).

In the course of evolution, the ***limbic system*** gradually separated from the olfactory system. Unlike the latter, however, it did not remain in a primitive functional state but continued to evolve and assume higher functions in the sensory system. Today the limbic system is thought to play a central role in the experience of personality, memory, and an individual's basic emotional attitude. The olfactory system and all other sensory systems are connected to the limbic system. As a result, it is often assumed that the limbic system "tinges" our sensory perceptions, mingling them with emotions. Although feelings certainly do not originate in the limbic system, it does represent a bridge of sorts between the inner world and conceptual activity. This bridging function, which is especially evident with regard to the chemical senses, allows us to become conscious of emotional elements in the perceptual process. Olfactory or gustatory substances often affect digestive processes directly—for example, by triggering saliva flow, gastric secretions, insulin release, or in some instances even nausea or vomiting. Conversely, digestive disorders can also cause qualitative changes in the perceptions of the chemical senses, which are also affected by the overall status of the metabolic system (as in malnutrition, for example). Examples include increased sensitivity to specific missing nutrients (salt cravings, protein cravings, etc.). Thus smell and taste reach deeply into the material world of the body, with the limbic system playing a central role as mediator between consciousness and the unconscious.

In the course of evolution, the limbic system was forced downward and inward as the cerebral cortex increased greatly in size. In humans, all that remains of the limbic system are narrow, arching strands located above and below the corpus callosum on the inner surface of the cerebrum and temporal lobe (Figure 205). We call this the archicortex or "ancient brain." It is connected to the rhinencephalon or paleocortex, which is the very oldest part of the brain. In humans, the "old parts"

of the brain include the fornix and hippocampus, which run under the corpus callosum, and the indusium griseum, which lies above it (Figure 205). Collectively known as the limbic system, these portions of the brain not only connect the telencephalon to even deeper structures in the brain (hypothalamus, midbrain, etc.) but are also connected to the other sensory systems and especially to the cerebral cortex.

After separating from the olfactory system in the course of evolution, the limbic system became increasingly independent within the brain. In humans, the olfactory system (paleocortex) has regressed but the limbic system has continued to evolve, ultimately forming a link between the highly developed cerebrum (neocortex) and the brain stem, which is connected to the spinal cord (Figure 205). The brain stem includes the reticular formation, a network of nerve cells and fibers that extends from the spinal cord to the hypothalamus in the interbrain.

Because of its close connections to the reticular formation and the autonomic nervous system, the limbic system will be described in detail in a later section.

Surface Sensitivity (The Skin Senses)

The skin is the surface separating the body from the outside world. More than just a protective covering, it serves many different functions such as respiration, elimination, thermoregulation, and immunological defense. Sensory functions are also a central task of the skin. The skin includes sense organs that serve three major groups of sensory processes:

1. Organs for sensing varying degrees of ***warmth*** in our surroundings. These organs inform the body about outside temperatures and allow it to adapt by setting regulatory mechanisms in motion to maintain a constant body temperature.

2. The skin houses many different types of sense organs that convey **sensations of touch**. Through touch, we experience other bodies and our own body. Through our major sense organs (eyes, ears), our consciousness lives entirely in external space, which is filled with light and air. Through touch, we become aware of corporeality as such for the first time, although initially only on a superficial level.

3. The organs of **deep sensitivity** located in our muscles and joints allow us to experience our own body as a moving body grappling with gravity. Kinesthetic and proprioceptive sense organs make us aware of the position of joints and the location of our limbs in space, while our sense of strength makes us conscious of muscle activity. Thus the skin senses and senses located in the muscles have to do with experiencing space. This experience can become conscious either outwardly (through touch) or inwardly (through our muscle senses or deep sensitivity).

The Sense of Warmth or Temperature

The sense of warmth occupies the upper end of the range of sensory organs related to our experience of space. Warmth (fire) disintegrates solids and guides space-bound forces back into the non-spatial realm. Our sense of warmth allows us to perceive the temperature of bodies in our surroundings (and thus also their inner activity) and to compare it to our own body temperature. Perception of warmth is thus very closely related to thermoregulation and, ultimately, with our experience of self. In the course of evolution, an experience of personal identity became possible only after the evolution of warmbloodedness—the organism's ability to maintain a constant body temperature.

The human body maintains a core temperature (essentially, the temperature inside the visceral cavities) of 37.1° C (Figure 206). Temperatures on the body's periphery (skin and limbs) fluctuate

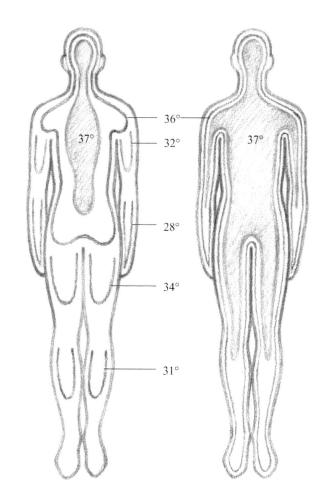

Fig. 206. **The body's temperature field**. *Body temperature is constant only in the visceral cavities (core temperature). As external temperatures increase, the layered warmth zones expand into the limbs. In other words, axial and radial gradients develop.*

in order to serve thermoregulation, which is based on subtle interactions between the core and the periphery that resemble a feedback loop. The mediating element here is the blood. When external temperatures rise, the body radiates more heat, or warmth is removed from its surface through evaporative cooling as perspiration dries. When outer temperatures decrease, the amount of heat lost to radiation is reduced—especially from the extremities (hands and feet)—by reducing circulation.

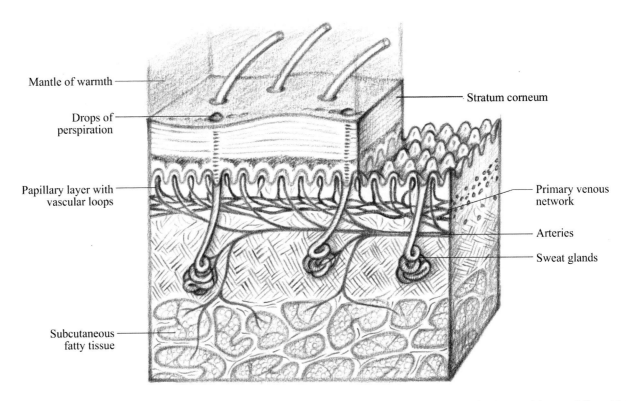

Mantle of warmth

Drops of perspiration

Papillary layer with vascular loops

Subcutaneous fatty tissue

Stratum corneum

Primary venous network

Arteries

Sweat glands

*Fig. 207. **The skin as an organ of temperature regulation**. The stratum corneum (outermost layer of the skin) and hairs retain warmth that radiates from the capillary loops of the papillary layer, creating a mantle of warmth over the skin. The primary venous network plays a major role in thermal regulation.*

The skin has at its disposal an extensive venous network that lies directly under the epidermis. From this network, numerous looplike capillaries extend into the papillary layer (Figure 207). Special vascular mechanisms such as arteriovenous anastomoses permit rapid increases and decreases in circulation in the skin (especially in fingers and toes) and corresponding changes in heat loss.

Blood is the most important organ for transferring heat into and out of vessels in the skin. Thus thermoregulation is first and foremost a circulatory problem. Circulation of blood and warmth is influenced from two sides, by the metabolism (especially in the muscles, where warmth is produced) and by the nervous system, which perceives and regulates heat status. The hypothalamus of the diencephalon contains neurons that can measure blood temperature and trigger the appropriate circulatory responses. Sensations from the skin also contribute to thermoregulation. Impulses from thermoreceptors are fed into the hypothalamus and the circulatory centers of the brain stem (in the medulla oblongata and midbrain) via the spinothalamic tracts of the spinal cord. The nervous system cannot influence warmth circulation directly but indirectly affects warmth radiation by regulating vasodilation, which alters the perfusion of various body parts. The nervous system ascertains the status of internal (blood) temperatures and sets appropriate regulatory processes in motion to ensure a constant core temperature.

Temperature perception takes place primarily in the skin, through several different types of ***thermoreceptors***. Cold and heat receptors have

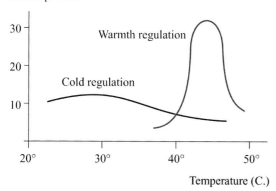

Fig. 208. **Cold and warmth receptors differ in their excitability.** *The frequency of action potentials of cold receptors increases when temperatures sink, that of warmth receptors, when temperatures rise, especially in the 35-50° C range (81).*

different attributes. On the basis of the behavior of the respective efferent nerve fibers, it is possible to conclude that cold receptors, which respond to sinking temperatures, are more numerous in the skin and cover a wider range of temperatures, whereas heat receptors are stimulated by rising temperatures, especially in a higher range (Figure 208). The body cannot register absolute temperatures, however, but produces a graded response to movements of warmth between the outer environment and its own core.

Here we see again the same general principle that we recognized with regard to the major sense organs, namely, that our sense organs dismantle the contents of the outside world into individual elements that are never reassembled into a coherent whole in the nervous system. The same principle is still more evident in the other skin senses (see below).

Although thermoreceptors are very simple in structure, warmth perception plays a decisive role in the human organism because of its importance for homeothermia and "I"-consciousness. The consequences of including soul-spiritual processes in our reflections on thermoregulation are far-reaching indeed. Our muscles and metabolic organs engage the

soul-spiritual aspect of our being in the material realm so that our will can unfold. This is where energy conversions occur, binding the soul to the physical element. This energy can also be released, in internal processes of "combustion" and excretion, so that soul elements can be experienced.

How strongly the soul can influence the skin's perfusion (and therefore also its warmth) is immediately obvious whenever we observe a sudden blush or pallor as feelings of shame, fear, or anger flood the soul. Conceivably, the flows of warmth circulating in the blood constitute the bridge between the soul-spiritual aspects of our existence and the living body. It is also conceivable that we use the element of warmth to transform the physical body or, conversely, to transform physical elements into soul-spiritual ones (see p. 184). We will return to this subject later (see p. 410).

The Organs of the Sense of Touch

The sensations transmitted by the skin are qualitatively very different from those of the other dominant sense organs (eye, ear). When we touch, we experience not only the material aspect of the surrounding world but also ourselves. Touching an object is what makes us believe it really exists. Through our sense of touch, we come in actual "contact" with other bodies for the first time. Thomas, the doubting apostle, believed in the reality of the Resurrection only when he had touched the Christ. Blind people who have cultivated their sense of touch and raised it to a higher level of consciousness often have a much stronger awareness of the reality of the objects around them than do sighted people. Normally, our sense of touch is relatively dull and underused. We barely notice how many different sensory processes it encompasses. Human skin contains many sensory organs of very different types. For the most part, their structure and functioning have been well researched (Figure 209).

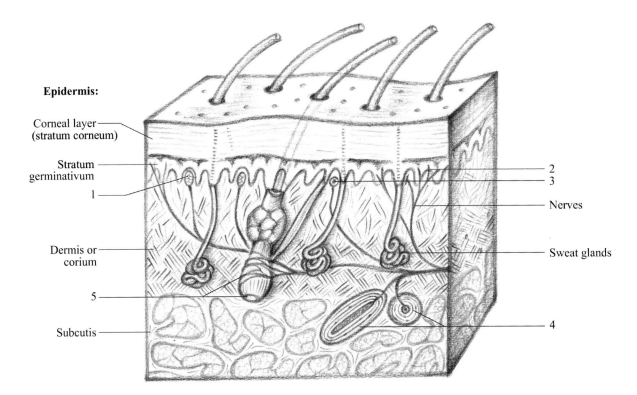

Epidermis:

Corneal layer (stratum corneum)

Stratum germinativum

1

Dermis or corium

5

Subcutis

2
3

Nerves

Sweat glands

4

Fig. 209. **Layered structure of the skin, showing locations of the most important skin organs** *(1-5). The sense organs of the skin are located either on the boundary between the dermis and the epidermis (e.g., Meissner's corpuscles, 1) or on the boundary of the subcutaneous tissue (e.g., Pacinian corpuscles, 4). Free nerve endings (thermoreceptors, nociceptors, etc., 2) infiltrate the epidermis in some cases or form organized nerve complexes (Ruffini corpuscles, 3; Merkel cells, etc.) directly below it. The hair follicles are also surrounded by dense neural networks, 5, which are very important for the sense of touch.*

We must make a fundamental distinction between free nerve endings in the epidermis and more complex, encapsulated sensory organs. Examples of encapsulated **cutaneous sensory organs** are the Ruffini and Krause corpuscles, which consist of delicate neuronal networks surrounded by "sacks" of nonneuronal cells (Figure 209). More complexly structured sense organs include Meissner's corpuscles and Pacinian corpuscles. Meissner's corpuscles are usually located in the papillae, i.e., directly under the epidermis. They look like tiny pinecones. Each Meissner's corpuscle is a stack of wedge-shaped nonneural cells interspersed with very delicate, pressure-sensitive nerve endings and enclosed in a capsule of connective tissue. In Pacinian corpuscles,

which are relatively large (1-2 mm in length), the encasing cells are like layers of an onion, and the nerve fibers are all located in an elongated inner chamber that runs the length of the corpuscle. Hair follicles, each of which is surrounded by a network of very delicate nerve fibers, are also sensitive to tactile stimuli (Figure 209).

Based on the pattern of excitation of afferent nerves, modern physiology distinguishes three basic sensory modalities in the skin, defining the type of stimulus in purely physical terms:

1. **Intensity detectors** are tactile receptors that respond only to pressure stimuli (free nerve endings, Merkel cells, or Ruffini corpuscles).

2. **Speed detectors** are receptors that

register pressure per unit of time (Meissner's corpuscles and neural networks at the bases of hair follicles).

3. *Acceleration detectors* are receptors that register the acceleration of incoming pressure stimuli in addition to pressure and time. They are complicated mechanoreceptors such as Pacinian corpuscles, whose onionlike layers of casing cells serve as filters so that the nerve endings in the inner chamber register only the vibration, not depth of pressure. For the most part, these organs convey impulses of tactile sensation and vibration.

Connections to the central nervous system. Neural impulses originating in various receptors in the skin reach the spinal cord via the posterior roots of the spinal nerves. After crossing to the other side, they are conducted via the anterior and lateral spinothalamic tracts and the thalamus to the postcentral gyrus of the cerebral cortex (Figure 210). In the brain stem, the spinal pathways are joined by the trigeminal nerves, each of which conducts sensations from the surface of one side of the head to the postcentral gyrus on the opposite side. Thus the surface of the brain reflects the body's entire surface, only upside down, mirror-image reversed, and severely distorted. Much larger areas of the brain are occupied by the functionally most important areas of skin (lips, fingers) than by relatively insensitive areas such as the torso (see the sensory homunculus, Figure 210).

In the spinal cord, impulses from various skin receptors are sorted by modality (pressure, contact, vibration, pain, temperature; see Figure 210) and conducted *separately* to the brain stem, where decussation occurs as needed, and then to the cerebral cortex, where consciousness of tactile sensations develops. It is interesting to note that sensations in the postcentral gyrus are not consolidated into coherent "images" according to their body parts of origin; the different modalities are kept separate for further processing. With regard to the sense of touch, we encounter a familiar riddle: how can coherent or holistic sensory experiences possibly develop, since the

neurological channels for different modalities are always kept separate throughout the nervous system?

On the soul level, we experience *tactile sensations* as a unitary process. Different parts of the body's surface vary greatly in their degree of sensitivity. Highly sensitive areas (fingers, lips, the tip of the tongue, the outer genitals) are contrasted with relatively insensitive zones (the skin of the back, or lower leg). Tactile sensations can be extremely complex, ranging from crude perceptions of an object's surface (rough, smooth, sticky, velvety, etc.) to detailed perceptions of its three-dimensional shape. A sensation of pressure due to a falling object may be relatively inconsequential, whereas a handshake may tell us worlds about a person's essential character. As we see, tactile experience is extremely varied and differentiated. But just as the plethora of visual perceptual possibilities is based on the activity of four types of receptors in the eye, ultimately only the three above-mentioned modalities underlie all the complex events of tactile sensation. In touching an object or another person, however, we experience significantly more than just these three physically defined stimuli. Touching tells us not only the surface character of another body but also something of its inner nature. The reverse is also true and is an important phenomenon: With our touch, we also convey something of ourselves. Think of the caressing or consoling hand of a lover, the blessing hand of a priest, or the healing hand of a physician. As with other sensory processes, touching must include not only an afferent, perceptive process but also an active, efferent, outward-radiating process. In psychological terms, we are again dealing with *will processes* here. The morphological foundations of these will processes, however, are still largely unknown. Skin tension, circulation, and the connective and vascular tissues surrounding the organs of tactile sensation may play important roles here. When we consider that tactile experience is inextricably bound up with space and that every instance of pressure makes an "indentation" on a

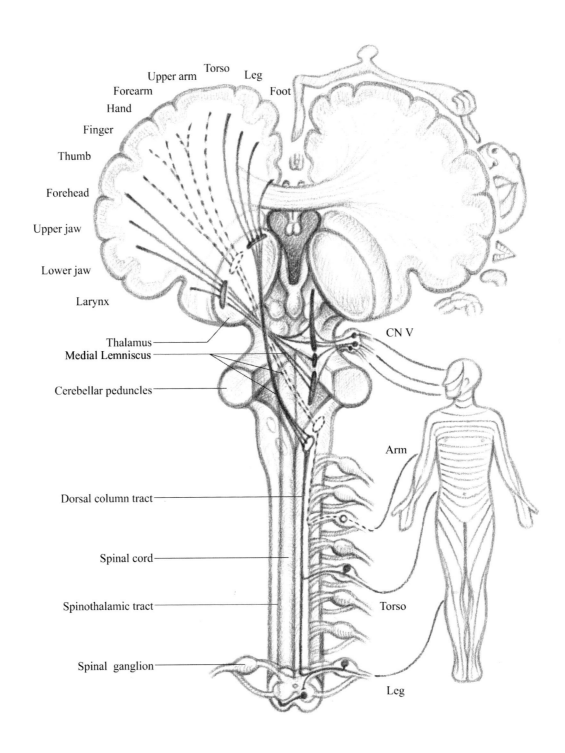

Fig. 210. **Major sensory pathways to the cerebral cortex**. *The posterior column pathways, which carry conscious sensations from the respective areas of the skin to the cerebrum, cross to the other side in the so-called medial lemniscus at the level of the rhomboid fossa. They are then joined by the trigeminal nerve (CN V) coming from the head. In the thalamus, these pathways are routed toward the postcentral gyrus of the cerebral cortex, where the body's surface is reflected in extremely distorted form on the basis of the functional importance of its parts (the so-called sensory homunculus, above right).*

spatial body, reducing its volume slightly, it is not difficult to imagine that reversing the indentation and restoring the body's original form are of central importance in experiencing the nature of what caused the pressure. Through indentation and restoration, two three-dimensional bodies actively meet, and the possibility of recognizing the being of the other arises.

The Sense of Pain

In a certain respect, the sense of pain can also be included in the skin senses, although perception of pain (nociception) is unique among the senses. We distinguish between dull and sharp or stabbing pains and between "first" pain (fast and transient) and "second" pain (slow and persistent) after an injury. But in spite of these distinctions, pain is always rather undifferentiated, a sensation bordering on the pathological. We usually feel pain either after tissue damage or as a consequence of extreme irritation of other sense organs. The phenomenon of pain probably evolved as the first of all senses, in response to outside forces encroaching on the body; further differentiation of this sense with regard to the type and scope of the encroaching forces then resulted in specific sense organs. If this is true, pain is the archetypal sense and can appear in a great variety of different ways. Pain impulses coming from the skin are transmitted to the brain along the pathways of the sense of touch (spinothalamic tracts); like sensations of touch, pain also becomes conscious in the cerebral cortex (Figure 210). But sensations of pain often undergo further processing in the spinal cord or the brain stem (especially in the thalamus), usually resulting in defensive or counterregulatory reflex responses that often do not become fully conscious.

A noteworthy phenomenon is the pronounced sensitivity of the serous membranes lining the **body cavities** (pleura, peritoneum, etc.). During the embryonic period, body cavities develop specifically where the formation of space-filling substance (for example, through proliferation of embryonic connective tissue or mesenchyme) does not occur. The absence of matter-filled space gives rise to cavities in which the organs are then able to develop. The inner linings of the chest, abdominal, and pelvic cavities, as well as the cranial cavity, are exceptionally richly innervated and highly sensitive to pain. In contrast, the organs (including the brain) that are housed in these cavities are almost totally insensitive. In this instance, nature constructs protective walls around the organs to separate them from outside influences so that their vital functions can take place undisturbed, obeying laws of their own in the body's dark, silent internal cavities. Wherever space is "created" inside the body to make room for the organs (viscera), the sense of pain stands guard, protecting the organs' mysterious and vital activity. This phenomenon also sheds light on the sense of pain in the skin, which also protects normal life functions and draws attention to itself only when destructive pathological processes "make themselves felt."

Deep Sensitivity (The Muscle Senses)

Even with our eyes closed, we can estimate the **angles** of our joints and the **positions** of our limbs in space—a hand gesture, the location of an arm or leg, or where our fingers are in relationship to each other. If we use two hands to compare the weight of two objects (such as two matchboxes of the same size but with different contents not visible from the outside), it is always astonishing to discover how precisely we can determine the difference in weight. While comparing weights, we usually move our hands up and down a bit—in other words, we move our muscles rhythmically. The different degrees of muscle tension caused by different weights are perceptible and allow us to determine which object is heavier. This is known as a **"muscle sense."**

The muscle sense and the sense of position in the joints are components of so-called deep sensitivity. As we learned in the chapter on sensory-motor systems (Figure 167), muscles contain very delicate sense organs (muscle and tendon spindles). Stimuli from the spindles are routed first into sensory-motor reflex circuits without becoming conscious, but we can also interpret them consciously, as we can the input of sensory organs in the joints (mechanoreceptors in the joint capsules and ligaments). The sum total of these inputs is "deep sensitivity."

Gravity affects the musculoskeletal system, and we come to grips with gravity every time we move. We become conscious of changes (contraction and expansion) in muscles and joints because the long spinal pathways (spinobulbar tract, posterior column pathways) rapidly convey stimuli from sensors in the musculoskeletal system to the brain via the medulla oblongata and thalamus (Figure 210). As a result, we "look inside ourselves," so to speak; our muscles allow us to experience not only the spatial world outside us but also our own bodies as objects moving in space. Heat dissolves bodies in space (through combustion or evaporation, for example). Through the muscle senses, however, we move in the opposite direction, into the depths of space. The resulting experience of space is of crucial importance not only for actual movement but also (especially in connection with the sense of equilibrium) for how we experience the world, i.e., for our sense of life or well-being and our self-confidence.

The Sense of Equilibrium

Muscle receptors allow us to perceive our bodily movements in three-dimensional space, but they must be complemented by the organ of equilibrium (labyrinth), which relates the body to the Earth's gravitational field—i.e., to the space around us—thus harmonizing our own movements with the forces of external space. We have already briefly discussed the structure of the organ of equilibrium in connection with the organ of hearing. The three endolymph-filled semicircular canals are located at right angles to each other, with each one representing one of the three planes of space. Each canal includes an ampulla with a sensory organ (the crista ampullaris and cupula). The otolith organs in the sensory terminals (acoustic maculae) of the utricle and saccule are directly affected by gravity (Figure 211A, and Figure 189 C, p. 265). Friedrich Husemann once described these receptors as "blind eyes" fixed on the Earth's center in order to determine the body's position in the Earth's gravitational field (123).

In the semicircular canals, movements in the fluid endolymph play a decisive role (Figure 211 B). When the body (or the head) moves in one of the planes of space, inertia causes the endolymph to move in the opposite direction, which in turn tilts the cupula, which stimulates the receptors and associated nerves.

Thus the organ of equilibrium separates the body's movements in space, which must be seen as a whole, into static and dynamic components. In terms of physics, the static maculae register linear acceleration while the ampullae register progressive acceleration. Within the petrous bone, the semicircular canals, instead of being aligned with the three planes that divide the body, lie at 45-degree angles to them (Figure 212). As a result, for example, the left anterior semicircular canal lies in the same plane as the right posterior canal and vice versa. Clearly, these sense organs "dissect" space into its individual elements rather than reproducing it exactly. Space is "dissolved," as it were; we must recreate it or put it back together (unconsciously,

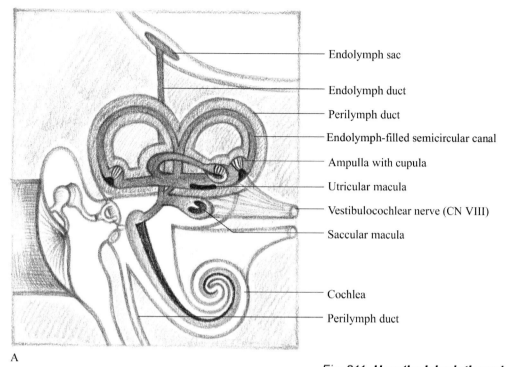

Endolymph sac

Endolymph duct

Perilymph duct

Endolymph-filled semicircular canal

Ampulla with cupula

Utricular macula

Vestibulocochlear nerve (CN VIII)

Saccular macula

Cochlea

Perilymph duct

A

Cupula

Perilymph
Receptor cells
Endolymph

Nerve

B

Fig. 211. **How the labyrinth works**.
A: Endolymph (red) fills the three semicircular canals, the utricle, and the saccule. Thus there are five sensory terminals (three ampullae and two maculae). The canals are surrounded by perilymph (blue) and stabilized with thin strands of connective tissue. The receptors in the semicircular canals are stimulated primarily by movements in the endolymph, those in the cochlea by movements in the perilymph.
B: Detail showing the ampulla of a semicircular canal. When the head is turned to the right, inertia of the endolymph causes the cupula to lean to the left (arrow).

of course) in order to experience it as a whole. Here we find again the same principle of analysis and resynthesis that we noted with regard to the other sense organs. Here, too, the physiological foundations of resynthesis remain a mystery, although of course the central nervous system plays a decisive role. As we mentioned earlier with regard to sensorimotor systems, the cerebellum is centrally important in regulating equilibrium. It is interesting to note that a three-dimensional cellular structure prevails in the cortex of the cerebellum: The neurons important

for regulating equilibrium are themselves located at right angles to each other. Like the primary motor and sensory cortex fields of the cerebrum, the cortex of the cerebellum also reveals a homunculuslike "map" of the body. Here, images of "internal space" (muscles, organs of movement) and external space (mediated by the labyrinth) come together and are compared. For human beings, this process remains completely unconscious.

All information from the peripheral nerves, the various sensory terminals of the two labyrinths,

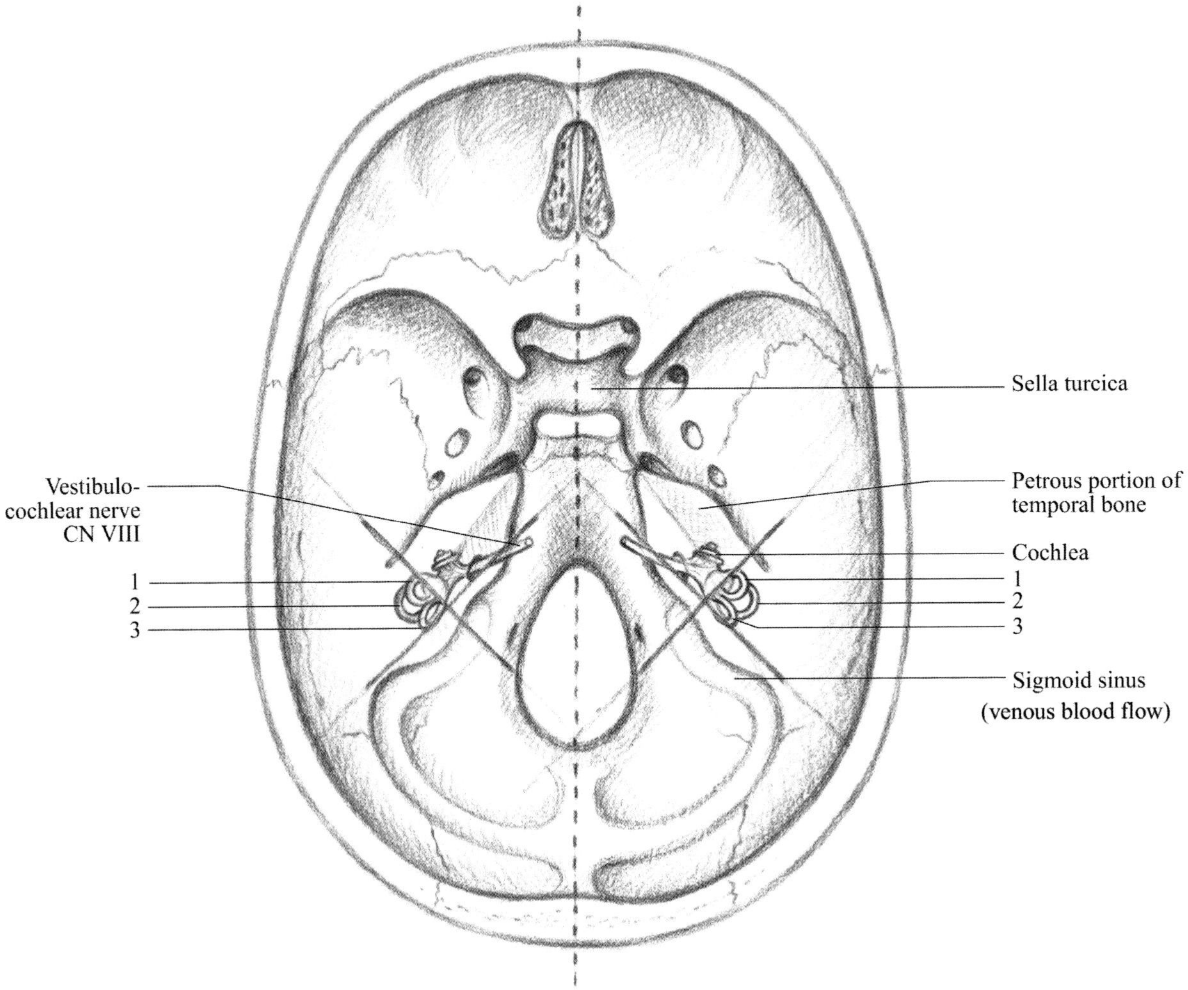

Vestibulo-
cochlear nerve
CN VIII

1
2
3

Sella turcica

Petrous portion of
temporal bone

Cochlea
1
2
3

Sigmoid sinus
(venous blood flow)

Fig. 212. **View of the base of the skull showing the location of the labyrinth in the petrous pyramid.** *As the red lines indicate, the left anterior semicircular canal (1) lies in the same plane as the right posterior canal (3); correspondingly, the left posterior canal (3) lies in the same plane as the right anterior (1). The entire system of semicircular canals stands at a 45-degree angle to the planes of the body. 2: lateral semicircular canal; CN VIII: eighth cranial (vestibulocochlear) nerve.*

and other input from the brain within the nervous system come together in the cerebellum, where they are offset and balanced against each other. Based on our previous observations, it is certainly safe to assume that something more than purely neural processes must be involved here.

The endolymph duct, which ends in a little sac on the back of the petrous pyramid under the dura mater (Figure 211A) is a counterbalance valve for endolymph oscillations in the semicircular canals. It has no significance for our perception of space. The perilymph duct (Figure 211A) does have a direct connection to the fluid-filled space surrounding the brain, allowing changes in pressure in the labyrinth's perilymph to be transmitted to the cerebrospinal fluid. As we can see, 1/6/16 the fluid system of the inner ear is linked on two sides to the brain's fluid system, whose buoyancy "lifts" us out of the experience of space, as we mentioned earlier.

These processes do not become conscious. When the functioning of the organs of equilibrium is disturbed, we lose our spatial orientation and normal body sensations. The result, as in seasickness, may be nausea, vertigo, and extreme discomfort. Thus the body's (unconscious) integration into space is a central experience intimately related to our existence. We need this constant but unconscious "feeling" of space in order to remain physically and psychologically in balance. The experience of space mediated by our sense of equilibrium radiates into the soul as an element of certainty without which our normal life on Earth would not be possible.

The Visceral Senses (Sense of Life)

The autonomic nervous system comprises the sum total of the delicate neural networks pervading all of the body's organs and tissues. Its organs include a great variety of receptors that register chemical stimuli (chemoreceptors), osmotic pressure in the tissues (osmoreceptors), and blood pressure (baroreceptors), to name just a few examples. In many cases, such stimuli are first processed locally, although they are also transmitted to the spinal cord and brain.

Blood-pressure regulation and respiratory regulation are especially well-researched examples of such unconscious sensory processes within the autonomic nervous system (Figure 213). The carotid body, located on the posterior wall of the bifurcation of the carotid arteries, is a sense organ that registers tension in the arterial wall (and therefore blood pressure). Neural impulses from the carotid body are transmitted through the carotid sinus nerve (a branch of the tenth cranial nerve) to the circulatory centers in the brain stem, which then set the appropriate autoregulatory

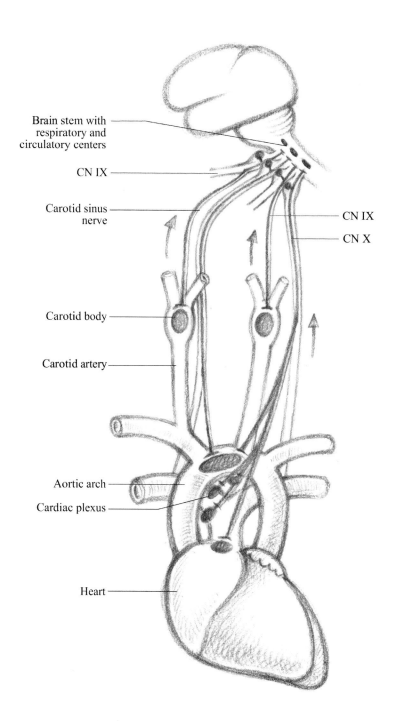

Fig. 213. **Blood pressure and respiration are regulated with the help of sense organs** *(chemoreceptors and baroreceptors) (red) located in the carotid artery, aortic arch, and base of the heart. Cranial nerves IX and X conduct impulses to the respiratory and circulatory centers in the brain stem. These regulatory processes are largely autonomic and unconscious.*

measures in motion. Other pressure receptors (baroreceptors) are located in the aortic arch and at the base of the heart. Impulses from these receptors are also conducted to the brain stem by branches of the tenth cranial (vagus) nerve (Figure 213). The carotid sense organs, however, are also chemoreceptors that aid in respiratory regulation by registering the blood's content of O_2, CO_2, and H^+ ions. This type of regulation is also autonomic and unconscious.

The exchange of information among different types of receptors within tissues and organs is extensive and highly differentiated, taking place on practically every level (molecular, cellular, neural), but it never achieves the level of consciousness. We experience only generalized sensations such as hunger, thirst, satiety, or urinary or fecal urgency. (Sexual sensations such as orgasm constitute an exception in that they may be dramatic in their intensity.) Rudolf Steiner coined the term "sense of life" to sum up all of the sensations originating in the internal organs (27). The sense of life conveys a generalized sense of well-being that is difficult to define in detail.

Afferent impulses from the viscera generally reach the brain via the spinothalamic tract in the anterior column pathway of the spinal cord (which also transmits sensations of pain) or via the tenth cranial nerve, but they are conducted only as far as the thalamus and limbic system (the so-called visceral brain), never reaching the cortex fields (postcentral gyrus, etc.) that are responsible for conscious sensation. For the most part, the circuits serving the sense of life are reflexive and unconscious.

The Sensory System as a Whole

Now it is time to take another look at the overall structure of the sensory world as it appears in our consciousness. In principle, we discovered the same basic structure in all sensory systems. Receptors, along with subsequent neural path-ways and sections of the brain, dissolve the sector of the world perceived by each individual system (sounds, images, tactile objects, etc.) into individual elements, which are transmitted to the nervous system (brain, etc.) along separate pathways. The image as a whole, which always constitutes a unity in our experience, never reappears on any level of the nervous system. The nervous system can analyze but cannot synthesize. Thus, as long as we consider only neural processes, just how we manage to experience a total image of a sensory phenomenon must remain a riddle. Other systems within the threefold organism, however, are also involved in perception as a matter of course, namely, the rhythmic system (blood circulation, respiration) and the metabolic system—the bodily foundations of processes of feeling and will, respectively. These forces are capable of recreating the unity of a sense impression that the nervous system has broken down into its component parts, thus making it possible for us to experience it in its entirety. Hence the perceptual image that becomes conscious in any given instance includes not only mental images produced by thinking but also emotional components and a volitional element corresponding to the qualities present in the perceived entity. We enter the reality of what we perceive only when we allow all three of these soul forces to play a part in perception.

At this point we might ask why nature chose this detour, "dismembering" each perceptual image and only secondarily putting it back together again in the human act of perception. (Evidently, the situation in animals is very different.) There are two answers to this question. From the perspective of the will, the possibility of "resynthesizing" an image that has first been analytically broken down results in the human *experience of freedom*. Depending on our level of consciousness, our image of reality is something we may need to struggle to achieve, rather than something that is passively "impressed upon" or "copied into" our consciousness. It comes about through the active participation of the human "I". As explained in detail in an earlier section, this does not mean that the perceptual process is inevitably subjective in character. From the perspective of thinking, the fact that the nervous system "fragments" the perceived image into myriad details creates the possibility of becoming conscious of what we perceive. The nervous system's job is to create consciousness. As a result, a disturbance in a neurological structure always leads to partial or total loss of consciousness in the respective sensory domain.

The level of consciousness achieved by perceptions of the outside world or of ourselves varies considerably, however (Figure 214). Through our senses of hearing and sight, we delve deeply into the being of the world that surrounds us. Smell and taste are similar, although on a somewhat lower level. With regard to our sense of warmth, our experience of the external and internal worlds is roughly equal in value. The cutaneous sense organs allow us to become conscious not only of the surface characteristics of spatial bodies (and to some extent also of their three-dimensional forms) but also of our own body as a space-filling organism. Temperature sensations and tactile impressions are central to the experience of the self (as a static body) but would normally not be possible without the presence of a touchable object. To an even greater extent, the muscle senses (Steiner's "sense of movement") also play a role in the experience of the self—as a body in motion, in this case. Through the muscle senses, an understanding of other bodies' movements in space also opens up for us. We do not become conscious of the functioning of the sense of equilibrium, which plays such a big part in incorporating our body into the world of space. We experience its processes only indirectly, through dizziness, nausea, or their absence. The senses active in the metabolic organs remain entirely below the level of consciousness. Here we are fully submerged in our own material nature, which we cannot influence directly.

Rudolf Steiner expanded the spectrum of sensory experience to include three additional "spiritual" senses, which he called the sense of word, the sense of thought, and the sense of ego (27, 76). The senses of word and thought are said to make it possible for us to delve fully

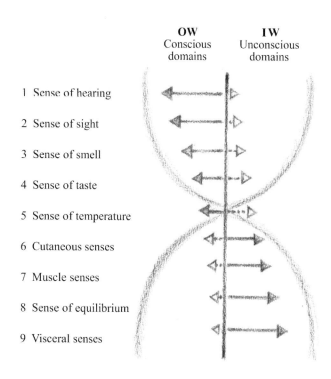

1 Sense of hearing

2 Sense of sight

3 Sense of smell

4 Sense of taste

5 Sense of temperature

6 Cutaneous senses

7 Muscle senses

8 Sense of equilibrium

9 Visceral senses

*Fig. 214. **Relationship of the different sensory systems to conscious experience**. The unconscious domain expands increasingly in the lower senses. OW: outside world; IW: internal world.*

consciously into the essential nature of a word or thought, respectively. The "sense of ego" is by no means identical to our experience of our own "I"; it allows us instead to gain a real experience of the nature of another individuality.

In Steiner's view, therefore, there are twelve sensory systems. They are easiest to understand if arranged in a circle or spiral (Figure 215). The series from 1 to 12 represents increasing levels of consciousness, through which higher or more profound aspects of the outer world are revealed to us. Because our degree of alertness and cognitive penetration of what we perceive are greatest in them, Steiner calls the four highest senses (the sense of hearing through the sense of ego) the actual cognitive senses (27, 76). In contrast, the more unconscious senses (visceral senses, deep and surface sensitivity) are called the will senses. Here, the bodily and material aspects of space are dominant. Between these two groups lie the

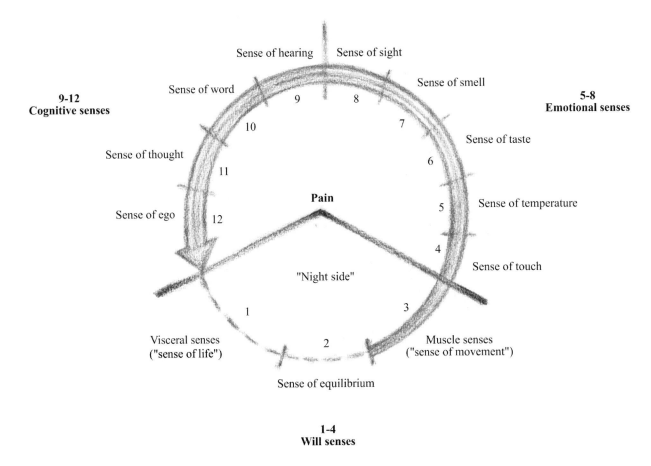

Fig. 215. **Attempt at a functional subdivision of the sensory systems,** *including the three higher senses described by Rudolf Steiner (the senses of word, thought, and ego). In this circular (or spiral) arrangement, the twelve senses follow a path of increasing differentiation and consciousness (arrow), and three larger groupings become apparent (will senses, emotional senses, and cognitive senses).*

"emotional senses" (the senses of sight, smell, taste, and temperature). These emotional senses are dominated by rhythmical movement between the interior and exterior, between the object of attention and the self, an interplay that gives rise to inner sensations and feelings.

In spite of such subdivisions, we must not forget that the sensory systems taken together constitute a whole. In reality, the separate systems we have considered overlap, and in some cases a true integration of sensory domains (synesthesia) occurs.

The Autonomic or Vegetative Nervous System

The autonomic nervous system (ANS) is the polar opposite of the central nervous system, which is centered in the skull-encased brain. The center of activity of the ANS is located on the periphery, in the numerous plexuses of the abdominal cavity, such as the solar plexus and the many neural networks known as intramural plexuses that serve the internal organs, including the enteric nervous system. These networks always include ganglion cells, usually in aggregations (ganglia), so that neural switching can also occur within the organs. Thus we see that the same kind of neural synaptic circuitry that we found in the cerebral cortex also occurs on the periphery in the autonomic nervous system—now in the organs themselves—but without any involvement of consciousness. If all the autonomic nerve cells and their dendrites and axons were removed from the viscera and weighed, we would find that they are approximately as heavy as the brain itself (16). This observation not only points to the structural polarity between the central nervous system (brain) and the peripheral, autonomic nervous system, but to the functional polarity as well.

The ANS is an exceptionally important subset of the nervous system and essential to vital organ functions. Within it, three major functional domains can be distinguished (Figure 216; Rohen, 2001, 16). The highest control centers are located in the brain, particularly in the hypothalamus-pituitary system or axis (HPA) and in the limbic system. The peripheral domain includes the plexuses within the organs (intramural plexuses), which are usually rich in neurons. Because of their complex

circuitry, these plexuses are to a considerable extent functionally independent of higher centers. Between these central and peripheral domains lies a middle domain of the ANS that is at least in part rhythmically or segmentally structured and consists of two major systems with antagonistic functions, namely, the sympathetic and parasympathetic tracts (shown in red and blue respectively in Figure 216). The sympathetic system's cells of origin lie in the spinal cord, primarily in the segments (C_8–L_3), and are connected by way of the spinal nerves to the segmentally structured sympathetic trunk or chain, which in turn is connected to the major ganglia of the periphery by many fine nerves. The parasympathetic system also spans the middle domain. Its nerves run from above (cranial) and below (sacral) directly to the peripheral ganglia in the body cavities. This subdivision of the middle domain into sympathetic and parasympathetic portions with antagonistic effects reveals the rhythmic principle that predominates in this central part of the body.

This threefold structure of the autonomic nervous system is also expressed in the way its different organizational levels function. The effects of peripheral autonomic nerves are local, extending into the membrane activity of individual cells. In the hypothalamus, centers that often consist of only a few neurons control higher functions of the system as a whole, such as thermoregulation, sugar metabolism, water balance, etc. In the middle (rhythmical) organizational domain, individual functions (such as contraction of smooth muscle cells or secretion from individual glands)

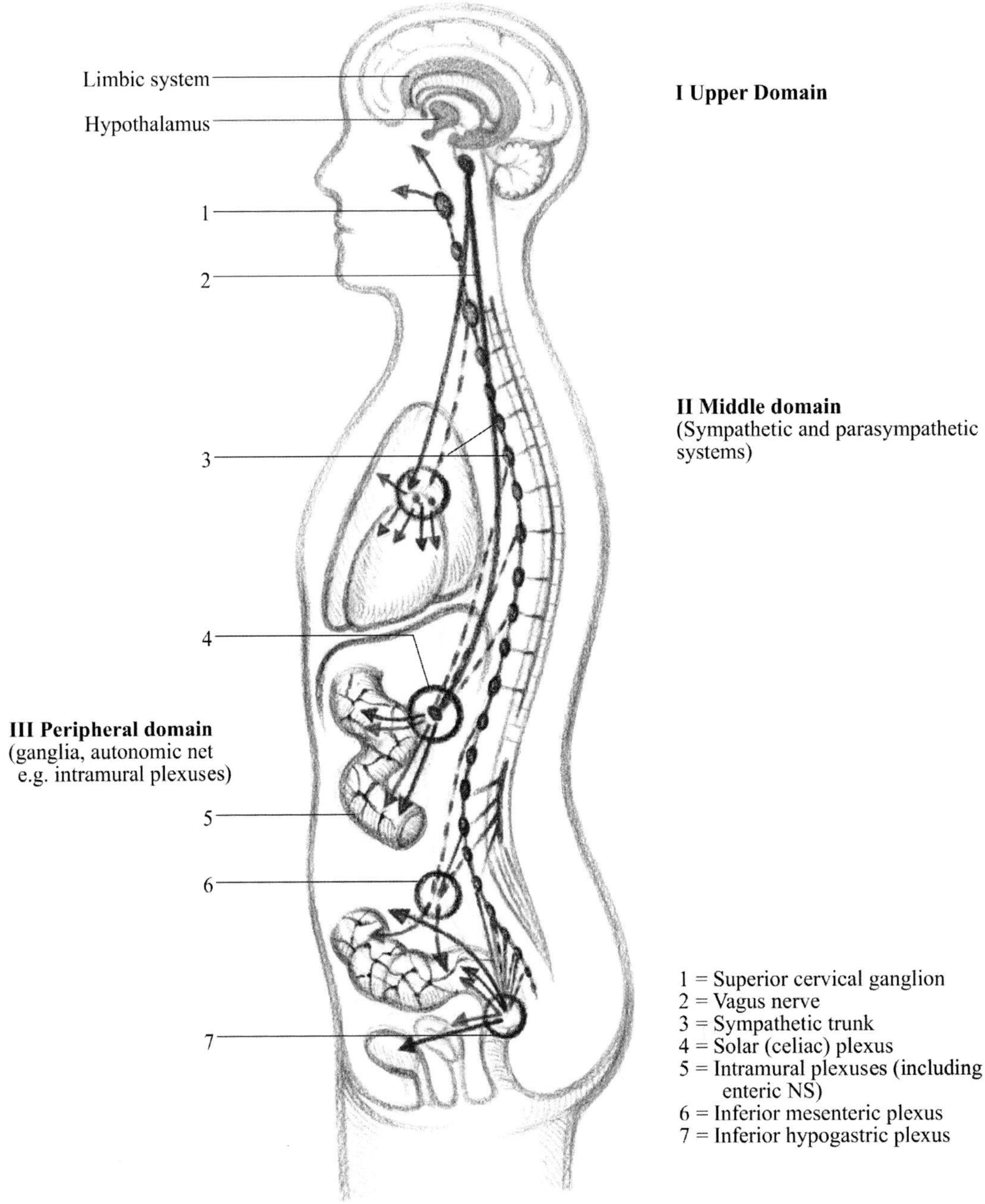

Limbic system

Hypothalamus

I **Upper Domain**

1

2

II **Middle domain**
(Sympathetic and parasympathetic systems)

3

4

III **Peripheral domain**
(ganglia, autonomic net e.g. intramural plexuses)

5

6

7

1 = Superior cervical ganglion
2 = Vagus nerve
3 = Sympathetic trunk
4 = Solar (celiac) plexus
5 = Intramural plexuses (including enteric NS)
6 = Inferior mesenteric plexus
7 = Inferior hypogastric plexus

Fig. 216. **Subdivision of the autonomic nervous system** into three functional domains. The upper domain (limbic system and hypothalamus, green) is located in the brain and serves control functions. The middle domain creates connections among autonomous peripheral plexuses within the organs and is centered in the spinal cord and brain stem. It is partially rhythmic/segmental in structure and consists of two functionally different elements, the sympathetic system (red) and the parasympathetic system (blue). The peripheral domain encompasses the intramural plexuses (circles), which are located in the organs and are served by the major ganglia in the body cavities, such as the solar plexus, etc. In the peripheral plexuses, sympathetic (red) and parasympathetic (blue) nerves mingle with various switching elements to form a complex network with a high degree of functional independence.

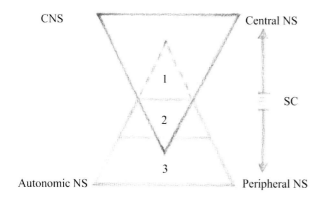

CNS

Central NS

1

2

SC

3

Autonomic NS

Peripheral NS

Fig. 217. **Diagram of the different emphases of the central and autonomic nervous systems,** *showing the threefold subdivision of the autonomic nervous system into upper (1), middle (2), and lower (3) portions, with increasing decentralization toward the periphery. The broad bases of the pyramids indicate concentrations of neural tissue, found on the periphery in the ANS and in the head in the CNS.*
SC: Spinal cord; NS: Nervous system.

still play a role, but always in connection with a global function such as recovery, regeneration, or increasing bodily activity. On this level, the actions of the sympathetic and parasympathetic systems are always antagonistic, whereas in the upper domain, in the hypothalamus, they are synergistic.

In contrast to the central nervous system, the most essential functions of the autonomic system (along with the bulk of its neurons) are peripherally located (Figure 217). Thus these two systems are polar opposites in terms of their organization and structure.

The Peripheral Organizational Level (Intramural System)

All organs are densely laced with autonomic nerve fibers. Intramural plexuses also contain ganglia, where synaptic switching occurs. In the duodenum, for example, Auerbach's plexus lies between the inner and outer muscle layers and under the mucosa. Very fine nerve fibers run from such plexuses to glands, blood vessels, and the mucosal epithelium. The entire intestine is densely laced with nerve fibers and ganglion cells. Where these collections of cells are located varies tremendously, however, depending on the functions of the organs they serve.

How Autonomic Nerves Work

In sensorimotor systems, nerve fibers are always in direct contact with organs (e.g., through motoric end plates in the case of striated muscle fibers). In contrast, autonomic nerves usually do not actually touch the cells whose activity they influence (smooth muscle cells, gland cells, etc.), tending instead to affect groups of cells through neurotransmitters, which are received by specific receptor molecules in the cell membranes (Figure 218). For example, a group of cells in the smooth muscle of a blood vessel is "bathed" in chemicals released by autonomic nerves. When the concentration of chemicals becomes high enough, it effects a change in the contractive state (tone) of the muscle cells. Extensive peripheral vascular contractions can increase blood pressure, while extensive dilations reduce it. In this way, peripheral vegetative responses also work back on the entire organism. Of course this is also true of other vegetative reactions such as glandular secretions (e.g., perspiration in connection with thermoregulation, etc.).

But we must always keep in mind that organ and tissue functions are largely independent of the nervous system. Cellular regeneration and metabolism, glandular secretion and muscle contractions also occur without neural "impulses." The organs function independently and autonomously, according to their own inherent laws.

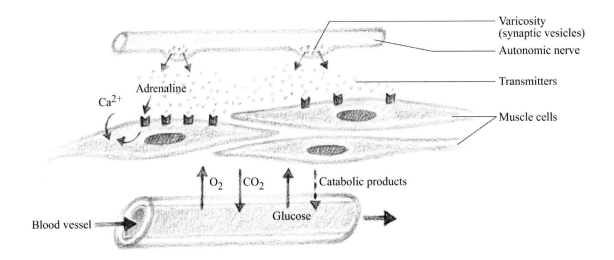

Fig. 218. **Interaction of a smooth ("involuntary") muscle with the vascular system and autonomic nerves.** *The varicosities (nerve terminals) of the autonomic nerves release chemical transmitters that influence the contractive state of smooth muscle cells by changing their membrane permeability (calcium influx, etc.). Chemical conversions within the muscle cells (the "will" aspect) are regulated by blood vessels (gaseous exchange, glucose supply, and metabolic waste removal). Note that autonomic nerves lack any structures (equivalent to motoric end plates in striated muscles) that contact muscle cell membranes directly.*

The autonomic nervous system simply serves the function of "information exchange" *among* organs. In anthropomorphic terms, it makes sure that the organs "communicate with each other" so they can fine tune their activity. Reallocation of resources is one example: one organ's energy supply may need to be restricted in order to increase another organ's output. The autonomic nervous system ensures that functionally related organs are harmoniously linked. Such interlinking can occur even at the local level, although of course we remain completely unconscious of this under normal conditions. Information exchange that affects the organism as a whole is under parasympathetic or sympathetic control at higher levels of the autonomic nervous system (as noted below).

Structure and Function of Autonomic Reflex Loops

The autonomic and central nervous systems work in fundamentally different ways. One characteristic difference is that the efferent branch of an ANS reflex loop consists of at least two neurons (one preganglionic and one postganglionic neuron) instead of only one, as is the case in sensorimotor systems (e.g., the motoric anterior horn cell in the spinal cord). In the sympathetic division, for example, the cell bodies of first-order (preganglionic) "visceromotor" neurons are located in the spinal cord, but those of second-order neurons are located in the peripheral paravertebral or prevertebral ganglia. Furthermore, their branching terminals do not contact individual muscle cells directly. Instead, the axon branches develop many little "varicosities" (beadlike swellings) consisting of numerous synaptic vesicles that release

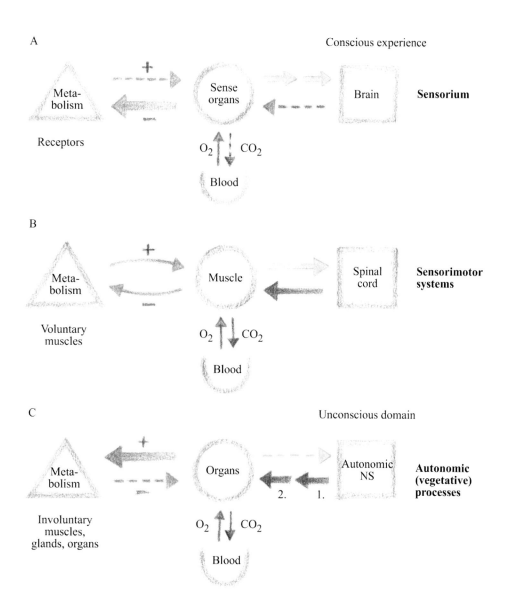

Fig. 219. **Comparing the three major functional domains of the nervous system** and their relationships to the metabolic system and to blood-mediated respiratory processes (cellular gaseous exchange). A: Sensorium, CNS; B: Sensorimotor systems; C: Autonomic nervous system.

transmitters such as epinephrine or acetylcholine into the surrounding tissue. If a smooth muscle cell, for example, is equipped with the appropriate receptors, the transmitter binds with the receptor, triggering intracellular reactions (such as calcium influx) that ultimately lead to contraction of the cell (Figure 218).

Here too, as with striated muscles, efferent nerves cannot be considered conductors of will impulses. Analyzing nerve–smooth muscle interaction leads to deeper insights if we consider it against the background of the threefold organization of the organism as a whole (Figure 219). Of course, as is also the case with striated muscles, contraction of smooth muscle cells depends on energy conversions within the cell (ATP to ADP, etc.), which then affect the contractile filaments (actin/myosin filaments). In smooth muscles, the filaments are not arranged as regularly as they are in striated muscles, but their tone is equally dependent on intracellular calcium concentrations. Even without neural stimuli, a living cell can alter its calcium concentration and thus also its contractile state (tone) by adjusting its membrane permeability to calcium ions. This is an autonomic process and depends on the availability of energy and oxygen. Like all cellular systems served by the autonomic nervous system, smooth muscle cells are dependent on three different functional systems: the respiratory and circulatory system (for intratissue O_2/CO_2 exchange), the metabolic system (for conversion of energy sources, such as glucose, ATP, etc.), and the nervous system (for release and breakdown of transmitters). Each of these systems obeys its own laws and functions relatively independently. The nervous system plays an important role by coordinating the interactions of these functions. This is an *organizational role*, not a will-initiating activity. Metabolic activity provides the physical basis of the will, while respiratory activity underlies feeling. Only the "conceptual" or informational element is based on neural activity (Figure 219).

None of this activity reaches our consciousness under normal physiological conditions, however. The working of our organs remains unconscious and takes place automatically. Presumably, this phenomenon is related to the fact that autonomic reflex loops (which, like reflex loops throughout the nervous system, consist of afferent and efferent branches) are dominated by the *efferent* branch, while reflex loops in sense organs are dominantly *afferent*. Afferent and efferent branches are more or less in balance only in sensorimotor systems. Of course this does not mean that afferent or efferent neurons are numerically equivalent or more numerous, as the case may be. We are talking here about their relative functional importance. In the autonomic nervous system, for example, the number of afferent neurons is unusually high, but functional activity is largely determined by efferent neurons. In sensory systems, the reverse is true (Figure 219).

A corresponding asymmetry is also evident on the metabolic side (Figure 219). Catabolism dominates in sensory systems. Impressions coming into the body from the outside world first trigger catabolic processes, which must then be counteracted by regenerative processes in the blood. The reverse is true in the autonomic nervous system. Anabolic processes predominate, stimulated by substances coming from the outside (nutrient and fluid intake, respiration, etc.). In this case, catabolism is secondary. Only with advancing age does it begin to have more effect on autonomic processes.

This asymmetry is also pronounced with regard to consciousness. In sensory systems, a one-sided differentiation of afferent neurons is also the reason for the one-sidedness of sensory perception (our consciousness focuses entirely on the outside world). In contrast, the one-sided differentiation of the efferent branch of reflex loops in the autonomic nervous system (development of preganglionic and postganglionic neurons, translocation of motor neurons into the peripheral ganglia, etc.) also seems to be why the body's internal activities remain unconscious and elude voluntary control. The higher brain centers of the cerebral cortex cannot directly influence the autonomic domain. We can influence our circulation and other responses (blood pressure, metabolic activity, etc.) only indirectly, through emotional agitation or the like (blushing, perspiring with fear, etc.)

The Middle Organizational Level (The Sympathetic and Parasympathetic Systems)

The middle level of organization is subdivided into two antagonistic parts, the sympathetic and parasympathetic systems, and represents the rhythmic element within the autonomic nervous system. The cells of origin of this level are located in the spinal cord and brain stem, in a netlike mass of nerves called the reticular formation. The nerve fibers leaving these cells follow the

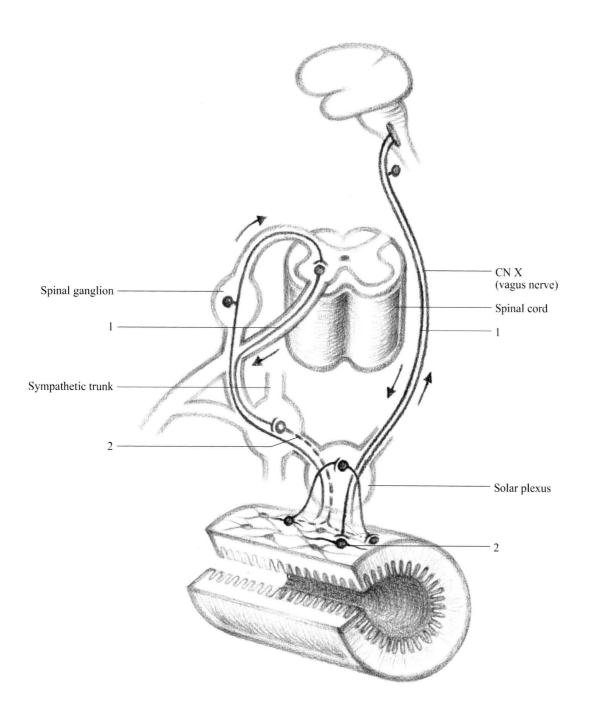

Spinal ganglion

1

Sympathetic trunk

2

CN X
(vagus nerve)

Spinal cord

1

Solar plexus

2

Fig. 220. **Connections between the peripheral autonomic plexuses and the spinal cord**. *Structure of a typical autonomic reflex arch. In contrast to the reflex arches of striated muscles, which have only a single efferent neuron, the efferent branch of an autonomic reflex arch always consists of two efferent neurons, the preganglionic (1, solid red line), and postganglionic (2, red dashes), shown here as an example of the sympathetic system.*
CN X: the vagus nerve as a representative of the parasympathetic system (afferent neuron in blue, efferent neuron in black). 1: Preganglionic neuron; 2: Postganglionic neuron.

spinal nerves to the periphery of the body and the sympathetic chain to the major ganglia complexes of the chest and abdominal cavity. From there, vegetative nerves finally enter the effector organs themselves (Figures 216 and 220). The gesture of the sympathetic system is one of spreading out from spinal centers, while the parasympathetic system displays more individualization. In the sympathetic nervous system there are more postganglionic fibers compared to preganglionic fibers than in the parasympathetic system (16). The cells of origin of the sympathetic system are limited for the most part to the thoracolumbar segments of the spinal cord (C_8–L_3). By way of the sympathetic chain, their fibers reach upward to the head and downward to the pelvic organs (genitals, rectum, etc.), following the arteries instead of developing peripheral nerve tracts of their own. In contrast, the cells of origin of the parasympathetic system are located in the head (cranial autonomic system) and in the sacral portion of the spinal cord (S_2–S_4, sacral autonomic system) and either follow cranial nerves (CN III, VII, IX) or develop nerves of their own such as the tenth cranial (vagus) nerve, which bridges the major gaps between the chest segments and runs through the chest cavity to the solar plexus in the abdominal cavity (Figures 216 and 220).

The **neuronal structures** of the sympathetic and parasympathetic systems are also very different. The parasympathetic system usually has very long preganglionic neurons reaching all the way to the organ plexuses, where the second set of postganglionic efferent neurons begins. In contrast, the preganglionic neurons of the sympathetic system are significantly shorter: In the chest, they are switched in the ganglia of the sympathetic trunk, in the abdomen only in the prevertebral ganglia (solar plexus, hypogastric plexus, etc.) (Figure 220). The two systems also differ in the transmitter substances secreted by their nerve endings. Sympathetic nerve fibers on the periphery usually secrete epinephrine or norepinephrine, while parasympathetic fibers secrete acetylcholine. These transmitters increase or inhibit the activity of the cell groups they affect.

When we consider the **effects** of sympathetic and parasympathetic stimulation in detail, they initially may seem contradictory and unrelated.

Sympathetic stimulation, for example, leads to contraction of the smooth muscles of the vascular system (vasoconstriction), relaxation of the smooth muscle cells of the bronchi or gastrointestinal tract, contraction of splenic muscles, and an increase in heart rate.

In the metabolic system, sympathetic stimulation leads to release of glucose from the liver and a subsequent rise in blood sugar level. Parasympathetic stimulation, on the other hand, leads to glycogen formation in the liver and decreases in blood sugar.

A unified picture does emerge, however, when we classify these individual effects according to functional perspectives. After all, the body's general reaction status always alternates (rhythmically) between two basic tendencies, namely, between an activity-oriented, energy-consuming state of receptivity to the environment on the one hand, and a more self-directed state of disengagement that is antagonistic to activity on the other. The sympathetic nervous system is the "**activity nerve**" (ergotropic reaction state). It consumes the body's energy reserves, raises blood pressure, increases heart rate, and enhances physical or mental performance, but it also "switches off" the metabolic organs (e.g., intestinal activity, glycogen storage in the liver). Extreme increases in activity under the influence of the sympathetic system cause "stress" and (ultimately) pathological reactions (heart attack, blood pressure crises, etc., 132, 133). Sympathetic stimuli also increase the activity of the brain and sense organs, thus enhancing wakefulness and response times.

In contrast, the parasympathetic system is the "**restorative nerve**" (trophotropic reactions). It ensures that energy sources (glycogen, fats) are resynthesized in the liver and muscles. It restarts intestinal activity, accelerates absorption of nutrients, reduces blood pressure and blood sugar, and—if needed—produces restorative sleep (see Table 26).

Clearly, the rhythms of human life—inasmuch as they involve the autonomic nervous system—are reflected in these reactions. It is equally clear, however, that sympathetic and parasympathetic nerves do not "cause" vegetative rhythms (in the

Organ	Adrenergic effects of the sympathetic system	Cholinergic effects of the parasympathetic system

Eye
  Iris
  Ciliary muscle
	Dilation
	Nonaccommodation
		Contraction
		Accommodation

Heart
  Frequency
  Contractile strength
  Rhythm
 	
  Conduction time
	Accelerated
	Strengthened
	Ventricular extra systoles, Tachychardia, Fibrillation
	Shortened
		Slowed
		–
		Bradycardia, AV block
		Vagal cardiac arrest
		Lengthened

Blood vessels
  Coronary vessels
  Muscle vessels
  Intestinal vessels
	Dilation
	Contraction
	Contraction
		?
		–
		–

Lungs
  Bronchial muscles
  Bronchial glands
	Bronchodilation
	?
		Contraction
		Secretion

Gastrointestinal tract
  Peristalsis
  Sphincters
  Glandular secretion
	Decreased
	Contraction inhibited
	?
		Increased
		Relaxed
		Promoted

Extrahepatic bile ducts, Gall bladder	Relaxation	Contraction
Spleen (muscles)	Contraction	Relaxation
Salivary glands	Secretion (thick fluid)	Secretion (thin fluid)
Pancreas Islets of Langerhans		Insulin secretion
Liver	Glycogenolysis	Bile secretion
Adrenal medulla	Secretion of adrenaline and noradrenaline	

Bladder
  Muscles
  Sphincter
	Relaxation
	Contraction
		Contraction
		Relaxation

Cerebral cortex	Generalized activation, increase in consciousness	Inhibition, reduction in consciousness
General reactive state	**Ergotropic "activity nerve"** Waking	**Trophotropic "restorative nerve"** Sleep

Table 26. Main effects of the sympathetic and parasympathetic systems on the functions of different organs.

sense of "motor" nerves). They simply adjust the organs' inherent, autonomous vital processes, coordinating and harmonizing them to adapt the body's reactive status to current environmental conditions.

Adaptation and regulation extending beyond local processes take place in higher vegetative centers in the brain stem, especially in the medulla oblongata and in the tegmentum of the midbrain. In the skull, in the domain of the central nervous system, the spinal reticular formation expands, resulting in an extensive reticular neural mass housing many autonomic centers at the base of the rhomboid fossa and in the midbrain (Figure 221). Vitally important centers that regulate respiration and circulation are located in the medulla oblongata, along with the parasympathetic nuclei of origin of the seventh, ninth, and tenth cranial nerves (the facial, glossopharyngeal, and vagus nerves). Higher centers responsible for inhalation, exhalation, heart rate, etc., are located in the tegmentum. Today we know that spontaneous discharges of specific cell groups in the tegmentum regulate all peripheral events necessary for the movements of inhalation, while other groups are responsible only for the movements of exhalation.

As we see, the second organizational level of the autonomic nervous system serves to rhythmicize, harmonize, and balance the peripheral processes of the intramural nervous system and those of the central nervous system. The sympathetic and parasympathetic systems, which are polar opposites in both morphology and function, form a middle, rhythmical link between organ functions and the "head" of the autonomic system (i.e., the hypothalamus and the adjacent limbic system).

The Upper Organizational Level (Hypothalamus and Limbic System)

The Hypothalamus

The reticular formation of the spinal cord extends into the midbrain and hindbrain and is continuous with the hypothalamus (Figure 221). Relatively well-defined nuclei, which perform higher control functions for the entire autonomic nervous system, develop within this netlike mass of nervous tissue. Here, the contrast between sympathetic and parasympathetic systems no longer plays a role. Instead, global autonomic functions as such come to the fore: water balance, homeostasis, reproductive rhythms (menstrual cycle), regulation of metabolic processes during pregnancy and birth, intake and processing of nutrients (hunger and thirst centers), etc.

From a functional perspective, the hypothalamus always "keeps an eye" on activity that affects the entire body. When increased activity exhausts the body's energy reserves, sensations of hunger and thirst appear, stimulating intake of food and water. The hypothalamus then ensures that the body's water balance is reestablished and that the liver's energy reserves are replenished. W. R. Hess made the important discovery that many types of biological regulation (especially in reproduction but also in mineral and water balance, thermoregulation, respiration, food intake, etc.) are linked to specific behaviors. In animals, for example, certain regulatory processes involved in feeding (e.g., pecking order), reproduction, or elimination of feces or urine are associated with species-specific behavior patterns. Behavioral reflexes come about because the hypothalamus also has connections to sensorimotor systems, especially the subcortical motor systems.

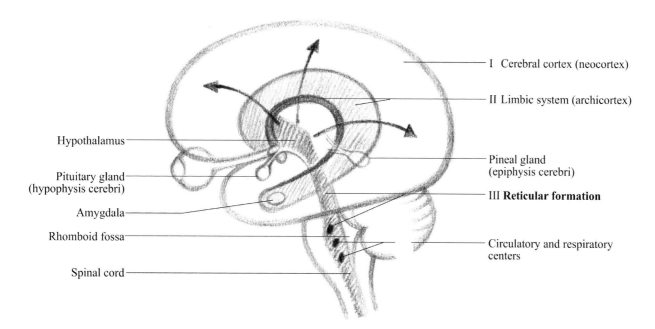

Hypothalamus

Pituitary gland
(hypophysis cerebri)

Amygdala

Rhomboid fossa

Spinal cord

I Cerebral cortex (neocortex)

II Limbic system (archicortex)

Pineal gland
(epiphysis cerebri)

III **Reticular formation**

Circulatory and respiratory
centers

Fig. 221. **Location of the reticular formation** *(blue)* **in the brain.** *The reticular formation forms a coherent, netlike mass of neural tissue that extends from the spinal cord through the hindbrain and midbrain to the interbrain (hypothalamus). The vitally important centers of the autonomic system (respiratory and circulatory centers, etc.) are located in the reticular formation of the brain stem. Signals (arrows) relayed to the cerebral cortex by the reticular formation arouse the cortex to waking consciousness.*
I – III: Structures serving the brain's three levels of consciousness (cf. Table 27, p. 318).

The hypothalamus also has important connections to the limbic system (Figure 205), the arch-shaped structures that surround the interbrain inside and beneath the cerebrum (especially the temporal lobe). The limbic system includes the hippocampus, induseum griseum, fornix, etc. (see Figure 221). On the other hand, the hypothalamus also has extensive connections to the *reticular formation* of the midbrain and hindbrain, where the higher sympathetic and parasympathetic centers are located. Via the groups of nuclei in the reticular formation, the hypothalamus influences the entire peripheral autonomic system, including respiratory, circulatory, thermoregulatory, and metabolic functions (see Figure 221).

But the hypothalamus also plays a special role in the *rhythm of sleeping and waking*. It was formerly believed that narcotics work by paralyzing the cerebral cortex, thus inducing sleep (or narcosis). We now know, however, that many narcotics act primarily on the reticular formation

and affect the cerebral cortex only indirectly. Normally, impulses (arousal signals) from the reticular formation stimulate the cortex (see Figure 221). In dangerous situations, "alerting reactions" produce unusually intense stimulations, triggering a state of enhanced alertness. The hypothalamus and the diencephalon regulate the sleep-wake rhythm through a rhythmic alternation of cortical stimulation and coordinate all vegetative functions involved in the transition from waking to sleeping and vice versa. This example clearly illustrates the central importance of the hypothalamus for the entire autonomic nervous system.

But the reticular formation receives regulatory/controlling impulses not only from the hypothalamus but also from the sensory systems. Ultimately, therefore, sensory activity also affects the autonomic nervous system. The connections are especially well researched with regard to the visual apparatus. The optic nerve has a direct connection—the retinohypothalamic optic nerve tract—to reticular formation via the hypothalamus, thus allowing the eye to influence vegetative processes, especially the circadian (twenty-four hour) rhythm of metabolic processes such as liver function, blood formation, etc. The optic system serves as a timer, adjusting autonomic circadian rhythms to the 24-hour solar cycle. The pineal gland, which produces the light-dependent hormone melatonin, is known to play a major role in regulating the body's circadian rhythm.

And finally, the hypothalamus influences the secretory activity of the pituary gland (hypophysis) and therefore plays a central role in regulating the entire hormonal (endocrine) system. The base of the hypothalamus elongates into a pointed "pocket" (the infundibulum), which is contiguous with the *neurohypophysis*, and unites with the anterior hypophyseal lobe (which develops from the roof of the pharynx) to form a single organ, the hypophysis (pituitary gland, Figure 222).

The anterior and posterior lobes of the hypophysis are also of different origins. The anterior lobe is an endocrine gland. The posterior lobe is part of the interbrain—or more specifically, of the hypothalamus. Through its connection to the anterior hypophyseal lobe, the hypothalamus is able to influence the body's entire hormonal system because the anterior lobe is the endocrine system's highest regulatory organ. The hypothalamus is connected to the anterior lobe by a special vascular system that is similar to a portal vein system and is used to transport hypothalamic hormones (liberines) to the hypophysis, where they trigger release of the anterior hypophyseal lobe hormones known as releasing hormones. Because the interbrain is affected by the cerebrum, the endocrine system is subject to central nervous regulation.

Certain nuclei in the hypothalamus also produce hormones, which are transported to the posterior hypophyseal lobe for release (neurosecretion). This activity will be described in greater detail in a later section.

The Limbic System

The limbic system is the bridge connecting the hypothalamus (as the "head" of the autonomic system, i.e., the highest center of vegetative nuclei in the reticular formation) with the cortex. As described in a previous section, the limbic system increasingly freed itself from the olfactory system in the course of evolution and continued to differentiate (Figure 205). Although in a certain sense it is part of the "old brain" or archicortex, which was forced to the interior and underside of the brain as a result of the overwhelming development of the cerebrum (neocortex), the limbic system still occupies a relatively large amount of space. The commissural pathways between the right and left hemispheres increased greatly in size along with the neocortex; in a longitudinal section, they appear as the corpus callosum in Figure 222. As a result, the cortex areas of the old brain are split into two groups of structures, one above the corpus callosum and one below. The group above the corpus callosum includes the cingular gyrus, which extends into the hippocampus, and the so-called indusium griseum, which extends into the dentate gyrus. The fornix runs below the corpus callosum in a great spiraling arch (Figure 222).

On the one hand, the complex, arch-shaped limbic system is connected with the "visceral brain" (hypothalamus and reticular formation), but it also continues into the neocortex (cingular gyrus/hippocampus). The cortex of the hippocampus is still archaic in structure in that it has only three layers (allocortex), whereas the neocortex has developed the more complex six-layered structure of the isocortex.

Thus the limbic system serves as an intermediary between the unconscious (vegetative) functions of the hypothalamus and reticular formation and the fully conscious functions of the cerebral cortex. Although it stands at the threshold of the neocortex, its functions are still played out largely unconsciously.

Animal experiments have shown that stimulating the limbic nuclei (especially the amygdala complex, located in the temporal lobe

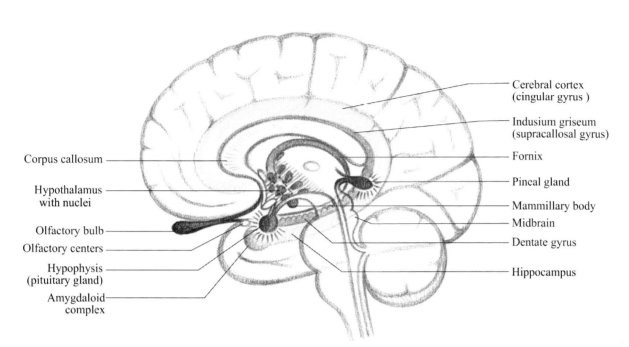

*Fig. 222. **Medial cross section of the brain, showing the hypothalamus and limbic system**. The cingular gyrus (which continues into the hippocampus) and the indusium griseum (which continues into the dentate gyrus) run along the top of the corpus callosum. Below the corpus callosum is the fornix, which extends as far as the mammillary body.*

in front of the hippocampus) produces reactions that are heavily emotionally tinged, such as aggressiveness, hypersexuality, fits of rage, etc. In most cases these responses are also associated with changes in vegetative functions (increases in blood pressure and heart rate, more rapid respiration, changes in glandular functions, etc.). It has also been suggested that the limbic system *emotionally "tinges"* sense perceptions. In addition, it also plays a very important role in regulating sleep-wake rhythms. The limbic system is constantly sending stimulating impulses to the cerebral cortex to increase consciousness and/or maintain a state of wakefulness (Figure 221). During REM sleep, periodic stimulation of the central nervous system is accompanied by eye rolling, reductions in muscle tone, erections, etc. Quite possibly, the limbic system (which sits on the threshold between the two worlds of our consciousness) asserts itself more strongly than usual in REM phases of sleep, which is known to be frequently associated with dreaming.

Meanwhile, the limbic system has been shown to be centrally important to the human *capacity for memory*. Located at the very threshold of (cortical) waking consciousness, the limbic system retrieves images or experiences that have been "forgotten" and have sunk down into our subconscious. Apparently, emotional stimulation plays an important role in this process.

As mentioned in a previous section, these responses must not be attributed one-sidedly to the nervous system. The entire organism is always involved, not only in sense perception itself but also in the related act of remembering. Neural centers simply serve to make us conscious of these psychological processes. Related circulatory and metabolic processes are the actual physical foundations of feeling and willing, respectively.

The Nervous System and Consciousness

The Brain as the Organ of Consciousness

The brain can be subdivided into three major functional domains that differ greatly in their levels of consciousness. The hypothalamus and the reticular formation of the brain stem (Figure 221) represent the "vegetative" portion of the brain. For the most part, they control autonomic functions. Toward the periphery, they merge with the body's autonomic nervous system via the reticular formation of the spinal cord. Functions that run their course within this system are largely reflexive and unconscious.

In contrast, the limbic system represents an intermediary stage of consciousness. As already mentioned, this is where sensory experiences are given an "emotional tinge." The limbic system is also where memories appear and are fixed, at least in the short term. As the functional bridge between vegetative neural functions and the cerebral cortex, between unconsciousness and full consciousness, the limbic system may be prerequisite to our experience of personality. It may also be important for imagination and dreaming. On the whole, therefore, it represents an intermediary dimension in our consciousness.

The third and highest level of functioning and consciousness is achieved only in the cerebral cortex (neocortex). The cortex is not only the basis of waking consciousness resulting from sensory activity but also (ultimately) the place where memories become conscious and can be stored for the long term. "Blueprints" for movements and conceptions that guide our entire motor system are also related to functions of the cortex (in this case primarily of the frontal lobe).

Subdivision into lobes. The human brain can be subdivided into four major lobes, which are separated by deep grooves (central sulcus, lateral sulcus, etc.; see Figure 223). It is interesting to note that the cortex areas of these lobes are associated with major higher function complexes. For example, the frontal lobe serves motor functions, the parietal lobe sensory functions, and the temporal lobe primarily memory functions. At this point, it is tempting to bring up the general concept of the three basic human soul forces (thinking, feeling, and willing). If we avoid the assumptions that "willing" proceeds from the brain and that memory is based entirely on neural activity, this basic outline certainly remains justifiable in certain respects. By now, the "doctrine of centers" in its original form has been largely dismissed. Nonetheless, areas within the cerebral cortex are dominated by specialized functions, so the cortex as a whole is a highly diversified structure.

The *frontal lobe* houses primarily cell systems related to the body's voluntary movements. Several decades ago, when lobotomies were still being performed on patients with severe neurological disorders, it was discovered that patients who had undergone frontal lobotomies (separation of the frontal lobe from the rest of the brain) experienced radical changes in personality. They lost all initiative, becoming lethargic and immobile. (This is why these operations were discontinued.) Today, the most frequently cited functions of the frontal lobe include "planning future actions, initiative, a feeling of strength, consequences of motor actions, endurance, the social ego, the experience of personality (as it relates to motor activity)," etc. (126). It is clear that the anterior, phylogenetically most recently developed sections of the human frontal lobe are not "motor centers" as such but places where will intentions emerging from the entire body are organized, coordinated, and finally become conscious.

The polar opposite of the frontal lobe is the *temporal lobe*, which also achieved its present size only at the end of the evolutionary process. Today the temporal lobe is said to be the area where neuronal activity from the entire system is stored for the long term, again with the cautionary note that memory is not simply a neural function but involves the entire human body and that specific brain areas are simply where memories become conscious.

The *parietal lobe* is generally described as the "sensory cortex." It is where sensations coming from skin and muscle receptors become conscious. Higher functions related to these areas include distinguishing right and left, local memory, kinesthetic sensations, tactile recognition of objects, recognition of motor and mechanical actions, etc. Here, general sensory functions overlap with more specific ones that originate in the major sense organs (eye and ear).

The *occipital lobe* primarily houses the cortex areas that serve visual processing as well as related higher functions such as symbol recognition ("reading center," "optical speech center"), image recognition and recall, and spatial experiences.

Areas for auditory perception and processing are located in the upper portion of the temporal lobe and in the insular lobe (Figure 223).

Lateralization of the Hemispheres

The basic structure of the cerebral cortex is the same on both sides. Although it has been known for quite some time that certain functional areas (such as Broca's speech center) develop only on one side, the realization that the two halves of the brain serve very different functions in humans (and essentially only in humans) is relatively recent and based on psychological investigations of "split-brain" individuals whose corpus callosum had been severed (Sperry et al., 86 and 87). Normally, in right-handed people, the left hemisphere is dominant. (Because of the crossing of neural pathways, the left hemisphere is connected to the right side of the body.) Right-handed people use the left hemisphere not only for dominantly right-handed motor activities but especially for analytical, mathematical, and abstract thinking. The left hemisphere is also the verbal hemisphere. In other words, the motor mechanisms of speech are heavily dependent on the functioning of the "motor" speech center in the left frontal lobe. Victims of left hemisphere strokes usually lose the ability to speak. It is interesting to note that left-hemisphere dominance develops only after the first year of life, in connection with learning to walk and talk. By age five, the left hemisphere has completely assumed leadership.

The right hemisphere, however, is by no means inferior or insignificant. When we consider the human being as a whole, right-hemisphere functions are more comprehensive or "higher" than left-hemisphere functions. The right hemisphere plays a major role not only in our experience of space but also in artistic, synthetic, and holistic thinking. Understanding an image or a complex of sounds as a whole is possible only with the help of the right hemisphere. The left hemisphere allows us to distinguish optical details, as well as individual tones or quantitative differences. To oversimplify, the left hemisphere sees individual trees, while the right hemisphere sees the forest as a whole. Clearly, polar differentiation of the two brain hemispheres provides the human individuality with a radical key to the mysteries of

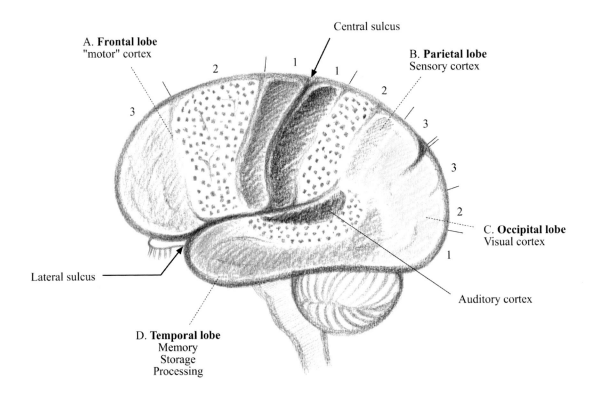

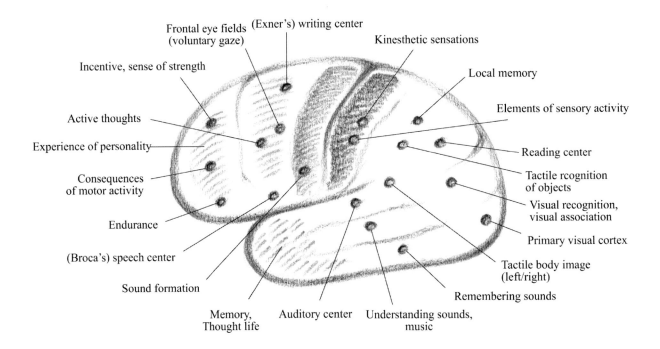

*Fig. 223. **Functional subdivision of the cerebral cortex**. Upper illustration: Subdivision into four lobes bounded by the primary sulci (central sulcus, lateral sulcus, etc.). 1: primary; 2: secondary; 3: tertiary brain centers. Lower illustration: Location of the most important cortex fields, based on clinical experience (adapted from Kleist, in Rohen, reference 16).*

the universe. Humans are always able to become conscious of any object or being from both an analytical and a synthetic perspective. When we enhance the analytical aspect, we become aware of numerical laws, quantitative details, and individual facts but often lose sight of the whole and the spiritual element that unites these details. When we emphasize the synthetic aspect, we become aware of higher connections, creative possibilities, and the spiritual context in which individual details are embedded. Of course words no longer play a role in the world of the right hemisphere. Recognizing forms, images, and their spiritual foundations transcends verbalization and conceptualization. The right hemisphere is nonverbal.

Consciousness and Subconsciousness

The cerebral cortex is our "upper chamber," so to speak. With its help, we become conscious of what happens inside ourselves (although only to a limited extent) and in the world outside us. One of the greatest wonders of human existence is our *ability to learn.* The will or motivation for learning comes from the "I". For example, when we want to master new movement patterns (such as a sport or playing an instrument), we must repeatedly make ourselves aware of the status quo with the help of the cerebral cortex, which reflects the whole process. The fact that new neural connections (synaptic modifications) are created in this process illustrates only the physical, material aspect of learning. Once we master the new movement pattern, the details disappear from our consciousness, and the movement occurs almost unconsciously and automatically. Experienced pianists are no longer really aware of notes, fingers, or keys—their fingers seem to "move themselves." In morphological terms, the "program" shifts to a *subcortical* level. In the case of motor activity, it shifts to the so-called basal ganglia (caudate

nucleus, lenticular nucleus, etc.) at the transition from the pyramidal to the subcortical motor system. This shift frees up the cortex and makes it available for new learning. Nietzsche once spoke of forgetting as a blessing, and in fact we would not be able to continue to develop if past accomplishments continued to burden our consciousness instead of sinking down into our subconscious.

Of course this applies to sensory learning as well as motor learning. There are also nerve centers that process impulses coming from sensory systems and "store" them in ways that remove them from consciousness. But they can be retrieved from storage—i.e., remembered—through a process whose morphological foundations remain unexplained, even today. We do know, however, that the hippocampus plays a major role in short-term memory (Figure 222). In any case, in certain diseases such as Alzheimer's, degenerative changes occur in these nuclei, usually concurrently with memory loss. Memory, however, is a process that involves the entire human body rather than merely the cerebral cortex. Nerve tissue is simply responsible for making us conscious of our experience, not for the experience itself. First and foremost, recalling something we have forgotten requires a will effort, which probably reaches the brain via the metabolism and the blood.

In summary, we can say that three major levels of consciousness are present in the brain. Normal waking consciousness is based primarily on the cerebral cortex (neocortex), whereas processes in the brain's interior (reticular formation, hypothalamus) essentially run their course unconsciously and can be influenced only indirectly, by way of precise ideas. The limbic system (archicortex) serves as an intermediary between these two poles, and its reactions become partially conscious by way of emotions and feelings. In principle, however, these three levels of consciousness are not clearly delineated. The unconscious can become conscious; conscious experiences can be forgotten and sink into subconsciousness. These domains are linked in both directions by numerous pathways.

I. Upper level	Cerebral cortex (neocortex)	Waking consciousness (conscious processing of sensory stimuli, movement, executive functions, memories)
II. Middle level	Limbic system (archicortex)	Transitional function (semiconscious), dreaming, emotional tinging of sensory stimuli, control of vegetative processes
III. Lower level	Hypothalamus and reticular formation	Unconscious functions, regulation of vegetative processes, sleep/wake rhythm, connecting the autonomic nervous system with the endocrine system

Table 27. Levels of consciousness in the brain and associated structures (see also Figures 221-223).

The Nervous System as the Foundation of the Human Soul and Spirit

In conclusion, let's consider the nervous system again in its entirety, especially in terms of its relationship to the human soul and spirit. The basic soul forces—thinking, feeling, and willing—differ not only qualitatively but also in their degrees of consciousness, with thinking (conceptualizing) and willing constituting a polarity. In conceptualizing, we achieve the highest degree of consciousness currently accessible to us. In contrast, our will functions completely unconsciously. Feeling mediates between these two extremes.

The nervous system consists of networks of highly differentiated neurons linked by synapses. In morphological terms, learning is the development of new interneuronal connections and the dissolution of old ones. Thus the human brain is very flexible. Nerve fibers (usually found in white matter) serve to conduct impulses. So do neuron cell bodies (mostly located in gray matter), but their chief function is the overall maintenance and regeneration of neurons.

As mentioned earlier, if we follow Rudolf Steiner's line of thinking, we can see metabolic processes as the basis of the will, circulatory and respiratory functions as the basis of feeling, and neural processes only as the basis of conceptualization (18). Ultimately, however, all three of these basic principles play a role in every type of tissue. Nerve tissue would be unable to survive without metabolic activity, and in fact neurons are extremely metabolically active. Circulation is also very important. Consequently, if we attempt to associate psychological processes with physiological events, we must keep in mind that only the membrane activity of nerve fibers and cells is truly informational in character and thus corresponds to the psychological activity of conceptualization. In the neuron cell bodies, which are usually located in gray matter, metabolic processes are especially dominant. In other words, this is a place where will impulses could intervene.

Modern methods such as PET scanning have revealed major increases in metabolic activity in corresponding areas of the cortex upon completion of specific purposeful tasks (counting, reading, speaking, etc.). Thus it is quite conceivable that will impulses reach the brain by way of the blood and circulatory system, especially in the case of memory processes. If this is so, the activity inside neuron cell bodies is not limited to regeneration but also includes a life process that serves the capacity for memory. Similarly, synaptic activity may be related to the alternation between sympathy and antipathy in emotional processes. But "feeling in thinking" means understanding. As mentioned previously (p. 227), Goethe once wrote, "If you do not feel it, you will never get it." Although it is always possible to explain any logical connection in purely abstract terms, real, "substantial" understanding always presupposes some emotional activity, an inner experience of truth or evidence that touches the very core of our being. This is more than just pure "information."

Within the head and central nervous system, therefore, we find ***three basic functions:***

1. Pure conceptualization, which mirrors the world and the ideas that live in it but does not achieve the character of being.

2. Understanding thoughts and images (rhythmic activity in breathing/feeling, formation and dissolution of synaptic connections); and

3. Remembering (the development of memory and ideas retrieved from blood-mediated willing with the help of cytoplasmic metabolic processes in neuron cell bodies).

Ultimately, these three basic processes shape and maintain consciousness. But how are they played out in the middle (spinal) and lower (autonomic) domains of the nervous system?

We might imagine that the autonomic nervous system makes it possible for us to perceive the events and processes of our own internal world, similarly to the way the central nervous system and associated sense organs allow us to perceive the world outside us—in other words, that in both instances we gain sensations and ideas through the activity of our organs. However, we know that this is not the case; we remain unconscious of organ activity. Conceivably, the autonomic nervous system might even serve the opposite function—to prevent consciousness of organ activity instead of enabling it, as Rudolf Steiner once put it (65).

Of course the basic soul processes of "thinking, feeling, and willing" also play a role in the autonomic nervous system, but because afferent functions are outweighed there by efferent functions, organ processes remain unconscious except during illness, when they rise to consciousness in the form of pain, nausea, or pathological dream images.

Thus the morphological threefold subdivision of the nervous system corresponds to a threefold division in consciousness (88). The central nervous system (brain) supports daily waking consciousness. The autonomic nervous system in the viscera does not convey any sensations that become conscious; this is the domain of the unconscious or subconscious (sleep). A zone of intermediate consciousness appears only in the nervous system's middle domain—characterized in this book as the spinal domain and consisting primarily of sensorimotor systems, which also extend all the way to the cortex. This zone is responsible primarily for reflexive processes, which are comparable in some respects to the dreaming state. They become increasingly conscious in areas closer to the brain and gradually merge into unconscious and automatic functions as they approach the periphery.

Rudolf Steiner expanded on the functional threefoldness of the nervous system to include psychopathological manifestations. To my knowledge, Steiner's suggestions for understanding psychiatric illness were the first attempt to use the nervous system's functional threefoldness as the basis of a "functional psychiatry." In cases of illness, the three domains of the nervous system affect different members of the human constitution and release different forces. Thus the manifestations of psychiatric illness are different on each level.

The Endocrine System (Hormonal Glands)

The hormones of the endocrine system radically extend the scope of the informational system's monitoring and control, altering the vital processes of cells and organs with great precision. Because endocrine hormones are distributed via the bloodstream rather than through nerve tissue, they are available to cells located anywhere in the body as long as those cells have the appropriate receptors. This link to blood circulation and thus to the metabolic system adds a deeper dimension to the autonomic system and makes it supremely effective.

The significance of this added dimension becomes obvious when we consider the intermediary stages (Figure 224). As discussed in the previous chapter, the efferent branch of an autonomic reflex arch consists of one preganglionic and one postganglionic neuron, and the endings of the second neuron release messenger substances (such as adrenaline, noradrenaline, acetylcholine, etc.) into the surrounding tissue (Figure 224A). If the second neuron, instead of producing dendrites, develops into a gland cell from the very beginning (as is the case in the adrenal medulla), the resulting structure is called a paraganglion (chromaffin body). Paraganglia serve endocrine functions by releasing messenger substances or neurotransmitters (in the case of the adrenal medulla, adrenaline and noradrenaline) directly into the blood (Figure 224B). If the first neuron also produces hormones in its cell body, they are transported to the nerve endings and then released into the vascular system (neurosecretion, Figure 224C). For example, hormones from the neurosecretory neurons of the hypothalamus enter the blood via the posterior lobe of the pituitary gland. The anterior pituitary lobe, however, contains true gland cells whose hormones affect cellular metabolism either directly, or indirectly by stimulating other hormonal glands (Figure 224D). The resulting cascades of hormonal effects are not unlike the nervous system's neuronal chains, and they form similar feedback loops. In the final stage of differentiation, endocrine cells or groups of cells (organs) release their hormones directly into the blood and reach their target organs via blood circulation (Figure 224E). The sum total of all of these organs makes up the system of endocrine glands.

When we consider endocrine activity on the **cellular level**, we discover a distinctly threefold arrangement of different types of hormones. A "lower" group consists of the steroid hormones, which are active in reproduction. Steroids are lipid hormones, and cell membranes (which contain no lipids) present no barriers to them. They work inside cells in the nucleus and in protein biosynthesis, which takes place partly in the nucleus and partly in the cytoplasm. The thyroid hormones making up the "middle" group are derived from the amino acid tyrosine. They work in the cytoplasm, where they intensify mitochondrial respiration and accelerate energy transfers (ATP, etc.). In the body as a whole, their activity is expressed in an increase in basal metabolism. It is interesting to note that the thyroid gland, which produces the hormones that regulate cellular respiration, is located close to the respiratory tract—specifically, directly in front of the trachea.

In addition to the tyrosine derivatives ("middle") and steroids ("lower" hormones), there is also an "upper" group, the peptide hormones, which represent the informational element in this threefold

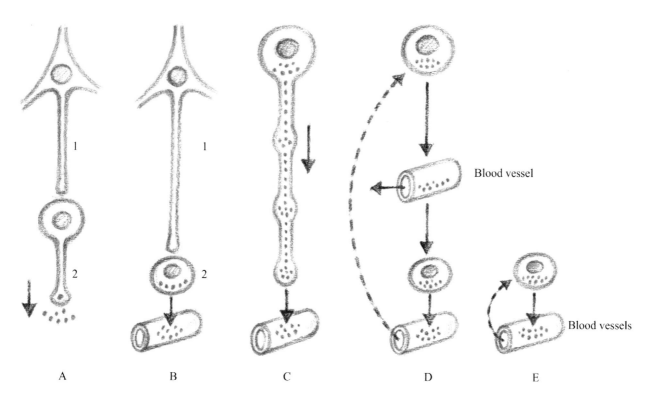

Fig. 224. *Different stages of differentiation in the development of neuroendocrine pathways*.
A: Two neurons (preganglionic, 1, and postganglionic, 2) in the efferent axon of an autonomic reflex arch in the spine;
B: In the adrenal medulla, for example, the postganglionic neuron (2) is transformed into a gland cell;
C: In the neurosecretory cells of the hypothalamus, for example, the neuron itself becomes a hormone-producing cell;
D: Endocrine cells form "effector pathways" via the blood circulation (with positive and negative feedback loops);
E: Peripheral endocrine cells affect organs either directly or indirectly via the vascular system.

system. Peptides, which cannot penetrate cell membranes, work on metabolic activity through receptors located on the outer surface of target cell membranes. Most anterior pituitary hormones are peptides. They are secreted into the blood, where they circulate and affect other hormonal glands (thyroid, adrenals, gonads).

Because the secretions of peripheral hormonal glands also work back on the pituitary, especially via hypothalamic input, feedback loops develop, often with specific rhythms. For example, blood cortisol levels fluctuate in a characteristic twenty-four hour pattern (73). Secretion of reproductive hormones and their regulation by the pituitary gland also display a typical periodicity. Temporal limitation of functions, however, is different in each subsystem of the endocrine system (see below).

Development and Function of the Endocrine Organs

In addition to the anterior pituitary lobe, five other endocrine glands develop: the thyroid gland, the parathyroids, the islets of Langerhans in the pancreas, the adrenals, and the gonads. Since all of their hormones are released into the blood, the location of their glands seems unimportant at first glance. From an abstract point of view, they could be located anywhere. But on closer examination, their location contributes a great deal to understanding their essential character and points to processes that define their development. Their very locations are archetypal phenomena.

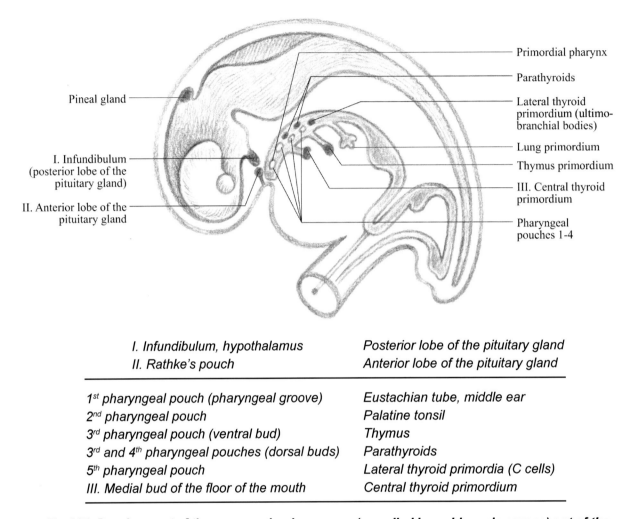

I. Infundibulum, hypothalamus	*Posterior lobe of the pituitary gland*
II. Rathke's pouch	*Anterior lobe of the pituitary gland*

1st pharyngeal pouch (pharyngeal groove)	*Eustachian tube, middle ear*
2nd pharyngeal pouch	*Palatine tonsil*
3rd pharyngeal pouch (ventral bud)	*Thymus*
3rd and 4th pharyngeal pouches (dorsal buds)	*Parathyroids*
5th pharyngeal pouch	*Lateral thyroid primordia (C cells)*
III. Medial bud of the floor of the mouth	*Central thyroid primordium*

*Fig. 225. **Development of the upper endocrine organs (so-called branchiogenic organs) out of the pharyngeal or branchial apparatus**.*

The Pharyngeal Organs: Thyroid, Parathyroids, and Thymus

First, let's consider the branchiogenic organs, i.e., the endocrine organs that develop out of the embryonic "branchial apparatus" (pharyngeal pouches). These are the thyroid, parathyroids, and thymus (Figure 225).

At an early stage in human embryonic development, as described in a previous chapter, pharyngeal arches and pouches reminiscent of the gills of aquatic vertebrates appear. The pharyngeal pouches are four or five lateral bulges on the pharynx primordium, each surrounded by pharyngeal arteries. The pharyngeal (or branchial) apparatus originally evolved to serve respiration alone, but in humans and other higher vertebrates who developed lungs for breathing, it undergoes a change in function. Instead of simply degenerating, it is incorporated into other, higher functional systems that are also related to respiration. In humans, this system gives rise to organs that receive sound (auditory ossicles, middle and outer ear) on the one hand, and to organs that produce sound (larynx, lower jaw including the jaw joint and jaw muscles) on the other. But organs that initially seem to have nothing to do with air or the gaseous element (thyroid, parathyroids, and thymus; Figure 225) also develop out of the lower pharyngeal pouches (3rd–5th). The thyroid bud develops in the middle, not far from the lung primordium. Initially, it resembles an exocrine gland. Along with the pulmonary bud, it grows downward in the direction of the chest cavity. The parathyroids split off from both sides of the third and fourth pharyngeal pouches and grow downward together with the primordial thyroid, forming four individual glands (two upper and two lower) located behind the thyroid. The thymus, which develops out of anterior buds on the third pharyngeal pouch, moves down into the chest cavity until it comes to rest above the heart. Finally, the fifth pharyngeal pouch forms another small bud that is incorporated into developing thyroid tissue as the lateral thyroid primordium. It gives rise to the C cells of the thyroid, which produce the hormone calcitonin.

The thyroid gland. In adults, the thyroid is located below the larynx and in front of the trachea (Figure 226). It produces thyroxine (T_4), which contains four iodine atoms. Inside cells, thyroxine can be transformed into highly active triiodothyronine (T_3) by splitting off one iodine atom. Throughout the body, but especially in the brain, T_3 promotes growth and maturation by stimulating protein synthesis. Beginning in the eleventh week of gestation, thyroid hormones stimulate growth of the body and ensure rapid differentiation of the nervous system and sense organs. In adults, these hormones increase tissue consumption of O_2 and raise basal metabolism and body temperature. Sympathetic stimulation of the thyroid enhances alertness and readiness for action, increases the heart rate, and intensifies general activity.

Along with the lungs, the thyroid gland develops out of the pharynx primordium, and its location in front of the trachea at the upper end of the respiratory tract reveals its functional connection to the respiratory system. The thyroid becomes the organ that expedites an individual's incarnation into his or her physical organism. The

blood absorbs oxygen in the lungs and carries it to the tissues, where it is used to produce energy in cellular metabolism. Thyroid hormones "kindle" this internal "combustion" process, increasing oxygen consumption and enhancing cellular activity. In general terms, increased availability and consumption of oxygen mean increased activity and—in the brain—greater alertness and intellectual performance. This is why hyperthyroidism can cause sleeplessness and incoherent thinking, while hypothyroidism can cause stupor and mental deterioration (myxoedema, cretinism). Pulmonary respiration makes us citizens of the Earth. All of our physical and mental activity is made possible by oxygen. Thyroid hormones with their light-absorbing iodine mobilize the "inner light" in the metabolic system to make it available in the head for mental and spiritual activity or in the metabolism itself for realizing will intentions (89).

Iodine appears to play an important role in this internal "***light metabolism.***" Iodine is reused repeatedly in the body, so only very small amounts (0.15 mg/d) need to be absorbed from food. In the thyroid, iodine atoms released in the conversion of T_4 to T_3 are used to make more thyroxine (T_4). Any excess hormone is bound to a protein and stored in the thyroid follicles as thyroglobulin. T_4 release and storage (functions similar to exhalation and inhalation) are regulated by the anterior pituitary lobe. A thyroid-stimulating hormone (TSH) is the anterior pituitary hormone that promotes thyroxine release. It is interesting to note that T_4, which is relatively inactive in tissues, serves as the messenger substance in the feedback loop to the pituitary gland, whereas highly active triiodothyronine has almost no effect on the pituitary.

The parathyroid glands and thyroid C cells. The thyroid gland functions on the boundary between the domain of life and the human soul and spirit. Growth and basal metabolism, as expressions of the tendency of soul-spiritual forces to incarnate into the physical, characterize the functional domain of thyroid hormones. In the parathyroid glands and thyroid C cells, this "incarnation process" takes

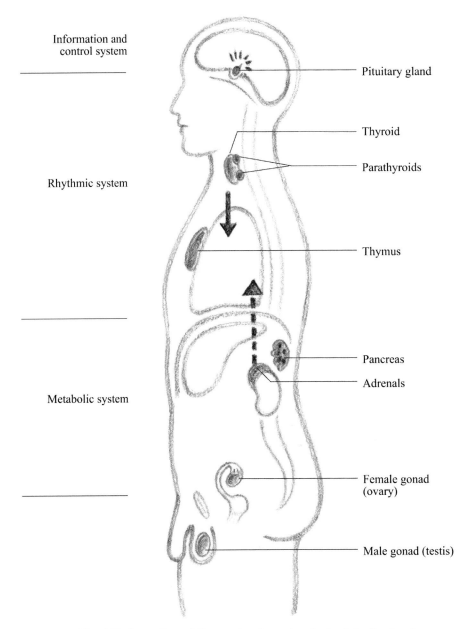

Information and
control system

_____

Rhythmic system

_____

Metabolic system

_____

Pituitary gland

Thyroid

Parathyroids

Thymus

Pancreas

Adrenals

Female gonad
(ovary)

Male gonad (testis)

Fig. 226. **Location of the endocrine glands** *(red)* **in the body.**
Arrows indicate directions of "radiating energy," i.e., supersensible forces.

place on the deeper level of bone mineralization and blood calcium and phosphate levels. Blood levels of calcium and phosphate are almost constant, fluctuating only within very narrow limits. Functions essential to our physical life depend on these electrolytes, and the body is extremely sensitive to disturbances in their balance. Calcium (Ca^{2+}) and phosphate (HPO_4^{2-}) are deposited in bones in the form of hydroxylapatite, which gives the bones their solidity. Calcium, however, also plays important roles in the structures and functions of many cells. By regulating ion transport, calcium channels in cell membranes affect cellular exchange processes and states of excitation. This is especially important in nerve cells, which is why a reduction in blood calcium levels (hypocalcemia) can cause overexcitability, muscle tremors, or even spasms (tetany). On the other hand, phosphorus (which means "light-bearer") serves the buildup of energy sources (such as ATP) in cells and is therefore intimately connected with essential life functions.

To a significant extent, therefore, the material existence of the physical human body as an entity that occupies space depends on incarnation into the solid element (Ca) and on its polar opposite, dissolution into "process" and energy (P). The near constancy of calcium and phosphate blood levels is an expression of the tenuous balance between these two tendencies. The hormones of the C cells in the thyroid and parathyroid glands regulate this balance precisely.

It is interesting to note that light also plays a role in a third element involved here, namely, vitamin D (calcitriol), a steroid hormone. When blood calcium levels drop, PTH (parathyrin) immediately mobilizes cells that break down bone, releasing Ca^{2+} into the blood. The C cell hormone calcitonin has the opposite effect, increasing Ca^{2+} deposition in bones and lowering blood calcium levels. To this balance, which is regulated entirely by blood calcium levels, vitamin D metabolism adds a connection to the outside world and the influence of light. Normally, the amounts of P and Ca circulating in the body are constant, and 100 percent of the calcium absorbed from the intestines is excreted. But when the body needs calcium salts (for example, during growth or after calcium losses), the hormone vitamin D causes increased calcium absorption and raises blood calcium levels. Vitamin D_3 (cholecalciferol) is the most important representative of the D vitamins. It forms in the skin through UV radiation of 7-dehydrocholesterol, a provitamin, and is then converted to vitamin D hormone (calcitriol) in the liver and kidneys. Calcitriol causes changes in the intestinal epithelium that allow more calcium ions to enter the bloodstream. This calcium can then be incorporated into bones or used in other parts of the body. In rickets, a vitamin D deficiency disease, bones are not sufficiently calcified and the child's soul falters in its incarnation into the body.

The *thymus*, the third branchiogenic organ (Figures 225 and 226), allows the "I" itself to establish a foothold in the body and to assert itself in its surroundings as an independent being with its own unique, personal physical body. After birth, the thymus becomes the central organ of the immune system. It is the "school" where white blood cells (lymphocytes) produced in the bone marrow "learn" to distinguish between self and nonself. In other words, they become immunocompetent cells that immediately recog-nize and destroy foreign cells not belonging to the self. The immune system ensures the individual's material integrity so that the spiritual "I" can rely on the body into which it incarnates. Because proteins often serve regulatory functions in the body, it is essential to prevent foreign proteins from entering the body and subjecting it to exogenous influences.

Thus the branchiogenic endocrine glands have intimate functional connections to processes that take place in the organs of the chest. The endocrine glands support respiration and blood circulation in ways that facilitate the incarnation of the human soul-spiritual entity (respiration, thyroid, O_2/CO_2 conversion, "light of thinking," etc.) into the living physical body (bone forma-tion, parathyroids, external light). Finally, on the immunological level, the individuality defends the unique character of its body against that of other bodies (thymus). It is interesting to note that lymphocytes migrating into the thymus "withdraw" from the context of the body as a whole as they take the decisive step of "learning" to distinguish between self and nonself. Immature pre-T cells are "imprisoned" in large reticular cells (nurse cells) in the thymus cortex, where they are shielded from all environmental influences. Most of them die, but the survivors, who have "learned" to distinguish endogenous from exogenous proteins, migrate into the lymphatic organs, where they continue to replicate.

Immunomaturation in the thymus is quali-tatively very different from the activity of the thyroid and parathyroid endocrine subsystems. It takes place internally and in darkness, in stark contrast to the air and light that play such a role in the other two subsystems.

The Abdominal Endocrine Glands: Pancreatic Islets of Langerhans and Adrenals

From a functional perspective, the thyroid, parathyroids, and thymus belong to the chest cavity, which houses the organs of the rhythmic system, while the adrenals and pancreas belong to the abdominal cavity, which houses the metabolic organs. As a result, the abdominal endocrine glands are more involved in metabolic processes (Figure 226).

The *adrenals* consist of two parts, which have different origins. The adrenal cortex develops out of the epithelium of the abdominal cavity itself (coelom epithelium), while the adrenal medulla develops out of the neural crest, the primordium of the nervous system. As development proceeds, these two parts come to rest alongside each other and fuse to form a single organ, but they continue to serve very different functions. The adrenal medulla is a paraganglion belonging to the sympathetic portion of the autonomic nervous system. Medulla cells synthesize adrenaline and noradrenaline, the primary hormones of the sympathetic nervous system (Figure 224B). In contrast, the adrenal cortex is a true endocrine gland that produces many different hormones, the most important of which are glucocorticoids. While thyroid hormones have an anabolic effect, stimulating protein synthesis, the effect of adrenal cortex hormones (specifically, cortisol) is catabolic and inhibitory. Adrenal cortex hormones also inhibit both immune and inflammatory responses. In the body's tissues, they inhibit filament formation (collagen synthesis), decrease the rate of growth, and break down bones. Under the influence of cortisol, amino acids produced through protein breakdown are synthesized into glycogen in the liver. In fatty tissue—one of our major energy reserves—cortisol breaks down fat (lipolysis) and inhibits fat storage (lipogenesis).

When we survey this great variety of hormonal effects, a basic "excarnating" tendency becomes evident. Thyroid hormones support the incarnation of the soul-spiritual entity into the physical body by promoting growth, increasing basal metabolism, increasing oxygen consumption, etc. Conversely, adrenal cortex hormones support the release of soul-spiritual forces from the realm of the living, so it makes sense that they should also be active in the nervous system, where they enhance our capacity for perception (which is based on catabolic processes), and accelerate the aging process.

The location of the adrenals at the upper end of the kidneys is no mere coincidence; it points to their dramatic inner functional connection to the kidneys. The adrenals, or "upper kidneys," are also functionally related to the gonads, which could be described as "lower kidneys" in this context. On different levels, all three are organs of excretion or release. The gonads "excrete" gametes, the kidneys chemicals for elimination in the urine, and the adrenals "life forces" (through catabolism).

Pituitary control. Unlike the parathyroids and the pancreatic islets of Langerhans, which are connected only to the bloodstream (Figure 227), the thyroid and the adrenal cortex are connected to the nervous system via the anterior pituitary lobe. Thyroid hormones drive life forces into the body, whereas adrenal cortex hormones free them from the body. Anterior pituitary hormones regulate these holistic processes, which are also connected to the central nervous system via the hypothalamus and thus influenced by consciousness. Hormones secreted by the thyroid and adrenals work back on the anterior pituitary lobe, which can also enhance the glands' secretory activity through specific (glandotropic) hormones—TSH in the case of the thyroid, ACTH in the case of the adrenal cortex (Figure 227). The resulting feedback loops are quite similar to the multilink functional systems of neuronal feedback in the CNS. When the glands produce too many hormones, increased blood levels inhibit the pituitary gland; when they produce too little, the pituitary is stimulated to produce more TSH or ACTH. Through specific releasing factors, the pituitary gland adjusts the set point of these

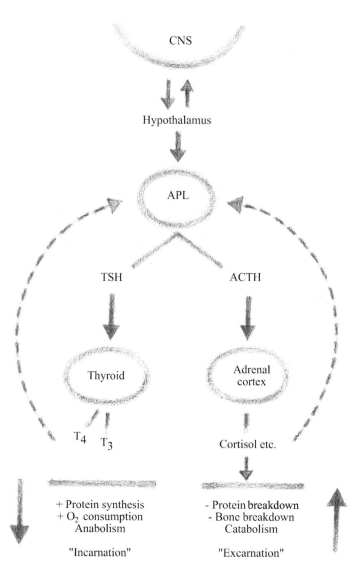

CNS

Hypothalamus

APL

TSH   ACTH

Thyroid   Adrenal cortex

T_4 T_3 Cortisol etc.

+ Protein synthesis
+ O_2 consumption
Anabolism

"Incarnation"

- Protein breakdown
- Bone breakdown
Catabolism

"Excarnation"

Fig. 227. **Hormonal feedback loops controlled by the anterior pituitary lobe** *(APL).*

feedback loops. In other words, like a higher nerve center, it adjusts the entire system's level of functioning.

In this way, thyroid and adrenal cortex functions, which are polar opposites in many respects, become fundamental to the life processes of the organism as a whole.

In contrast, the **pancreatic islets of Langerhans** and their hormones are linked directly to the blood rather than incorporated into the nervous system's feedback loops. The central energy source for all of the body's metabolic and life processes is sugar (glucose), whose "combustion" in the presence of oxygen makes energy-rich phosphates (ATP, etc.) available in the cells. The islets of Langerhans produce two hormones that affect blood sugar levels, namely, **insulin**, which lowers glucose levels, and **glucagon**, which raises them. Secretion of these hormones is directly triggered by sugar levels in circulating blood, which are "perceived" by pancreatic cells. The liver is involved in regulating these events. Insulin promotes the synthesis of glycogen from glucose in the liver, while glucagon breaks stored glycogen down into glucose again, which then circulates in the blood (Figure 228).

Similarly, thyroid C cell (calcitonin) and parathyroid (parathyrin) hormones work directly to maintain blood levels of calcium and phosphorus, with the kidneys rather than the liver playing the decisive role (Figure 228).

As with the pituitary-dependent glands, a functional polarity is also apparent on this level, in this case between "upper" processes (Ca/P regulation, bone/nerve), in which light plays a role and the kidneys are the central organ, and "lower" processes (glucose/energy conversions) in which warmth plays a role and the central organ is the liver (see Figure 228).

The intermediary between these polar processes is the blood. Blood composition is the decisive factor in the organism's central functions (energy conversion, thermoregulation, mineral balance). But nonpituitary-dependent endocrine glands are not completely independent in their connection to the blood. Experiments have shown that cells in certain hypothalamus nuclei perceive fluctuations in blood-sugar level, blood temperature, electrolyte concentrations, etc., and exert regulatory effects via the sympathetic or parasympathetic systems. This is probably also where circadian rhythms are synchronized with the rhythms of fluid and food intake. Ultimately, therefore, both the hypothalamus and the higher-ranking limbic system play decisive roles in regulating and harmonizing these vitally important functions.

The Pituitary as an Endocrine Organ

We have now become familiar with two major endocrine systems that control growth and metabolic functions through glandotropic pituitary hormones: the thyroid system, which serves anabolic (incarnation-promoting) metabolism, and the kidney system, which serves catabolic (excarnation-promoting) metabolism. There is also a third system, however, that allows the pituitary to intervene directly in metabolic activity through specific hormones that "bypass" the above-mentioned glands. The anterior pituitary lobe (APL) produces somatotropin (STH) or **growth hormone** (GH), a potent anabolic hormone that promotes protein synthesis. In the liver, STH stimulates anabolic activity by triggering the production of somatomedins. STH also increases the rate of mitosis in tissues and stimulates longitudinal bone growth in adolescents. Disturbances in hormone production can cause either pituitary dwarfism or gigantism during growth stages, as well as acromegaly in adults.

Pituitary STH production is also ultimately controlled by the hypothalamus, which affects the APL through its releasing hormones—somatoliberin (GHRH), which promotes STH production, and somatostatin (SIH), which inhibits it (Figure 229).

This anabolic subsystem, which also plays a role in work and stress, contrasts with the antagonistic functions of **posterior pituitary hormones**. Instead of the liver (an anabolic organ), the kidneys as organs of elimination are involved in this subsystem, whose central organ is the **posterior pituitary lobe** (PPL). The PPL, however, cannot produce hormones itself. They are produced in the hypothalamus—more specifically, in its paraventricular and supraoptical nuclei, whose cells develop long axons that extend all the way to the PPL. These axons transport hormones to the PPL, where they are released into the blood (neurosecretion). These hormones

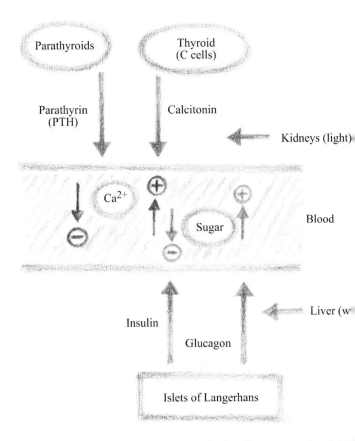

Fig. 228. **Hormonal regulation of blood sugar and calcium levels** by the islets of Langerhans (pancreas), thyroid, and parathyroids.

target elimination in the broadest sense. Oxytocin stimulates uterine contractions during delivery, and vasopressin (also known as antidiuretic hormone or ADH) supports urine concentration through resorption of water in the collecting tubules of the kidney. Disruptions in the production of this hormone can lead to diabetes insipidus, a condition in which the kidneys eliminate up to twenty liters of fluid per day.

Metabolic by-products (especially salts, but also urea as the end product of protein metabolism) are eliminated through a complex process that concentrates them into one to one-and-a-half liters of urine per day. Ultimately, the antigrowth process of releasing life forces from

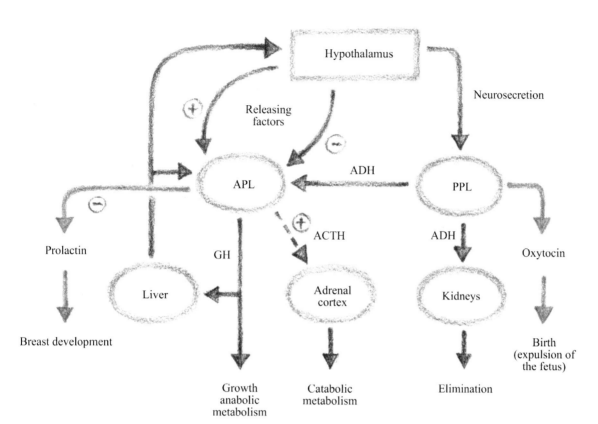

*Fig. 229A. **Effects of the hypothalamus** on the endocrine system via the anterior and posterior pituitary lobes (APL/PPL).*

the body ("excarnation"), which is promoted by the PPL hormone ADH, is made possible only by the kidneys' urine-concentrating activity. It is interesting to note that ADH has a side effect on the APL, where it stimulates ACTH production, thus indirectly promoting catabolic processes via the adrenal cortex. This phenomenon emphatically underlines the overall tendency that prevails on this side of the system (Figure 229A).

At this point, we might ask why the body needs a direct "track" from the pituitary itself. Why do growth and elimination also need to be controlled directly from "above," bypassing the polar systems of the thyroid and adrenals? The current assumption is that the hormones produced by peripheral endocrine glands are inadequate during postnatal growth or are too one-sided in their effects to control the complex

differentiation of the organism as a whole, especially its progressive maturation on the soul-spiritual level. In this context, a direct connection to the pituitary and hypothalamus certainly seems to make sense.

But another, very important functional connection becomes evident when we consider two other hormones produced along with STH and ADH, namely, prolactin (produced by the APL) and oxytocin (produced by the PPL). Oxytocin is central to the birthing process and milk secretion; prolactin promotes growth of the mammary glands during pregnancy and controls lactation. But prolactin is also active in growth and differentiation processes during puberty and later in the rhythmic processes of the reproductive system (menstrual and ovulation cycles). Reproduction is based on growth and differentiation processes that take place outside of the parental organism's own life processes. These "extra" processes serve the preservation of the species rather than the life of the individual. They obey different laws and—in the case of a pregnancy—may even push the body to the very limits of its existence. In a certain respect, therefore, the reproductive organs are kept structurally separate from the rest of the body. As a result, they need their own hormonal and neurological control mechanisms. In the context of gamete development and gestation, anabolic ("incarnation-promoting") and catabolic ("excarnation-promoting") life processes assume a different significance and cannot be allowed to disturb the corresponding endogenous processes. Perhaps this offers some explanation for the unique status of reproductive hormonal feedback loops (Figure 229A).

The Endocrine System and the Reproductive Organs

The reproductive organs make it possible for another being to incarnate into the physical world. For this purpose, the organism sets aside ("sacrifices") part of itself to make space for the incarnating being to develop. These processes are controlled by the embryo itself. The preparatory processes that make conception and early embryonic development possible are also controlled primarily by the gonads, not by the pituitary/hypothalamus system. The gonads serve as "timers" for periodic changes in the system as a whole, especially for the secretion of pituitary and hypothalamus hormones.

The **anterior pituitary lobe** produces two different hormones (gonadotropins) that affect the gonads, namely, follicle-stimulating hormone (FSH) and luteinizing hormone (LH), both of which are produced in the anterior pituitary lobe only after it is stimulated by gonadoliberin, a releasing factor from the hypothalamus, which

reaches the anterior pituitary lobe via the pituitary portal system. At sixty- to ninety-minute intervals, the hypothalamus releases gonadoliberin to the anterior pituitary lobe. Because the hypothalamus is highly sensitive to reproductive hormones, this rhythm is influenced by levels of circulating gonadal hormones (progesterone, estrogen, androgen). Thus the timing of gonadoliberin release is determined by the gonads themselves, not by the hypothalamus.

In functional terms, therefore, the extremely complex system of reproductive hormones is totally geared to conception and the development of the infant, with the gonads playing the leading role. The reproductive system is unlike any other endocrine regulatory system in that the pituitary/hypothalamus system plays a minimal role in it, serving only to coordinate it with other body functions and to harmonize the rhythmic life processes (along with anabolism and catabolism) within the reproductive system itself (Figure 229B).

The Pituitary/Pineal System

As we have already seen, the pituitary gland must be considered the uppermost center of the endocrine system. It is connected to the hypothalamus via the posterior pituitary lobe or neurohypophysis. In contrast, the pineal gland is part of the epithalamus, which forms a step "up" from the limbic system to the endbrain just as the pituitary is oriented "downward" toward the metabolic organs (Figure 222). These two polar organs, which represent the "upper" and "lower" levels of the control system, are central to the entire system's functioning and are located close together.

The pituitary lies in a goblet-shaped depression in the sella turcica at the point where the base of the skull curves and the anterior and posterior fossae meet in the angle of the clivus. As noted before (p. 66, see also p. 386), this angle is related to human uprightness, to the freeing of the human

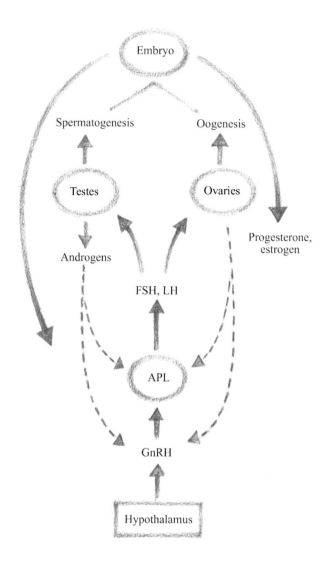

*Fig. 229B. **Endocrine control of embryonic development**. Feedback loops between the pituitary and the gonads develop independent of other endocrine pathways. (GnRH: gonadoliberin).*

body (especially of the head and its sense organs) from its surroundings, and ultimately also to the process of individuation. It is somehow archetypal that an endocrine gland in this particular location should be the "master gland" that controls the body's entire endocrine glandular system and links it to the brain's hypothalamus system.

The posterior pituitary lobe secretes two hormones (antidiuretic hor-mone and oxytocin) that are both related to "elimination" processes—elimination of urine (ADH) and stimulation of contractions that expel the infant from the uterus (oxytocin). These hormones are produced in specific nuclei in the hypothalamus and then transported to the posterior pituitary lobe, where they are released into the blood (neurosecretion). From the hypothalamus, however, they can also affect the nervous system itself (probably via the limbic system), thus influencing sensory alertness, emotional tinging of sense impressions, and memory.

Elimination (excretion) processes in the body always entail not only loss of substance but also the release of forces previously bound up with these substances. Urinary excretion is involved in mineral balances on the boundary between solid and liquid. Birth can be understood as the "excretion" or release of a newly developed body into its own life. In both cases, the hormones involved merely facilitate these functions, and their chemistry and effects say little about the processes themselves. The two posterior pituitary hormones are chemically very closely related and evolved from a common preliminary stage (vasotocin). ADH promotes water resorption in the kidneys (the antidiuretic principle), is a vasoconstrictor, and influences circulation of cortisol in the pituitary/ adrenal system. According to Rudolf Steiner, the regulation of elimination and circulation supports a flow of forces from the kidneys and reproductive organs to the head, ultimately releasing forces that serve sensory alertness and memory (65).

One level down from the activity of PPL hormones are the hormonal processes controlled by the **anterior pituitary lobe**. As we have already seen, many metabolic functions are controlled by hormones released into the blood by endocrine glands (thyroid, adrenals, etc.). By influencing organ metabolism, these hormones regulate formative processes in the body's material element. Thus the APL is primarily involved in life processes.

In contrast, the **epithalamus** and **pineal gland** are more closely connected to the central nervous system. Two long "reins" or habenulae secure the pineal gland to the thalamus (Figure 222).

Along with the epithalamus, the pineal gland belongs to the limbic system. If it is destroyed (by a tumor, for example) during childhood, puberty sets in prematurely. Consequently, it has been assumed to have functional (inhibitory) connections to the genitals. The only thing that seems certain today, however, is the function of this gland in regulating circadian rhythms. The body's twenty-four hour rhythm, an endogenous biological rhythm that reflects the sun's cycle, is essentially controlled by the hormone melatonin (the so-called "time-keeper hormone"), which is produced in the pineal gland. Melatonin reaches the internal organs via the bloodstream and regulates their circadian rhythms. The synthesis of melatonin in the pineal gland can be synchronized with daily and seasonal changes in light intensity through the visual system. In the area of the crossing of the optic nerves (optic chiasm), some fibers branch off from the optic pathway to a specific nucleus of the hypothalamus (suprachiasmatic nucleus), which, in turn, stimulates the pineal gland and the nuclei of the hypothalamus, thereby becoming a control center for the circadian rhythms of the organism (Figure 230). There is a great deal of evidence that the pineal gland plays a central role in an internal light metabolism of some sort.

According to Rudolf Steiner, a (will-based) stream of energy flows from the lower part of the human body to the head, accumulating in the pituitary gland where it meets up with a more "thoughtlike" stream of forces concentrated in the pineal gland (65). The meeting of these two contrasting force-streams, he says, produces a buildup of tension that, when released, causes remembered images to become conscious. If this is so, the pituitary/pineal system could form a crucial bridge between below and above, where life forces are released from the autonomic system to become conscious in the form of memories, while conceptual forces from the central nervous system sink down into the vegetative system and the subconscious (forgetting or suppression).

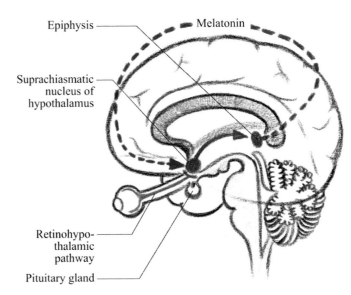

Fig. 230. **Feedback loop between the pineal gland and the hypothalamus nucleus for the control of day/night rhythm.** *The control center is the suprachiasmatic nucleus in the hypothalamus which is stimulated by the retinohypothalamic pathway (blue). Melatonin, produced in the pineal gland, functions as a "time-keeper hormone."*

Head Development
and Organ Metamorphoses

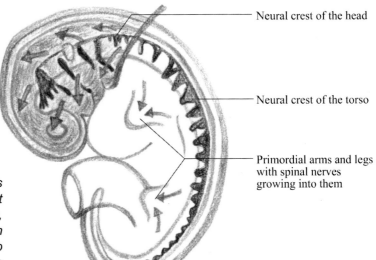

Neural crest of the head

Neural crest of the torso

Primordial arms and legs with spinal nerves growing into them

Fig. 231. **The head's neural crest** supplies substance not only for the cranial nerves but also for other tissues in the head (muscles, bones, cartilage, and connective tissue). In the rest of the body, these tissues develop out of mesodermal material. In the head, this primordial tissue is known as mesectoderm or ectomesenchyme (red).

Head Development
and the Integration Principle

The formation of the head occupies a unique and remarkable position within the overall development of the body. During the embryonic period, the primitive head not only differentiates more rapidly than the torso (and much more rapidly than the limbs) but also develops according to distinctly different laws. This "head problem" has been the subject of animated scientific discussion since Goethe's time. Goethe explored the possibility that the vertebrae metamorphose into the skull (analogous to his theory of plant metamorphosis) but was unable to arrive at a conclusive solution. Nonetheless, this idea stimulated the scientists of his time, especially the anatomist Lorenz Oken of Jena, to pursue the laws governing head development and to tackle a problem that is still discussed today, even in the context of genetics.

Clearly, the development of the human head presents a profound mystery, one that Goethe suspected but was not quite able to grasp. Today we know that the head develops according to fundamentally different principles from the torso and limbs, but we have not been able to solve the basic developmental mystery. Teichmann demonstrated that images in the Pharaohs' tombs express the ancient Egyptians' conviction that the head is a metamorphosis of the individual's torso from the preceding incarnation (91). In several different contexts, Rudolf Steiner described in great detail how the head emerges from formative forces and energies that worked in the torso and limbs in the previous life (92, 93).

First, however, let's consider the facts known to science today.

Head tissue does not develop according to the formative principles governing the rest of the body. In the torso, the basic tissue that gives rise to bones, connective tissue, muscles, and circulatory organs is **mesenchyme**. This mesenchymal tissue emerges from the mesoderm through disintegration of the somites, the primordial torso segments that develop at rhythmic intervals along the embryonic axis (chorda dorsalis). Since the chorda dorsalis ends at the base of the skull, the primordial head has no somites and therefore no mesenchyme. The bones of the head, along with its muscles and connective tissue, must develop in some other way.

It took a long time for scientists to prove that head mesenchyme emerges from primordial nerve tissue. The brain is derived from ectoderm, which invaginates to form the embryonic neural tube. A fault line along the edge of this invagination gives rise to the **neural crest** (Figure 231). Cells from the head's neural crest migrate throughout the head, forming reticular tissue that is very similar to the embryonic connective tissue in the rest of the body. Like the latter, it is also capable of producing a wide variety of tissues such as bone, muscle, teeth, and connective tissue. Thus the cells in the head's bones and connective tissue are **neurogenic** in origin. Close relatives of these cells develop into neurons and glia cells, which are functionally part of the body's information system. Because of its unique origin, the mesenchyme that appears in the head—and **only** in the head—has been called **mesectoderm** or **ectomesenchyme**. The entire primordial head—brain, sense organs, bones, teeth, and muscles—is ultimately derived either directly from ectoderm or from the embryonic neural tube, which is also of ectodermal origin. Endoderm and mesoderm are not involved in head development. As offspring of the information system, the brain, sense organs, and other formations in the head are incapable of developing blood vessels or blood and therefore become viable only after the vascular system grows into the head from below.

To better understand the phenomenon of head development, we must briefly review the unique situation of **nerve tissue**. The nervous system is fundamentally different from the body's other organ systems in that it has no real interstitial tissue and no extracellular space as such.

In the rest of the body, substances are almost always exchanged between blood vessels and organ tissues through the intervening extracellular space, which is capable of absorbing large amounts of fluid and thus functions as a buffer. The lymphatic vascular system exists specifically to drain this space, which is usually rich in proteins and other substances that enter it from the circulating blood. Extracellular space also includes connective tissue around organs as well as active immune cells and substances.

With all of its structures that surround and protect the organs, this extracellular space is extremely important in metabolic exchanges. It is totally absent in the central nervous system, where the transport of fluids, nutrients, and other substances is handled by a system of specialized cells (glia cells) that separate the blood vessels from actual nerve tissue. Because the informational processes of the nervous system take place on cell membranes at the synaptic cleft, the space between nerve cells and nerve fibers, although technically an extracellular space of sorts, cannot be involved in metabolic exchanges because any changes in ion concentrations and fluid volumes would immediately cause the collapse of membrane potentials, making the transmission of information totally impossible. Thus nerve tissue behaves similarly to plant tissues, which also have no extracellular space of the sort found in animal bodies. In plants, too, substances are transported through the cells themselves without any involvement of intercellular spaces filled with connective tissue.

The situation in the head is unique. In the facial skull, a type of interstitial tissue (mesectoderm or ectomesenchyme) does in fact develop out of neural crest cells, and the functions it serves in the metabolism of the head organs are similar to connective-tissue functions in the rest of the body. The head develops a "torso organization" of its own, so to speak, deriving the material for it from nerve tissue instead of from the primordial torso. The primordial head has access to formative forces that seem to have prior experience with mesenchymal organ development. As a result, they can produce practically the entire spectrum of differentiated tissues—from simple connective tissue cells to bone, muscle, and nerve cells—from a single source. Only the head's vascular system originates in the torso. The head's formative forces are simply not capable of producing blood. Unlike limb and torso bones, which develop out of richly vascularized mesenchyme, even the bones of the skull derive ultimately from neurogenic mesectoderm. To exaggerate slightly, we might call the head bones "nerve bones" and the bones of the rest of the body "blood bones." In the facial skull, extracellular space filled with connective tissue develops to serve torsolike metabolic exchanges, demonstrating that the head is capable of inducing a "torso process" of its own without the need for mesodermal and endodermal tissue. Obviously, the head obeys laws of its own, and its developmental processes must be seen as the result of earlier formative activity and events.

*Fig. 232. **Embryonic development of the long bones**. Bone is deposited from the outside onto an elongated section of cartilage, forming a collar.*
A: General view, showing layers;
B: Longitudinal section showing changes within the cartilage (calcium deposits, development of vesicular cartilage, etc.).

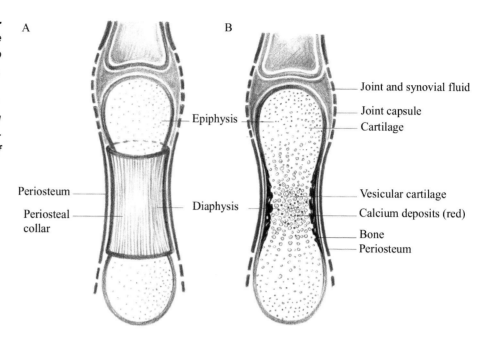

Development and Metamorphosis Of Bony Elements

Long bones develop on underlying cartilaginous models that are similar in shape to the mature bones, although somewhat less detailed. The cartilaginous parts of future bones grow relatively rapidly, and bone tissue suddenly begins to appear on the shank around the end of the second month of gestation. Initially, this bone tissue is deposited onto the cartilage *from outside* by the surrounding perichondrium. Thus the primary, cartilaginous skeletal element acquires a tube-shaped **collar of bone** that develops directly out of connective tissue and is therefore classified as membranous bone. With the development of this calcified collar, the perichondrium becomes periosteum, and thus the bony casing is called the periosteal collar of the diaphysis (Figure 232 A). The two epiphyses or terminal portions of the bone are usually somewhat broader. Initially, they have no bony collar, because in these locations

the periosteum (which later develops into the joint capsule) separates from the cartilage to bridge the joint space. The periosteum covers a series of cartilaginous elements and their primary joints like a sleeve that has thus far become ossified only in the diaphyses.

It has sometimes been argued that development of the periosteal collar from outside inhibits the nutrition and growth of the central cartilaginous elements, causing swelling and the development of enlarged vesicular cartilage cells in the interior of the shaft, accompanied by deposition of calcium salts in the cartilaginous matrix—in other words, cartilage degeneration (Figure 232B). This, however, is a legitimate physiological process that also occurs even without bone formation. It is possible that this phase of bone development reflects a global phylogenetic crisis that occurred during the Earth's evolution, since the development of vesicular cartilage with calcium deposition does display distinctly pathological traits. In any case, the embryonic cartilaginous skeleton as a whole is still crudely animallike and lacks the finely differentiated forms of the adult skeleton (Figure 233).

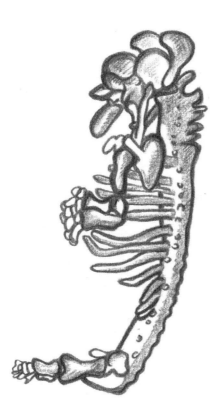

Fig. 233. **Reconstruction of the cartilaginous skeleton of a human embryo** *(end of week 7; adapted from W. Hagen, 141).*

Immediately after the onset of cartilaginous degeneration in the diaphysis of an embryonic long bone, mesenchyme and blood vessels begin to grow in the calcified vesicular cartilage of the interior (Figure 234). This new tissue also originates in the periosteum—specifically in its inner, well-vascularized cambium layer, which suddenly develops a bud of tissue that grows into the diaphysis, erodes the calcifying matrix, and releases the vesicular cartilage cells from their capsules, thus creating an irregular hollow space. This space, the ***primary marrow***, contains some tissue detritus but is mostly filled with actively growing embryonic connective tissue (mesenchyme) that is rich in blood and cells. The primary marrow grows rapidly in all directions but especially lengthwise, in the direction of the two epiphyses (Figure 234A). Initially, only an irregular scaffolding of cartilage remains around

the edges of the marrow cavity. This scaffolding then serves as a foundation for mesenchymal bone-producing cells (osteoblasts) that lay down new bone. Osteoblasts also settle in the remaining scaffolding of the original cartilage tissue, where they deposit initially uncalcified osteoid layers (Figure 234B). The result is a dense mesh of bony scaffolding, the so-called spongy bone, in the interior of the embryonic long bone. In addition to expanding lengthwise, the spongy bone ultimately also fills the hollow shaft and fuses with the bony collar deposited from the outside.

The periosteal collar develops via ***direct ossification***—i.e., out of the connective tissue of the periosteum, without any cartilaginous model. It supplies the compact bone of the future long bone, which is found mostly in the diaphysis. Continued deposition from outside increases the thickness of the shaft. Thus periosteal bone growth supports primarily ***lateral growth***.

Endochondral bone develops differently, through the ***indirect ossification*** of cartilage in the interior, which produces spongy bone. Even in the embryonic stage, the scaffolding of the spongy bone is adapted to future functional stresses, with its trabeculae exactly aligned with stress trajectories. This structure, which maximizes strength with a minimum of material (Figure 235), is not evident in the compact bone of the shaft, which needs to be more massively constructed to resist forces of flexion.

Thus the development of ***spongy bone*** is initiated by a well-vascularized mesenchymal bud that makes its way into the interior of the diaphysis, where it increases in length. Later, mesenchyme buds that erode cartilage and develop spongy bone tissue also appear in the two epiphyses (the future heads of the bone). These epiphyseal nuclei grow in all directions (i.e., spherically) until no cartilage remains except on the future joint surfaces and in the epiphyseal disks at the boundaries with the shaft (Figure 234B). Because cartilage cells in the epiphyseal disks continue to replicate, the bone continues to increase in length. Cartilage is constantly broken down on the boundary surfaces, however, so as such the

A

B

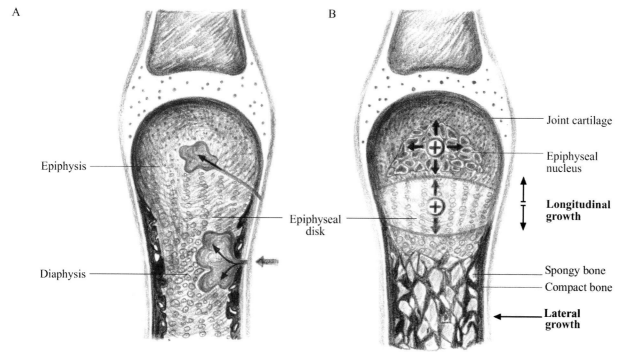

Epiphysis

Diaphysis

Epiphyseal
disk

Joint cartilage

Epiphyseal
nucleus

**Longitudinal
growth**

Spongy bone

Compact bone

**Lateral
growth**

Fig. 234. Above: **Later developmental stages in the development of long bones near the joints**. *Lateral growth results from deposition of bone tissue in the diaphysis (arrows), longitudinal growth from cartilage proliferation in the ephiphyseal disk. The well-vascularized mesenchyme that grows in from the periosteum (arrows in A) erodes cartilage and forms nuclei of spongy bone and marrow (for details, see text).*

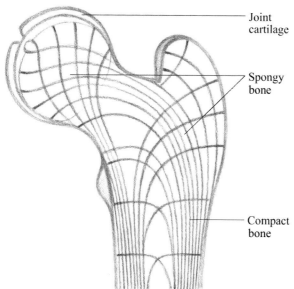

Joint
cartilage

Spongy
bone

Compact
bone

Fig. 235. Left: **Diagram of the head of the femur**, *showing the trajectorial arrangement of spongy bone trabeculae. This structure corresponds to the actual trajectories of forces pushing and pulling on the bone.*

epiphyseal plates never become significantly thicker. Thus endochondral growth, which produces spongy bone, supports *longitudinal growth*, while periosteal bone formation, which produces compact bone, supports lateral growth. These two processes are polar in character and relatively independent of each other. Periosteal ossification

involves peripheral, cosmic forces such as those involved in the development of the bones of the skullcap, while endochondral ossification is dominated by the central, Earth-related forces at work in the limbs. Here we find again the basic polarity between matter and form, blood and nerve (see Table 28.)

A. Direct (desmal) ossification	B. Indirect (endochondral) ossification
Ossification proceeds from connective tissue	Ossification proceeds from cartilage
Compact bone	Spongy bone
Compact structure, not trajectorial	Functional, trajectorial (cancellous) structure
Deposited from outside	Formed from the inside out
Periosteal, desmal ossification	Endochondral ossification
Peripheral forces	Central forces
Head-related ("conceptualization")	Limb-related (will)
Form pole	Matter pole
Lateral growth	Longitudinal growth

Table 28. Basic processes in limb bone development.

In this context, it is significant that the nuclei that produce spongy bone are later transformed into marrow, where blood cells develop. While the trabeculae with their trajectorial structure are fully incorporated into the Earth's gravitational field, blood (which develops out of the same mesenchymal tissue) frees itself from gravity to flow in an endless, living stream throughout the body, without ever assuming solid form. These are the functional elements of a motor system whose ever-changing form comes to grips with three-dimensional space on Earth in order to manifest an individual's will through movement.

In ***periosteal bone development*** in the shaft, as well as in the membranous bone layers of other bony elements such as the skullcap bones, the opposite pole of forces comes into its own and the element of form plays a major role. Compact bone, or cortical bone, gives bones their shape and solidity and serves as attachment points for muscles, thus making it possible to manifest in movement the formative impulses that are inspired by the nervous system and represent images or concepts of movements. This, therefore, is a formative element that has more to do with conceptualization than with the above-mentioned will.

Development of the Human Skull

It is interesting to note that these two types of bone development are also found in the skull. The large, flat bones of the calvaria (the frontal, parietal, and occipital bones and the squamous portions of the temporal bones) develop through direct (desmal) ossification that proceeds from the surrounding connective tissue. They are membranous bones, comparable to the periosteally ossified portions of long bones. In contrast, the bones of the base of the skull (the petrous, sphenoid, ethmoid, and occipital bones) develop on the basis of a cartilaginous skeleton (the chondrocranium) that is only secondarily transformed into bone through endochondral ossification (Figure 236).

Peripheral ("cosmic") forces are heavily involved in shaping the skullcap, as is evident in the almost crystalline formative tendencies in this domain (the desmocranium). Seen as a whole, the bones of the skullcap form a protective covering for the brain, but instead of coming about through tangential bone deposition from outside (as is the case with the sleeve of the long bones of the limbs), they originate in pointlike ossification centers. Two of these are found on the frontal bone, one on each of the parietal bones, and one on the occipital bone. Bony trabeculae develop out of each of these points in radiating patterns that remain in a single

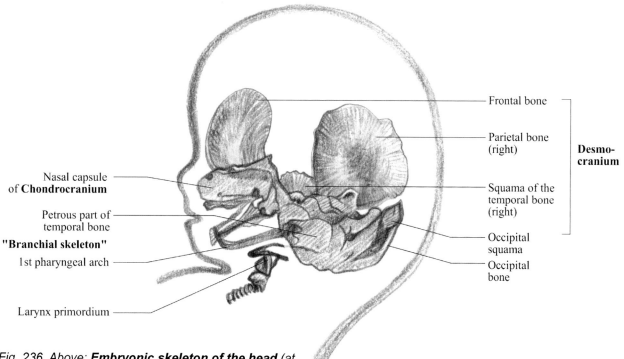

Nasal capsule
of **Chondrocranium**

Petrous part of
temporal bone

"Branchial skeleton"

1st pharyngeal arch

Larynx primordium

Frontal bone

Parietal bone
(right)

Squama of the
temporal bone
(right)

Occipital
squama

Occipital
bone

**Desmo-
cranium**

*Fig. 236. Above: **Embryonic skeleton of the head** (at approximately 3 months). Blue: cartilaginous chondrocranium of the base of the skull; gray: cartilaginous pharyngeal arches ("branchial apparatus"); yellow: membranous bones of the skullcap (desmocranium).*

*Fig. 237. Right: **Skull of a newborn**. The bony plates of the skullcap develop as trabeculae grow radially from five ossification points. The skull sutures, which also form the fontanelles, are also epiphyseal plates, where growth occurs. A: diagonal front view; B: view from above.*

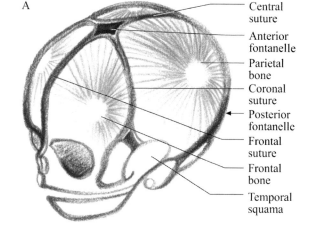

A

Central
suture

Anterior
fontanelle

Parietal
bone

Coronal
suture

Posterior
fontanelle

Frontal
suture

Frontal
bone

Temporal
squama

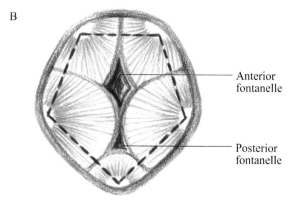

B

Anterior
fontanelle

Posterior
fontanelle

plane. As a result, the skullcap bones develop into bony plates that meet to form a pentagonal three-dimensional body—a fragment of a pentagon dodecahedron—augmented by the primordia of the two temporal squamae (Figure 237).

While the periosteal collars of the long bones are primarily radial in their orientation, like the orientation of the limbs themselves, periosteal growth in the skullcap is limited to surfaces. In other words, the trabeculae elongate as they radiate outward from their respective ossification

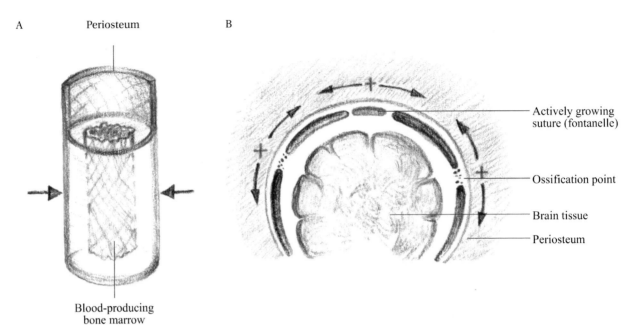

Fig. 238. Comparison of the developmental dynamics of long bones (A) **and skullcap bones** (B). *In the cranium, the life forces active in the interior of long bones (in blood formation, etc.) are transferred to the outside (red shading) in the form of thought forces. In the cranium, the centripetal bone-forming process that originates in the periosteum of long bones (from the outside, see arrows) is transformed into the radial growth of skull plates, which originates in the ossification points and produces a spherical three-dimensional body that increases in size at the actively growing sutures (epiphyseal cartilage, double arrows).*

points, forming bony plates that together define the skull cavity. Unlike the center of long bones, the skull contains no blood-forming tissue (marrow) but instead encloses the brain (Figure 237).

We can attempt to understand the developmental gesture of the skullcap not only as the polar opposite of long bone development but also as a **process of inversion (turning inside out) and integration**.

Long bones are shaped from the outside by periosteal collars, resulting in hollow internal spaces where blood-producing marrow can develop. The centripetal "dying off" process of bone formation is counteracted by the enlivening blood formation in the interior, a lifelong process of regenerating the body's vital and formative forces through the blood (Figure 238A).

In contrast, if we look at the configuration of forces in the head, we see an "inversion" of what

takes place in the long bones (Figure 238B). In the development of the skullcap, periosteal ossification produces a sphere instead of columnar structures. Here, too, a hollow space (the cranial cavity) develops, but instead of containing highly regenerative, blood-forming tissue, it houses nerve tissue, which (in adults) loses all of its regenerative powers (i.e., "dies") after differentiating into an extremely complex and delicate structure. But what happened to those regenerative forces? They now appear "outside" the enclosed cavity, in the surrounding sphere, in the form of forces of thought and conceptualization for which the brain provides a physical basis, just as muscles and blood circulation provide the basis for the will activity that moves the limb bones (Figure 238B). The formative forces at work in the limbs are "turned inside out" in their interaction in the head.

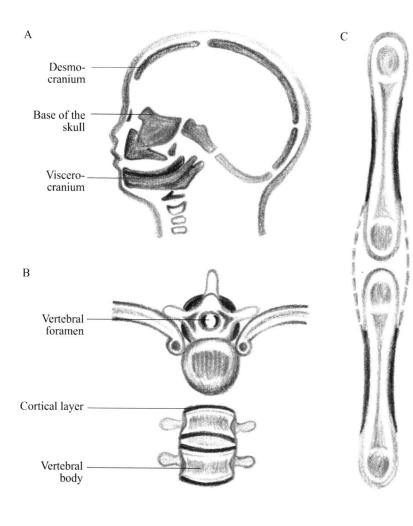

A

Desmo-
cranium

Base of the
skull

Viscero-
cranium

B

Vertebral
foramen

Cortical layer

Vertebral
body

C

Fig. 239. **Bone development in the three major functional domains of the human body.**
A: Spherically shaped head;
B: Rhythmically segmented torso (vertebrae and ribs);
C: Radially structured limb bones (adapted from Rohen, 15).

Red: Endochondral ossification;
Black: Periosteal ossification;
Gray: Cartilaginous preliminary stages.

Here, however, an additional process must also be taken into account, namely, the integration of a number of individual elements into a new, unitary whole. The development of the shape of the long bones is repeated throughout the limbs, always in the same way. In the skull, however, these separate developments are united into an **overarching whole**, which is why we can speak of integration as well as inversion. Later explanations of metamorphosed shapes will further clarify this process.

Development of the Torso Skeleton

With regard to their mode of ossification, the bones of the torso occupy an intermediate position between skull bones and limb bones. The characteristic structural elements of a vertebra are the vertebral body (anterior) and the neural arch with the spinous and transverse processes (posterior) (Figure 239).

The **vertebral body** takes shape primarily through endochondral ossification, i.e., from within, without the development of a periosteal collar. Thus the vertebral body is mostly spongy, consisting primarily of trajectorially arranged trabeculae, which elongate in all three dimensions of space, forming star-shaped patterns.

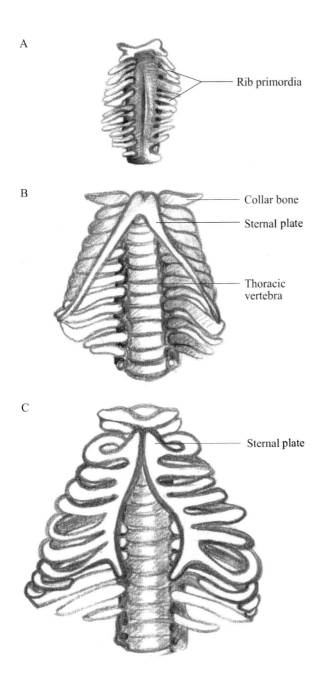

A

— Rib primordia

B

— Collar bone

— Sternal plate

— Thoracic vertebra

— Sternal plate

C

— Sternal plate

*Fig. 240. **Reconstruction of the cartilaginous rib-cage in various stages of embryonic development** (adapted from Charlotte Müller, 1906). The ribs of each side are connected by a sternal plate. The two plates then fuse from top to bottom to form the sternum.*
A: 13-mm long embryo (Day 40)
B: 15-mm long embryo (Day 44)
C: 23-mm long embryo (Day 50)

Longitudinal (vertical) growth of the vertebral body occurs in a disc of cartilage at each end, comparable to the epiphyseal disks of long bones. Externally, a periosteal collar develops only secondarily and never thickens significantly. It serves only to develop a thin, stabilizing cortical layer (Figure 239).

Ossification of the ***vertebral arch***, however, is primarily periosteal. The cartilaginous primordial neural arch ossifies from the outside, through a periosteal collar that develops out of connective tissue. The neural arch, which protects the spinal cord, resembles the membranous bone of the skullcap bones or the periosteal collar of limb bones. Continued growth is supported by secondary development of epiphyseal cartilage from cartilage remnants, primarily on the ends of the processes. In contrast to the vertical growth of the vertebral body, the direction of growth in this case is primarily horizontal, and the developmental gesture is one of surrounding the central hollow space.

Thus the same two modes of ossification that form limb bones are also at work in the ***vertebral column***, but in separate locations. Endochondral ossification, associated with the central forces of the blood—i.e., with the matter or will pole—dominates in the vertebral bodies, while periosteal ossification, associated with forces that work from outside—i.e., the nerve, form, or conceptual pole—dominates in the neural arches, although secondary endochondral bone development also appears there, as does secondary periosteal ossification in the vertebral bodies. Here we are attempting to characterize only the dominant process in each instance, which will suggest the respective formative principle.

The ***ribs***, which are attached to the front of the vertebrae, are completely independent structures and develop more or less like the long bones of the limbs.

It is interesting to note that the mesenchyme that appears on the anterior ends of the ribs and develops into the primordium of the breastbone belongs primarily to the ribs. Fusion of these blastemas (sternal bars) on either side results in what is known as the ***sternal plates*** (Figure 240).

As the ribs lengthen and the thorax grows, these two crests grow closer together and ultimately fuse (from the top down) to form the breastbone (sternum).

The **sacrum** develops out of five fused vertebrae whose development is no different in principle from that of the other vertebrae. The lateral portions of the sacrum, which develop out of primordial rib material, increase greatly in size and make up most of the mature bone. The neural arches are transformed into the posterior sections of the sacrum and the vertebral bodies into the anterior sections. Even in the adult sacrum, the structural elements of the former vertebral primordia are clearly recognizable.

The Skull as a Metamorphosis of the Torso and Limb Skeleton

As mentioned earlier, Goethe was the first to recognize that individual skull bones could be seen as metamorphosed vertebrae. In 1790, he described organ metamorphosis in plants and applied it to understanding the essential nature of plants. The obvious next step was to attempt to apply the idea of metamorphosis (so closely related to the theory of evolution, which had recently surfaced for the first time in human history) to a deeper understanding of the forms of animal and human bodies. Goethe describes pulling a battered sheep skull from the sand dunes in the Jewish cemetery near Venice in 1790. He immediately recognized that skull bones are metamorphosed vertebrae. As if touched by a higher spiritual reality, Goethe found himself deeply moved and disturbed by this thought, as he promptly reported to friends. He kept the idea to himself, however, pondering it in silence, until Lorenz Oken, professor of anatomy at the University of Jena, suddenly went public with it, causing Goethe considerable agitation. Here are Goethe's own words from his collected scientific writings (94):

The second part of my Morphology recounts how I had the opportunity to examine and recognize first three, then six vertebrae. In this observation I found hope and the prospect of great reassurance. I considered the development of this thought in detail, but without arriving at anything conclusive. Finally I spoke about it confidentially among friends, who agreed thoughtfully and followed my line of thinking in their own way.

In 1807 this tenet was sprung upon the public tumultuously, in incomplete form, and in a way that inevitably produced much controversy and some acclaim. How much damage was done by the premature nature of the presentation will be left to history to decide, but the worst was its false influence on a worthy and magnificent work. Unfortunately, this harm will become more and more apparent in the aftermath.

Oken's publications made a very strong impression on the scientific community of the time and—as mentioned at the beginning of this chapter—initiated awareness of the so-called "head problem." As a result, the development of the vertebrate head has been the repeated subject of scientific studies. Today an abundance of detailed information is available, but the problem of Goethe's skull metamorphosis cannot be considered solved. In fact, Rudolf Steiner emphasized that it could never be solved without reference to reincarnation (65). From this perspective, it makes sense that Goethe was unable to come to terms with vertebral metamorphosis during his lifetime. Although he was familiar with the idea of reincarnation and convinced of its truth on a spiritual level, he was not yet fully able to grasp its scientific implications. Hence his reluctance to approach this problem scientifically.

Later research took a different direction, and the profundity of the problem was increasingly forgotten as scientific analysis brought more details to light. In the section that follows, we will attempt to speak as frankly as possible about the actual phenomena.

Vertebral Metamorphosis

The spine consists of thirty-one to thirty-three vertebrae (seven cervical, twelve thoracic, and five lumbar vertebrae, plus the five fused vertebrae of the sacrum and three to six coccygeal vertebrae). The vertebrae are securely stacked, separated only by their intervertebral discs. Posterior articular processes (Figure 241A and B) allow a certain degree of mobility. All **vertebrae** share a basic structure but differ considerably in their structural details, depending on where they are located in the spine. Each vertebra consists of an anterior vertebral body and a posterior neural arch with a total of seven processes—four articular processes and three that serve as points of attachment for muscles (Figures 241A and B). The locations of the processes reflect the three dimensions of space: the articular processes are located on the vertebra's upper and lower surfaces, the spinous process is posteriorly located, and the transverse processes are laterally located. The vertebral body, a massive, unarticulated structure, is bean-shaped in the lumbar region, triangular in the thoracic region, and trapezoidal in the cervical region (Figure 242). The vertebral body decreases consistently in size from the bottom to the top of the spine and is totally absent in the first cervical vertebra (atlas). Instead, the second cervical vertebra (axis) has a "tooth" (dens) or upright peg around which the atlas (and with it, the entire head) can rotate.

The **vertebral processes** also become smaller and more delicate toward the top of the spine and are reduced to mere stumps in the atlas and axis (Figure 242). The atlas is a relatively shapeless ring with a minimum of distinguishing features. The ribs are fully differentiated only in the thoracic segments. In the cervical region, they appear as little extra prongs (anterior tubercles) on the transverse processes; in the lumbar region, the rudimentary rib is identical with the transverse process, which in this case is also called the costal (rib) element (cf. Figure 11). Thus the rib element is not totally absent in the spinal segments above and below the ribcage. From bottom to top, variation in the size of the rib elements results in two cycles of expansion and contraction in the vertebrae. In

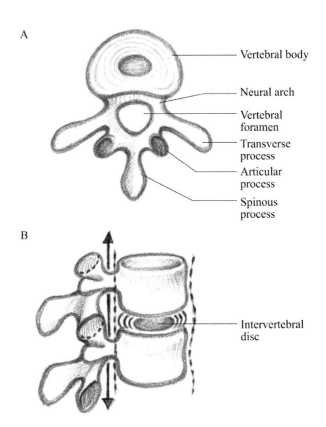

Fig. 241. **Structure of the vertebrae and spine**.
A: *Structural elements of an individual vertebra (here, a lumbar vertebra viewed from above);*
B: *Connection between vertebrae (side view of two lumbar vertebrae).*
Arrow: vertebral canal (foramen).

the sacrum, the rib element expands dramatically and constitutes most of the bone mass (lateral mass) of the sacrum. In the lumbar vertebrae, the "ribs" are reduced to delicate processes. In the thoracic region, twelve pairs of true ribs develop, forming the ribcage. In the cervical region, the rib elements are again reduced and are restricted to the anterior portions of the transverse processes. In the atlas, they disappear almost completely. We might expect to find a renewed expansion of this structural element in the head (Figure 11, p. 30, and Figure 242).

Similar rhythmic changes are also evident in the two other vertebral structural elements. The **vertebral body** becomes smaller toward the top of the spine. Ultimately, in the axis and atlas, the

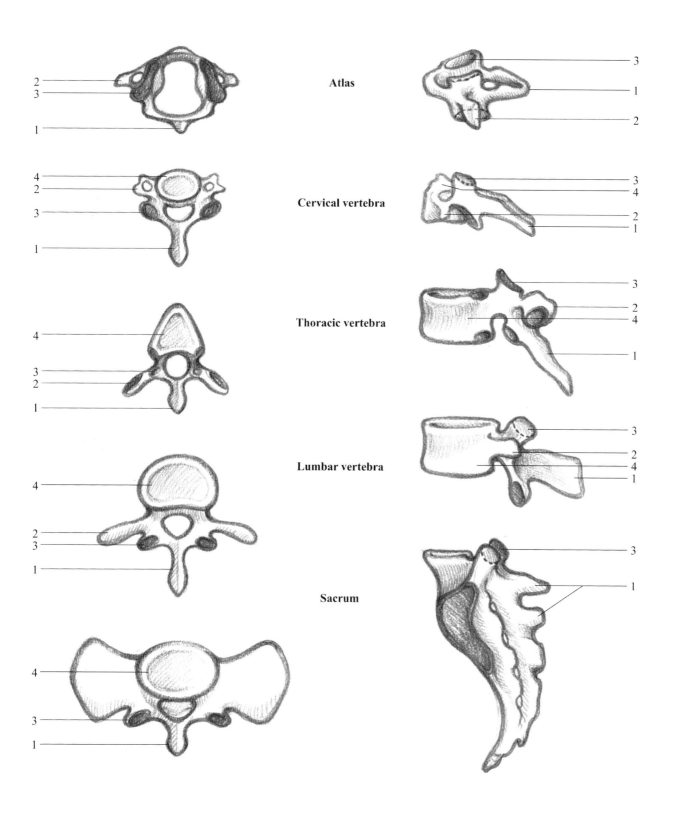

Fig. 242. **Changes in the shape of the vertebrae within the spine**.
Left column: View from above; right column: Side view from the left; blue: Articular surfaces.
1: Spinous process; 2: Transverse process; 3: Articular process; 4: Vertebral body.

A

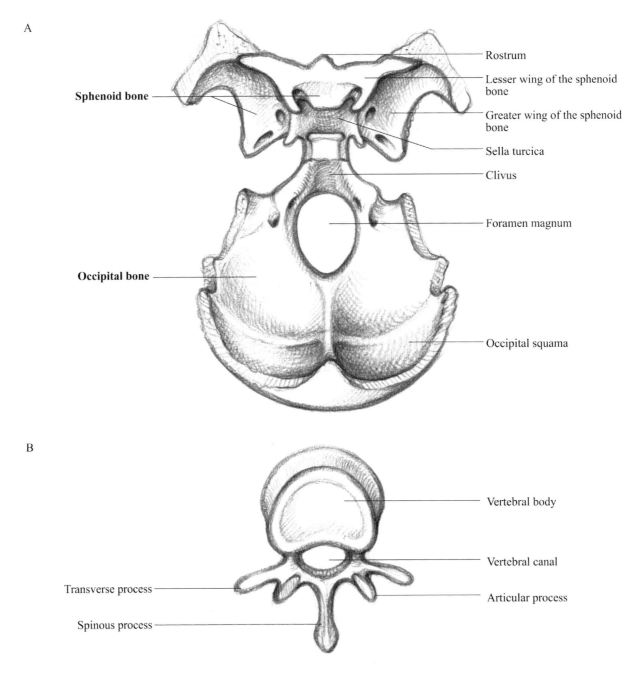

Sphenoid bone

Rostrum

Lesser wing of the sphenoid bone

Greater wing of the sphenoid bone

Sella turcica

Clivus

Foramen magnum

Occipital bone

Occipital squama

B

Vertebral body

Vertebral canal

Transverse process

Articular process

Spinous process

Fig. 243. **Metamorphosis of a vertebra into the skull.** *Comparison of a lumbar vertebra to the bones of the base of the skull.*
A: Os basilare, which consists of the sphenoid and occipital bones;
B: a lumbar vertebra (both viewed from above).

To metamorphose into the base of the skull, the vertebra must rotate in the front/back dimension and undergo further transformations in its shape (for details, see text).

weight-bearing masses shift to the sides and nothing remains of the anterior portion except a ring of bone that is remarkably similar to the posterior neural arches. The vertebral processes also grow smaller toward the top of the spine. In the lumbar vertebrae, the spinous process is broad and substantial and extends straight back. In the thoracic vertebrae, it "droops" diagonally downward, and in the cervical region it begins

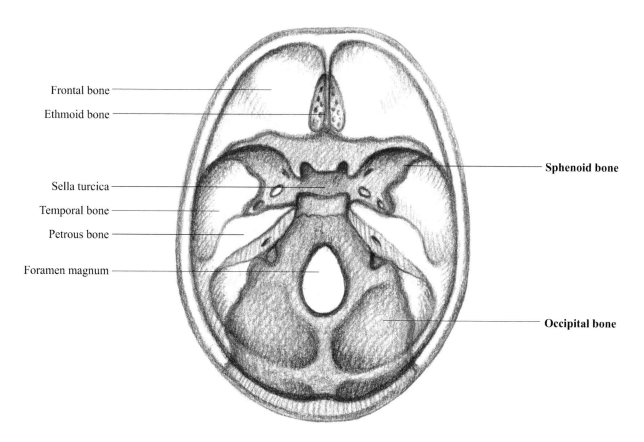

Frontal bone

Ethmoid bone

Sella turcica

Temporal bone

Petrous bone

Foramen magnum

Sphenoid bone

Occipital bone

Fig. 244. **Base of the skull** *(view from above). The os basilare (red), which consists of the anteriorly located sphenoid bone and the posteriorly located occipital bone, is the "foundation" of the base of the skull. It represents the metamorphosed spine, or Goethe's "vertebra of the head."*

to "fly," separating into two parts that spread out like wings. In the atlas, the spinous process is reduced to a very small appendage. In the thoracic spine, the articular processes, which are vertically oriented in the lumbar spine, shift toward the front and their articular surfaces become nearly horizontal. In the cervical spine, they shift almost to the sides of the vertebrae; in the axis, they form a horizontal surface next to the vertebral body to support the atlas.

If we pursue these metamorphosing forms still farther, into the base of the skull, we discover two closely associated bones (the sphenoid and occipital bones) that together exhibit all the structural elements of a vertebra, but with front and back reversed (Figure 243). The seven posteriorly

located vertebral processes correspond to the seven anterior processes, some of them wing-shaped, that emerge from the body of the sphenoid bone: the lesser wings above, the greater wings to the side, the pterygoid processes below, and in front the rostrum, which is oriented toward the nasal septum. The anteriorly located body of the vertebra corresponds to the similarly undivided, bowllike occipital bone with its two lateral portions surrounding the foramen magnum. The sphenoid and occipital bones (collectively called the *os basilare*) are surprisingly similar in structure to a vertebra (such as the lumbar vertebra shown in Figure 243). But we must avoid the purely analogous thinking of Mees, for example (95). The structural metamorphoses (in the front/

A

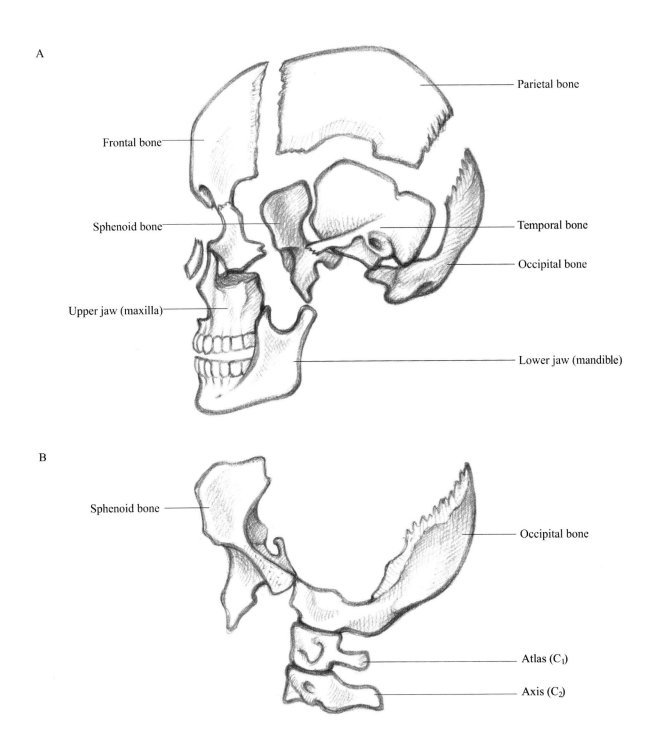

Frontal bone

Parietal bone

Sphenoid bone

Temporal bone

Occipital bone

Upper jaw (maxilla)

Lower jaw (mandible)

B

Sphenoid bone

Occipital bone

Atlas (C₁)

Axis (C₂)

Fig. 245. **The disassembled skull** (side view).
A: location of the base of the skull (os basilare, red), which consists of the sphenoid bone (anterior) and the occipital bone (posterior). The temporal bone fits into the gap between the sphenoid and occipital bones.
B: the "head vertebra" (sphenoid and occipital bone), isolated and viewed from the side, together with the first two cervical vertebrae (atlas, C_1, and axis, C_2).

back dimension, for example) that we have just attempted to describe indicate that even deeper mysteries lie concealed here.

We cannot simply consider the os basilare the "vertebra" of the skull. In this bone we can see not only a metamorphosed individual vertebra but also a formation that encompasses the structural elements of ***all vertebrae*** in idealized form. ***The os basilare integrates the entire spine into a single ideal structure. This principle of integration is the real mystery of vertebral metamorphosis***. At the level of the atlas, a null point is reached. A complete reversal of front and back occurs. But the form also enters a new space, where it manifests uninfluenced by the Earth's gravitational field. This is the only way to explain the wonderful winged shape of the os basilare, the skull's "foundation" (Figures 244 and 245).

It is difficult to imagine a complete reversal of this type taking place during embryonic development simultaneously with integration into a more highly differentiated structure, especially since head formation outpaces the development of the torso and limbs. For this reason, Rudolf Steiner always viewed the development of the head as "proof" of his theory of reincarnation (65).

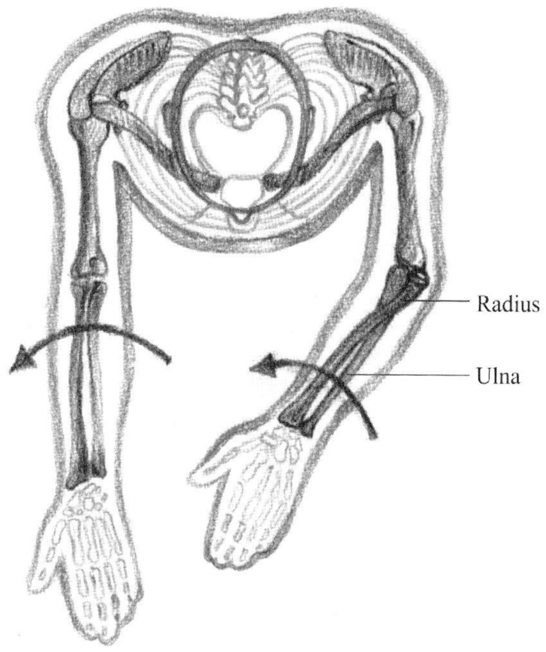

*Fig. 246. **Arm bones and pectoral girdle**, showing supination (right arm) and pronation (left arm). Inward rotation (arrow) causes crossing of the two lower arm bones (radius and ulna), which are parallel in the supination position (arrow).*

Upper Limb Metamorphosis

The principle of integration also helps us understand how limb bones metamorphose into the skull. Because the bony elements of limbs are all relatively similar in shape, the search for analogous individual elements does not lead very far in this instance (95). We can approach the essential nature of a limb only by attempting to grasp the dynamics of its movements and tracing them back to their archetypal images.

The upper limb belongs to the torso's midsection. The pectoral girdle rests on top of the ribcage, and arm movements take place primarily in the horizontal dimension. Uprightness frees the upper extremity to move between above and below (cosmos and Earth). All arm movements are based on two archetypal gestures that are apparent from the very structure of the hand.

One gesture involves pronation (inward rotation) and the opposability of the thumb. This gesture turns the hand into a grasping organ. Closing the hand to make a fist or take hold of a tool or other object is the archetypal gesture of creative activity in earthly space—in other words, of transforming will into deeds (Homo faber). The opposite gesture results when the hand is opened, the thumb returns to its original position, and the arm turns outward (supination, Figure 246). This is a gesture of receptivity, submission, or openness to something higher or nonearthly—i.e., to the cosmos (Homo sapiens). It is also the gesture of prayer, pleading, or quiet listening to inspiration from above. In contrast, a clenched fist has always been the gesture of work or of militant (even revolutionary) will. In fact, the entire anatomy of the upper limbs can be deduced from this polarity in their movements.

A

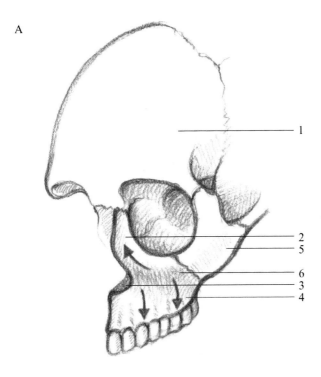

*Fig. 247. **Structure of the upper jaw and its location in the skull.***

A: Diagonal front view of a partial mosaic of the facial bones showing the upper jaw, zygomatic bone, and frontal bone. Arrows (red) indicate the opposing dynamics of the upper jaw's frontal and alveolar processes. The palatine process, a balancing element, runs horizontally.

B: Front view of the facial skull. The two upper jawbones surround the entrance to the nasal cavity. Together with the zygomatic bones, they make up the central portion of the facial skeleton and define individual facial expressions. Red arrows: Directions of movement of the four maxillary processes.

1: Frontal bone
2: Frontal process ⎫
3: Palatine process ⎬ of the upper jaw
4: Alveolar process ⎭
5: Zygomatic bone
6: Zygomatic process of the upper jaw

B

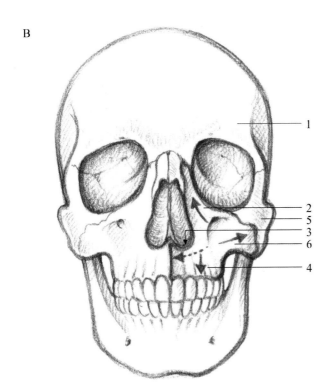

In Leonardo da Vinci's **Last Supper**, the Christ demonstrates the active gesture (pronation) with his right arm and the receptive gesture (supination) with his left. It is interesting to note that all of the disciples on his right are gesturing in pronation, those on his left in supination. In a brilliant artistic expression of these archetypal arm movements, Leonardo illustrates the position of the human being between above and below (or cosmos and Earth), as well as the central position of the Christ between two extremes.

In the mosaic of the skull, the shape of the **upper jaw** (**maxilla**, Figure 247) expresses the polarity of these movements. The upper jaw has four processes that extend outward from the body of the bone, which encloses the maxillary sinus. The delicate frontal process swings upward in an elegant gesture. Together with the nasal bone and the frontal bone, it forms the root of the nose. The greatest concentration of "I" consciousness is possible in this point, which the Brahmans of India emphasize with a red dot. The frontal processes of both halves of the upper jaw surround the nasal cavity, revealing their relationship to the rhythmic (respiratory) system (Figure 247).

Below the frontal process, the alveolar process develops. This portion of the bone holds the teeth. It is also involved in the structure of the oral cavity, where chewing reduces food to small pieces and initiates the body's involvement with solid earthly matter. In the alveolar process, the arm gesture of pronation or making a fist is again visible (Figure 247).

Two other processes—the lateral zygomatic process and the inward-directed palatine process—occupy intermediate positions between the upward-sweeping frontal process and the alveolar gesture of gripping the teeth below (Figure 247). The palate separates the oral and nasal cavities. It is the "diaphragm" of the head, so to speak. Instead of separating disparate elements, the zygomatic process joins them. It links the braincase (which houses the brain and the organs of hearing and equilibrium) to the facial skull, which is more closely related to metabolic and respiratory functions.

Thus the shape of the upper jaw expresses the dynamic of the upper limbs in archetypal form. As is also true of vertebral metamorphosis in the skull, however, the upper jaw does not repeat the structural details of the arm but sums them up in a single *integrated, all-encompassing form*.

The Zygomatic Bone and the Frontal Bone

The human arm's extensive range of motion is due to two features. The clavicle (collarbone) holds it away from the ribcage and the scapula (a flat bone that slides within large loops of muscles) allows it to move freely above the torso. Similarly, the upper jaw's integrative expressiveness in the facial skull is possible only because it is supported from above by the frontal bone and from behind by the zygomatic bone in the base of the skull. Like the scapula, the frontal bone is a flat bone originally consisting of two parts that fuse at an early stage of development (Figure 237). The frontal bone is a plate that is bent at a right angle, forming the roof of the eye socket. Its brow ridges

and the shape of the root of the nose (glabella) contribute a great deal to the signature of an individual face (Figure 147). Just as the mobility of the scapula (especially its ability to rotate) allows the arm to access the "heavenly space" above the horizontal, the frontal bone reflects the individual's "I"-being, which grapples with the forces of the "heavenly" or spiritual world in thinking.

Through their roles in shaping the bony eye socket, both the frontal bone and the zygomatic bone are significantly involved in the location of the eye, our light-sensing organ (Figure 247). In lower vertebrates, the eyes are located laterally, in the temporal region, rather than frontally (Figure 40C). In humans, the eyes shift to the front and the direction of their longitudinal axes changes, allowing us to experience the spatial world through binocular vision. (This shift is associated with uprightness and the development of a more spherical head.) The zygomatic bone, which forms the sidewall of the eye socket, plays a significant role in separating the socket from the temporal cavity (Figure 40D). The trident-shaped zygomatic bone also links the upper jaw, temporal bone, and frontal bone into a stable, expressive structure and is thus a determining factor in the physiognomy of the face, i.e., in the visage of the "I" or individual. Together with the opposable thumb and the lower arm's ability to rotate, the pectoral girdle (collarbone, scapula, and shoulder joint) of the upright human being creates the freedom of movement that makes possible an infinite variety of body language, technical accomplishments, and—ultimately—cultural achievements.

We sense that the initiative for arm movements always emanates from a point on the back between the scapulas. Similarly, along with the brow ridges and the zygomatic bone as a link to the back of the skull, the human forehead with its "I point" at the root of the nose is a telling expression of the essential being and character of a human individuality and its past.

Lower Limb Metamorphosis

Are integrative formative principles also apparent in the metamorphosis of the lower limbs in the head, as is the case with the upper limbs? To begin, let's observe the unique functions of the lower limbs. Here, too, we find two basic functions:

1. Support of the vertically balanced, upright body while walking;

2. Locomotion, primarily in the horizontal plane.

Maintaining support and balance while freeing one leg from the Earth's gravitational field is a prerequisite of locomotion. To serve this purpose, the lower limbs develop arching structures at all essential points—for example, in the pelvic ring, the arches of the feet, and the hip joints. Like the arches in Romanesque cathedrals or the more utilitarian Roman structures such as aqueducts, which are especially suited to supporting heavy weights, the skeletal structure of the lower limbs also manifests a static principle capable of supporting the body's weight elegantly and harmoniously (Figure 248). The human body is adapted but not subordinated to the Earth's gravitational field. The almost weightless stability of beautiful Romanesque domes is also discernable in the arrangement of our lower limbs.

An arch encompasses both integration into gravity and release from gravity. The weight-bearing columns of the leg bones are constructed to resist longitudinal forces (push and pull). Their spongy tissue is trajectorial in structure. Through arching structures, especially in the feet, the legs free themselves from the ground and become mobile in three-dimensional space. Each leg serves alternately as the supporting leg and the free leg. Unlike our arms, which can be independent of each other in their movements, our legs are dependent on each other for their movement. They form a functional unity because they always have to work together.

The second major complex of functions involves locomotion. Here, the principle of the angle

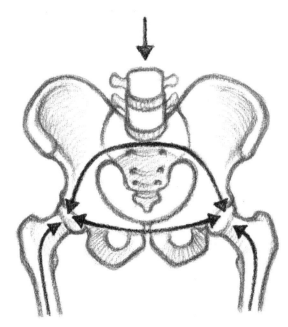

Fig. 248. ***Arched structure of the pelvis****. The pelvic arch transmits the downward thrust of the lumbar spine (vertical arrow) to the heads of the femur. Crossbracing is provided by the arch of the pubic bone.*

lever plays a role. The foot and lower leg form a right-angled lever that is moved by muscles pulling on tendons, some of which are very long. The principle of the angle lever is also realized in the movement of the knee and hip joints. In locomotion, flexion and extension are the chief movements. Rotation is generally avoided and is possible only in the free leg.

Now that we have grasped the basic dynamic of the lower limbs, metamorphic correspondences also become apparent in the head. In the ***lower jaw***, which represents a metamorphosis of the lower limbs, the angle lever appears in perfect form. The body of the lower jaw is attached to the ascending ramus, which ends in two processes—the coronoid process, which serves as a point of attachment for muscles, and the condylar (articular) process. Initially separate in embryonic development, the two halves of the jaw later fuse into a single bone so that the functional collaboration present only on a dynamic level in the legs becomes a definitive, unified structure in the lower jaw.

The basic structure of the lower jaw is the ***basal arch***. The alveolar process and teeth perch on top of it as if on a balcony (Figure 249). Together, the basal arch, alveolar process and teeth form the body of the lower jaw, which does the actual work of chewing—biting off and grinding bits of food. This, however, is the exact opposite of what takes place in the lower limbs. In the lower jaw, instead of integration into three-dimensional space, we find three-dimensional bodies being broken down to begin the digestive process. Essentially, chewing and liquefying food signifies that solid matter is entering the fluid phase, beginning the digestive process of releasing the forces inherent in matter.

But the second function of the lower limbs, locomotion (in which the angle lever plays such an important role), is also evident in the lower jaw. We have already mentioned the lower jaw's angled shape. Its ascending branch terminates in the condylar process, which articulates with the temporal bone to form the ***jaw joint*** (***temporomandibular joint***). We might expect to find the lower limbs' dynamic of locomotion reflected in the lower jaw, but here again circumstances are reversed in the head. It is interesting to note that the mechanical work of chewing is not accomplished by putting strain on the jaw joint. On the contrary, the joint is largely relieved of the mechanical stresses of chewing (pressure, tension, etc.). Nature accomplishes this stratagem by lengthening the angle lever. If the ascending branch of the jaw were very short, the result would be significant pressure on the joint, but in humans the relatively long ascending branch reduces the pressure to almost nothing, as photoelastic stress analysis confirms (120), and the joint moves relatively freely. In humans, although not in animals, the jaw's range of motion is so great that we might speak of a natural, physiological dislocation. Whenever the mouth is opened wide, the head of the jaw slides out of its socket. The cartilaginous articular disk of the jaw joint then allows both parts of the joint to be used in a variety of ways, making even more movement combinations possible.

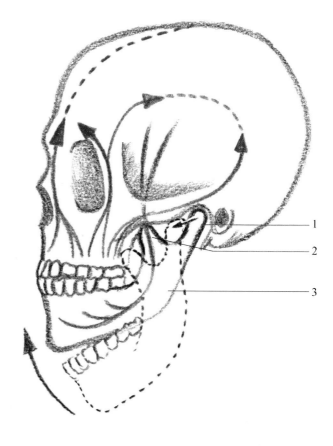

Fig. 249. ***The skeleton of the jaw***, *showing the trajectories that dissipate the force of chewing. The jaw joint is largely relieved of the pressure of chewing.*
1: Articular (condylar) process; 2: Muscle (coronoid) process; 3: Basal arch.

Like the femur neck angle in the leg, the ***angle of the lower jaw*** changes over time. (In the jaw, the change is due to functional demands on the chewing apparatus and changes in dentition.) In the jaw, however, unlike the leg, the result is the release of the joint from the confines of three-dimensional space, leading to an unusually great variety of new movement possibilities. This development occurs only in humans. Its prerequisites are complete bodily uprightness, the angle at the base of the skull, and the inhibition of jaw growth in the front-back dimension. (In human evolution, a right-angled lower jaw is one of the most important features distinguishing Homo sapiens from apes or early hominids.) This development helped make speech possible. In addition to a harmonious, closed row of teeth, a mobile tongue, and a descended larynx, speech also requires a delicate jaw joint relieved of most pressure. When we speak, however, we always imprint something of a spiritual character on a spatial formation of air and warmth that never achieves full material reality. The lower limbs' movement in space thus undergoes a metamorphosis in the lower jaw, which is freed from mechanical stresses in order to serve as the foundation for reshaping spatial forces into speech and song. We will return to this subject when we discuss the temporal bone in relationship to the ear.

Temporal Bone and Pelvis

In comparing the scapula and pelvis, we saw that the pelvis has a double, lemniscatic framework with the hip joint located in its crossing point (Figures 56 and 57). The upper framework, the ilium, forms the greater or true pelvis. The lower framework (ischium and pubic bone), which develops out of vertebral processes, makes up the lesser or false pelvis, which houses the genitals. Together with the sacrum, these bones develop into the solid body of the pelvis, which provides a stable foundation for the upright torso on the one hand and for the moving legs on the other (Figure 250). Thus the pelvis exhibits a polarity of formative gestures—on the one hand the upward-directed, expansive tendency of the ilium and on the other the downward-directed thickening of the ischium (Figure 250). Thus the pelvis mediates between the two poles of our existence, between above (uprightness, levity, release from space) and below (integration into space, stasis, solidification). As such, it is the keystone of the entire skeleton, which it constantly keeps in balance.

In the head, the ***temporal bone*** exhibits a similar dynamic in its form (Figure 251A). In the course of development, four different bones fuse to form the temporal bone. Let's consider its most important elements.

The squama is a membranous bone that develops in the same way as the flat bony plates

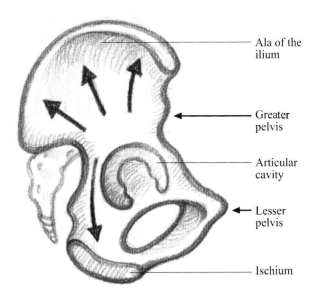

Fig. 250. ***The double framework of the pelvic bone****. Polar formative gestures—upward expansion of the flat surface of the ilium (arrows) and thickening of the downward-directed, radial ischium (single arrow) are apparent here, as they also are in the temporal bone.*

of the skullcap. As it develops, the squama grows outward in all directions (radially) from a point more or less on the level of the external auditory canal. As it grows toward the skullcap, it slides over the lower edge of the parietal bone.

The developmental gesture of the petrous portion of the temporal bone, often referred to here as just the "petrous bone," is very different. This pyramidal section of bone inserts itself like a wedge between the sphenoid bone and the occipital bone (Figure 251B). It develops on a cartilaginous foundation and soon encloses the labyrinth capsule (which contains the organ of balance and the inner ear) as well as the middle ear. Together with the mastoid process, the petrous bone forms a drop-shaped protrusion of bone that juts out at the bottom. Structurally, the petrous bone is the polar opposite of the squama. The delicate zygomatic process (which is horizontal and forward-directed in its orientation) holds the balance between the two (Figure 251A).

Comparing the embryonic pelvic bone to a side view of the temporal bone reveals distinct

A

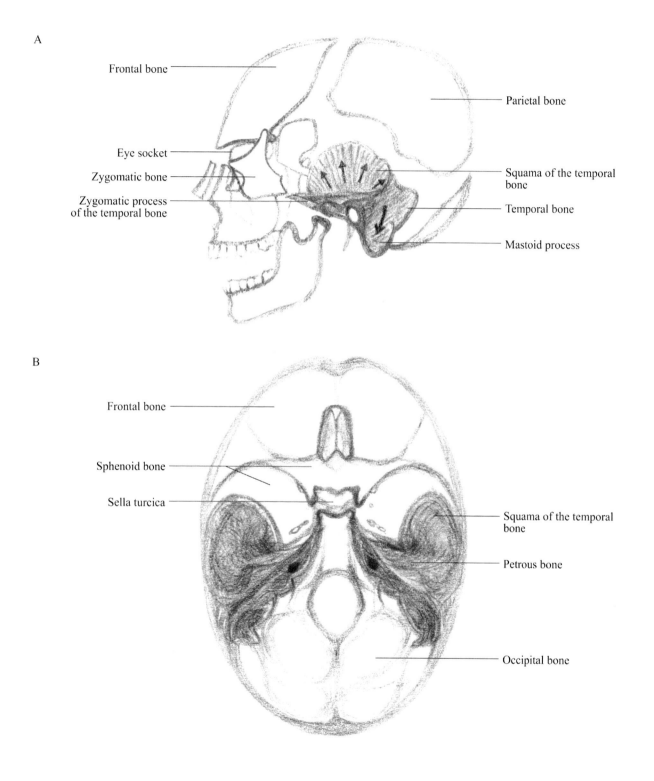

Frontal bone

Parietal bone

Eye socket

Zygomatic bone

Zygomatic process
of the temporal bone

Squama of the temporal
bone

Temporal bone

Mastoid process

B

Frontal bone

Sphenoid bone

Sella turcica

Squama of the temporal
bone

Petrous bone

Occipital bone

Fig. 251. **Position of the temporal bone** (red) **in the mosaic of the skull.**
A: The skull disassembled.
B: The base of the skull as seen from above. The temporal bone fills the gap between the sphenoid bone and the occipital bone. The petrous bone, which is part of the temporal bone, extends all the way to the sella turcica.

structural similarities. The flat, expansive ilium corresponds to the squama of the temporal bone, the zyogmatic and mastoid processes to the processes of the hip bone that develop into the pubic bone and ischium. In the center of these two opposing formative tendencies lie the acetabulum (in the leg) and the jaw joint and auditory canal (in the temporal bone). But no matter how convincing it may be at first glance, this formal analogy leads us no farther. We must consider the inner, functional dynamic in order to truly understand the metamorphosis.

The *pelvis* is the resting base from which all movement of the lower limbs originates, beginning with the hip joint. In the context of the whole, therefore, the pelvis is the foundation for creating and maintaining a balance between movements above and below it. Our limbs extend outward into space in the process of turning our conceived movements into deeds.

In contrast, the wedge-shaped *petrous bone* retreats into the skull (Figure 251B). Through hearing, the inner ear (housed in the petrous bone) makes us conscious of the inner nature of the spatial world. The outer auditory canal is a gateway to the inner world, while the acetabulum leads to the outer world. In the former, we experience the architecture of matter through hearing; in the latter, we experience the world of space directly and actively through our movements. The female pelvis provides a space where a new being can incarnate out of the spiritual world into a body. The petrous bone creates space for the organs of hearing and equilibrium. The organ of equilibrium allows three-dimensional space as such to become manifest through sensory activity; the organ of hearing does the same for the spatial world's internal architecture as expressed in different frequency ratios. In order to serve this function, the petrous bone must renounce any life of its own. As described in an earlier section, it develops out of blood and connective tissue through endochondral ossification but loses its blood-producing marrow at an early stage of development, "dying off" to become the hardest, most calcified bone in the body. Other bones that develop through endochondral ossification are rich in spongy tissue and remain capable of alteration

and adaptation for a lifetime. In other words, they are relatively alive and capable of regeneration. This is not the case with the petrous bone. During the first few years of life, its marrow is replaced by air-filled hollow spaces (pneumatization), making later internal modifications impossible.

The *pneumatization of the petrous bone*, which makes the middle ear functional as an organ of sound conduction, is a very mysterious process. It begins around the eighth month of gestation, when an epithelial bud grows into the middle ear, which is still completely filled with loose-meshed mesenchyme. The epithelial bud grows rapidly, displacing mesenchyme, until the ossicles finally lie free and exposed, covered only with mucous membrane, in the hollow space of the middle ear (cf. Figure 183). At birth, pneumatization is complete in the middle ear but still continues in the inner ear, displacing the blood-producing marrow of the petrous bone's spongy bone and transforming it into air-filled "mastoid cells" (Figure 183). In the process of pneumatization, the petrous bone almost completely loses the cell-rich marrow tissue needed for regeneration and adaptation. As a result, it becomes the only bone in the body that can no longer be modified. Thus our ability to hear is purchased at the expense of the petrous bone's life and ability to regenerate. The name "petrous," which derives from the Greek for "stone," is thus completely justified.

The Principle of Formative Integration in Tooth Development

Human teeth are not uniform rods inserted into the jaw with no relationship to each other. Instead, they reveal characteristic individual elements, and the principle of integration is as apparent in their structure and development as it is in the upper and lower jawbones whose alveolar processes hold the teeth.

Baby teeth (the first dentition) include three distinct groups of teeth: incisors, canines, and primary molars. Each incisor is chisel-shaped,

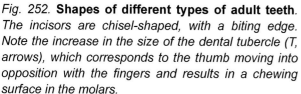

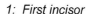

1: *First incisor*
3: *Canine tooth*
5: *Second premolar*
6: *First molar*

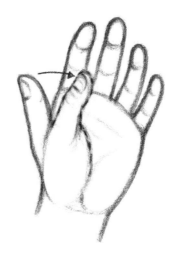

Upper jaw

Lower jaw

Fig. 252. **Shapes of different types of adult teeth**. *The incisors are chisel-shaped, with a biting edge. Note the increase in the size of the dental tubercle (T, arrows), which corresponds to the thumb moving into opposition with the fingers and results in a chewing surface in the molars.*

with a shallow concavity facing the oral cavity and the merest trace of a dental tubercle. This shape is comparable to an outstretched hand in the supination position, as in a gesture of receiving or entreating (Figure 252). The slightly concave inner surface of the tooth corresponds to the palm of the hand, the biting edge to the fingers and thumb held side by side, and the dental tubercle to the ball of the thumb.

In the canine teeth, the biting edge becomes pointed and the tubercle more prominent. In the primary molars, a horizontal chewing surface emerges for the first time as the tubercle develops into an independent cusp. In comparison to permanent teeth, the first primary molar is shaped like a premolar, the second more like a molar. The primary molars are actual functional molars, capable of crushing and grinding food. They do most of the actual work of chewing. Incisors can bite food into pieces but cannot chew effectively. Hence the primary molars with their two cusps are much more comparable to a grasping hand with its opposable thumb. Chewing surfaces develop because the palatine cusps increase so greatly in size in the molars. The gesture of this metamorphosis is similar to what happens

when the thumb moves into opposition with the other fingers, shifting the hand from the receptive position to the grasping position adapted to earthly work (Figure 252). The molars, therefore, are the teeth most closely related to metabolic tasks, while the incisors, which receive food without processing it, are more outward directed and serve a senselike function. The canine teeth occupy an intermediate position between these two polar groups (Figure 252).

In considering how the arms metamorphose in the head, we must not immediately compare nails to teeth when we look for correspondences (95). Although it is true that five baby teeth develop in each side of the upper jaw—exactly as many as the fingers or nails of our hands—we have already seen that individual limb elements do not reappear in the metamorphosis of limbs into the head. Instead, the dynamic principle of the limbs as such assumes a permanent form in the head. Similarly, the shape of the teeth expresses in an ***integrative*** manner the entire dynamic of movement between the polar "upper" (cosmic/peripheral) and "lower" (centralized/earthly) elements. In each individual tooth, this integration into a whole is repeated, each time with a somewhat different emphasis.

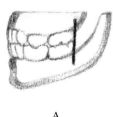 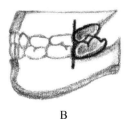 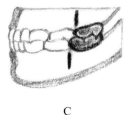

A   B   C

Fig. 253. **Alignment of the six-year molars at the beginning of the second dentition.** *Displacement of the upper and lower first molars (red) allows cusps and grooves to mesh in a normal adult bite (occlusion) without requiring any change in the size of the dental arch of the first dentition (adapted from Korkhaus 137). A: A three-year-old child; B and C: A six-year-old child.*

With regard to the organism as a whole, the incisors tend toward the nerve/sense aspect, the molars more toward the metabolism and limbs, and the canine teeth toward the harmonizing middle. This ***threefoldness in dentition*** is also confirmed by specialized dentition patterns in animals and by the unique ***physiognomic features of human teeth*** (cf. also Figure 44). Rodents (rats, rabbits, etc.) have pronounced incisors that continue to grow as long as the animal is alive. As a rule, rodents are nervous, restless animals with acute senses. In contrast, molars predominate in the dentition of ruminants, which devote themselves peacefully to their metabolic activity. And finally, all the teeth of carnivores resemble canine teeth. In carnivore species, the middle system is emphasized one-sidedly and both metabolic activity and sensory processes are more restrained.

Human teeth also reflect a similar trend. Individuals with strongly developed, rodentlike, or protruding incisors are usually alert, lively, extroverted characters who are quick to grasp outer events but often process them only superficially. As a rule, people with sharp, prominent canine teeth are active, flexible personalities, easily emotionally stimulated. In contrast, individuals with dominant molars and less prominent incisors and canines are often more introverted, and metabolic and will

processes are emphasized in them. Teeth say a great deal about a person's character because they are one of the most highly formed elements in the head. Scientific dental physiognomy, however, is still in its earliest stages, as is also true of the physiognomy of the face, ear, and other parts of the body.

Second dentition. Until now, we have been talking primarily about the baby teeth, which are later replaced by permanent teeth. The second dentition begins with the eruption of the first molar between the sixth and seventh years of life. This tooth is the cornerstone of the permanent teeth (Figure 253).

The rhombic shape of the crown of the first upper molar staggers the spacing of the teeth so that each successive emerging tooth rests in the space between the two teeth above or below it. (This is a change from the situation in the first dentition, where the primary molars are vertically aligned). Exact vertical alignment of permanent teeth would mean that a normal, characteristically human adult bite (occlusion) could not develop. Thus we can see that the architecture of the permanent teeth is built up from the back of the mouth to the front. The front section of the arch of the first dentition remains unchanged in size, although the space available for individual teeth is adjusted (Figure 253).

The skeletal system plays a decisive role in this process. Two forces work together in the eruption of a tooth:

1. The tooth primordium with its root blastema. This is the actual driving force behind the eruption of a tooth, because the proliferation of the mesenchyme of the dental papilla and dental follicle lead to a rapid increase in size in the root, which forces the primitive tooth out of the alveolus (socket).

2. The reshaping of the bony alveolus in which the primitive tooth is embedded. As the tooth emerges, local buildup and breakdown of bone constantly reshape the alveolus, thus altering the tooth's direction of growth.

This process can be compared to firing a gun. The "powder" (root blastema) provides the needed force, and the barrel of the gun determines the bullet's direction. Thus the bone of the jaw is the deciding factor in the positions and spatial relationships of individual teeth within the whole (Figure 254). When we consider that osteoblasts (bone-building cells) and osteoclasts (bone-resorbing cells) both originate in the blood-producing mesenchyme of the bone marrow, the holistic character of tooth development immediately becomes apparent.

The harmonious arrangement of human teeth (closed row, normal occlusion, similar tooth lengths) is primarily a result of bone growth (Figure 254). Development of the baby teeth (first dentition) is associated with a maturation process that involves the entire body and is completed at the end of the first seven years of life, when the child is ready for school. In the child's sixth or seventh year, the body—including the teeth, the body's hardest structures—has developed to a point that allows formal learning. School readiness means simply that bodily forces once involved in growth and development are now released from that "commitment" and can be applied to thinking and learning.

The second dentition, which usually occurs between a child's sixth or seventh and twelfth to fourteenth year, is again linked to the more

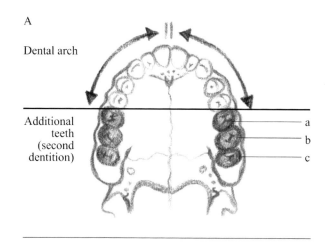

a: First molar, 6 -7ᵗʰ year of life (school readiness)
b: Second molar, 12-14ᵗʰ year (sexual maturity)
c: Third molar, 18-20ᵗʰ year (social maturity/"coming of age")

a: First molar, 6 -7th year of life (school readiness)
b: Second molar, 12-14th year (sexual maturity)
c: Third molar, 18-20th year (social maturity/ "coming of age")

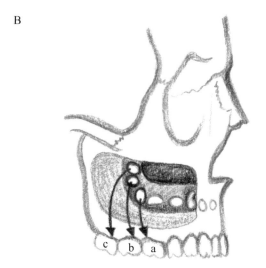

Fig. 254. **Changes in the growth of the upper jaw during the second dentition.** *The dental arch of the primary teeth remains largely unchanged in size. The jaw expands toward the back as additional teeth (molars) break through. At the end of each seven-year-period, one molar shifts into the plane of occlusion. A: Upper jaw (view from below); B: Upper jaw (side view).*

Seven-year period	Width/length (dominant direction of growth)	Age in Years		Maturational phases
		Male	Female	
I	Width	0-3	0-3	
	Length	3-6	3-6	←——— School readiness
II	Width	6-10	6-9	
	Length	10-14	9-13	←——— Sexual maturity
III	Width	14-18	13-17	
	Length	18-21	17-20	←——— Social maturity

Table 29. The first three seven-year periods of life and their relationships to human maturational phases.

general maturation of the body. Puberty (sexual maturity) sets in at the end of the second seven-year period. At this point, soul forces are "set free" to be expressed in human interactions, especially interactions between the sexes.

Bone growth, however, is not yet complete. The wisdom teeth (third molars) have yet to emerge, which they usually do around age twenty-one, at a time when the overall growth of the limbs is coming to a halt. This final reshaping of the body involves not only the teeth and long bones but also all organ systems, including the brain. Only when this process is complete does the person become a fully conscious, mature, and self-determining individuality, or in other words, an "I"-being.

Even from these brief reflections on developmental physiology, it is clear that the two dentitions are different. The first falls into the first seven-year-period, during which "life forces" are released from the physical body to serve thinking (school readiness). The second dentition rounds out the second seven-year period, which ends with the maturation of the endocrine system and genitals. As a result, soul forces are "released" from the body to serve a more individualized feeling life (puberty).

The final stage of growth, however, is completed only when the third molars have emerged (often a difficult process) and bone growth in general is completed. At this stage, the "I", the individuality itself, comes of age (Table 29).

The Threefoldness of the Facial Skeleton and the Physiognomy of the Human Face

The skull metamorphosis outlined above also opens up a new understanding of the physiognomy of the human face. As Rudolf Steiner once put it, the human face is like a living imagination that becomes visible. It is a direct manifestation of an individual's essential being.

If the lower limbs metamorphose into the lower jaw and help form the oral cavity and chewing apparatus, what we see there is the organism's material aspect. Correspondingly, the mouth and lower jaw express the individual's will nature.

The upper limbs, which are functionally more closely related to emotional activity and to the body's middle (rhythmic) system, metamorphose into the upper jaw. The collarbone (clavicle) is transformed into the zygomatic arch, the portion of the face that most strongly expresses the emotional aspect of human soul life. In a certain sense, the ear is derived from the world of matter or will, and it is located on the boundary between the lower jaw and the cranium. The eye, which develops out of the world of feelings but is closely associated with conceptual activity, is located on the boundary between the upper jaw and the cranium. The upper jaw area is bounded above by the frontal bone, which is incorporated into the desmocranium and therefore belongs to the world of thinking. Thus the shape of an individual's forehead reveals a great deal about the thinking aspect of that person's essential being.

Because the basic forces of human soul activity (thinking, feeling, and willing) are reflected in the successive formations in the head (Figure 255), the threefold structure of the facial skull can serve as the basis of a *functional physiognomy*. The uppermost portion includes the forehead and eyes, which tell us a great deal about a person's intellectual capabilities. The middle region (nose, upper jaw, and zygomatic bones) belongs to the rhythmic system and reflects emotional capabilities or feeling. The mouth, lower jaw, and chewing muscles are strongly related to the individual's will activity and represent the metabolic domain. A person's "strong-willed" chin and mobile lips, along with how the chewing muscles move, can tell us a lot about that person's will activity and metabolic constitution.

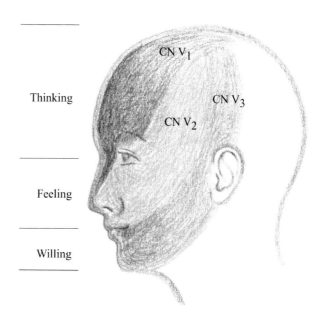

Fig. 255. *The three branches of the trigeminal nerve (CN V$_1$, CN V$_2$, CN V$_3$) serve the three main regions of the head.* From the physiognomic perspective, these regions are related to the three soul forces of thinking, feeling, and willing.

The Integrative Arrangement of the Cranial Nerves

The arrangement of the cranial nerves (and especially of the trigeminal or fifth cranial nerve) illustrates the principle of integration especially well.

In the torso, one pair of nerves is associated with each vertebra/rib segment. On either side of the spinal column, a spinal nerve exits each segment through holes in the vertebra. A spinal ganglion is incorporated into the posterior root of each of these nerves (Figure 256). After birth, as the torso's longitudinal growth continues, the segments of the spinal cord and their associated spinal nerves shift upward, since postnatal growth of the spinal cord is minimal. This shift, however,

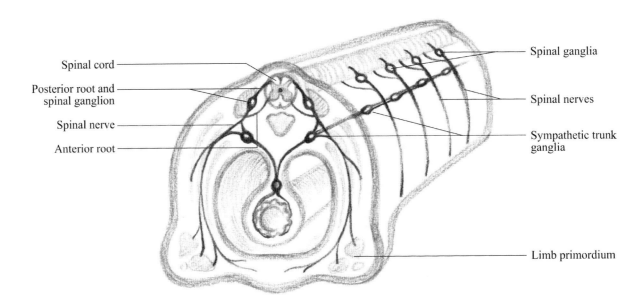

Fig. 256. **Embryonic torso segments**. *In each segment, a spinal nerve develops out of an anterior and a posterior root. The spinal nerves innervate the torso wall and limbs.*

does nothing to alter the architecture of the segments themselves.

In the head, muscles, bones, and nerves are no longer separated into segments. Instead of many spinal nerves, a *single* major cranial nerve (the *trigeminal or 5ᵗʰ cranial nerve*) develops and subsumes *all* of their functions (Figure 257). The ganglion belonging to the trigeminal nerve is located on the anterior surface of the petrous pyramid. Although structured like a spinal ganglion, it is not comparable to any single spinal ganglion but only to the sum total of *all* spinal ganglia. The trigeminal ganglion is incorporated into the sensory portion of the trigeminal nerve, which serves the same function as the posterior root of the spinal nerves but is responsible for the entire head instead of only a single segment. It is interesting to note that the three branches of the sensory portion of the trigeminal nerve correspond to the threefolding of the facial skull, which we previously described as resulting from limb metamorphosis and in relationship to the physiognomy of the human face (Figure 255).

The first branch of the trigeminal nerve is the ophthalmic nerve, which serves the forehead and the bridge of the nose. The second branch (the maxillary nerve) serves the area between the upper jaw and the palpebral fissure, and the third branch (the mandibular nerve) serves the lower jaw and temples (Figure 257). It is interesting to note that each branch subdivides into three subbranches. In each case, one subbranch leads inward to the mucosa, one outward to the skin, and one (the central branch) to the organ in question.

Spinal nerves have connections to the sympathetic trunk and thus to the autonomic nervous system (Figure 256). The sympathetic trunk runs parallel to the spinal column and has a ganglion for each segment. The trigeminal nerve has similar connections to the autonomic nervous system. Each of the three major trigeminal branches includes a vegetative (parasympathetic) ganglion that serves one of the three regions of the face. The ciliary ganglion belongs to the ophthalmic nerve (CN

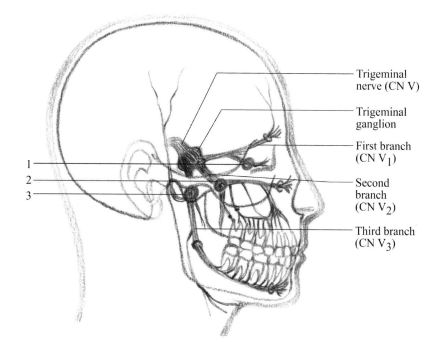

Fig. 257. **Branching pattern of the fifth cranial (trigeminal) nerve.** *Its three main branches, which emerge from the trigeminal ganglion, serve the upper (forehead, eyes), middle (nose, upper jaw), and lower (oral cavity, lower jaw) regions of the face. 1-3: Autonomic ganglia of the three main trigeminal branches.*

Labels in figure:
Trigeminal nerve (CN V)
Trigeminal ganglion
First branch (CN V_1)
Second branch (CN V_2)
Third branch (CN V_3)

V_1), the pterygopalatine ganglion to the maxillary nerve (CN V_2), and the otic ganglion to the mandibular nerve (CN V_3) (see Figure 257). The motor portion of the trigeminal nerve serves the chewing muscles associated with the jaw joint, the muscles of the floor of the mouth, and the tensor tympani muscle in the middle ear.

In a certain respect, therefore, the trigeminal nerve represents the integration of *all* of the sensory portions of the spinal (torso) nerves. In the head, these spinal innervation patterns have been realized in their ideal form.

The **other cranial nerves** are also in no way comparable to the rhythmically arranged spinal nerves of the torso. Instead, integrative formative principles are evident in all of them. The cranial nerves have individualized as a result of concentrating on specialized functions (cf. reference 16). For example, the seventh cranial (facial) nerve innervates the muscles of facial expression, the twelfth cranial (hypoglossal) nerve the tongue. As a cranial nerve develops, a spinal-type ganglion may even appear (as in

the hypoglossal nerve), but it later disappears. The tenth cranial (vagus) nerve becomes the primary nerve for the parasympathetic portion of the autonomic nervous system; it extends all the way to the abdominal cavity. The three ocular muscle nerves (CN III, IV, and VI) specialize in specific eye movements, and the ninth cranial (glossopharyngeal) nerve concentrates primarily on perceptions of taste.

Each spinal nerve encompasses all of these different groups of neural functions, but each group is integrated into only one of the twelve cranial nerves, which has specialized in the corresponding function. Describing all of these specialized functions in detail is beyond the scope of this book.

Organ Metamorphoses

The head does not consist entirely of skeletal elements but also houses soft tissues and organs. If there is any truth to the metamorphic principle of integration, it should also be apparent in these other parts of the head, and in fact it is. First, let's consider the major sense organs (eye and ear), which in many respects are determining factors in human head formation.

Kidney/Eye Metamorphosis

A structural comparison of the eye and the kidney reveals a similar underlying principle, namely, cup formation.

In the kidney the renal corpuscles form a cup-shaped structure; in the eye, it is the embryonic optic cup, which gives rise to the tissues most important for vision (retina, pigmented epithelium, etc.; see Figure 258). Renal corpuscles—approximately 1.2 million per kidney—are distributed regularly throughout the renal cortex. The visual system has only two comparable organs, namely, the two eyes. In the metamorphosis of the body into the head, each kidney's many renal corpuscles are integrated into one of the eyes (a single but highly differentiated organ).

When we compare these organs' cup-shaped structures, which are their actual functional elements, the integrative formative principle is clearly discernable. In the renal corpuscle, the interior wall of the cup invaginates to receive the many vascular loops of the glomerulus (Figure 258A2). The neighboring system of renal tubules represents the connection to the outer world. Now let's imagine that the glomerular vessels are forced out of the cup, forming an external mantle of vessels around it, and that an indentation develops on the opposite side where the renal tubule attaches. The result is the archetypal form of the embryonic optic cup, where the lens develops through invagination from outside (Figure 258B). At a certain point during the embryonic period, a vascular network (the hyaloid vessels) actually does exist inside the optic cup, but it degenerates before birth, leaving behind only the central vessels of the retina. As a result of our imagined metamorphosis, the basic cup structure turns completely inside out, and a major integration and concentration occurs, reducing a large number of small organs (in the kidney) to a single unified organ (in the eye).

The cup-shaped **renal corpuscles** are arterial organs oriented toward the inner world of the body. Their vascular loops empty large amounts of blood plasma (150-180 liters per day) into the cup. As this fluid is resorbed in the neighboring renal tubules, it is examined and its salt content monitored "from outside," so to speak. The kidneys are organs that "look" inward, not outward. They "sense" the body's fluids and dissolved solids. Elimination via the kidneys, however, releases inner light forces that radiate into the head, where our thinking concentrates them into concepts.

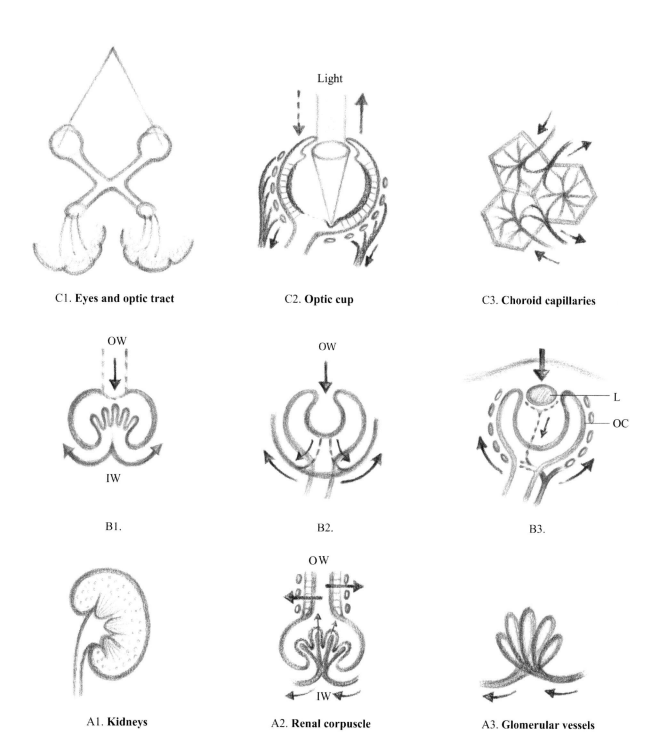

C1. **Eyes and optic tract**　　　　C2. **Optic cup**　　　　C3. **Choroid capillaries**

B1.　　　　B2.　　　　B3.

A1. **Kidneys**　　　　A2. **Renal corpuscle**　　　　A3. **Glomerular vessels**

Fig. 258. ***Kidney/eye metamorphosis****. The renal cortex (A1) contains approximately 1.2 million renal corpuscles (A2), cup-shaped structures that surround the vascular loops of the glomeruli (A3). The eyes (C1) also emerge from cup-shaped structures (optic cup, C2), but in this case the cups are surrounded on the outside by vessels that form flat, polygonal capillary fields (C3) instead of three-dimensional loops. B illustrates hypothetical intermediary stages in kidney/eye metamorphosis. B1: The glomerular capillaries (connected to the inner world, IW) withdraw from the cup and form an external vascular covering. B2: The renal tubules (connected to the outer world, OW) begin to invaginate, turning the original cup inside out. B3: Out of this stream of forces, the lens (L) develops, providing the optic cup (OC) with a connection to the outer world. The vascular covering develops into the choroid.*

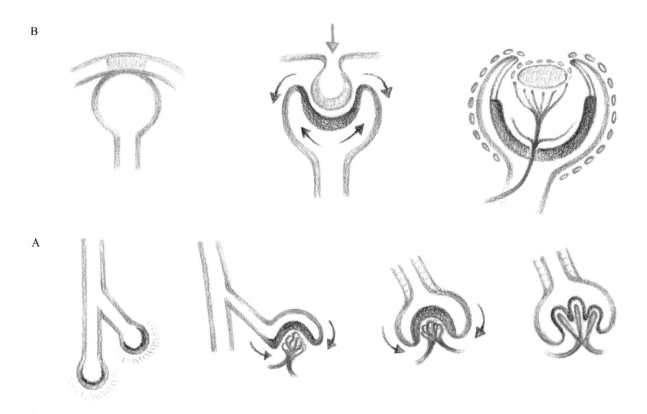

In contrast, the **eye** is totally outward-directed in its functioning. It opens itself up to light, which falls on the retina, inducing a neural process that ultimately allows us to become conscious of what we see. But we perceive objects as existing outside of us, not inside our brains. The blood-based functions that probably have to do with "projecting" images into the outer world emanate from the choroid's massive capillary network (the choriocapillaris), which surrounds the optic cup. This is also where the forces are released that we use to perceive objects in the outside world. The vascular system of the choroid is conspicuously different from that of the renal corpuscles. The choroid vascular network develops in the form of polygonal fields with centrally located arterioles that look as if the blood were trying to gush out of them. Drainage of venous blood occurs through large vortex veins on the eye's equator. The intensity of blood-related functions in the eye is illustrated by the fact that the outer wall of the optic cup is also involved in the organ's functions, whereas the outer wall of a renal corpuscle is nothing more than a structural covering. In the eye, the outer wall develops into an exceptionally active cell layer, the retinal pigmented epithelium, which is involved in almost all of the retina's metabolic exchanges and serves as a mediator between the blood and nervous tissue. In the eye, the retina integrates the processes of ultrafiltration and resorption (which are divided between the glomeruli and the renal tubules in the kidney) into the cup itself. As a result, the eye achieves a higher level of development as an organ.

Unique aspects of kidney/eye metamorphosis also become apparent when we consider the **developmental history** of both organs. It is interesting to note that the embryonic eyes and kidneys emerge from structures that are similar in shape (Figure 259). In the case of the kidneys, spoon-shaped formations appear first, becoming more and more cup-shaped as they develop into the renal corpuscles (Figure 259A). Initially, the inner lining of the cup consists of tall, cylindrical epithelial cells, which become progressively flatter as they contact the glomerular vessels.

*Fig. 259. **Embryonic development of the renal corpuscles and the eye.***
A: Sequential development of a renal corpuscle and its glomerular loops, which move into the cup as it develops out of a spoon-shaped structure. The cup develops through invagination (arrows).
B: Development of the optic cup is the result of growth from the inside out (arrows) and invagination of the lens vesicle from the outside in (blue arrow).

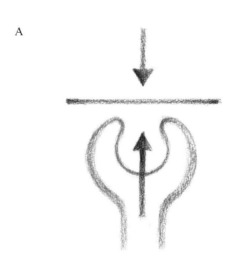

As if nature had "learned" from the development of the kidneys, eye development begins immediately with a ***single*** vesicle (instead of many), which develops into a cup. This vesicle, however, develops out of the inner layer of the optic cup—in other words, it is a primary formation, not a secondary one, as in the kidneys. The lens vesicle, which develops out of ectoderm, is pulled into the outward-directed "invagination" of the cup from outside (Figure 259). Thus the inner layer of the optic cup, the future retina, is the active element here, "sucking" in the lens vesicle. It also draws blood vessels into the interior of the cup, where they nourish the rapidly growing lens and retina. This unique development is made possible by a retardation of the growth of the lower portion of the optic cup's inner layer. A deep channel (fetal sulcus) develops, which serves as a pathway for the blood vessels and as a bridge to the optic nerve for the growing nerve fibers. In the eye, the renal corpuscle's vascular bundle is transformed into the highly developed vascular network of the choroid, which surrounds the optic cup on all sides and thus makes possible the first actual sensory processes between the blood and the receptors.

In the eye, the kidney's convoluted and protracted sequence of developmental stages becomes straightforward, and a higher level of structural integrity is achieved immediately.

We find ***opposing formative processes*** (arrows in Figure 260) at work in both the eye

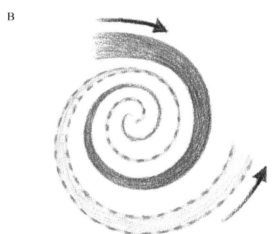

*Fig. 260. **Contrasting formative gestures in the eye (A) and ear** (B), corresponding to antipathy (A) and sympathy (B) on the psychological level. For details, see text.*

and the kidney. In psychological terms, we would call these processes "antipathetic." Antipathy is always necessary if consciousness is to come about. The meeting and touching of opposing forces contributes to consciousness. From this perspective, the kidney as well as the eye is a sense organ or organ of perception, even though its functions reach deep into the metabolic domain.

Upper Abdomen/Labyrinth Metamorphosis

The interaction of forces is very different in organs such as the liver, which deal directly with material processes such as the synthesis and breakdown of compounds. In psychological terms, this domain is characterized by sympathy, not antipathy (Figure 260). In the abdominal organs we find a functional gesture of the spiral, which is also seen in the liver and (in the broader sense) the spleen; in the head, the spiral as a structural principle underlies the labyrinth, along with the cochlea and semicircular canals. In this metamorphic sequence, we must focus on the problem of space, since these organs all relate to the matter that fills space, determines metabolism, and accounts for the organism's physical makeup.

Through the *labyrinth* and associated areas of the brain, we relate to our own physical nature or to that of our surroundings. The semicircular canals and maculae allow us to experience space and the dimensionality of the material world from outside. But we also experience the material world's formative forces (in the form of sounds and tones) from within, through the ear. The "architecture" of corporeality as expressed in sounds is the "inner aspect" of the space we experience from outside through the semicircular canals. The endolymph in the perpendicularly arranged semicircular canals is the only body fluid that is moved by the outer world instead of by endogenous flows. As it moves (passively) in one of the three planes of space, it registers the body's (or, more precisely, the head's) movements in space. In contrast, the maculae, which contain tiny crystals (otoliths) that are affected by gravity (also a unique situation in the body!) "register" the Earth's center in relationship to the body's position. Here we experience matter-filled space as such (i.e., statically), not as a corollary of movement (Figure 261). Normally, we are unconscious of the activity of these sense organs and associated parts of the brain (the vestibular system of the cerebellum), which serve to maintain equilibrium. Conscious

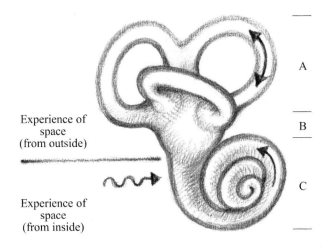

Experience of space (from outside)

Experience of space (from inside)

Fig. 261. **Diagram of the labyrinthine apparatus.** *In the semicircular canals, fluid movement is related to experiencing space. In the cochlea, it relates to experiencing sound (i.e., the material nature of space as experienced from within).*
A: Semicircular canals; B: Static organs (utricle, saccule); C: Organ of hearing.

sensations such as dizziness, nausea, or a feeling of being annihilated (depending on the degree of disturbance) appear only in pathological situations.

The *auditory process* is very different (Figure 261). Within the ear, sound waves die away, so to speak. As they move from air to water to solid (bending of the hair cells), the physical process comes to a standstill in a null point where an inner (neural and mental) process takes over. The very form of the spiraling cochlea symbolizes this process. Hearing entails internally reproducing an incoming sound that expresses certain inherent qualities of the material world. The sound that spirals inward to the null point is followed by "listening" that travels the same path in reverse; the inward (passive) spiral is followed by an outward (active) spiral.

The process of Inspiration in spiritual (supersensible) perception must be imagined similarly. In Inspiration, imaginative images are first produced and then "extinguished" from within, in a listening process of sorts (13).

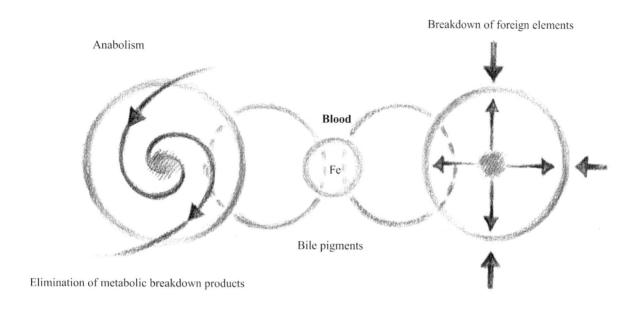

Anabolism

Breakdown of foreign elements

Blood

Fe

Bile pigments

Elimination of metabolic breakdown products

Fig. 262. **Basic functional processes in the hepatobiliary system** *(left)* **and in the spleen** *(right) are linked by the blood and by iron conversion in particular. For details, see text.*

In observing the three upper abdominal organs—*liver, gallbladder, and spleen*—we discover the same functional processes again, but this time on the purely material level.

After birth, the *liver* develops a functional architecture of polygonal lobules. The basic structure of the lobules is radial, as is the flow of blood, lymph, or gall within them, which always moves from the periphery to the center or vice versa. In functional terms, this is another double spiral (Figure 262). We might say that the liver stands on the threshold of the space the organism occupies as a material body. The liver takes "building blocks" flowing in from the intestine and enlivens and synthesizes them in a way that makes them suitable for the body. The liver is responsible for building up the substance of the body, i.e., for "bringing it into space." Unusable matter such as toxins, metabolic breakdown products, etc., are excreted into the intestine. Building up endogenous substances and eliminating wastes are two opposing processes. When we consider that most of

the matter in the body—primarily proteins, of course—is constantly being monitored, broken down, and resynthesized by the liver, it is easy to conceive of this process as "listening" on the material level. In this instance, the inward and outward spirals take place in the world of matter and physical bodies.

The *spleen* serves very different functions. This is where matter in the body is observed "from outside." The main issue here is immunological: does a particular substance belong to the body itself or to the outside world? The last immunological monitoring of matter in the blood takes place in the spleen as a means of safeguarding the body's internal milieu as distinct from the environment. This process is the material counterpart of what happens in the labyrinthine apparatus, where space-filling matter is also perceived from outside.

But the spleen is also involved in equilibrating blood flows within the body. Through its storage function, it regulates the amount of blood in circulation.

Between the liver and the spleen lies a third functional domain that also has to do with space but tends to remain more of a process, developing a certain organic foundation only through the **biliary system**. In a certain respect, this element is related to the static organs of the inner ear.

How do we actually become and remain connected to our space-filling bodies? In other words, how do we become earthly human beings? The primary factor in this process is the **iron** in our blood, which transports oxygen and thus makes energy transfers possible within the body. Iron is incorporated into prophyrin molecules (heme) and bound to proteins (globin) to form hemoglobin. In the bone marrow, hemoglobin is incorporated into red blood cells (erythrocytes), which circulate in the blood and handle the transport of gases (O_2/CO_2). Each erythrocyte contains approximately 30 picograms of hemoglobin. (In other words, 100 ml of blood contains approximately 15 grams of hemoglobin.) Because erythrocytes have a life span of only 100 to 120 days, hemoglobin turnover is very high; eight to nine grams of it are broken down and resynthesized every day. It is interesting to note that 95 percent of the iron from hemoglobin breakdown is reused, so some of the iron present in the body at birth is still present at death (61). Most hemoglobin breakdown occurs when erythrocytes are broken down in the spleen. The porphyrin ring is split apart and converted into bile pigments (biliverdin or, later, bilirubin), which are channeled into the liver through the portal vein and then released into the intestine in the bile. In the colon, intestinal bacteria reduce bilirubin to urobilinogen and stercobilinogen, which are eliminated in the feces. But a portion of these compounds (approximately ten to twenty percent) is reabsorbed from the intestine and transported back to the liver (enterohepatic circulation). The iron released through erythrocyte breakdown is transported in a protein molecule called transferrin, which consists of twenty-four polypeptide chains in the form of a pentagon dodecahedron with two iron molecules in its center (61).

The resulting picture is highly dynamic. The spleen breaks down erythrocytes and sends the products of hemoglobin breakdown (bile pigments, globin, iron) to the liver. With the help of transferrin, iron is transported to the bone marrow where it is again incorporated into the hemoglobin of red blood cells. Under normal circumstances, buildup and breakdown are in balance but take place at very rapid rates. Iron binds the human "I" to its physical nature because earthly life can be maintained only through oxygen transport. If breathing stops, life is extinguished and death sets in. Ultimately, this signifies excarnation from the world of space, a vertically oriented process. Moving earthward (centripetally) or toward the Earth's center signifies incarnation, whereas heavenward (centrifugal) movement signifies excarnation. In the sensory domain, these metabolic processes are transformed into static spatial orientation (perception of up and down, etc.) as made possible by the maculae.

Thus it becomes apparent that (metabolic) liver processes are similar to processes taking place in the organ of hearing, while spleen processes correspond to those of the semicircular canals and the processes of the iron-blood-bile system correspond to those of the maculae. Thus it is quite possible to imagine how these three metabolically active organs of the upper abdomen (liver, gallbladder, spleen), which people of ancient times related to the planets Jupiter, Mars, and Saturn, are transformed into the organs of hearing and balance as the body metamorphoses into the head.

Head Development
and the Disintegration Principle

Head formation, as we have investigated it up to this point, appears twofold: the head seems to be put together out of two major sections—the cranium (desmocranium), which includes the skullcap and cranial cavity and houses the brain, and the facial skull (viscerocranium), which encloses the viscera of the head and includes the oral and nasal cavities. In many respects, these two sections are polar opposites. The facial skull is the basis of individual physiognomy, a visible image of the person's essential being. The cranium protects the brain, where images of the world are formed.

The situation in the limbs is quite different. In the organs of movement, these two polar modes of being are still intimately connected, and we find two different types of bone development, endochondral (indirect) and periosteal (direct) ossification. Endochondral ossification takes place from within; it is built on a cartilaginous model and produces spongy bone tissue, whose interstices contain the marrow that produces blood. Periosteal ossification takes place from outside; it begins with connective tissue and produces compact bone, which is massive and contains no marrow. As we saw in a previous chapter, these two types of development are manifestations of different, even polar opposite, processes (Figure 263).

The **compact bone** of the long bones is what gives individual bony elements their shape. It is where muscles attach; functionally, therefore, it is especially closely related to the movement system. The compact bone has no trajectorial structure. Its

mass resists the changing stresses (flexion, weight-bearing, etc.) that occur during movement or impact. If the bracing effects of muscles did not counteract many of the forces applied to bones, the compact bone would have to be many times more massive than it actually is. Thus muscles and bones combine to form a functional system. Muscles do more than simply produce movement. To a considerable extent, they also regulate strain on the compact bone. As a result, the human skeleton is much more delicate than the actual impacts on it would suggest. Ultimately, therefore, bone thickness is determined by muscles. As a tensioelastic system, the muscles, along with the bones' outer supporting structural layer (cortical bone or compact bone), represent the form element in the movement apparatus. They are what determines—from outside, as it were—the appearance of the movement apparatus at any given moment.

In contrast, the **spongy bone**, which develops through endochondral ossification, has more connections to the vascular system and the body's metabolic processes. Red blood cells produced in the marrow of the spongy bone circulate in the body's blood vessels. The trabeculae of the spongy bone are trajectorial in structure, i.e., adapted in every detail to static stresses on the skeletal system. The arrangement of the trabecula reflects spatial forces that work from the Earth into the skeletal system. These are central, terrestrial forces, not the cosmic, peripheral forces we find reflected in the compact bone. The reticular tissue of marrow is involved not only in building up and breaking down bone (which allows the spongy

Fig. 263. **A comparison of the formative principles in limb bones (A) and skull bones** *(B). The limbs' endochondrally developed spongy bone (the "blood" or "material" aspect) metamorphoses into the facial skull, while the periosteally developed compact bone (the "form" or "nerve" aspect) is transformed into the skullcap (calvaria). The former is terrestrial, the latter cosmic in orientation (arrows). The base of the skull forms a "joint" of sorts between these two domains.*
1: The sella turcica on the base of the skull.

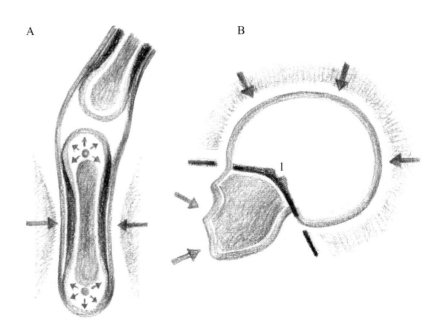

bone to adapt to changing stresses) but also in the metabolism of the organism as a whole. Both osteoblasts (bone-producing cells) and osteoclasts (bone-resorbing cells) are able to mobilize mineral salts from bone tissue as needed, releasing them into the bloodstream and making them available to organs. Thus bones are the body's most important mineral repository, where all of the important elements (calcium, magnesium, phosphorus, trace elements, etc.) needed for metabolism are deposited, as they also are in the depths of the earth. To date, not enough research has been done on the extent of the relationship between the intensity of blood production and blood movement—important elements in circulation as a whole—and metabolic processes in the spongy bone (cf. also reference 68). In any case, in the contrast between spongy bone and compact bone or endochondral and periosteal ossification, we again encounter the polarity of matter and form, of metabolic and informational processes that shapes the body as a whole (cf. Table 28, p. 340).

To understand how these forces metamorphose in the head, we must realize that they are distributed among different parts of the head instead of working together as they do in the limbs. We will call this the **principle of disintegration.**

In the limb bones, cosmic/peripheral and terrestrial/central forces work together, and every movement includes both elements. But in order to move, we need not only bones and muscles but above all, joints. **Joints** are the element that mediates between the two poles (Figure 263). Joints allow any movement to come to rest—that is, to be fixed in a specific position. This is the form aspect of joint function. Conversely, joints also allow new movements to be realized through the will; this is the material aspect. Metabolic (material) processes that take place in muscles produce energy and alter the position of joints, while patterns of innervation proceeding from the nervous system serve to coordinate movements (a form-giving function within the musculoskeletal system). The polar opposite forces of the blood/metabolic system on the one hand and the form-giving informational system on the other ultimately also determine the details of movements.

In the **head**, however, few limblike movements are possible because everything has hardened into form. The movements we observe in the jaw joint (chewing muscles) and around the orifices (mimic muscles) are specific in character and qualitatively very different from limb movements. Only the bones of the base of the skull, which can be understood as a metamorphosis of vertebral elements of the torso, are derived from cartilage. The forces of form and matter that shape the dynamic of the limb system have become separated in the head. As a result, form forces predominate in the development of the skullcap (desmocranium), whereas the individualizing forces of matter and blood are more evident in the development of the facial bones (viscerocranium) (see Figure 263).

As we described in a previous chapter, the **skullcap** consists of flat bones that develop directly out of the skinlike covering of the neurocranium (i.e., through intramembranous ossification). These bones, like the compact bone of long bones, are shaped from outside. The trabeculae radiating from the five ossification points produce pentagonal shapes, so that skull formation becomes almost crystalline in character—a clear expression of the dominance of form forces, which display almost no individual traits (Figure 36, p. 67, and Figure 237, p. 341).

The situation is completely different in the **facial bones**, where bone morphology is largely determined by personal forces belonging to the individual. The structure of these bones is a pictorial, almost symbolic expression of the person's individual character—a phenomenon that is further enhanced by facial expressions. In the limbs, will forces are expressed in movement and allow the individual to acquire individual experiences by resisting the earthly element. In the face, these same forces manifest directly in the shape of the facial bones. The "spongy bone" or "blood and will" aspect of the movement apparatus appears in metamorphosed form in the facial portion of the head (Figure 263).

Now let's take a somewhat closer look at the **development of the calvarium** (skullcap). Here, bones do not develop in the same way as the periosteal collar of the long bones. Instead, as illustrated in Figure 237, pointlike ossification centers develop, followed by trabeculae that radiate out from them. This type of development more closely resembles endochondral ossification in the limbs, where bony nuclei develop and

radiate outward in all directions, forming spherical bony elements, especially in the **caputs**. Thus the development of the skullcap, although it takes place in one plane and never achieves three-dimensionality, exhibits some characteristics of endochondral ossification. Of course the fact that bones of the skullcap include some spongy bone (diploe) that contains blood-producing marrow does not mean that the skull can be seen as a will-influenced organ of movement. In the sphere of the head, will forces metamorphose into the forces of thinking, which we need for perception, conceptualization, and memory. As such, these forces surround the skull bones on the **outside** and must be reflected inside it, in the brain, in order to become conscious. In effect, this means that **the limbs are turned inside out as they metamorphose into the head** (Figure 238, p. 342 and Figure 263).

In the bones of the **facial skull**, the situation is somewhat different. Here the will-related and metabolic forces at work in the interior (spongy bone) of the long bones are more dominant. Consequently, we might expect facial bones to be derived from cartilage and well supplied with marrow, but this is not the case. Instead, they develop directly out of the head's embryonic connective tissue (mesectoderm or ectomesenchyme), usually without any cartilaginous intermediate stages. Later, they are often partially pneumatized, i.e., their scattered marrow spaces are replaced by air-filled chambers such as the maxillary sinuses. In the facial skull, the centripetal formative process penetrates into the interior of the bony elements, which is not yet the case in the skull bones, with the exception of the frontal bone. (In the anterior portion of the frontal bone, which extends into the face, the spongy bone is replaced by the frontal sinuses.)

In the face, therefore, the (compact bone-related) "forces of form" work from the outside in to shape the bony elements, but the structures themselves are associated with spongy bone-related (material) forces coming from within. It is therefore possible to imagine that these structures, the actual individual aspect of the shape of the head, reflect the destiny of a past life.

But the facial skull and skullcap, which are in many respects polar opposites, are connected by a third element, namely, the **base of the skull** with the sella turcica in its center (Figure 263). Here, the base of the skull functions somewhat like joints in the limbs. It forms the boundary between the brain and the head's "metabolic domain." Through the brain, forces rising up out of the metabolism are transformed into the movements of mental images. Conversely, thought forces sink down into the metabolic domain (the unconscious) where they can become life processes. As a boundary region, the base of the skull becomes a "joint" of sorts for the movement of forces between these two major portions of the head.

The base of the skull, however, is more than just a "joint" between the cranium and facial skull. It conceals more profound mysteries. Most of the base of the skull (the chondrocranium) develops out of cartilage, ossifying only secondarily. Like the spinal column and ribcage in the torso, the base of the skull incorporates formative laws that can be ascribed to both domains of the head. Even with regard to the structure of its bones, therefore, the base of the skull can be seen as a connecting element between the cranium and the facial skull. As a result of the disintegration principle, the two great polar principles manifest separately in the head, in contrast to the limbs, where they work together. The face is entirely devoted to physiognomy, i.e., to outward-directed individual expression, while the brain becomes the basis for internal individual mental activity. These two domains would remain unconnected were it not for the base of the skull, which is not a solid boundary but has openings and channels that serve functional as well as physical connections. We get the impression that nature has applied (or in certain respects, "invented") the disintegration principle in the structure of the head in order to insert a third, linking, "middle" element between polar domains, just as in the torso the organs of the chest are inserted between "upper" and "lower" elements.

The facial part of the head, as we have seen, is threefold in its structure (Figure 255). The upper portion is shaped by the forehead and eyes. The optic nerves carry the world of light into the nervous system through channels in the base of the skull. But the eyes, along with the muscles of the forehead and eyelids, are also an important element in the individuality's outward-directed physiognomic manifestation.

The middle portion of the face, which is more closely associated with feeling, is the site of the nasal cavity, which has connections to the cranium through the cribriform plate of the ethmoid bone. An aspect of reality that relates to the element of air is revealed to us through the organ of smell. On the other hand, the cribriform plate presumably also transmits respiratory rhythms to the cerebral fluid, superimposing them on its rhythmic fluctuations in pressure and thus influencing the more subtle sensing processes that occur in the nervous system.

And finally, the lower portion of the facial skull includes the oral cavity, which enters into connections with the organs of speech via the trachea and esophagus. Here the sense of taste is the dominant element with links to the cranium. In addition, this part of the skull includes the organ of hearing, deeply embedded in the base of the skull, and the organs of speech, which allow the individual's intentions to flow out into the outside world. Through the sensory nerves that lace the base of the skull, the brain is informed about the surrounding world. Especially through speech, but also through facial expressions and respiration, the individuality works back on its surroundings.

The base of the skull, with the sphenoid and ethmoid bones and the sella turcica in its center (Figure 263), is where these opposing forces ebb and flow.

The Respiratory System of the Head

In the facial skull, the two halves of the nasal cavity not only serve respiration but also provide the olfactory system with deep-reaching connections to the nervous system, particularly the limbic system. Through the development of the paranasal sinuses, the "air element" in the head is also involved in physically shaping the face and thus the physiognomy of the individual. To a certain extent, it even reflects maturational rhythms in the first three seven-year periods of development. The vocal apparatus, another important insertion between the facial and cranial parts of the head, develops as a result of interaction between the respiratory system and the oral cavity. A crucial evolutionary prerequisite to this development is the functional transformation of the "branchial apparatus," exclusively devoted to respiration in aquatic vertebrates.

Let's begin by considering the skeletal elements of the head's respiratory system, particularly the ethmoid bone and the paranasal sinuses.

The Ethmoid Bone and the Paranasal Sinuses

The ethmoid bone lies in the base of the skull but serves as the "cornerstone" of the facial skull; the upper jaws and the frontal, palatine, and lacrimal bones all attach to it (Figure 264). It is a T-shaped skeletal element that forms the upper portion of the nasal cavity and the inner (medial) wall of the eye socket. The cribriform plate provides the olfactory nerves with a connection between

the cranial cavity and the olfactory mucosa in the roof of the nasal cavity. The lateral masses of the ethmoid bone contain air-filled spaces (the ethmoid air cells). The ribcage, which is of central importance to the respiratory system in the torso, provides the foundation for the pectoral girdle and arms. Similarly, the complex ethmoid bone provides a foundation for the neighboring bones (upper jaw, etc.) that represent the metamorphosis of shoulder and arm bones in the facial skull. Furthermore, the ethmoid bone with its specialized mucosa plays a central role in channeling airflow in the head. Its two pairs of nasal conchae direct incoming air toward the olfactory mucosa in the roof of the nasal cavity or toward the respiratory tract. As air passes over the conchae, it is moistened, warmed, and monitored for odors by the olfactory nerves.

The function of the ***ethmoid cells*** has not yet been fully explained, but the postnatal growth spurts that the paranasal sinuses as a whole undergo suggest that more profound connections are involved, possibly related to a spiritualized respiratory process of incarnation and excarnation.

Ultimately, not only inhalation and exhalation but also incarnation and excarnation are made possible by the movements of the ribcage. Death is the last great exhalation, birth the first deep inhalation. It is surprising to note that the major human developmental and maturational phases (school readiness, puberty, etc.), which can also be understood as respiratory processes, are accompanied by structural changes not only in the face but in the paranasal sinuses as well (Figures 265 and 266).

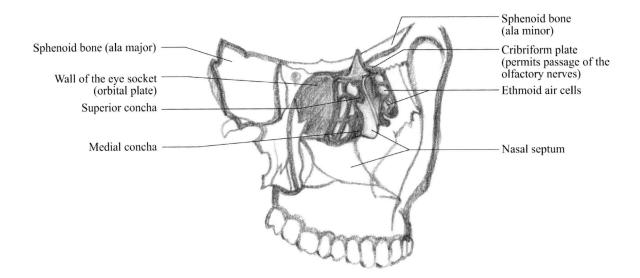

Sphenoid bone (ala major)

Wall of the eye socket (orbital plate)

Superior concha

Medial concha

Sphenoid bone (ala minor)

Cribriform plate (permits passage of the olfactory nerves)

Ethmoid air cells

Nasal septum

Fig. 264. Above: **Location of the ethmoid bone in the facial skull** *(as seen from the right front). The upper jaw is transparent in the illustration. The ethmoid bone is connected to the anterior body of the sphenoid bone and forms the bony base of the nasal cavity. The ethmoid air cells are pneumatized. The superior and medial concha arch forward into the nasal cavity. The lateral orbital plate forms most of the interior wall of the eye socket.*

Fig. 265. Below: **Location of the paranasal sinuses in the skull** *(front view). The paranasal sinuses develop out of the nasal cavity and remain accessible from it (arrows). The entrance to the frontal and maxillary sinuses is located below the medial concha.*

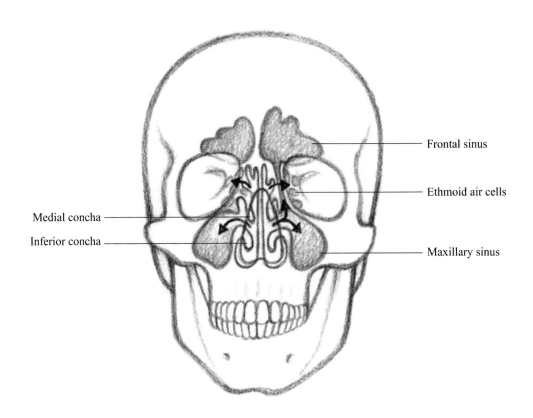

Medial concha

Inferior concha

Frontal sinus

Ethmoid air cells

Maxillary sinus

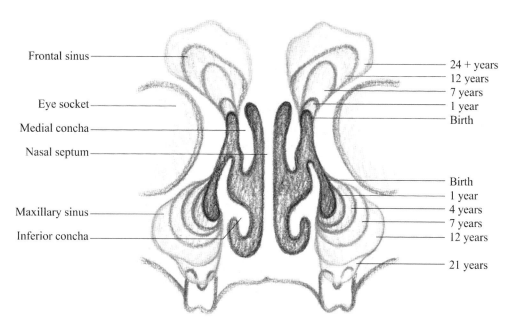

Fig. 266. **Postnatal development of the frontal and maxillary sinuses.** *Development proceeds from the middle nasal passage, located below the medial concha. Expansion of these two sinuses occurs in spurts paralleling the body's phases of growth and maturation.*

The Paranasal Sinuses

The paranasal sinuses emerge from the nasal cavity and develop into hollow, air-filled spaces in the large bones of the face. The maxillary sinus lies in the upper jaw, the frontal sinus in the frontal bone, and the sphenoid sinus in the sphenoid bone. The ethmoid bone contains many little air-filled chambers, the ethmoid air cells (Figure 265).

The sinuses develop out of the nasal cavity when buds of nasal mucosa grow into the neighboring bones. As a result, these bones develop mucosa-lined hollow spaces in place of hematopoietic marrow spaces (Figure 266). Thus the facial skeleton is largely pneumatized, i.e., it contains many air-filled cavities. Not involved in respiration as such, these cavities have been thought to serve as resonance chambers for speech and song, and mechanical functions such as reducing the weight of the skull have also been

considered. To date, however, none of these theories has proved conclusive, so the actual significance of the sinuses remains obscure.

A phenomenon that points toward the true nature of these air-filled spaces is the fact that they develop and grow in spurts synchronized with postnatal maturational phases. Although present in primordial form in the embryo, the sinuses begin to develop only after birth and achieve their full size between the third and twenty-first years of life (Figure 266).

The sinuses and human maturational phases. Most impressive is the development of the two maxillary sinuses. They increase greatly in size during the second dentition (ages six through twelve) but only slightly after puberty. Development of the frontal sinuses stops later, between the ages of twenty and twenty-four, when growth of the sphenoid sinus is also complete.

Children undergo three major phases of postnatal growth and maturation, each of which encompasses six or seven years. After the first seven-year period, girls complete these maturational phases somewhat earlier than boys do. In modern times, an as yet unexplained acceleration has occurred, shortening these phases to six or even five years in both sexes.

Each seven-year period begins with an "expansive" phase of weight gain, increase in bone width, etc., and ends with a phase of longitudinal growth and shape accentuation. These subphases are approximately equal in duration (3–3.5 years; see Table 29, p. 362).

At the end of the *first seven-year period* (ages zero through six), a child is ready for school, meaning that his or her body has matured enough to make sufficient forces available for learning. After uprightness is achieved and the first dentition is complete, life forces are released and made available for mental activity. Often this inner shift takes place within just a few months and is very apparent to those close to the child.

The *second seven-year period* (ages seven through thirteen) ends with puberty, which sets in earlier in girls than in boys. Puberty entails more than sexual maturity alone. At puberty, the entire body has undergone a major growth spurt, the second dentition is complete, and the structure of the musculoskeletal system has been solidified. The forces that are released and become available to the young person at this point are not life forces but primarily soul forces. These psychological forces beg to be shaped by the "I", which is often still fragile—a frequent cause of problems in the educational and social lives of adolescents.

The young person becomes "ready for life"— that is, in full possession of his or her "I", the core of an individual personality—and ready to act on the basis of independent judgment only upon conclusion of the *third seven-year period* (today, usually as early as age eighteen). Long-term relationships and life-shaping career decisions often begin at this age. All this is possible because the forces now freed up in the body are forces the "I" can take hold of and shape independently.

The development of the paranasal sinuses is synchronized with these rhythmic waves of growth, and the release of the aforementioned forces is clearly reflected in the shaping of pneumatic spaces in the head. Respiration proceeding from the lungs is significantly involved in producing the lower body's substance. In the head, the role of the respiratory system is reversed—i.e., it is involved in removing substance through pneumatization. In this process, it is possible that organic forces are released and made available for soul-spiritual activity. The fact that the sinuses enlarge during rhythmic maturational spurts suggests that they are associated with "inner respiratory processes" of this sort.

The Olfactory System

The roof of the nasal cavity is lined with olfactory mucosa, which contains receptors whose axons project through the cribriform plate into the cranial cavity, where they connect first to the brain's olfactory centers and then to the limbic system (Figures 202 and 205), thus ensuring that olfactory experiences reach the personality's emotional domain and the gateway to the subconscious. As described in an earlier chapter, respiration and feeling (emotional responses) are closely related. Our sense of smell reveals the inner nature of a substance or another living being and makes us conscious of it. This is the inward-directed path of the respiratory system in the head.

Furthermore, the rhythm of respiration is probably transmitted to the brain's fluid system via the olfactory region and the cribriform plate. In cases of injury, cranial fluid has been known to flow out the nose. In the area of the cribriform plate, the fluid-filled space surrounding the brain is in close contact with the nasal mucosa. The rhythmical movements of respiration therefore also influence the cerebral fluid and its rhythmicity.

The respiratory system of the head is also involved in the development of speech. To understand this, we must first consider the transformation of the "branchial apparatus" during embryonic development.

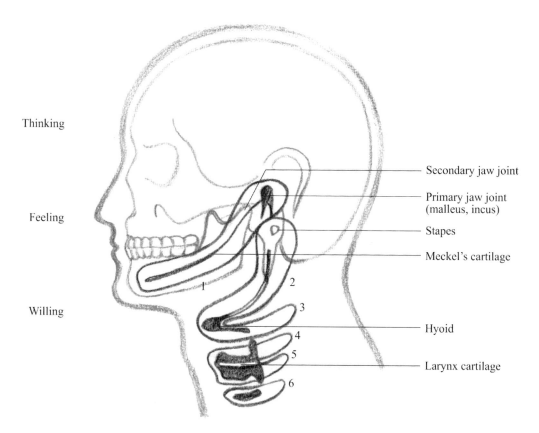

Fig. 267. **The human visceral skeleton (branchial apparatus).** *Five to six pharyngeal arches (1-6) appear in the embryo. They undergo a change in function into the organs that conduct (auditory ossicles) and produce (larynx) sounds.*

The Branchial Apparatus (Branchial or Pharyngeal Skeleton)

In the human embryo, the branchial skeleton consists of four to six pharyngeal arches and an anterior connecting link (copula). Each branchial (pharyngeal) segment is equipped with a pair of muscles, a pair of blood vessels, and a pair of nerves, revealing a metameric principle similar to that in the torso. The branchial apparatus, which is devoted to respiration in fishes, becomes superfluous in terrestrial vertebrates and undergoes a profound change in function. During human embryonic development, the branchial skeleton is transformed into bony elements that serve the organs of hearing and speech (Figure 267).

The first pharyngeal arch (known as Meckel's cartilage) induces the development of the lower jaw and then promptly disappears, leaving behind only two of the auditory ossicles, the hammer and the anvil. Thus the primary jaw joint between the hammer and the anvil is incorporated into the sound conduction apparatus, while a new (secondary) jaw joint forms where the lower jaw meets the temporal bone (Figure 267). The second branchial segment (the hyoid arch or Reichert's cartilage) gives rise to the stirrup, the styloid process of the temporal bone, the stylohyoid ligament, and the lesser horns of the hyoid bone (the third pharyngeal arch provides the greater horns). The body of the hyoid develops out of a ridge (the copula) that links the second and third pharyngeal arches. The anterior portions of the fourth and fifth arches fuse to form the thyroid (larynx) cartilage (Figure 267).

The bridge formed by the auditory ossicles transmits airborne sound waves from the eardrum to the inner ear—an essential prerequisite of hearing. In the development of speech, the larynx produces vibrations in the outgoing stream of air, which are then shaped into speech sounds in the oral cavity. In phylogeny, therefore, purely respiratory organs (gills) evolved into the organs that produce and perceive sound. Conceivably, in the metamorphosis of the torso into the head, the skeletal elements that serve respiration are transformed into the branchial skeleton and thus become the organs of hearing and speech. In other words, instead of simply producing regular, rhythmical air movements (respiration), they now produce frequency modulations in airflows, as required for speaking, singing, or hearing.

Metamorphosis of the Reproductive Organs into the Organs of Speech

As described in a previous chapter, the **genital organs** are unique in that they create a space within the body where a different being can incarnate. The primordial germ cells migrate into the genitals where they mature, isolated from the activity of the other organs. Here, the individual organism creates space for activity that is totally separate from other body functions. Even though the fertilized ovum is a "foreign body" with regard to its genes and protein structure, it implants in the uterus without triggering any immune responses. Why this is possible remains a largely unsolved riddle in reproductive biology.

When viewed as a qualitative process, it seems possible that the metamorphosis of reproductive functions produces the **speech organs**, which are connected to the respiratory system (airways). The

larynx releases small quantities of air (together with moisture, warmth, etc.) that are then shaped into formations (speech sounds or tones) into which ideas or thoughts "incarnate." Language embodies a person's ideas, making them apparent to others so that they can be understood. This is a creative process not unlike physical conception in the lower part of the body.

The signature shape of both the female genitals and the speech organs is a basic Y-shaped structure. The two main bronchi unite to form the trachea, whose upper end develops into the larynx (Figure 268). The stream of air, which is interrupted by the vocal cords in the larynx, can be shaped into a word or tone in the oral cavity. A decisive factor in this process is the narrowing of the airway accomplished by the ring of sphincter muscles around the larynx. Animals often have two complete sphincters, one inner and one outer. In humans, the inner sphincter has been transformed into the functionally very important muscles that move the vocal cords. The pair of arytenoid cartilages incorporated into the inner ring of muscles makes it possible to change the width of the glottis and tense the vocal cords. The sensitive interior of the larynx is surrounded and protected by the thyroid cartilage, whose broad, elegantly curved shape is reminiscent of the pelvis.

The **uterus**, which provides the hollow space where the offspring can develop, is surrounded and protected by the bones of the pelvis. The anterior symphysis and the posterior sacral bone link the pelvic bones into a three-dimensional body in which the uterus is securely suspended, supported by its own ligaments and by the muscular pelvic floor. Similarly, the soft tissue of the larynx is suspended in the ring of thyroid cartilage. Unlike the larynx, however, the pelvic ring is closed at the back. The sacral bone, which consists of five fused vertebrae, forms a downward-pointing triangle, symbolizing the descent of the vertebral element into earthly gravity, so to speak. At the lower end of the spine, the vertebrae sacrifice all possibility of movement to support the upright, walking human being and to create the basis for physical and spiritual mobility in the upper spine

A

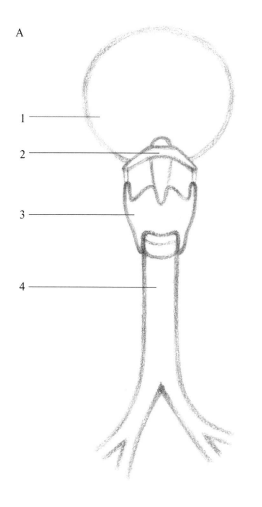

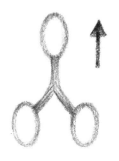

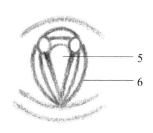

A
Speech organs:
1: The head inasmuch as it is involved in producing speech (oral and nasal cavities)
2: Hyoid
3: Larynx (thyroid cartilage)
4: Trachea
5: Glottis
6: Inner larynx muscles (the muscles surrounding the glottis; vocal cord muscles)

B

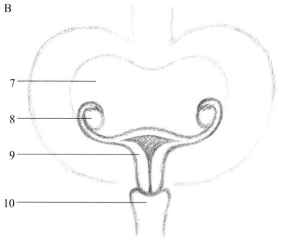

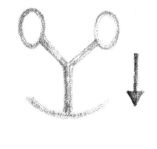

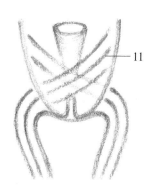

B
Genital organs:
7:   Pelvic cavity
8:   Ovary
9:   Uterus
10: Vagina
11: Spiral muscles in the cervix

Fig. 268. **Metamorphosis of the female genital organs (B) into the organs of speech (A).**

and in the base of the skull. Perhaps people had this connection in mind when they named this bone "the sacred bone" (***os sacrum***). When we view the sacrum anteriorly and in relationship to the two pelvic bones, a different signature becomes apparent (Figure 269). The impressive posterior "wedge" is conspicuously absent in front, where the pubic angle of the symphysis forms an open, inverted triangle. The result is a regular hexagram reminiscent of a Star of David. The sacrum (posterior) thrusts downward into space from above, while the anterior pelvic triangle, which houses the outer genitals, "steps out of space" to allow a different being to incarnate from (spiritual) nonspace into (earthly) space in the act of conception.

In the female, the basic structure of the ***internal reproductive organs*** is also Y-shaped. The vagina and uterus, together with the two fallopian tubes that connect them to the ovaries, form a Y. Its vertical axis points downward, however—the reverse of the Y formed by the larynx, trachea, and bronchi (Figure 268). The uterus also has sphincter muscles, but unlike those of the larynx, they form a double helix (Figure 268).

The muscles surrounding the ***uterus*** expand during pregnancy to allow more space for the developing fetus, but the sphincterlike muscular rings of the cervix remain closed, opening only during delivery, when the uterine muscles begin to contract rhythmically.

Here again, a metamorphosis is evident. The uterus receives incoming matter that then takes shape in the hollow interior in a way that

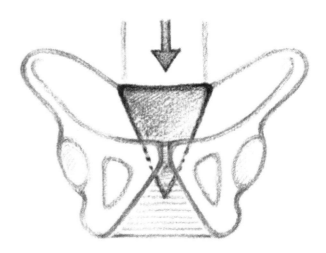

Fig. 269. ***The human pelvis*** *(seen from the front and above). The triangular sacrum (dark gray) is inserted into the ring of the pelvis from above like a wedge-shaped keystone. In the front, under the pubic symphysis, another triangular space is left free (red) to permit the conception and birth of a new human being.*

is determined by the incarnating being. Spiral muscles intervene in the material stream of development when the infant is born into external space. On a higher level, something similar takes place in the ***speech organs***, where an "etheric stream" of air, ultimately derived from the entire organism, is dissected into air quanta by ring-shaped sphincter muscles, producing vibrations that are "molded" into words or tones by the oral cavity and then become audible. Here, a more subtle and highly evolved "birth" takes place.

The Pituitary/Pineal System

The metamorphosed respiratory system occupies a relatively large amount of space in the head. In contrast, the cardiovascular system—so central to human existence—seems totally absent at first glance. This is a fundamental mystery waiting to be solved, but to find the first clue, we must start by venturing farther afield.

If the entire torso metamorphoses into the head, the gastrointestinal tract must also undergo a metamorphosis. The only possible result is the central nervous system. The brain and gastrointestinal tract display the same basic subdivision into five functionally distinct sections. The gastrointestinal tract processes the material aspect of the world, the brain its sensory, nonmaterial (informational) aspect. Perhaps it is no coincidence that the intestines and brain often use the same messengers (neurotransmitters) in their functional processes.

During embryonic development, the colon wraps around the convolutions of the small intestine, forming a large spiral. The colon is open to the outside world and takes in bacteria from outside, and the intestinal flora even produce substances that the body needs but cannot produce itself. Sporadic cessation of peristaltic contractions allows the colon to "view" its contents and decide what should be eliminated and what should be reabsorbed.

These functions reappear on a higher level in the cerebrum. Instead of taking in part of the outside world on the material level, the brain takes it in on the mental or informational level, "digesting" impressions and deciding which to eliminate and

which to admit. Like the colon, the embryonic endbrain (telencephelon) grows in a large spiral, superimposing itself on the other, subordinate parts of the brain (interbrain, midbrain, etc.), which process and internalize neural impulses important for movement and vital functions. The activity of the small intestine could be seen as the material correlate of this unconscious neural activity. In contrast, the stomach's role is to mediate between the upper and lower sections of the digestive tract. On a higher level, the midbrain serves similar functions.

Discovering such connections is a slow process, more intuitive than factual. This is true especially with regard to the workings of the heart.

Let's look again at the polarity between the facial and cranial parts of the skull, which are connected by the skull base (Figure 263). The facial skull is outward-oriented and individualized, reflecting the person's character. Through sense impressions (upper portion, eye), respiration (midsection, nose, sense of smell), food intake, and speech (lower section, oral cavity, sense of taste), the facial skull is actively involved in grappling with the outer world, right down to the material level. In contrast, the cranium houses the central nervous system (cerebrum, brain stem, cerebellum, etc.), which is buoyed up by cerebral fluid and rests almost weightlessly on the base of the skull with the sella turcica in its center. Through the brain, experiences of the outer world can be processed, recalled, or used internally to control life processes.

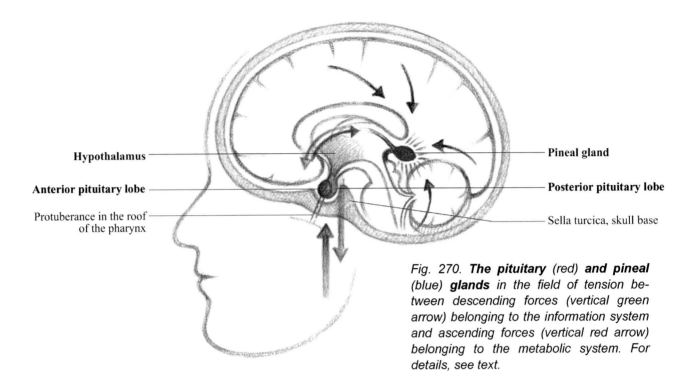

Hypothalamus

Anterior pituitary lobe

Protuberance in the roof
of the pharynx

Pineal gland

Posterior pituitary lobe

Sella turcica, skull base

Fig. 270. **The pituitary** *(red)* **and pineal**
(blue) **glands** *in the field of tension be-*
tween descending forces (vertical green
arrow) belonging to the information system
and ascending forces (vertical red arrow)
belonging to the metabolic system. For
details, see text.

The outward-oriented forces of the face and those of the actual interior (cranium) must somehow be connected by a "spiritual-physical middle" realm. Rudolf Steiner discovered these connecting forces in the pituitary/pineal system (65). For example, he described a buildup of tension that is suddenly released (like an electrical spark leaping a gap) and assumes form whenever a mental image emerges from memory.

The **pituitary gland** lies in the sella turcica in the skull base, surrounded by a dense network of veins (the cavernous sinus). During embryonic development, the anterior pituitary lobe develops out of a bud of tissue that emerges from the stomodeum (Rathke's pouch). In other words, the anterior pituitary develops like an exocrine gland with no outlet duct. This developmental gesture illustrates how intimately this gland is still related to the lower section of the facial skull (oral cavity, etc.). The entire pituitary system as a whole gains access to the interbrain via a stalk of gray matter (the infundibulum) that connects the interbrain and

the posterior pituitary lobe. This connection allows the pituitary (a glandular organ that develops out of the roof of the pharynx) to work together with the hypothalamus, a part of the interbrain that plays a central role in regulating body functions.

The pituitary is the "queen" of the endocrine glands. Together with the hypothalamus, it directs all *internal* life processes (water balance, thermo-regulation, circulation, growth, etc.). As a result, streams of forces from the body's interior can be concentrated in this spot on the skull base.

In a notable archetypal phenomenon, the sella turcica, which houses both pituitary lobes, achieves its central, "elevated" location in the base of the skull only in humans. This phenomenon is related to uprightness and the increased size of the human cerebral hemispheres (cf. Dabelow, 96). The angle in the skull base at the sella turcica (clivus angle) can therefore be seen as a typical structural attribute of the uprightwalking, "I"-endowed human being. In mentally handicapped people, the "I" cannot incarnate completely, and the skull base is often flattened, making the clivus angle more obtuse. In such cases, the sella turcica and pituitary are not elevated (96).

Unlike the pituitary, the **pineal gland** or pineal body (Figure 270) rests on the roof of the midbrain. Like a rider firmly in control of galloping horses, the pineal gland is secured to the thalamus nuclei by two strong "reins" (habenulae). Through the nuclei of the habenulae, the pineal gland influences the activity of the hypothalamus and limbic system. By producing melatonin through its connections to the visual system, the pineal gland is also heavily involved in regulating the sleep-wake rhythm and other circadian rhythms in the body. In all likelihood, the internal "light metabolism" that develops here, on the boundary between waking consciousness (cerebral cortex) and unconsciousness (limbic system, ANS), plays a role in the formation of memories.

As described in a previous chapter, however, memory as a storage process is not purely neuronal but involves the entire organism. In the head, forces released through the elimination of matter (in the kidneys, for example) are consciously experienced as "primary light" in the form of remembered images. The pineal gland may play a decisive role in shaping these images out of the stream of light coming from below. If this is so, the pineal gland reveals itself as the principle that provides the form, while the pituitary provides the material or content.

If we consider the heart's function in the organism from the same perspectives, it is clear that pituitary-pineal interaction is similar on a higher (metamorphosed) level to cardiac activity in the rhythmic system. The pituitary-pineal system, however, is concerned not only with respiratory processes but with actual streams of substance that are profoundly related to the problem of space and of matter itself.

In a previous chapter, we learned that the **heart** is intimately involved in spatial processes. Incarnation and excarnation are constantly occurring in the heart in rhythmic alternation.

Streams of blood, some of which have received lymph from the thoracic duct or cerebral fluid from the brain, flow into the atria under the sign of the cross (i.e., through crossing veins). In the atria, these streams come together, bringing with them their "experiences" in different parts of the body. At this point, however, the streams still run parallel, as if unrelated to each other, and substance-filled space as such is still experienced from outside.

In the ventricles, however, these streams come to a standstill for a fraction of a second, change their direction, and are mingled in a vortex of sorts. As the blood is mingled and compressed and its flow interrupted by the heart's rhythmic action, forces bound up with the bloodstream are loosened. As these life forces are released, the blood is "etherized" (in Steiner's words) and released from space ("excarnated") (67). The opposite process is also possible. Especially during sleep, the streams of forces we experience in thinking can stream "from above," via the nervous system in the head, into the heart, where they are united with the blood and then move out into the body (the subconscious).

The release of forces (as a prerequisite to conscious experience) and their transition to unconsciousness (through being bound up again with the earthly element) could be seen as a higher metamorphosis of the heart's rhythm. In the head, all that remains of this rhythm is the pulsing of forces between the pituitary/hypothalamus system on the one hand and the pineal/epithalamus system on the other.

To cast this phenomenon in mythological imagery, we might say that the sella turcica in the base of the skull, along with the pituitary and the surrounding blood vessels, is a "Holy Grail" filled with life-giving forces that stream into it from above (i.e., from the spiritual world) through the mediation of the pineal gland (Figure 270).

Much more investigation remains to be done, however, before the veil that conceals these mysteries can truly be lifted.

Evolutionary Aspects of Human Development

"The human being is the ultimate product of a constantly self-enhancing Nature."

From Goethe's essay on Winckelmann (Weimar edition, W46/29)

"The god had become human
in order to raise human beings to the level of the gods.
We glimpsed the most exalted grandeur
and thrilled to the highest beauty."

J.W. v. Goethe, in commemoration of the statue of Zeus at Olympia
(Weimar edition, W46/30)

The Physiological Foundations of Freedom

In the vast majority of our actions, we human beings are dependent on inner or outer circumstances and are therefore unfree. Through our thinking, however, we have access to the world of ideas. When we derive the impetus for our actions from this world through creative thinking (e.g., through Intuition), we are in no way dependent on our physical organization, and especially not on the brain, whose functioning has nothing in common with the *essential nature* of ideas. Thus we are truly free in this respect—and in this respect only (2).

Freedom, however, depends on more than just thinking. Does free will also have physiological foundations? A person who is paralyzed may be able to derive motives for independent action from intuitive thinking, but bodily limitations will make these intentions impossible to realize. And do our organ functions truly allow any of us the latitude needed to realize new, creative ideas? It is well known that animals do not have this option. As a rule, animals remain capable of learning only for a short time after birth (the imprinting phase) and not out of their own initiative. Later, they become completely fixed and inflexible.

In the early years of our life, we humans are also heavily influenced by environment, education, and predispositions, but later our individual freedom increases. This process actually begins when we acquire *uprightness*. Mastering an upright, bipedal gait is our first victory over dependency on our environment. As a result of uprightness, our upper extremities are freed from the constraints of reflexes and locomotion and can be used for new, individual, and (eventually) freely invented movements. Uprightness is also

crucially important to the form and functioning of the human head. Balanced freely atop the spine, the head acquires tremendous mobility, especially with regard to the sense organs. When we take the human head's increased range of motion into account, our visual field expands to almost 300 degrees. Increased eye mobility further increases our visual field in almost all directions and permits individualization of visual perception. An upright human being's field of binocular vision is very large compared to an animal's and makes space perception possible. Along with binocular vision, we gain the ability to distance ourselves from our surroundings. Binocular vision, therefore, is an essential physiological foundation for the beginnings of "I" experience (cf. especially reference 54).

In addition, human beings have a tremendous *capacity for learning*, which persists for most of our life span and is based on the unique adaptability of our nervous system, among other things. Even elderly people can still learn a foreign language or new manual or intellectual skills, although not with the same playful ease as children.

The human musculoskeletal system allows us a surprising degree of latitude. Our ability to learn new movement combinations—whether in a wide variety of sports, in acrobatics, gymnastics, or dance, or in playing a musical instrument—is tremendous (especially in our younger years, of course).

In addition to vision and learning, a third area of freedom—"free space," so to speak—that is virtually nonexistent in animals is the field of *speech and language*. According to Chomsky, the basic mechanisms underlying the ability to

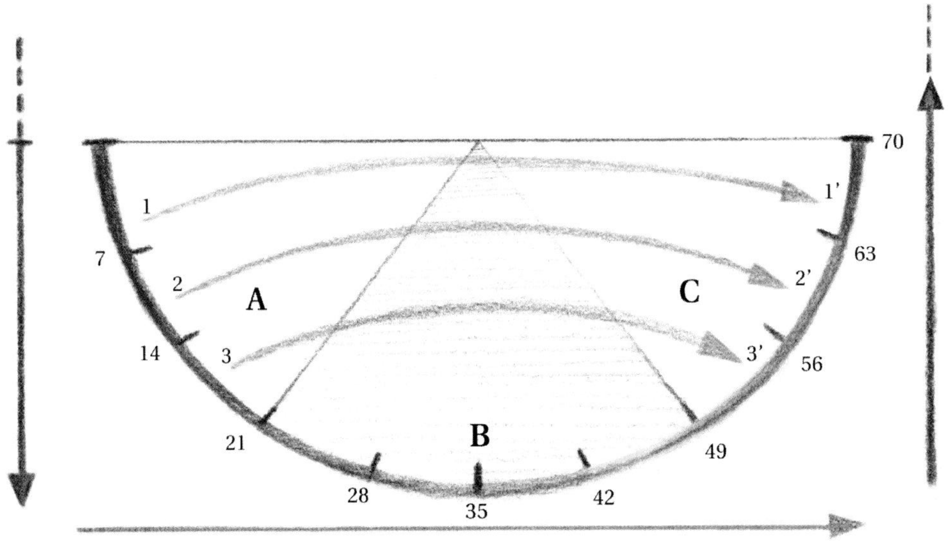

Fig. 271 A. **Seven-year periods in human biography**. Three basic, major sections can be distinguished. In the last century, the phase of youth (A) has become significantly shorter through acceleration, while the phase of aging (C) has become significantly longer. Thus incarnation and excarnation processes (arrows) are polar opposites. The first three seven-year periods (1–3) all end in decisive morphological transformations (1: school readiness; 2: sexual maturity; 3: social maturity), which are reflected in corresponding periods of gradual excarnation during the aging phase (1'–3'). Phase B (age 21–49) is characterized by full engagement in external life.

speak seem to be inherited, at least to some extent (97). Nonetheless, speech as a means of conveying or exchanging ideas is something we achieve individually, something we each take hold of and shape for the purpose of freely unfolding the intentions of the "I". The ability to speak develops only as the result of interrelationships among free individuals. People who are totally isolated from their fellow human beings do not develop coherent speech.

It is not for nothing that Goethe characterized conversation—that is, the exchange of ideas made possible by speech—as the highest human good (98). In his tale of the Green Snake and the Beautiful Lily, the Gold King asks, "What is more splendid than gold?" "Light!" is the answer. "And what is more enlivening than light?"

"Conversation!" In this context, and in view of our earlier discussion of the metamorphosis of the speech organs, it seems safe to assume that the capacity for speech will reveal untold possibilities as human evolution continues.

The experience of freedom, however, is also dependent on an individual's **physical, social, and cultural milieu** as well as on his or her degree of development and maturity, which changes significantly over the course of a lifetime. At different stages of life, the body supports the individuality in very different ways. In other words, each of the developmental phases that succeed each other at approximately seven-year intervals creates a phase-specific freedom in which the "I" can unfold the intentions it has acquired through Intuition.

Rhythms in Human Life

Development over the course of an individual human lifetime is neither uniform nor linear. It takes place in spurts that often involve dramatic crises in addition to structural changes. As in many other biological processes such as growth and regeneration, these changes occur at roughly seven-year intervals (109, 110). The first major transformation is accomplished after seven years of life and coincides with school readiness. The second, accomplished after fourteen years of life, coincides with puberty, the third (twenty-one years) with social maturity. In many respects, the similar but less incisive intervals that mark life's final stages are the mirror image of the developmental phases of childhood and adolescence. In the past few centuries, however, adolescent maturation has become compressed or accelerated while aging has become protracted. For example, the average age of menarche in girls was seventeen in 1840 and fifteen in 1900, but it is closer to twelve today. On the other hand, human life expectancy has increased significantly over the last century; centenarians are no longer a rarity in our society (Figure 271A).

The most dramatic morphological changes occur during the first seven-year period. Approximately one year after birth, a child begins to stand upright and walk unsupported. Next, speaking develops through imitation, followed by independent although initially imperfect conceptualization, which develops on the basis of imitative speech and perception. In physiological terms, these first few years of life are dominated by brain development (Figure 271B). To a large extent, the number of neurons in the cerebral cortex is fixed at birth, and it remains constant for the rest of the person's life, but the number of dendrites and thus the number of connections between neurons (synaptic contacts) increases dramatically. The structural maturation of the brain is not yet completed by age five or six. At this point (school readiness), formative forces are released from the activity of brain development and can be applied to conscious learning. This first intellectual awakening coincides with the beginning of the second dentition.

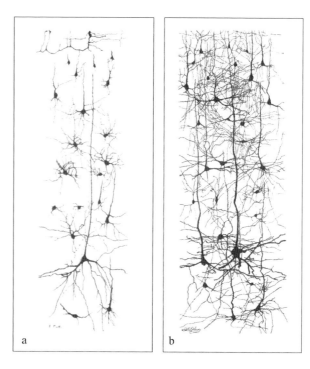

Fig. 271 B. **Structural changes in the visual cortex of the cerebrum in the first two years of life.**
a: Newborn; b: Two-year-old. The number of neurons does not change, but the numbers of dendrites and connections between cells increase greatly (from Per Brodal, The Central Nervous System, Oxford University Press, 1992).

The permanent teeth continue to erupt throughout the second seven-year period, which ends in another major morphological transformation (puberty). This developmental period is characterized by the increasing movement of individualizing formative forces from the head into the rest of the body. The preadolescent growth spurt (between the ages of nine and twelve) results in a great increase in height. Anatomical investigations confirm that bone is also being transformed, becoming denser and harder (Haversian transformation). To a certain extent, the same is also true of tendons and muscles. In essence, the second dentition is also based on a bone-forming process, because the crowns that determine the actual shape of the teeth are completed long before their actual eruption, which is based primarily on growth of the roots and metamorphoses in the jawbones (see pp.

360-62). All of these morphological changes are related to the beginning of sexual differentiation. The endocrine glands (gonads, adrenals, pituitary, etc.) commence production, and the body begins to assume its typical female or male form. Secondary sex characteristics appear (facial hair, pubic hair, changing of the voice, etc.), and bones and muscles grow stronger. A decisive transition ("crossing the Rubicon," in the parlance of Waldorf teachers) occurs around age nine, when the organs of the middle system have largely matured. For example, the final number of pulmonary vesicles (280×10^6) is achieved during the ninth year of life. Their later development is limited to increases in size, which effectively increase respiratory surface area. No further structural changes occur in the lungs.

Recent research has shown that the brain also undergoes decisive structural changes at puberty (an overview is given in reference 131). These changes affect especially the frontal lobe (volitional movement, sense of self, etc.), the temporal lobe (verbal comprehension, interpersonal relationships), and the limbic system (emotional center), whereby the pleasure-reinforcement system with dopamine as neurotransmitter plays an important role. In these areas of the brain, large numbers of cell systems are not only eliminated but also newly established. The myelination of axons and the creation of new synapses are intensified. Young people now learn to focus their concentration, to evaluate their experience more effectively, to regulate their sleeping patterns (which are initially often very arhythmical), and to control their feelings.

Taken as a whole, the morphological and neurological transformations during this period are dramatic. On the psychological level, they are often associated with instability and uncontrolled reactions (the crisis of puberty).

As has been recently shown (138 and 139), young people are most at risk for engaging in violent behavior between the ages of 15 and 22.

The forces that are freed up once the body has been largely transformed are primarily soul forces, which can then be used by the individuality—now consciously manifesting—to shape his or her own life. Thus the third seven-year period (years fourteen to twenty-one) stands decisively under the influence of the individuality itself. Once reproductive maturity is achieved, a self-directed, independently responsible capacity for loving develops, often resulting in partnerships that may last a lifetime. In this phase, bodily changes are centered on developing the final forms of all the body's details—not only limbs, bones, and muscles but also internal organs, and above all, the blood. The blood's hemoglobin content increases significantly, hematopoietic bone marrow reaches maximum capacity, and the efficiency of the heart and lungs increases. The organs of the head (brain, sense organs, etc.) mature during the first seven-year period, the metabolic organs (bones, muscles, endocrine glands, etc.) during the second. Now the individuality must work out of the center to establish a balance between these poles, and so the heart (together with the circulatory system) becomes the center of the human body (cf. reference 111 and 135). On the soul level, idealism, courage, religious feeling, and the capacity for devotion and self-sacrifice may develop during this phase, but lack of direction and violent tendencies may appear if the individuality's harmonizing, centripetal forces are not strong enough.

In the phase of mature life that follows (roughly between the ages of twenty and fifty; B in Figure 271A), acquired capacities are applied to the individual's working life. If social circumstances permit, freely choosing and shaping a career allows the individuality to mature further by realizing its youthful ideals.

In a certain sense, the third and last major stage of life (beginning around age fifty; C in Figure 271A) represents an excarnation process that is the polar opposite and mirror image of the incarnation process of youth. During the first seven-year period of this stage (approximately years forty-nine to fifty-six and now more commonly fifty to sixty), the individual's soul and spirit begin to free themselves from the body. This phase stands under the sign of declining fertility (menopause, etc.), which often leads to midlife crises and health problems. On the positive side, the development of a cosmopolitan capacity for love that transcends the individual now becomes possible. For the first time, the individuality begins to loosen its grip on the immediate circumstances of its life, to process its experiences and to gain a certain distance from its previous activity. Spiritual experiences and insights can now be transformed into forces of love that are directed toward the world instead of toward one's own "I", as was the case in youth.

The second phase of aging (years fifty-six to sixty-three and now usually sixty to seventy) is a metamorphosis of the second phase of childhood (years seven to fourteen), when children undergo the change of teeth and the profound bodily changes that culminate in sexual maturity. This phase of aging, in which the soul slowly begins to free itself from the body, may be accompanied by serious problems. Retirement brings radical changes in lifestyle and habits, and this is the phase when cardiovascular and metabolic disorders (osteoporosis, rheumatic disorders, gout, arteriosclerosis, etc.) most often appear. In his pedagogical lectures, Rudolf Steiner mentions repeatedly that placing excessive demands on the memory and intellect of children during the second seven-year period deprives the developing body (especially the skeletal system) of life forces and predisposes these individuals to sclerotic disorders during the corresponding phase of aging. If such connections prove true, it is conceivable that the increasing intellectualization of children in our society will have very serious consequences indeed. On the positive side, the "release of soul forces" during the second phase of aging can also lead to new, creative impulses enhanced by life experience that ray out into the world with healing and helping effects.

From the perspective of biology, there is no logical reason for aging (Hayflick, reference 30). Animals in the wild do not age to the same extent as humans. Maturation and aging are specifically human phenomena; their meaning is found in the spiritual enrichment of the world by individuals who have developed radiant forces of love through bodily metamorphoses and life experience.

Especially in great individuals, these forces may be enhanced to the point of wisdom during life's final years. This wisdom can bear profound and lasting fruits for the world and for younger people in particular (cf. reference 112). On the negative side, this final period of life often entails staggering physical decline, dementia, memory loss, and the breakdown of perceptual abilities (deafness, blindness, etc.) During the first seven-year period, the brain is being built up and developed and the development of sensory organs and memory is completed. In the mirror image of this period in the last phase of life, all these may degenerate, but they may also be transformed into higher faculties (wisdom, creative power, and the capacity to bestow blessing).

In conclusion, it is important to emphasize once again that the ages cited here represent nothing more than a general pattern, because acceleration in adolescence and increasing longevity have significantly stretched the boundaries of the classical phases of development and maturation. Nonetheless, these seven-year rhythms represent real spiritual laws, and understanding them can reveal deep secrets of nature and human evolution.

Evolutionary Principles
and the Genesis of the Modern Human Form

In previous chapters, evolutionary principles were described in relationship to individual organ systems, in some cases in great detail. At this point we will simply attempt to summarize our conclusions as a basis for tackling a final, very complex series of issues.

Since Darwin's time, biologists have essentially held only two factors (selection and mutation) responsible for the progress of evolution. The genetic material (genome) of organisms is constantly undergoing (random) transformations. Some of these mutations (and the resulting bodily changes) are minor, some major (Schindewolf, 100). The altered structures are then subjected to environmental selection and either eradicated or preserved through inheritance. In the tension between inner (genetic) changes and external influences (selection), more highly evolved life forms are said to emerge exclusively on the basis of the laws of coincidence, and the result is said to be optimal adaptation of species to their appropriate habitats.

Today, these principles have been confirmed through so many examples that their existence can no longer be doubted. However, they represent only the analytical or mechanical aspect of the overall process and account for only a portion of the relevant phenomena. As we saw in an earlier chapter, there are also other, parallel principles at work. On closer inspection, these principles prove to be the exact opposite of the analytical principles in evolution.

Our discussions in previous chapters revealed three major, distinct groups of evolutionary principles (Table 30, p. 404):

1. *The orthogenetic principle*, which keeps the entire stream of evolution directed toward its ultimate goal (the human being). Modern animal species are side branches or end stages that are no longer capable of evolving. As the only vegetative bud on the "Tree of Evolution" that is capable of continued physical and spiritual evolution, the human race is full of unimagined evolutionary potentials. Coincidence, although undoubtedly also necessary in evolution, works against the orthogenetic principle. Orthogenesis makes use of the genetic diversity resulting from chance mutations to give direction to the stream of evolution.

2. *Adaptation and antiadaptation*. These processes relate to a "coming to grips" with the environment. Animal species emerging from the orthogenetic stream of evolution are subjected to specific environmental conditions. Through adaptation, these species often develop surprisingly one-sided and highly differentiated specialized organs that allow them to survive but also make them incapable of further evolution. Adaptation, which produces differentiation and one-sidedness, is counteracted by the retarding principle of antiadaptation, which avoids one-sided specialization and preserves the capacity for further evolution. Only the continued presence of

nonadapted, "primitive," flexible organisms within each structural model guarantees that evolution will continue.

3. The third group of factors is related to the *empirical principle*, which also has its counterpoint, the principle of selection. The process of adaptation still contains certain "creative elements" in that it permits further evolutionary steps toward perfect adaptation to specific (and always very restrictive) environmental conditions. Strictly speaking, selection means simply the destruction of the unfit (the dying-off of imperfect organs or organisms) and is essentially negative in character.

On a different (spiritual) level, however, coming to grips with the environment results in "experiences" that then flow into further evolution, leading to new structural models. This is the empirical principle. There can be no doubt that such "experience" occurs, but it leads to conclusions that are applied not to already existing, adapted organisms but to new, "primitive" life forms that are still capable of adaptation and evolution. These new forms serve as the germ of a whole new class of organisms with an altered, completely new, but always inherently harmonious structural model. It is possible that many "major mutations" actually belong in this category.

A more detailed discussion of these principles follows.

Adaptation and Antiadaptation

Through chance mutations and selection, organisms become increasingly adapted to their habitat, but their evolution becomes more and more of a dead end. The differentiations they achieve often lead to extreme specialization, which persists for millions of years in many cases, leaving no room for further evolution. A classic, much-discussed example is limb evolution in equine species, which transformed the original four-toed *Eohippus* into modern, solidungulate horses (see Figure 38). This transformation was accompanied by corresponding changes in the skull and chewing apparatus. Many such one-sided adaptations can be found in the animal kingdom. We might even say that the emergence of specialized, one-sided species is characteristic of animal evolution as a whole.

In contrast, the evolution of the human body is characterized by an avoidance of specialization. At every evolutionary stage, the human form remained flexible and capable of further evolution, as recently documented in detail by Verhulst (52). In the chapter on skull development, this phenomenon was discussed at greater length. The spherical shape of the human *skull* was not derived in stages from the tube-shaped, elongated skulls of reptiles and lower mammals. On the contrary, the spherical form is the primary form, the one that remains capable of further evolution. It is the original from which tube-shaped specialized forms can be derived. We recognize the same phenomenon in the shape of the dental arch. Mammals develop one-sided shapes adapted to chewing specific foods, whereas the human dental arch is regular, harmonious, and not adapted to one specific mode of mastication, which would have made the development of speech impossible. Incidentally, the same is true of the oral cavity. Here, too, specialized evolutionary adaptations in the development of the tongue, the roof of the palate, the uvula, etc., were avoided in the context of developing the capacity for speech.

On the other hand, this "restraint" in the development of the jaw and face also had consequences for brain development. The human cranium (desmocranium) remains flexible and capable of expansion for a long time, allowing the brain to continue to grow. It is also significant that the development of the cerebral cortex does not involve neuronal specialization. Large portions of the cortex remain undifferentiated and impressionable. This is especially true of the brain's most recently developed sections, the frontal and temporal lobes.

Human limbs also retain many embryonic traits such as the five digital rays of the hand and foot, as well as the shape of the limbs themselves. In the human digestive tract (stomach, colon), major adaptations to one-sided and highly specialized diets are also conspicuously absent. Aided by their intelligence, human beings can make almost any foods digestible and thus avoid specialization of the digestive organs.

Antiadaptation is especially apparent and impressive in the relatively long period of *postnatal development* in humans. As Kipp pointed out, protracted childhood and adolescence are specific to humans (54). A long postnatal developmental period, in which children are almost totally dependent on their mothers and incapable of surviving on their own, is in effect a significant extension of the embryonic period (Portmann, 56 and 66). In these early stages of development, human beings are enormously impressionable and capable of learning—a unique situation in the postnatal development of animal species.

We have listed phenomena that illustrate the retardation of adaptive processes through negative adaptation or antiadaptation. Antiadaptation, however, appears as a positive element in evolution. In many cases, instead of simply avoiding a particular direction, it means going in a very different or even opposite direction (positive adaptation). For example, this is the case in the development of the *five-fingered hand* with its opposable thumb. The shortening of the first digital ray, the development of the saddle joint at the base of the thumb—in short, differentiation of the hand into an organ suited to grasping and manipulating objects—is a process that cannot be seen simply as retardation. In fact, it describes a progressive differentiation, one that opens up new functional possibilities. A hand suitable for grasping permits not only tool use but also countless artistic activities—basic prerequisites for cultural development. In the evolution of the human hand, differentiation does not mean becoming one-sided through adaptation to a specialized function. Instead, it unlocks a multitude of new functional possibilities.

The same principle plays a role in the development of the *lower limbs* and pelvis. The evolutionary significance of the elongation of the femur, the reshaping of the pelvis, and the development of the arched structure of the foot has been hotly debated, but there can be no doubt that these developments made upright walking possible, along with the independent mobility of the human arms and retention of the spherical shape of the head (cf. also reference 52).

Similarly, higher differentiation of the *cerebral cortex* in humans is also more than just an adaptation to the more complex movements of upright walking. Cortical differentiation permitted further differentiation and additional functional possibilities. Antiadaptation of this sort accomplishes more than simply avoiding differentiation or adaptation; it unlocks new possibilities.

Another example of positive antiadaptation is the development of the *organs of speech and communication*. Instead of simply being held back at early stages in their development, the larynx, oral cavity, muscles of facial expression, soft palate, etc., also differentiate, but in a direction that makes speech possible. Like the development of the cerebral cortex or of hands suited to grasping, the ability to produce many different sounds also opens up an almost infinite range of new functions for the activity of the human "I" and is therefore an essential prerequisite to the development of human culture.

Ultimately, antiadaptation produces an organism that frees itself from its habitat instead of being held captive by it. The freedom the human species gained as a result of antiadaptive processes made possible the incarnation of an independent, creatively active individual or "I". Thus the principle of antiadaptation can also be described as the principle of individuation.

The Empirical Principle

It has often been said that nature learns only from its successes, not from its failures (49). In other words, positive adaptations are preserved, while others (the "failures") are eradicated in the process of selection. Only the best adapted survive (Darwin's "survival of the fittest," 99). The one-sidedness of this train of thought has been severely criticized, quite convincingly by Norman Macbeth (50).

On closer observation, it becomes evident that evolution does indeed learn from its so-called failures. With regard to the **evolution of the heart**, we saw that the "mistakes" of one level no longer appear on the next level. The new model incorporates "experience" gained on the previous level, as if nature had indeed "learned from its mistakes." For example, incomplete cardiac septation is not repeated in the next structural model; from the very beginning, a fully septated heart appears. The heart is a very good example of how evolution perfects an organ one step at a time, from one level or structural model to the next, until the separation of systemic and pulmonary circulation is finally achieved, along with warm-bloodedness. Admittedly, this principle becomes fully comprehensible only when seen in connection with the orthogenetic principle—in other words, when we admit that evolution has a goal "in mind."

Phylogenetic changes in the **fetal membranes** also illustrate that "learning" of this sort occurs (Figure 272). The eggs of fishes and amphibians develop in the water, without the benefit of specialized membranes. In reptiles, the amnion, yolk sac, allantois, etc., develop secondarily, as folds that grow up and around the embryonic disk until it is enclosed. In mammalian embryology, these fetal membranes are a primary development, and the amniotic cavity develops directly in the embryoblast through the formation of gaps between the cells (Figure 272). As if

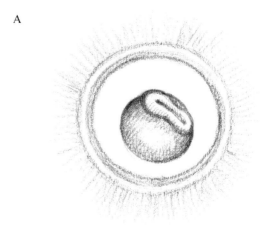

Fishes, amphibians

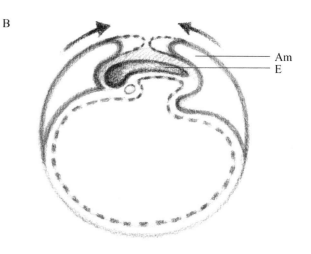

Reptiles, birds

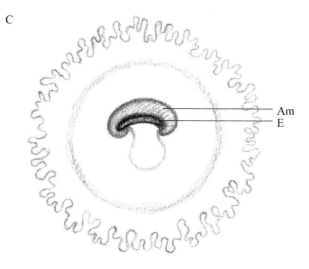

Mammals, primates, humans

*Fig. 272. **Evolutionary changes in vertebrate embryology**. In lower vertebrates (fishes, amphibians; A), the embryo is totally exposed to the natural world, protected only by the egg's mucous membrane and the surrounding water and air. Birds and reptiles (B) lay eggs that enclose the developing embryo. The folds that become the fetal membranes (Am: amnion, etc.) develop only secondarily (arrows). In mammals, primates, and humans (C), the amniotic cavity is a primary development, present before embryonic development begins. E: embryo.*

nature had again "learned" from previous levels, mammalian embryonic development does not proceed directly to germ formation but begins with the development of the fetal membranes. The fact that embryonic development shifts to the interior of the mother's body can be seen as a continuation of the individualizing tendency, that is, the tendency to separate from and become independent of the outside world. Eggshell and uterus are manifestations of this tendency on successive levels. The individualizing tendency is accompanied by longer gestation periods, which enhance antiadaptation and result in greater development of organs that need a long time to mature, such as the brain. The "invention" of intrauterine development can be seen as the result of a learning process, as a logical next step after egg deposition.

Such steps in learning are also apparent in the evolution of individual organ systems. In our discussion of **kidney development**, we pointed out that the mammals abandon the sauropsid portal system. Instead, they develop a glomerular filtration system from the very beginning and are therefore able to control the balance of water and salt in their bodies.

Exactly how the empirical principle takes effect in evolution remains an open question. However, it is not too difficult to imagine this principle in action, if we consider animal organisms not only as biological "machines" but also as living, ensouled beings that incarnate into their bodies as humans do, although it seems appropriate to think that each animal species has a "group soul" instead of each individual having a soul of its own (14).

Orthogenesis

Without the orthogenetic principle, the empirical principle or "principle of experience" has no meaningful reality. For biological experience to result in successive steps toward perfection, evolution must be aiming at a specific goal. The goal, however, is the human being—the last to appear on Earth but present from the beginning of evolution as a "plan," that is, as a spiritual being. Without this "goal," the rungs of the evolutionary ladder make no sense.

The effects of the orthogenetic principle first became apparent when we considered the **development of the speech organs**. The crossing of the trachea and the alimentary canal, which already became an accomplished fact at the amphibian stage, was consistently preserved and refined at successive levels of vertebrate evolution (in spite of attendant complications for respiration and ingestion) until the oral cavity could finally be placed at the service of speech. (In vertebrates, this structural development was so disruptive that it forced the emergence of many complex, compensatory control mechanisms.) The crossing of respiratory and alimentary passages in the pharynx made sense only because it would permit the acquisition of a completely new faculty (speech) at a much later stage of evolution. In other words, the "plan" or potential to develop into an organism with the capacity for speech was inherent even at the amphibian level (Figure 45).

The **development of the heart** reveals another example of orthogenesis. Once lower vertebrates had made the transition to terrestrial life and pulmonary respiration, the pulmonary veins became connected to the heart for the first time. As a result, arterial blood entered the cardiac chambers, and the separation of venous and arterial blood became necessary. This phenomenon makes sense only when the heart's central location in the human body and its functional significance in the dimensions of space are factored into the equation. Complete cardiac septation is a complex process achieved only over several successive stages. Together with the transformation of the chambers through the process of concentration, septation produced an organ structure in which the three-dimensionality of space can be reflected in its true character, so that the heart can convey the experience of space and nonspace. In this respect, humans are unique in the animal kingdom. The tendency for the heart to become such a central organ in the body was evident from the very beginning of evolution, but the "plan" was fully implemented (after many false starts and intermediary stages) only in the human body.

Brain development is an example of a somewhat different sort. It is always surprising to realize how consistently brain development proceeded in the course of evolution. A cerebral vesicle (telencephalon) is present even in lower vertebrates, where it serves almost no purpose. This primordial organ begins to make sense only in humans, where a huge increase in its surface area (through gyrification) transforms it into the foundation of self-aware, conscious thinking. Even in higher apes, large portions of the cerebral cortex either serve no purpose or are not used to capacity. Steadily increasing cortex size conveyed no selective advantage for many species and can be understood only in reference to humans, who appeared much later and took advantage of the presence of the many available "brain centers" to develop the almost boundless capacity for learning that is so central to human individuality. The fact that the human brain still has many areas with no assigned functions is an important indication that the human race will continue to evolve to higher levels in the future.

We must see the evolutionary transformations of the skull, the characteristic shape of the human head, and the development of the visual system in the same context. For example, the ***visual nerves cross*** even in lower vertebrates, but this arrangement becomes functionally significant only in humans, where the partial crossing of the optic nerve fibers in the optic chiasm, the connection of visual projection fibers to the cerebral cortex, and the increased size of the binocular field of vision (which results when the eyes shift from the sides to the front of the head) permit an individual experience of space. (Like the differentiation of the cerebral cortex itself, this new experience of space makes a significant contribution to self-consciousness. These structures are all present as potentials even in lower vertebrates but are "intended" for a being—the human being—that appears only at the end of a lengthy process of vertebrate evolution, not to mention prevertebrate evolution.

Human and Animal Evolution

As we see, the "idea" of the human being underlies evolution as a whole. Animal species separated off from the mainstream prematurely and discovered suitable, often very narrowly defined environmental niches through adaptation (sometimes extreme adaptation). The ancestors of the human race, however, remained pliable and capable of further evolution. They passed through all the structural stages of the vertebrate series without ever incarnating completely. In other words, human ancestors were present on Earth in real bodies even among the most primitive vertebrates, but these forms were never able to fully incorporate the monumental human soul and spirit. Nonetheless, these life forms did guarantee the bodily continuity of the evolutionary stream whose goal was the human being. So we must not imagine that human souls spent all of evolution slumbering in the "bosom of the gods" and appeared on Earth only at the very end. In fact, the human soul is the driving (orthogenetic) force behind the entire evolutionary tree, while animal species are merely its branches (Figure 273). Apes, therefore, are descendants, not ancestors, of human beings (cf. also reference 52). Ape species cut themselves off from the progressive, "human" stream of evolution prematurely. In the same sense, all other vertebrates (and probably all other animals as well) are descended from humans—not from human bodies in their present form, of course, but from previous forms of human existence that, although animallike, never differentiated into lasting animal forms. Perhaps these human life forms can be imagined as embryolike, soft, malleable, and undifferentiated living things surrounded by tremendous auras of spirit and soul. These life forms preserved all the potential to become human but were not able to realize that potential at those early stages. Thus the "archetypal human being" is not something that lay dormant in the "other world" and had no relationship to the evolution of animals (with the possible exception of primates or anthropoid apes in the final stages), as some accounts would have it (53). Instead, the archetypal human element was fully integrated into animal phylogeny. We might even say that it fought its way from one structural model to the next, as the driving force behind the three major evolutionary principles, until it was finally able to unite with a suitable bodily nature and appear in physical form as the earthly human being, the "I"-imbued personality.

From this perspective, we suddenly gain a new relationship to animals. We must not see them merely as one-sided evolutionary "mistakes" or tragic deviations from the central, archetypal evolutionary stream. Rather, they played an important, even essential, role in the entire process of our becoming human. If we really take the empirical principle seriously, animal souls incarnating into earthly surroundings provided the basis for gaining experience on Earth. Ultimately, these experiences led to changes in the next model or level. We might formulate it like this: Animals "sacrificed" themselves so that the human race could come about. On the one hand, the (orthogenetic) mainstream of evolution was "purified" and freed of "brutish animal characteristics" as animal species split off from it. On the other hand, emerging animal species "experimented" with specific environmental circumstances and allowed this experience to be processed on a "cognitive" level. The fruits were then incorporated into further evolution, immensely enriching the overall process. To put it simply, we might say in all modesty that we ultimately owe our current human form to animals, and they must see us as their ancestors.

The Washing of the Feet

I give you thanks, cold, silent stone
And bend in quiet awe before you;
From you the plant in me has grown.

I give you thanks, green grass and flower
And bend in reverence before you;
You let me win the beast's swift power.

I thank you all, plant, beast, and stone
And bow in gratitude before you;
You helped me come into my own.

You child of Man, we thank you too
And kneel before you piously
Because we all exist through you.

With thanks resounds all life divine,
Resounds from beings, one and all.
Through thanks all beings intertwine.

By Christian Morgenstern

Summary

In vertebrate (and perhaps also invertebrate) evolution, three pairs of factors work together, each based on different physical-spiritual processes (Figure 273, Table 30). The basic biological processes underlying the analytical factors (mutation, adaptation, and selection) are relatively well known today, but the physical foundations of their (synthetic) counterparts (orthogenesis, antiadaptation, and empiricism) remain essentially unexplained. Ultimately, however, all of these processes are spiritual in character. For example, the laws of coincidence or chaos (mutation) are as deeply rooted in the spirit as are the laws of order or purposefulness (orthogenesis). Something similar is true of the two other pairs.

If we examine our own soul activity, the essential nature of these evolutionary factors

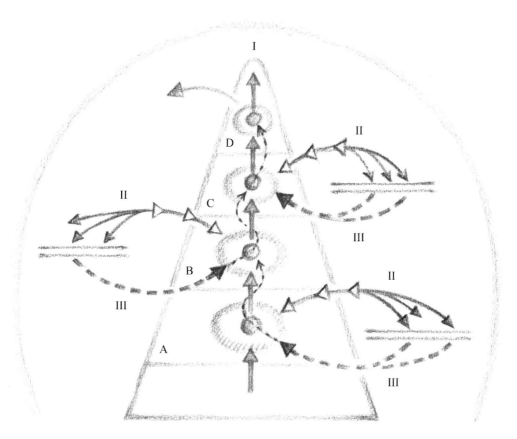

Fig. 273. **Fundamental evolutionary processes**. *The diagram shows four successive stages of vertebrate evolution, each higher than the last (A – D). Each stage emerges from an embryogenetic field (shading) that remains flexible and capable of further evolution. I: The orthogenetic principle (red); II: The principle of individuation (adaptation and selection—solid-headed arrows; antiadaptation—hollow-headed arrows); III: The empirical principle (blue)—forces of experience that then contribute to the ongoing process of evolution (I).*

becomes accessible, and we discover fundamental forces related to the forces of evolution. For example, we can relate the orthogenetic factors to our will, the empirical group of factors to perception and conceptualization, and the processes of adaptation and antiadaptation to the activity of feeling. The "desire to adapt," to develop specialized organs in response to specific environmental circumstances, is clearly related to sympathy. Conversely, antiadaptation—refraining from responding to environmental circumstances—contains an element of antipathy. These are the two primary factors in our emotional life (Table 30).

The **orthogenetic principle** is the creative will element in evolution. It keeps the process in motion by constantly striving toward the human being as the ultimate goal. In terms of the quality of the dimensions of space, this is the vertical or up-down dimension. In terms of processes, incarnation and excarnation are in the foreground here.

In contrast, the **empirical principle** is related to experiencing and recognizing functional connections and becoming conscious of them. Ultimately, therefore, this principle is related to visualization and thinking. Here we are dealing with the right-left dimension, which is expressed in the bilateral symmetry of the human form.

	Synthetic factors (positive components)	Analytical factors (negative components)	Psychological Corollaries	Dimension of space
I	Orthogenetic principle (goal-oriented)	Mutation (coincidental)	Willing	Up-down
II	Antiadaptation Individuation (retarding, conserving development)	Adaptation (differentiating) (restricting further development)	Feeling	Front-back
III	Empirical principle (experience; oriented toward the inner world)	Selection (habitat-oriented)	Thinking	Right-left

Table 30. Principles of evolution and their physical and psychological corollaries.

And finally, the **principle of antiadaptation or individuation** is characterized by constant alternation between the inner and outer worlds. This is a balancing, intermediary domain, where evolution not only moves forward but is also held back. The corresponding psychological domain is feeling, the corresponding bodily domain the front-back dimension. Thus the activity of adaptation and antiadaptation constitutes evolution in the narrower sense (Table 30, Figure 273). This is where an organism's inner world confronts the environment and thus where evolution on the material level actually takes place.

But we must not ignore the analytical forces (selection, mutation, etc.), which are the most discussed today. They are just as important as the three above-mentioned principles, which are more synthetic and spiritual in character. Without chance occurrences, there can be no purposeful movement; without chaos, no order. These factors, like thesis and antithesis, are inseparably connected. The principle of selection is indispensable in allowing issues to be experienced in the material world. Many current evolutionary hypotheses are based on principles that are not inherently false but have simply been applied one-sidedly. Only through a synopsis of all of the principles described in this book, we believe, is it possible to approach an understanding of evolution in its entirety and in depth.

The Future of Human Evolution and the Problem of the Resurrection Body

If the modern human body does not represent the end stage of evolution, several questions arise: Where will further evolution take us? What goals remain for the orthogenetic stream of evolution to achieve? Is the human race still capable of evolution? Haven't we reached a dead end or even a descending branch? There is much that speaks in favor of the idea that our bodily organization is degenerating rather than progressing: declining fertility rates (at least in industrialized nations), increases in degenerative diseases (often even in adolescents), declining memory (even in young people), and so on. According to Rudolf Steiner, the more technology and automation progress, the more our ability to read, write, and do arithmetic will decline (101). Today we can already note a decline in creativity and—what's worse—decreasing interest in our surroundings and our fellow human beings. People are becoming less and less interested in everything around them and increasingly numb and indifferent.

On the other hand, we can also observe a gradual change in consciousness and increasing involvement in contemporary problems, although initially only on the part of a small number of people. In this connection, it is worth reviewing a relatively long period of human history. People of earlier cultures, such as the Egyptian-Babylonian or Greco-Roman periods, experienced the world very differently from the way we experience it today (102, 103). They were still totally embedded in their tribes or ethnic groups and were on intimate

terms with their gods, whom they experienced as realities, either in dreams or through an instinctive clairvoyance that was still available to many people. Even as late as the Middle Ages, people were still more strongly rooted in faith than in thinking, and individual, scientific, objective thinking was still more the exception than the norm. Some great personalities who had already begun to develop this modern, independent way of thinking were ostracized, accused of heresy, or even burned at the stake. A dramatic shift—that is, a radical change in consciousness—set in at the beginning of modern times. Increasingly, individuals began to depend on their own judgment, shake off centuries-old traditional opinions, and develop a world view based exclusively on direct experience. Galen's views on cardiac function and circulation had remained unquestioned for centuries before William Harvey published his ideas on the circulation of the blood and Andreas Vesalius picked up a scalpel and tweezers to look at the structures of the human body and its organs for himself (104, 105).

This scientific and social shift at the beginning of the modern era is easy for us to survey today. It is a classical example of a ***change in consciousness***. (We are experiencing something similar in our own times, although it is taking a very different form.) Do these shifts affect only how people think and experience personal identity, or are bodily changes also involved? We know, for example, that the Mayas of Mexico bound the skulls of infants between two boards in an attempt to prevent impending changes of consciousness by inhibiting frontal lobe development. A swinging rubber ball was also suspended in front of the babies' eyes to force them to cross their eyes, which dampened the reality of space perception. Similar practices appeared during the late (already somewhat decadent) stages of Egyptian culture (127).

It is very likely that radical spiritual-physical changes, especially in the nervous system, took place in Europe during all major historical transitions, from megalithic culture to antiquity to the Middle Ages and finally to modern times. These changes gradually led to object-oriented, rational thinking supported by a strong sense of personal identity. We can be certain that other organ systems, such as the cardiovascular system, also underwent functional changes. Although little is known of such changes, they may have been responsible for altering how people behaved and experienced themselves during major cultural shifts.

Today we still know very little about the human potential for further development, but we can be certain that it exists. We will begin by exploring only two questions, which we will approach with great caution, restraint, and reverence: Did any evolutionary event (such as the "*Fall of Man*" as described in the Bible) ever radically change the human form? Was the Mystery of Golgotha, which took place at the beginning of the Christian era, important not only for the ensuing spiritual development of humankind but also for the ongoing evolution of the human physical body?

The Old Testament tradition describes the Fall primarily as an "expulsion from Paradise." In the previous chapter, we concluded that the ancestors of human beings must have been flexible, undifferentiated, unadapted animallike beings surrounded by huge auras of spiritual and soul forces. We can imagine that the soul-spiritual aspect of these beings could not yet identify with their physical bodies, that their consciousness identified much more closely with their soul-spiritual auras, and that they spent much of the time (especially at night) in the light-filled domain of the "gods." If this is so, then physical incarnation—

along with the simultaneous shrinking of the soul-spiritual aura and subsequent dimming of clairvoyant consciousness—can indeed be understood as an expulsion from Paradise. The Bible says "Their eyes were opened" and "You shall be like God." These statements may describe the first dawning of "I"-consciousness and the accompanying change in sensory functioning, i.e., the shift to consciously experiencing the surrounding world (79). The Bible goes on to say that henceforth women would bear children with great pain and that human beings would have to earn their daily bread with the sweat of their brows. On the north portal of Chartres Cathedral, where human evolution is illustrated in imposing pictures, we see Adam with his spade in hand, digging in the soil. This is the new, "post-Paradise" human condition as it was understood in a time when most physical labor was still devoted to procuring food. For the ancestral humans who lived primarily in soul-spiritual spheres, "embodiment" may also have entailed changes in their metabolic organs and mechanisms of reproduction (such as the transition to intrauterine gestation).

To a certain extent, the **structural changes in the nervous system** that resulted from the Fall can be traced and reconstructed. In a previous chapter, we described the three main functional domains of the nervous system: the sensorium (the sense organs and related portions of the brain), the sensorimotor systems, and the autonomic nervous system, which is located primarily in the viscera (i.e., on the periphery, as opposed to the "central" nervous system). In at least two of these domains, a certain functional imbalance or "shift" is evident—afferent systems dominate in the senses and efferent systems in the ANS. Afferent and efferent neural tracts are more or less in balance only in sensorimotor systems. If we observe how the major sense organs function, the nature of this "shift" immediately becomes clear. The outside world works directly on the sense organs through the medium of light (sight) or air (hearing), but awareness of the existence of objects, instead of developing internally, in the sense organ itself, is "projected" back out onto the perceived objects. In experiencing perception, we step outside of ourselves and approach the external objects we perceive with our senses. Their images in our consciousness do not remain inside us (in the retina or the inner ear, for example) where the forces of the outer and inner worlds meet. Our eyes have been opened; in awakening to the outer world, our consciousness has been externalized in a certain sense.

It is quite possible that an opposite shift occurred in the autonomic nervous system, where efferent activity dominates and afferent impulses arising out of the internal organs do not become conscious. As a result, our metabolism sinks down into the unconscious. In earlier times, metabolic forces were often experienced (usually in dream states) as demonic distortions—frightening, snakelike figures such as the head of the Gorgon Medusa, whose powers were banished by the reflective shield of Pallas Athena, the goddess of clear, self-aware thinking. Losing awareness and voluntary control of previously consciously experienced life processes is the flip side of awakening to the outer world through the higher senses (sight and hearing) and the cortical nervous system. Sensory-cortical activity presents us with a meaningless world whose reality we recognize only through the involvement of fully conscious thinking, which usually requires considerable deliberate effort. Here we get a first inkling that the purpose of these "shifts" in levels of consciousness may have been to endow human beings with the possibility of freedom.

But the above-mentioned **shifts in organ functions** were almost certainly also reflected in organ systems other than the nervous system and sense organs (cf. reference 79 in particular). We can observe that emotional excitement, instead of remaining self-contained, tends to affect glands and other organs. When we cry, for example, our lacrimal glands produce more fluid than usual, although there is no functional need for this. In this instance, glandular activity prevails over soul processes, asserting its independence, so to speak. Similarly, when we perspire in fear, our sweat glands step up their production even though the increase serves no thermoregulatory (i.e., biological) purpose. Many other such imbalances

occur in the body when one or the other system of forces predominates. For example, visualization is often enough to trigger sexual secretions or increases in blood pressure. Urinary urgency increases with excitement; saliva flow and secretion of appropriate gastric juices increase when we simply imagine certain foods.

When we discussed the metabolic and urinary organs, we saw that organ processes are designed primarily as harmoniously balanced feedback loops. In the kidneys, for example, approximately 99 percent of the fluid that exits the blood vessels is reabsorbed. In cellular metabolism, almost all of the amino acids released during protein breakdown are reused in protein synthesis. For some reason, only very small amounts cannot be reused but are eliminated from the body. These small amounts must then be replaced with amino acids from digested food. This is the "Achilles heel," so to speak, of metabolic activity. The imbalance or functional shift on this level is related to the appearance of disease or ultimately—through increasing accumulation of unusable residues—aging and death.

At this point, perhaps we can attempt to apply what we have learned to the problem of the **resurrection body** (the body of the resurrected Christ that first appeared to Mary Magdalene on Easter Sunday). Is it conceivable that it is biologically possible to overcome death? Was what happened in Palestine at the beginning of the Christian era actually a radical new step in evolution? Have we simply failed to grasp its substance, accustomed as we are to a faith based on feeling? This perspective could result in a completely new understanding of the Christ.

Let's first consider a few preliminary issues. Is it altogether possible for the "I" to influence or alter organ activity? We will begin by looking at the development of consciousness as such. Schooling our thinking with the help of specific concentration and meditation exercises can lead to a clairvoyant expansion of consciousness that allows us to perceive the spiritual realities "behind" the sense-perceptible world (13, 14). Clairvoyance appears when outward-directed forces are retained in the sense organs and are experienced in and around the organs themselves. In other words, the shift of perception into the outer world, as described above, is reversed. Since ancient times, this has been called the **gnostic path** of initiation (65).

On the other hand, systematic meditative exercises can also intensify feeling and willing in the vegetative domain to such an extent that the inner world of the unconscious is reillumined. In other words, metabolic organ functions can again be perceived by afferent autonomic nerves. In the opposite of what happens in the senses, the nerves that convey consciousness must here enter into direct contact with vital processes and become more involved in them. This reverses the shift in this system, too, and infinitely broadens the horizons of our perception. In ancient times, this was called the **mystic path** of initiation. It depends on intensifying feeling and willing rather than thinking (65).

But in addition to expanding its consciousness through systematic training, a self-aware individual can also alter organ processes themselves. In the history of India in particular, but also in Europe, there are many examples of spiritual paths that succeed in influencing and altering not only consciousness but also the body's life processes and organ systems. Just as the shift of processes in the nervous system can be overcome or reversed through conscious training, it is quite conceivable that the above-mentioned imbalances between life processes and soul processes inside the body could be balanced out and harmonized through an evolutionary process over a long period of time. Admittedly, overcoming our imprisonment in the material world and thus also the shifts and imbalances in our fundamental functions would require the involvement of an organ that we have not yet considered in this context, namely, the **blood**. Blood circulates through all the organ systems, linking the "upper" processes of the sense organs and nervous system with the "lower" processes of the metabolic system, muscles, etc. The blood binds functionally very different domains together. It is the organ that allows a person's free, self-determining "I" to influence and transform organ functions and to balance out the above-mentioned shift of functions as needed.

The essence of all this, of course, involves coming to grips with matter and overcoming the **problem of matter-filled space**. In previous chapters, we described qualitative differences in the three dimensions of space and how they work in shaping the human body. The human body is completely pervaded by the qualities of the right/left, up/down, and front/back dimensions. But Rudolf Steiner describes a space that is free of these forces, an almost cubical space in the chest, bounded by the sternum, the spine, the diaphragm, and the base of the skull (22). This space houses the heart and lungs. An earlier chapter in this book attempted to describe how the dimensions of space are "reversed" in the heart, thus making possible a transition from the spatial to the nonspatial domain or, vice versa, allowing nonspatial soul-spiritual forces to enter into and transform the spatial, matter-filled body (cf. pages 183-84 and 389). Related processes are also found in the respiratory tract. We can now imagine that the blood flowing through the heart brings new life forces such as those kindled by love from the nonspatial realm into the organs of the physical body. Through the cardiovascular system, it could thus actually be possible to transform the body into one that is freed from matter and consists entirely of life processes.

Love is the creative force that flows outward from the heart, transforming the body. In the future, it will become the central force in profoundly reshaping functional systems and reversing their shifts. Today we think of love almost entirely in the context of relationships between the sexes; we are almost totally unfamiliar with it as a force that moves worlds. Interactions between the sexes often have more to do with egotism than with love and not infrequently lead to disappointments and inner emptiness. True love is pure, radiant giving; it begins only when we stop expecting anything at all for ourselves. As soon as we count on even the slightest profit or aim for even the smallest personal gain, our love is no longer pure and unself-serving and becomes ineffective. How often do we simply beg for personal benefits when we pray? How many of our gifts and sacrifices are aimed at achieving personal salvation or performed in the expectation of thanks and approval? True love bestows no benefits on the giver; it is pure devotion and self-sacrifice, as demonstrated by the Christ's path to Golgotha. By meditating on the seven stages of Christ's passion, from the washing of the feet to the crucifixion and resurrection, we can experience for ourselves the incredible scope of the forces of love. Many years of intensive meditation of this sort lead to what has been called Christian or **Rosicrucian** initiation—ultimately, to direct personal/empathetic experience of the resurrection. If ancient documents are to be trusted, some saints experienced at least the beginnings of this bodily transformation. For example, it is reported that Nicholas of Flüe, the patron saint of Switzerland, ate nothing during the last twenty years of his life. Like a transfigured sage, he radiated love, wisdom, peace, and healing into the political confusion surrounding the emergence of the Swiss nation-state.

But of course the most important example is the **Christ** himself. Is it conceivable that what we call the power of Christ, for lack of a better term, changes not only our inner experience but also our very physical nature, allowing what St. Paul called the "new Adam," the reversal of the expulsion from Paradise, to become a reality? Love is the opposite of hate. Just as hatred brings coldness, contraction, and egotism, love brings radiating warmth and light, like the radiant light and warmth of the life-giving sun. If we assume that this superdimensional, almost cosmic power of love dwelled in the Christ and was carried in his blood, and if we also assume that the heart keeps a gate open between space and nonspace in the torso, it seems quite possible that Christ's resurrection body actually reversed the functional shifts discussed above. This would make it possible for bodily functions to continue as before, but unencumbered by matter and with their original harmony restored. For example, buildup and breakdown would continue in the metabolic system but would produce no wastes requiring elimination. The kidneys would continue to filter and resorb the body's fluids, monitoring and regulating internal life processes (the "water of life"), but no unusable residues would be eliminated. Reproduction, instead of taking place in utero through incarnation into matter, would happen through incarnation into the etheric formation of the spoken word (logos), and the function of the uterus would be transformed into that of the larynx (79). Without material "impurities" and through reversal of the above-mentioned shifts, the new body would have won back all of its essential functions and would manifest in radiant purity, as pure process.

According to Emil Bock's description, after the body of Christ was laid in the tomb, the particles of matter ("ash") may have been shaken out of his body (possibly with the help of an earthquake) so that only its form or configuration of forces persisted, with newly arranged and restructured functions (106). One term Steiner used for this is the **spirit body** (107). This may have been what appeared on the third day as the radiant resurrection body, initially "unfinished"—which is why Mary Magdalene was told "noli me tangere" (do not touch me)—and then in stabilized form, so that one week later, the doubting disciple Thomas was actually permitted to place his hand in the wound in the Risen One's side.

It will still take centuries before humankind has even an inkling of what happened in Palestine, and particularly on Golgotha, at the beginning of the Christian era. Christianity will remain meaningless as long as it is seen as a doctrine of faith. It will have to be understood in its reality, as ongoing evolution and transformation—also on the bodily level. Quite probably, the prototype of a new human body really was "born" then. If this is so, then the crucifixion was not a death but an initiationlike birth, an evolutionary process of transformation extending even to the physical level (108).

Final questions. If, from this perspective, the events of Golgotha did nothing more than reverse the Fall, why was it necessary for humankind to make this long journey through evolution's "earthly vale of tears"? Why couldn't the first human beings simply have stayed in Paradise? This question is actually about the meaning of evolution altogether. The human "I" developed out of freedom and hard-won insight, and this development would have been impossible without the descent into earthly space and the experience of the darkening of "paradisiacal" consciousness, which did not yet include individual self-awareness. In the future, the fully evolved human being will carry independent "I"-consciousness into the spirit world as a gift of love from the Earth. This consciousness can be acquired only through sunlike, all-encompassing love. But when love becomes manifest, a mystery is revealed. What happens when we sacrifice everything we have without asking for anything, without gaining anything, without desiring anything? When our forces ray outward in devotion, in the service of others, as if from a little sun, we experience a miracle: we become richer, not poorer, as a result. In times long past, wisdom became a fundamental component of our universe. In the future, perhaps, the tremendous, sunlike power of love will pervade our cosmos and provide it with new formative impulses.

This may well have been the vision of the writer of the Apocalypse when he described the further development of humankind as a battle between hatred and hardening on the one side and love and devotion on the other. Good people ("the blessed") who follow the progressive path of development receive new, white garments washed clean in the blood of Christ (i.e., they take love into themselves). Their foreheads are marked with the seal of the Angel of the Lord (the archangel Michael), meaning that their new bodily nature has been freed from the world of matter and hatred and made invulnerable. In contrast, fire and catastrophes destroy those who are filled with hatred and lag behind, clinging to the Earth and sacrificing to demonic beasts. And finally, in a shattering example of realistic esotericism, the writer of the Apocalypse describes the good souls fighting and begging, out of pure and selfless love, for those left behind, so that they too may ultimately enter the new world of the future.

Many esotericists suggest that in the future, humankind will divide into a progressive, evolving branch and a degenerating, descending branch that refuses to develop the potential of the higher "I" and therefore loses any potential for freedom

it once had. It is said that this branch of humanity will produce animallike forms. Here we can recognize the same evolutionary principles that we found in earlier stages of human evolution.

The egotistical, illusory "I" is centered in the head and lives in the brain's abstract, intellectual thinking, but the new, higher "I" will have its seat in the middle system, which gives rise to all harmonizing and balancing rhythms, i.e., to all further evolution. The "I" of the new human being, which radiates freedom and love, will have its center in the heart, in the interior of the (cubic) space that surrounds the thorax. From this center, the human aura will shine out into the spirit world that was once lost. Matthias Grünewald's painting of the resurrection, part of the Isenheim altar, is an incomparable image of this new, heart-centered "I".

It seems quite symbolic that the holy of holies in Solomon's temple was a cube and that the curtain in front of it was ripped apart during the events of Golgotha. The sentence "You are the salt of the earth," however, resounds with the message of the pure flame of love, which discards the ashes of earthly remains while preserving and redeeming the form-giving (saltlike) forces in order to guide Mother Earth into a new future.

This is what the old Germanic myths wished to express when, for example, they provided Siegfried, the sun initiate, with forces through which he was able to conquer the dragon. Bathing in the dragon's blood made him invulnerable, just as the sealing of the blessed in the Apocalypse conveys upon them not only protection but also a new form of existence. But Siegfried succumbed to death because he had not yet fully developed the radiant power of love. He died of a wound to that cubic space in the chest where the cross was centered and where the forces of resurrection have to be developed out of the heart. Parsifal, however, overcame his passions and found the grail through selfless love (in the Icelandic legend, the grail is called Ganganda Greida—transformative food for the journey). It is the grail from which the forces emanate that transform and renew the human being and ultimately lead to the attainment of the resurrection body.

References

1. Herbert Hensel, Allgemeine Sinnesphysiologie, Hautsinne, Geschmack, Geruch. In: *Lehrbuch der Physiologie,* W. Trendelenburg und E. Schütz, ed., Springer Verlag, Berlin, 1966.

2. Rudolf Steiner, *Intuitive Thinking as a Spiritual Path,* (GA 4). Anthroposophic Press, Great Barrington, Mass., 1995.

3. R. Steiner, lecture of 6.28.1914, in *Architecture as a Synthesis of the Arts,* (GA 286). Rudolf Steiner Press, London, 1999.

4. R. Steiner, lecture of 4.12.1922, (GA 82). (Not available in English.)

5. Helmut Kiene, *Grundlinien einer essentialen Wissenschaftstheorie.* Verlag Urachhaus, Stuttgart, 1984.

6. R. Steiner, *The Riddles of Philosophy,* (GA 18). Anthroposophic Press, Spring Valley, New York, 1973.

7. R. Steiner, *Truth and Knowledge, Introduction to "Philosophy of Spiritual Activity,"* (GA 3). Steinerbooks, Blauvelt, New York, 1981.

8. R. Steiner, *The Science of Knowing—Outline of an Epistemology implicit in the Goethean World View,* (GA 2). Mercury Press, Spring Valley, New York, 1996.

9. R. Steiner, *Goethe's World View,* (GA 6). Mercury Press, Spring Valley, New York, 1985.

10. Gerhard Wehr, *Rudolf Steiner, Wirklichkeit, Erkenntnis und Kulturimpuls.* Aurum Verlag, Freiburg/Br., 1982.

11. Henri Bortoft, *The Wholeness of Nature.* Lindisfarne Books, Great Barrington, Mass., 1996.

12. Arnold Gehlen, *Der Mensch, seine Natur und seine Stellung in der Welt.* 13th edition, Aula-Verlag, Wiesbaden, 1986.

13. R. Steiner, *How to Know Higher Worlds: a Modern Path of Initiation,* (GA 10). Anthroposophic Press, Great Barrington, Mass., 1994.

14. R. Steiner, *An Outline of Esoteric Science,* (GA 13). Anthroposophic Press, Great Barrington, Mass., 1997.

15. Johannes W. Rohen, E. Lütjen-Drecoll, *Funktionelle Anatomie des Menschen.* 11th edition, Schattauer, Stuttgart, 2006.

16. J.W. Rohen, *Funktionelle Neuroanatomie.* 6th edition, Schattauer, Stuttgart, 2001.

17. Johannes W. Rohen, E. Lütjen-Drecoll, *Funktionelle Histologie.* 4th edition, Schattauer, Stuttgart, 2000.

18. R. Steiner, *Riddles of the Soul,* (GA 21). Mercury Press, Spring Valley, New York, 1996.

19. John C. Eccles, *Mind and Brain.* Paragon House Publishers, New York, 1985.

20. Ernst Kretschmer, *Körperbau und Charakter.* 26th edition, Springer Verlag, Berlin, 1977.

21. *The Portable Plato: Protagoras, Symposium, Phaedo, and the Republic,* complete, in the English translation of Benjamin Jowett, by Plato, Benjamin Jowett ed., Viking Press, New York, 1948.

22. R. Steiner, lecture of 11.21.1914, *The World as Product of the Working of Balance,* (GA 158). Rudolf Steiner Publishing Co., London, 1948.

23. Gunther Hildebrandt, Zeiterleben und Zeitorganismus. In: G. Kniebe, ed., *Was ist Zeit,* pp. 163–197. Verlag Freies Geistesleben, Stuttgart, 1993.

24. W. Menzel, Clinical roots of biological rhythm research (chronobiology). In: G. Hildebrandt, R. Moog and F. Raschke (eds), *Chronobiology and Chronomedicine «Basic Research and Applications»,* pp. 277–287. Frankfurt, 1987.

25. Robert Aaron, *Die verborgenen Jahre Jesu.* p. 53 ff. Deutscher Taschenbuch Verlag, München, 1973.

26. St. Augustine, *Confessions.* J.W. Edwards, Ann Arbor, Mich., 1946.

27. R. Steiner, lecture of 8.22.1919. In: *The Foundations of Human Experience,* (GA 293). Anthroposophic Press, Great Barrington, Mass., 1996.

28. Novalis, *Gesammelte Werke,* Vol. II, Nr. 848. Carl Hanser Verlag, München, 1978.

29. R. Steiner, lecture of 5.17.1923. In: *Life Beyond Death,* (GA 226). Rudolf Steiner Press, London, 1995, p.59.

30. Leonard Hayflick, *Auf ewig jung? Ist unsere biologische Uhr beeinflussbar?* Vgs Verlagsgesellschaft, Köln, 1996.

31. L. Hayflick, The cell biology of aging. *J.Invest. Dermatol.* 73, p. 8 -14, 1979; s.a. *Antecedents of cell aging research, Exp. Gerontol.* 24, pp. 355–365, 1989.

32. Wilhelm Roux, Beiträge zur Entwicklungsmechanik des Embryo II. Ges. Abh. II, pp. 256–276. *Breslauer ärztl. Z.,* 1884.

33. Hans Driesch, "Entwicklungsmechanische Studien I," *Z. Zool. 53,* 1891.

34. Hans Spemann, *Experimentelle Beiträge zu einer Theorie der Entwicklung.* Springer Verlag, Berlin, 1936.

35. H. Bautzmann, Die Problemlage des Spemannschen Organisators. *Verh. Ges. Deutsch. Naturforsch. Ärzte, 98. Vers.,* Freiburg i. Br., 1955.

36. Keith L. Moore and T.V.N. Persaud, *The Developing Human: clinically oriented embryology.* Saunders, Philadelphia, 1998.

37. Dietrich Starck, *Embryologie*. 3rd edition, Thieme Verlag, Stuttgart, 1975.

38. Klaus V. Hinrichsen, ed., *Humanembryologie, Lehrbuch und Atlas der vorgeburtlichen Entwicklung des Menschen*. Springer Verlag, Berlin, 1993.

39. Kurt Goerttler, *Entwicklungsgeschichte des Menschen*. Springer Verlag, Heidelberg, 1950.

40. J. W. Rohen und E. Lütjen-Drecoll, *Funktionelle Embryologie*. 4th edition, Schattauer Verlag, Stuttgart, 2012.

41. Ernst Haeckel, *Generelle Morphologie der Organismen*. 2 Vols, Berlin, 1866; also *Natürliche Schöpfungsgeschichte*. Berlin, 1875.

42. R. Steiner, lecture of 5.29.1907. In: *The Theosophy of the Rosicrucians*, (GA 99), lecture 5, Rudolf Steiner Publishing Co., London, 1953.

43. Friedrich Schiller, Über Anmut und Würde. In: *Sämtliche Werke*. Vol. V, pp. 231–285, Winkler Verlag, München.

44. Johann G. Herder, *Ideen zur Philosophie der Geschichte der Menschheit*—quoted in A. Gehlen, (46), p.33.

45. R. Steiner, lecture of 3.17.1921. In: *Anthroposophy and Science*, (GA 324). Mercury Press, Spring Valley, New York, 1992.

46. Arnold Gehlen, *Der Mensch, seine Natur und seine Stellung in der Welt*. 13th edition, p. 30 ff, Aula Verlag, Wiesbaden, 1986.

47. A. Gehlen, *Urmensch und Spätkultur*. Aula-Verlag, Wiesbaden, 1986.

48. Adolf Portmann, *Einführung in die vergleichende Morphologie der Wirbeltiere*. 5th edition, Schwabe & Co. Verlag, Basel, 1976.

49. Herbert Schriefers, *Was ist Leben?* Schattauer Verlag, Stuttgart, 1982.

50. Norman Macbeth, *Darwin Retried*. Gambit Incorporated, Boston, 1971.

51. Joachim Illies, *Der Jahrhundertirrtum, Würdigung und Kritik des Darwinismus*. Umschau Verlag, Frankfurt/M., 1983.

52. Jos Verhulst, *Developmental Dynamics in Humans and Other Primates—Discovering Evolutionary Principles through Comparative Morphology*. Adonis Press, Ghent, New York, 2003.

53. Hermann Poppelbaum, *Man and Animal, their Essential Difference*. Anthroposophic Publ. Co., London, 1960.

54. Friedrich Kipp, *Childhood and Human Evolution*. Adonis Press, Ghent, New York, 2005.

55. Ernst-Michael Kranich, *Thinking Beyond Darwin, the Idea of the Type as a Key to Vertebrate Evolution*. Lindisfarne Books, Hudson, New York, 1999.

56. Adolf Portmann, *Biologische Fragmente zu einer Lehre vom Menschen*. 3rd edition, p. 79 ff. Schwabe & Co. Verlag, Basel, 1969.

57. J. W. Rohen, *Anatomie für Zahnmediziner*. 3rd edition, p. 158 ff. Schattauer Verlag, Stuttgart, 1994. Also E. Lütjen-Drecoll und J. W. Rohen, *Fotoatlas der Anatomie, Der menschliche Körper und seine Funktionen*. 2nd edition, Schattauer Verlag, Stuttgart, 2000.

58. J. W. Rohen, Chihiro Yokochi, and Elke Lütjen-Drecoll, *Color Atlas of Anatomy, A Photographic Study of the Human Body*. 5th edition, Schattauer and Lippincott, Williams & Wilkins, Baltimore, 2002.

59. Armin Husemann, *Der musikalische Bau des Menschen*. 3rd edition, Verlag Freies Geistesleben, Stuttgart, 1993.

60. Wolfgang Schad, ed., *Die menschliche Nervenorganisation und die soziale Frage*. Vol. I and II, Verlag Freies Geistesleben, Stuttgart, 1992.

61. E. Buddecke, *Grundriß der Biochemie*. 9th edition, Walter de Gruyter Verlag, Berlin, 1994.

62. Otto Wolff, *Grundlage einer geisteswissenschaftlich erweiterten Biochemie*. Verlag Freies Geistesleben, Stuttgart, 1998.

63. Novalis, Klingsors Märchen im Romanfragment, Heinrich von Ofterdingen. In: *Gesammelte Werke*. Vol. I, p. 338 ff. Carl Hanser Verlag, München, 1978.

64. R. Steiner, lecture of 12.24.1919. In: *The Light Course*, (GA 320). Anthroposophic Press, Great Barrington, Mass., 2001.

65. R. Steiner, lectures of 3.20-28.1911. In: *An Occult Physiology*, (GA 128). Rudolf Steiner Publishing Co., London, 1951.

66. A. Portmann, Cerebralisation und Ontogenese. In: *Med. Grundlagenforschung*, Stuttgart, 1962.

67. R. Steiner, lecture of 10.01.1911. In: *The Reappearance of Christ in the Etheric*, lecture 9, (GA 130). Anthroposophic Press, Great Barrington, Mass., 2003.

68. Paolo Bavastro and H. Ch. Kümmell, *Das Herz des Menschen*. Verlag Freies Geistesleben, Stuttgart, 1999.

69. Andreas Rohen, Ontogenie und Phylogenie der Herzentwicklung. In: *Das Bild des Menschen als Grundlage der Heilkunst*. Friedrich Husemann, ed., newly edited by Otto Wolff, Vol. III: Zur speziellen Pathologie und Therapie. 4th edition, p. 96ff. Verlag Freies Geistesleben, Stuttgart, 1993.

70. Alfred Benninghoff, Das Herz. In: *Handbuch der vergleichenden Anatomie der Wirbeltiere*. L. Bolk, E. Göppert, E. Kallius and W. Lubosch, eds., Vol. VI, pp. 467–556, p. 525 ff. Verlag Urban & Schwarzenberg, Berlin, 1939.

71. R. Steiner, lecture of 9.17.1924. In: *Pastoral Medicine.* Anthroposophic Press, Hudson, New York, 1987.

72. Georg und Michaela Glöckler, Die Zahl 70 und ein musikalisches Geheimnis des Platonischen Weltenjahres. In: *Das Goetheanum,* Nr. 66, 4. 2. 1995, pp. 729–730.

73. Gunther Hildebrandt, Die Zeitgestalt des Menschen. In: *Tycho de Brahe Jahrbuch für Goetheanismus,* pp. 23–57. Tycho-Brahe-Verlag, Niefern-Öschelbronn, 1994.

74. H. Matthiolius, H.M. Thiemann and G. Hildebrandt, Wandlungen der rhythmischen Funktionsordnung von Puls und Atmung im Schulalter. In: *Der Merkurstab,* 48, Heft 4, pp. 297–312, 1995.

75. Friedrich Schiller, Über die ästhetische Erziehung des Menschen, in einer Reihe von Briefen. In: *Sämtliche Werke,* Vol. V, p. 311 ff. Winkler Verlag, München.

76. R. Steiner, lecture of 7.22.1921, *Man as a Being of Sense Perception,* (GA 206). Steiner Book Centre, N. Vancouver, 1981; and lecture of 8.08.1920. In: *Spiritual Science as a Foundation of Social Forms,* (GA 199). Anthroposophic Press, Hudson, New York, 1986.

77. Jacques Lusseyran, *And There Was Light.* Morning Light Press, Sandpoint, Idaho, 1998.

78. Helen Keller, *The Story of my Life.* Doubleday, Page & Co., New York, 1905.

79. R. Steiner, lectures of 12.27-31.1911. In: *The World of the Senses and the World of the Spirit,* (GA 134). Steiner Book Centre, North Vancouver, B.C.,1979.

80. R. Steiner, lecture of 4.03.1920. In: The *Warmth Course,* (GA 321). Mercury Press, Spring Valley, New York, 1980.

81. Reiner Klinke and Stefan Silbernagl, *Lehrbuch der Physiologie.* Verlag Georg Thieme, 2nd edition, Stuttgart, 1998.

82. G. Thews, E. Mutschler and P. Vaupel, *Anatomie, Physiologie und Pathophysiologie des Menschen.* Wissenschaftl. Verlagsgesellschaft, Stuttgart, 1999.

83. R. Steiner, lecture of 9.29.1920. In: *The Boundaries of Natural Science,* (GA 322). Anthroposophic Press, Spring Valley, New York, 1983.

84. R. Steiner, lecture of 3.17.1921. In: *Anthroposophy and Science,* (GA 324). Mercury Press, Spring Valley, New York, 1991.

85. Arthur Zajonc, *Catching the Light, the Entwined History of Light and Mind.* Oxford University Press, 1993.

86. Sally R. Springer and Georg Deutsch, *Linkes und rechtes Gehirn, Funktionelle Asymmetrien.* Verlag Spektrum der Wissenschaft, Heidelberg, 1987.

87. R. W. Sperry, Hemisphere Deconnection and Unity in Conscious Awareness. *Americ. Psychologist 23,* 723–733, 1968.

88. R. Steiner, Lecture of 1.14.1917. In: *The Karma of Untruthfulness,* Vol. 2, (GA 174). Rudolf Steiner Press, Forest Row, Sussex, 2005.

89. R. Steiner, lecture of 12.19.1920. In: *The Bridge between Universal Spirituality and the Physical Constitution of Man,* (GA 202). Anthroposophic Press, Spring Valley, New York, 1979.

90. R. Steiner, *Occult Seals and Columns,* (GA 284). Anthroposophical Publishing Co., London, 1924.

91. Frank Teichmann, *Die ägyptischen Mysterien, Quellen einer Hochkultur.* Verlag Freies Geistesleben, Stuttgart, 1999.

92. R. Steiner, lecture of 8.07.1916. In: *The Riddle of Humanity,* (GA 170). Rudolf Steiner Press, London, 1990.

93. R. Steiner, lecture of 11.11.1923. In: *Man as Symphony of the Creative Word,* (GA 230). Rudolf Steiner Press, Forest Row, Sussex, 1991.

94. *Goethes Naturwissenschaftliche Schriften.* R. Steiner, ed., Vol. I, p. 322, Dornach, 1975.

95. L.F.C. Mees, *Secrets of the Skeleton, Form in Metamorphosis.* Anthroposophic Press, Spring Valley, New York, 1984.

96. Adolf Dabelow, Über Korrelationen in der phylogenetischen Entwicklung der Schädelform. *Gegenbaurs Morph. Jahrbuch 63,* pp. 1–49, 1929, and *67,* pp. 84–133, 1932.

97. Noam Chomsky, *Knowledge of Language, its Nature, Origin and Use.* Greenwood Press, London, 1986.

98. J. W. Goethe, Das Märchen, mit einem Beitrag von Rudolf Steiner. In: *Goethes Geistesart in ihrer Offenbarung durch sein Märchen "Von der grünen Schlange und der schönen Lilie."* 9th edition, Verlag Freies Geistesleben, Stuttgart, 1989.

99. Charles Darwin, *The Origin of Species.* John Murray Ltd., London, 1859.

100. O. H. Schindewolf, Über den «Typus» in morphologischer und phylogenetischer Biologie. Akademie der Wissenschaften und der Literatur, *Abhandlg. d. mathem.-naturwissenschaftl. Klasse, Jg. 1969, Nr. 4,* pp. 57–131, 1969.

101. R. Steiner, lecture of 10.14.1913, *The Path of Christ through the centuries,* (GA 152). Anthroposophical Quarterly, Vol. 20, #2, pp. 26-32, Summer, 1975.

102. Frank Teichmann, *Die Kultur der Empfindungsseele, Ägypten, Texte und Bilder.* Verlag Freies Geistesleben, Stuttgart, 1990.

103. F. Teichmann, *Die Kultur der Verstandesseele, Griechenland, Texte und Bilder.* Verlag Freies Geistesleben, Stuttgart, 1993.

104. William Harvey, *Exercitio anatomico de motu cordis et sanguinis in animalibus.* 1628.

105. Andreas Vesalius, *De humani corporis fabrica.* 1543.

106. Emil Bock, *The Three Years, The Life of Christ between Baptism and Ascension.* Floris Books, Edinburgh, 2005.

107. R. Steiner, lecture of 10.10.1911. In: *From Jesus to Christ*, (GA 131). Rudolf Steiner Publishing Co., London, 1956.

108. R. Steiner, *The Fifth Gospel*, (GA 148). Rudolf Steiner Press, Forest Row, Sussex, 1995.

109. Ernst-Michael Kranich, *Anthropologische Grundlagen der Waldorfpädagogik.* Verlag Freies Geistesleben, Stuttgart, 1999.

110. A. Rohen, *Rhythmen im Lebenslauf.* 6th edition, published by the Verein f. anthropos. Heilwesen e.V., Bad Liebenzell-Unterlengenhardt, 1998.

111. R. Steiner, lecture of 5.26.1922. In: *The Human Soul in Relation to World Evolution*, (GA 212). Anthroposophic Press, Spring Valley, New York, 1984.

112. Romano Guardini, *Die Lebensalter.* Topos Taschenbücher, 4th edition, Mainz, 1992.

113. John Barnes, *Goethe and the Power of Rhythm, a Biographical Essay.* p. 83. Adonis Press, Hillsdale, New York, 2002.

114. Herbert Hensel, Karl E. Schaefer and Ronald Brady, Rhythmical-Functional Order, p. 15. In: *A New Image of Man in Medicine, Basis for an Individual Physiology.* Futura Pub. Co., Mt. Kisco, New York, 1977.

115. Keith L. Moore and T.V.N. Persaud, *The Developing Human.* 5th edition, W.B. Saunders Comp., Philadelphia, 1993.

116. William Harvey, *An Anatomical Disquisition on the Motion of the Heart and Blood in Animals.* J.M. Dent & Sons, London, 1935.

117. A. Benninghoff and D. Drenckhahn, *Anatomie.* Band I, Urban und Fischer, München, 2003.

118. Stefan Leber, *Die Menschenkunde der Waldorfpädagogik.* Verlag Freies Geistesleben, Stuttgart, 1993.

119. K.V. Hinrichsen, *Human-Embryologie.* Springer Verlag, Heidelberg, 1993.

120. B. Tillmann, F. Härle, and A. Schleicher, Biomechanik des Unterkiefers, Deutsche Zahnärztl. Z., 38, 1983, pp. 285-293.

121. Eckhart Buddeke, *Grundriss der Biochemie.* 7th edition, Walter de Gruyter Inc., Berlin, 1985.

122. W.J. Hamilton, J.D. Boyd, and H.W. Mossman, *Human Embryology.* W. Heffer & Sons, Ltd., Cambridge, 1962.

123. Friedrich Husemann, *Das Bild des Menschen als Grundlage der Heilkunst*, Band I, Zur Anatomie und Physiologie. Verlag Freies Geistesleben, Stuttgart, 1991.

124. Max Clara, *Entwicklungsgeschichte des Menschen.* Quelle und Meyer, Leipzig, 1940.

125. Karl Wittmaack, *Über die normale und pathologische Pneumatisation des Schläfenbeins.* Jena, 1918.

126. K. Kleist, *Gehirnpathologie.* Barth Verlag, Leipzig, 1934. See also: J.W. Rohen, *Neuroanatomie.* 6. Aufl., Schattauer Verlag, Stuttgart, 2001.

127. Sylvanus Griswold Morley, *The Ancient Maya.* 3rd edition, Stanford University Press, Stanford, California, 1958.

128. G. Adams and O. Whicher, *The Plant Between Sun and Earth.* Rudolf Steiner Press, London, 1980.

129. Goethe's essay "Nature." In: *Goethe Scientific Studies*, edited by Douglas Miller, p. 4. Princeton University Press, Princeton, New Jersey, 1995.

130. Christian Morgenstern, *We Found a Path.* Pegasus Publishing, 2001.

131. Barbara Strauch, *The Primal Teen, What the New Discoveries about the Teenage Brain tell us about Our Kids.* Doubleday Publ., New York, 2003.

132. David S. Goldstein, *Adrenaline and the Inner World.* Johns Hopkins University Press, Baltimore, 2006.

133. Jay Shulkin, *Rethinking Homeostasis, Allostatic Regulation in Physiology and Pathophysiology.* MIT Press, Cambridge, Mass., 2003.

134. T. Kohda, Japan. Journal Med. Science, Vol. 4, 1934.

135. R. Steiner, lecture of 10.04.1919, *Social Understanding through Spiritual Scientific Knowledge*, (GA 191). Anthroposophic Press, Spring Valley, New York, 1982.

136. C.A. May, W. Neuhuber, E. Luetjen-Drecoll, Immunohistochemical classification and functional morphology of human choroidal ganglion cells. Invest. Ophthalmol Vis Sci 45, 361-367, 2004.

137. G. Korkhaus, Ätiologie der Zahnstellungs- und Kieferanomalien, Fortschr Orthod 1: 136-142, 1931.

138. C. Ohder, *Gewalt durch Gruppen Jugendlicher.* Hitit-Verlag, Berlin, 1992.

139. W. Heitmeyer, *Gewalt, Schattenseiten der Individualisierung bei Jugendlichen.* 3. Aufl., Juventa-Verlag, München, 1998.

140. "Ludwig Robert Muller (1870-1962): a pioneer of autonomic system research." In: Journal of Clinical Autonomic Research, ISSN 0959-9851, Vol. 8, No. 1, Feb. 1998, pp. 1-5.

141. W. Hagen, Die Bildung des Knorpelskeletts beim menschlichen Embryo. Archiv f. Anat. u. Physiol., 1900.

Recent publications taking a Goethean approach to science include:

Henri Bortoft, *The Wholeness of Nature, Goethe's Way toward a Science of Conscious Participation in Nature*. Lindisfarne Books, Great Barrington, Mass., 1996.

D. Seamon and A. Zajonc, editors, *Goethe's Way of Science, A Phenomenology of Nature*. State University of New York Press, 1998.

Stephen Edelglass, G. Maier, et al, *The Marriage of Sense and Thought, Imaginative Participation in Science*. Lindisfarne Books, Hudson, New York, 1997.

Rudolf Steiner, *Nature's Open Secret, Introductions to Goethe's Scientific Writings*, with an essay on participatory science by John Barnes. Anthroposophic Press, Great Barrington, Mass., 2000.

R. Steiner, *Goethe's World View*. Mercury Press, Spring Valley, New York, 1985.

Nigel Hoffmann, *Goethe's Science of Living Form, The Artistic Stages*. Adonis Press, Hillsdale, New York, 2007.

Craig Holdrege, editor, *The Dynamic Heart and Circulation*. AWSNA Publications, Fair Oaks, California, 2002.

Friedrich Kipp, *Childhood and Human Evolution*. Adonis Press, Hillsdale, New York, 2005.

Jos Verhulst, *Developmental Dynamics in Humans and Other Primates—Discovering Evolutionary Principles through Comparative Morphology*. Adonis Press, Hillsdale, New York, 2003.

For further information on Goethe's scientific approach, see the website of The Nature Institute: www. natureinstitute.org.

Recent publications taking a Goethean approach to medicine include:

Ralph Twentyman, *The Science and Art of Healing*. Floris Books, Edinburgh, 1989.

G. Van der Bie and M. Huber eds, *Foundations of Anthroposophical Medicine*. Floris Books, Edinburgh, 2003.

A. Husemann and O. Wolff, *The Anthroposphical Approach to Medicine. Vols. I – III*, Anthroposophic Press, Great Barrington, Mass., 1982.

M. Evans and I. Roger, *Complete Healing*. Anthroposophic Press, Great Barrington, Mass., 1992.

Herbert Hensel, Karl E. Schaefer and Ronald Brady, *A New Image of Man in Medicine*. International Research Institute for Man-Centered Environmental Sciences and Medicine, Futura Pub. Co., Mt. Kisco, New York, 1977.

G.S. Kienle, H. Kiene and H.-U. Albonico, *Anthroposophic Medicine*. Schattauer, New York, 2006.

Publications of the Louis Bolk Instituut, Driebergen, Holland (www.louisbolk.org):

Anatomy—Human morphology from a phenomenological point of view
Guus van der Bie, M.D.
Publication GVO 03

Physiology—Organ physiology from a phenomenological point of view
Christa van Tellingen, M.D.
Publication GVO 04

Immunology—Self and non-self from a phenomenological point of view
Guus van der Bie, M.D.
Publication GVO 05

Pharmacology—Selected topics from a phenomenological point of view
Christa van Tellingen, M.D.
Publication GVO 06

Biochemistry—from a phenomenological point of view
Christa van Tellingen, M.D.
Publication GVO 02

Embryology—early development from a phenomenological point of view
Guus van der Bie, M.D.
Publication GVO 01

Index

Word listings are followed by page numbers, then by Fig. numbers and Table numbers.

Acetabulum, 92, 94, 95, Figs 55 and 56

Adaptive processes. see Evolution

Adrenals, 321, 326–27ff, Figs 224B, 226 and 227

Afferent neurons, 228–33ff, Figs 163, 165, 166 and 166B

Aging, 395

Allantois, 121, Fig. 75A

Amnion, 50, Fig. 23

Amniotic cavity, Figs 24, 25 and 27

Amphioxus (Brachiostoma), 44

Anabolic and catabolic processes, 116ff, Fig. 73ff

Anatomy, functional, systematic, and topographic, 13

Ancient Moon, 62–63

Ancient Saturn, 62–63

Ancient Sun, 62–63

Antiadaptive processes. see Evolution

Antibodies, 125, 128, 135ff, 143

Apes, higher, postnatal development of, 83

Appendix, 125, 140

Archenteron, 44

Archetypal phenomena, xv, 12, 114, 116, 117, 170, 182, 201, 206, 211, 243, 267, 271, 321, 386

Arm, bones of the, 98, 99, Fig. 59A

Arteries, 165–66, 176, 182, 196, 197, Fig. 107

—layered structure of, 166, Fig. 107

Atria, 165, 166, 176, 177, 180, 181, 185, 186, 191, 193, 195, Figs 115, 118, 123, 126, 127, 132, 138 and 140

Auditory

—centers, 259, 260, Fig. 187

—meatus, 155, 249, 255, Figs 181 and 183

—nerve, 257–60, Figs 185 and 187

—ossicles, 256–58, Figs 184–85

—pathway, 259–60, Fig. 187

—process, 260–61, 370, Fig. 185

Autonomic nervous system, 301–12

Balance, organ of (vestibular apparatus), 242, 294–97, Figs 211 and 212

Baroreceptors, 297–98, Fig. 213

Basilar membrane, 257, Figs 185–86

Bilateral symmetry, 26, 30–31, Fig. 10

Bile

—acids, 122, 129, 130, 143, Figs 82 and 92

—capillaries, 127, Fig. 80

—duct, 126, 130, 134, Figs 78 and 80

—pigments, 122–23, 132–34, 143–44, Figs 84, 85 and 92

Biliary system, 125, 126, 131, 142–44, Figs 78, 85 and 92

Bilirubin, 134

Bladder, urinary, 148, 150, 158, 159, Figs 102 and 103C, Table 26

Blastocyst, 47, 49, 56, 58, 59, Figs 21 and 22

—development of, 49, Fig. 22

Blastopore lip, 44, 45, Fig. 20

Blastula, 43, 44, 46

Blood, 169, 171–73ff

—coagulation of, 172, 173ff, Table 16

—etherization of, 183–84, 387ff, 408

—functional threefoldness of, 172, Table 16

—vessels, layered structure of, 166, Fig. 107

Blood pressure and respiration regulation, and sense organs, 297, Fig. 213

Bone marrow, 169–71, 339, 340, 342, 358, 361, 372, 373, 375, Figs 110, 234 and 238A

—primary, 338

Bones

—compact bone, 338–40, 373, Table 28

—embryonic cartilaginous skeleton, 337–38, Fig. 233

—flat bones, 340–41, Figs 236–39

—long bones, 337–40, Figs 232–35

—spongy bone, 338–40, 373, Table 28

—in the three functional domains of the human body, 343, Fig. 239

Brain

—as an organ of consciousness, 314–19

—auditory centers of, 257, 260, Fig. 187

—evolution of, 73, 82, Figs 39 and 46

—language centers of, 212–13, Fig. 153

—lateralization of the hemispheres, 315–17

—left cerebral hemisphere of, 238, Fig. 170

—left hemisphere with cortical fields, Fig. 193B

—maturation of, 393

—olfactory centers of, 282–86, Figs 202 and 204–5

—optical fields in occipital lobe, Fig. 193C

—subdivision into lobes, 314–15

—visual centers of, 5–6, Figs 3 and 4

Brain stem (reticular formation), 236–38, Figs 169 and 170

Branchial apparatus, 381–82, Fig. 267

Branchiogenic organs, 322, Fig. 225

Calcaneus (heel bone), 97, Fig. 58A

Capillaries, types of, 165–66, 168, Fig. 109

Carbohydrate metabolism, 130, Fig. 83

Cardiac rhythm, 209–10, Tables 18 and 19

—cardiac skeleton, 193–94, Figs 136 and 137

—cardiac tube, septation of, 178, Fig. 117

Cardiovascular system, embryonic development of, 59, 60, Fig. 31

Carotid sinus nerve, 298

Carpus, 97, Fig. 58B

Cell division, 43

Cellular defense, 135, 136, Fig. 86

—respiration, 203, Fig. 143

Cerebellum, 220, 221, 234, 239, 241, 242ff, Figs 157D, 171 and 172, Table 20

Cerebral cortex

—consciousness and, 316–18, Fig. 223, Table 27

—functional subdivision of, 316, Fig. 223

—sensory pathways to, 292, Fig. 210

Cerebralization, increasing, in vertebrates, 73, Fig. 39

Cerebrospinal fluid, 140

Cervical vertebrae, 30, Fig. 11

Chemoreceptors, 297–98, Fig. 213

Chest cavity, 89

Choroid, 266–68, 275, Figs 191–92 and 198, Table 22

Chromosomes, 38

Chronobiological rhythms, 208–11, Figs 147–49, Table 19

Chronobiology, 35, 46, 208–11, Figs 147–49, Table 19

Chyme, 122, 142

Circulatory system, 20, 21, 22, 24

—in amphibians, 187–88, Figs 127 and 128

—in birds and mammals, 190–91, Fig. 130

—evolution of, in fish, 185–87, Figs 124–26

—in mammals and humans, 191, Fig. 131

—phylogenetic development of, 185–94, Figs 125–37

—in reptiles, 188–89, Figs 128 and 129

—threefoldness of, 165–67, Fig. 108, Table 15

Clavicle (collarbone), 89, 91, 92, 94, 105

Cleavage, 43, 45, 48, Fig. 20

Clitoris, 159–62, Figs 103 and 106B

Coccygeal vertebrae, 30, Fig. 11

Cochlea, 259, 260, Figs 184–86 and 185B

Cochlear duct, 257–58, Figs 184–85

Cognitive process

—dual character of, 9ff

—in seeing, 4

Cold and warmth receptors, 289, Fig. 208

Colon (large intestine), 120–23, 125, 130, 134, 144, Figs 75–77, Table 13

Color vision, 274, Table 24

Compact bone, 170, 338–40, 372–75, Figs 110 and 234, Table 28

—metamorphosis of, in skull development, 373–76, Fig. 263

Conception, 37–42, Figs 17 and 18

Conduction system of the heart, 195, Fig. 138

Consciousness

—historical changes in, 405–7

—levels of, in seeing, 272–73, Table 23

Coracoid process, 92, 93, 94, Figs 54 and 56

Cornea, 266, 268, 278, Fig. 191, Table 22

Corona radiata, 39, Fig. 15

Coronary arteries, 196–97, Fig. 139

—vessels, 196–97, Fig. 139

Corpus striatum, 234, 238, 241, Figs 171 and 172

Corti, organ of, 257–60, Figs 184–85

Cranial nerves, 364–65, Fig. 257

Cranium, shape and size of, in higher apes and humans, 82, Fig. 46

Cuboid, 97, Fig. 58A

Cytoplasm, in egg cell, 37

Cytotrophoblast, 55, 56, 57, Fig. 28

Deep sensitivity (muscle senses), 244, 293–94, Fig. 173

Dental arch, 77, Fig. 42

Dental development in mammals, one-sided, 79, Fig. 44

Dentition, second, 361, Fig. 254

Dermatocranium, 74

Diaphragm, 174, 206–7, Fig. 146

Digestive tract, 115, 120–25, 139, Figs 75 and 76, Table 13

Ductus arteriosus, 178, 181, 182, 197, 198, Figs 140 and 141

Duodenum, 120–23, 126, 142, Figs 76 and 78, Table 13

Ear

—eardrum (tympanic membrane), 256–57, Figs 184 and 185

—inner, 256–57, Figs 184–86

—middle, 252–57

—outer, 251–52, Figs 179–80

—pneumatization of, 252–55, Fig. 183

—threefold division of, 256, Fig. 184

Earth evolution, 62–63

Ectoderm, 45, Fig. 20

Efferent neurons, 228–33ff, Figs 163, 165, 166 and 166B

Embryoblast, 47, 48, 50, 56, 58, Figs 22, 23, 28 and 29, Table 8

Embryology, 13

Embryological development, 31, 37–63

—blood, 171, Fig. 111

—ear, 249–54, Figs 177–83

—endocrine organs, 322, Fig. 225

—eye, 264–68, Fig. 225

—genitals, 156–62, Figs 102–6

—head, 335–43, Figs 231–33 and 236–237

—heart and circulation, 174–80, 197–99, Figs 111–19, 140–41

—of the intestinal tube, 120–21, Fig. 75

—of the kidneys, 150–52, Figs 97–99

—lungs, 204–5, Figs 144–45

—nervous system, 216–21, Figs 154–58

—in relation to the liver, 125

—stages of and the Earth's evolution, 62–63

—structural stages of, 43–60

—torso, 343, Fig. 240

Embryonic disk, 50, 51, Fig. 24

Endbrain/telencephalon, 220, 236, 238, Fig. 157

Endocrine glands, 321–30

Endocrine system, 320–33

—and reproductive organs, 330

Endoderm, 45, Fig. 20

Endometrium, 42, 49, 50, 55, 56, 58, Figs 21, 23 and 28

Energy conversion, 112, 117, 119, 130

Enterohepatic circulation, 129, 130, 133, 134, 144, Figs 82, 85 and 92

Epiphyseal plate, 100, 101, Fig. 60B

Equilibrium, sense of, 245, 262–63, 294–96, Figs 189, 211 and 212

Ethmoid bone, 377–78, Fig. 264

Ethmoid cells, 377, Fig. 264

Evolution

—adaptation principle in, 69–71, 84, 396–98, 404, Fig. 48, Table 30

—antiadaptation in, 69–71, 84, 396–98, 404, Fig. 48, Table 30

—of the circulatory system, 199–200

—empirical principle in, 397, 398–400, Fig. 272, Table 30

—of fetal membranes, 399, Fig. 272

—fundamental processes of, 403, Fig. 273

—future of, 405–11

—of the heart, 185–93

—human and animal, 401–2

—individuation principle in, 149–57, 404, Table 30

—of the kidneys, 153–55, Fig. 100

—of the limbic and olfactory systems, 286

—orthogenetic principle in, 81, 84, 396, 400–401, 404, Table 30

—of the speech organs, 211–12, Fig. 150

—vertebrate, 64–84

—of the vertebrate brain, 73, Fig. 39

Eye

—accommodation system (muscles) of, 277–78, Fig. 199, Table 25

—development of the visual cortex, 393, Fig. 271B

—embryonic development of, 264–68, 368–69, Figs 190 and 259

—five functional systems of, 268

—layered structure of, 266, 268, Fig. 191, Table 22

Eyelids, 278

Facial expression, muscles of, 76, 105–8, Figs 41, 67 and 68

Facial skeleton, 362–63

Facial skull, 78, 350, 375, Figs 43, 263 and 352

Fallopian tubes, 49, 158, 159, Figs 21 and 103C

Fate map, 44

Fat metabolism, 129, 130, Fig. 82

Fertilization, 42

Fetal circulation, 197, Fig. 140

Fibula, 98, 99, Fig. 59B

Fingers, 97, Fig. 58B

Flexors, digital, 105, Fig. 64

Fontanelles, 341, Fig. 237

Foot, bones of, 97, Fig. 58A

Foot, digital rays of, 97, Fig. 58A

Foot and hand, 96, 97, Fig. 58

Foramen ovale, 178, 181, 197, Fig. 140

Forearm, 98

Form perception, 274–75, Table 24

Fovea centralis, 4, 7, 268, 271, 273–74, Figs 4, 194 and 196

Freedom, physiological foundations of, 391–95

Frontal plane, 34, Fig. 9

Frontal sinus, 379–80, Figs 265–66

Front-back dimension, 28

—functional significance of, 119

Functional systems

—informational, 16

—metabolic, 17

—rhythmic, 17–19

Functional threefoldness

—of the blood, 172, Table 16

—of the cell, 22–23, Fig. 8

—of the circulatory system, 165–67, Fig. 108

—of the facial skeleton and physiognomy, 362–63, Fig. 255

—of the human body, 14–22, Figs 7A–C and 7D, Table 1

—of the human soul, 23–26, Table 4

—of the kidneys, 146, Fig. 93

—of the muscular system, 103–11

—of the musculoskeletal system, 233, Fig. 166B

—of the nervous system, 217–28, Fig. 159

—of the organs of hearing, 256, Fig. 184

—of the skeletal system, 87

—of the urogenital system, 222, Fig. 159

Gallbladder, 371–72

Gametes, 37, 38, 40, Fig. 17

Gastrula, 45, Fig. 20

Gastrulation, 43, 45, 46, 50, Fig. 20

Gender differentiation, 158

Genetic material, 38, 42

Genitals, external, 162, Fig. 106

Genitals, female, development of, 158–59, Fig. 103

Genitals, male, development of, 157–58, Fig. 102

Genome, 42

Germ cells, development of, 37, 38, Fig. 14

Germline, 160, Fig. 104

Glomerulus, 146–48, 366–68, Figs 93, 96 and 258–59

Glucagon, 327

Goethean scientific method, 10–12, 16

Gonads (testes, ovaries), 38, 42, Fig. 14

—development of, 160–62, Fig. 105

Greek gymnastics, 242

Gustatory system, 280–82

Hair cells, 257, 263, Figs 185, 189B and 189C

Hand, bones of, Fig. 58B

Hand, bones of, 97

Hand and foot, 96, 97, Fig. 58

Head, evolution of, 65–67, 74–82, Figs 40–46

—muscles of, 107, Figs 67 and 68

Head development

—and the disintegration principle, 373–76

—and the integration principle, 335–65

Hearing, organs of, 256–61, Figs 184–87

—process of, 260–61, Fig. 185

—threefold subdivision of, 256, Fig. 184

Hearing and balance, organs of, 249–64

Hearing and speaking, functional cycle of, 263–64

Heart

—crossing of veins in, 181, Fig. 121

—embryonic development of, 174–80, 198–99, Figs 112–19, Table 17

—evolution of, 185–93, Figs 124–35

—function of, 182–84

—layered structure of, 166, Fig. 107

—ontogenetic development of in relation to the dimensions of space, 174–82

—primordium of, 54, 60, 171, 174–80, Figs 27, 31, 111–13 and 115–119

Hematopoiesis, stages of, 171, Fig. 111

Hemoglobin, 131–34, 144, 394, Figs 84 and 85

—metabolism of, 133, Fig. 85

Henle, loop of, 146, 148, 155, Figs 93, 96 and 100

Hensen's node, 52, 53, Fig. 26

Hepatobiliary system, processes in, 371, Fig. 262

Hip bone, 95, Fig. 56

Human maturational phases, sinus development in, 379–80, Fig. 266

Humoral defense, 135ff

Hypothalamus, 301, 303, 310–12ff, 318, 319, 326–32, Figs 216, 221–22, 224–25, 229A, 229B and 230, Table 27

Immune system, 128, 134–36ff, 139, 141, 143–44, 145, 168, 169, 172, 173, Figs 86 and 88, Table 16

Implantation, 28, 42, 48, 55, 56, 58, 59, 63, Figs 23 and 28, Table 9

Individuation principle in evolution. see Evolution

Induction (of physiological development), 44

Information system, 14, Fig. 7D

—exchange of, basic functional processes in, 14, 16, 19, Fig. 6

Insulin, 327

Interbrain/diencephalon, 220, 236, 238, Fig. 157

Intestinal tube, 44, 45, 52, 120, 121, Figs 20 and 75

Intestine, small, 120–26, 130, 134, 139, 142, Figs 75–78

Intramural plexuses, 301–3, Fig. 216

Iris, 268, 277ff, Fig. 191, Table 22

Islets of Langerhans of the pancreas, 321, 326–27ff, Figs 226 and 228

Jaw, upper jaw/maxilla, 352–53, Figs 245 and 247

—joint of, primary, 381, Fig. 267

—joint of, secondary, 381, Fig. 267

—lower jaw, angle of, 355

—lower jaw/mandible, 354–56, Figs 245 and 249

—temporomandibular joint, 79, 355–56, Fig. 249

Joints, 88, 100, 101, 102, 374, Figs 50, 60B, 61 and 263

—locations of, 88, 102, Figs 50 and 61

—structure and growth of, 100, 101, Fig. 60B

Kidney/eye metamorphosis, 366–69, Figs 258–59

Kidneys, 145, 148, 149, 152, 156, Figs 97, 98, 101 and 229A

—evolution of, 152–55, Fig. 100, Table 14

—functional threefoldness of, 146, Fig. 93

—generations in the development of, 150, Fig. 97

Labyrinth, 256, 295, Figs 184 and 211

—development of, 249–50, 263, Figs 177–78 and 189

—location of, 296, Fig. 212

Lacrimal apparatus, 278

Larynx, 212, Fig. 151

Learning, 391

Leg, bones of, 98, 99, Fig. 59B

Lemniscate, 30, 31, 90, 95, 96, Figs 12, 51, 56 and 57

Lens, 266, Fig. 191

—development of, 264–65, Fig. 190

—vesicle of, 264–65, Fig. 190

Life, sense of, 297–98

Limbic system, 285–86ff, 302, 310, 312–13ff, 318, Figs 205, 216 and 222, Table 27

Lipid, 129, Fig. 82

Liver, 116–20, 122, 123, 125, 126, 128–31, 133–36, 138–40, 142–45, 371, Figs 78–83, 85 and 92, Table 26

—functional structure of, 127, Figs 79 and 80

—work rhythms of, 131

Love as a creative force, 408–10

Lower jaw, angle of, 355

Lumbar vertebrae, 30, Fig. 11

Lungs, embryonic development of, 204–6, Figs 144 and 145

Lymph

—nodes, 124, 125, 129, 135, 137, 138, 144, Fig. 87

—system, 61, 137, 138, 140, 144, Fig. 32

Lymphatic organs, 135ff, 137ff, Fig. 77

—associated with the digestive tract, 124, 125, 128, 134, 135, 137, 138, Figs 32, 77 and 88–90

—vascular system of, 138, 144, 168ff, Fig. 89

Macula statica, 263, Fig. 189C

Mastoid process, 252–53, 255, Figs 181–83

Maturational phases, human, 362, Table 29

Maxillary sinus, 379–80, Figs 265–66

Medulla oblongata/myencephalon, 220, 236, 237, Figs 157 and 169

Meiosis, 41, Fig. 18

Mesoderm, 45, 51, 53, Figs 20, 25 and 26

Mesonephros, 150–53, 157, 158, Figs 97–99, 102 and 103

Metabolic system, 17–19, 115–62, Fig. 7C

—the digestive organs, 115–34

—the immune system, 135–44

—the urogenital system, 145–62

Metabolism, 111, 115–17

—fundamental functional processes of, 14, 17, 19, Fig. 6

Metacarpus, 97, Fig. 58B

Metameric structural principle, 29ff

Metamorphosis

—kidney/eye, 366–69

—Kidney/eye, Figs 258–60

—of the lower limbs into the lower jaw, 354–56, Figs 248–49

—of the pectoral girdle into the pelvic girdle, 92, 94–96,

Figs 55–57

—of the pelvis into the temporal bone, 356–58, Figs 250–51

—of the reproductive organs into speech organs, 382–84, Figs 268–69

—of ribs and long bones, 90–92, Figs 51–52

—of the torso and limb skeleton into the skull, 345–63

—upper abdomen/labyrinth, 370–72, Figs 261–62

—of the upper limbs into the upper jaw, 351–53, Figs 246–47

—of the vertebrae, 346–47, Fig. 242

—of vertebrae into the skull, 348–51, Figs 243–45

—of a vertebra into a shoulder blade (scapula), 91–93, Figs 53–54

Metanephros, 150, 152, 153, 156, Figs 97 and 99

Metatarsus, 97, Fig. 58A

Midbrain/mesencephalon, 234, 236, 238, 239, 242, Figs 157 and 171–72, Table 20

Middle ear, 256–57, Figs 184–85

—pneumatization of, 252–55, Fig. 183

Morphology, 12–13

Morula, 43, 46, 48, 49, Figs 21 and 22

Motor end plate, 111, 112, Fig. 72A

Motor neurons, 228, 230–33, 236, Figs 163–64

Movement in space, experiencing, 68, Fig. 37

Müllerian duct, 157–58, 161, Figs 102, 103 and 105

Muscle

—cells, innervation of, 304, Fig. 218

—contraction, 112, 113, 131, 232, Figs 72 and 166

—fibers, 103, 112–14, Fig. 72

—senses, 287, 293–94, 299

—spindles, 111, Fig. 72A

Muscular system, 103

—functional threefoldness of, 103ff

Myofibrils, 103, 112, 113, Fig. 72

Navicular bone, 97, Fig. 58A

Nephrotome, 151, 153, Figs 98 and 99

Nerve fibers, 223–27ff, Figs 161–62

Nervous system

—basic morphological divisions of, 221–23

—development of, 216–21, Figs 154–58

—general, 14

—threefoldness of, 222–23, Fig. 159

Neural crest, 326, 334–36, Fig. 231

Neural tube, 44, 52, 217–19, 220, Figs 155B and 156–58

Neurocranium, 74

Neuroendocrine pathways, 321, Fig. 224

Neurons, 224ff, Fig. 160

Neurula, 44, 45, 47, Fig. 20

Nociception, 293

Notochord, 45, 51, 52, Figs 20, 24 and 25

Olfactory, system, 282–85, 380, Figs 202–5

—mucosa, 284, Fig. 203

—receptors, 282–85, Figs 202–5

Oogenesis, 37

Optic. see also Eye

—cup, 265–66, 366–69, Figs 190 and 258–60

—nerve, 268–69, Figs 191–92

—tract, 5–6, 269, Figs 3 and 193

Oral and nasal cavities, phylogeny of, 80–81, Fig. 45

Organizer, embryonic, or Spemann, 44

Organ metamorphoses, 366–84

Organ of Corti, 257–60, Figs 184–85

Organ systems, threefoldness in, 21

Orthogenesis, 81, 84, 400

Os basilare, 348–49, Figs 243A and 244

Osmoreceptors, 297

Ossification

—endochondral, 338–39ff, 340, 343, 344, 358, 373, Fig. 239, Table 28

—periosteal (desmal), 339–40ff, 342–44, 372, 374, Figs 232, 238 and 239, Table 28

Otoliths, 263, Fig. 189C

Ovaries, 37, 42, 158–59, Figs 103B and 103C

Ovulation, 39, Fig. 15

Ovum, 37–38

Pain

—perception of, 293

—sense of, 293

Pancreas, 326, Figs 226 and 228

Paranasal sinuses, 378–80, Fig. 265

Parasympathetic nervous system, 301–4, 306–10ff, 311, 328, Figs 216 and 220, Table 26

Parathyroids, Fig. 226

Pectoral girdle, 89, 92

—muscle loops of, 106, Fig. 66

Pectoral girdle and pelvic girdle, transformation of, 92, 94, 95, Figs 55 and 56

Pelvic girdle, 94, Fig. 55

Pelvis, 384, Fig. 269

—arched structure of, 354, Fig. 248

—formation of, 96, Fig. 57

—and legs, functional arches in, 103, Fig. 62

—and temporal bone, 356–58, Fig. 250

Penis, 157–58, 162, Figs 102 and 106C

Perceiving and thinking, 9–10

Perception, process of, 248–49, Fig. 176

Periosteum, 101, 170, 337–39, 342, Figs 60A, 60B, 110, 234 and 238

Petrous bone, 356ff, 358ff, Fig. 251

Pharyngeal arches, 381–82, Fig. 267

Pharynx, primordial, 322–23, Fig. 225

Photoreceptors, regeneration of, 275–76, Fig. 198

Physiognomy, 363, Fig. 255

Pigmented epithelium, 265, 267, 268, 275–76ff, Figs 190, 192 and 198, Table 22

Pineal gland, 312, 322, 330–32ff, 385–87, Figs 222, 225, 230 and 270

Pituitary gland, 320–23, 326, 330–32ff, 386ff, Figs 222, 225–27, 229, 230 and 270

Pituitary lobe

—anterior, 330

—posterior, 331

Pituitary/pineal system, 385–87

Placenta, 48, 56, 57, 59, 63

Placentation, 48

Pneumatization of the middle ear, 252–55, Fig. 183

Polarity, principle of, 28, 31–33, Fig. 10

Portal vein, 125, 127–31, 140, 142, 185, Figs 79, 81 and 83

Portal vein system, 125, 126, 142, Fig. 78

Primitive gut, embryonic development of, 121, Fig. 75A

Primitive streak, 50, 51, 54, 59, Fig. 24, Table 9

Protein metabolism, 128, 129, Fig. 81

Pulse-respiration ratio, 210

Pure perception, 272

Radius, 98, 99, Fig. 59A

Reflex arcs, 228–33

Renal

—corpuscles, 146–48, 153, 366–68, Figs 93–96 and 258–259, Table 14

—cortex, 146

—medulla, 146, 148

—papillae, 146, 148, 149, Fig. 93

—pelvis, 146, 149, Fig. 93

—tubule, 146, 148, 149, 153, 155, Figs 93–96

Reproductive organs

—female (internal), 159, 382–84, Figs 103 and 268B

—male, 157–58, Fig. 102

—metamorphosis of into speech organs, 382–84, Fig. 268

Respiration

—internal, 202

—rhythm of, 206–8

Respiratory system, 17, 20, 21, 22, 24, 201–14

—in the head, 377–82

—processes of, 202, Fig. 142

Resurrection body, 407, 409–10

Reticular formation, 306, 310, 311–12ff, 317–18, Fig. 221, Table 27

Retina, 4, 5, Figs 190–92ff, 194–96 and 198, Table 22

Reversal of structural principles in the human form, 31, 33–34, Fig. 13

Rhythmic system, 20, Fig. 7B

—basic functional processes of, 17, 20, Fig. 6

—blood and organs of circulation, 165–200

—respiratory system, 201–15

Rhythms in human life, 392–95, Figs 271A and 271B

Rib cage, development of, 344, Fig. 240

Ribs, 29, 90–92, Figs 51 and 52

Ribs, humerus, and femur, structural comparison of, 90, Fig. 52

Right-left dimension, 26ff

Rods and cones, 269–70, 274–76, Figs 192, 194 and 198

Sacrum, 89, 91, 96, 103, Fig. 57

—development of, 345

Sagittal (median) plane, 34, Fig. 9

Scaphoid bone, 97, Fig. 58B

Scapula (shoulder blade), 91, 92, 93, 95, 100, 104, Figs 53–54, 56 and 66

—and hip bone, transformation of, 92, 94, 95, Figs 55 and 56

—and thoracic vertebra, comparison, 91, Fig. 53

—and thoracic vertebra, transformation, 92, 93, Fig. 54

Schwann cells, 226, Fig. 162

Sclera, 266–67, Figs 191–92

Seeing, cognitive processes and, 4–8

—levels of consciousness in various modes of, 272, Table 23

—modes of and related soul activities, 275, Table 24

—the role of thinking and concepts in, 3, 4, 8–10, 272–73

Segmentation principle, 27, 29, 32–33, Fig. 9

Sella turcica, 357, 374, 376, 385–87, Figs 251, 263 and 270

Semicircular canals, 250, 256, 294–97, Figs 178C, 184 and 211–12

Seminiferous tubules, 38, Fig. 14

Sense of life, 297–98

Sensorimotor systems, 234–42

—overview of, 234, Table 20

Sensory systems, 243–300

—asymmetry of sensory reflex loops, 248–49

—functional subdivision and action of, 243–47, Figs 173–74, Table 21

—functional subdivision of, 300, Fig. 215

—overview of, 245, Table 21

—their relation to conscious experience, 298, Fig. 214

—threefold division of, 247

—as a whole, 298–300, Fig. 215

Sensory-nervous system, 19, 21, Fig. 7A

Sertoli cells, 37, 38

Seven-year rhythms in human development, 362, 392, Fig. 271A, Table 29

—sinus development and, 380

Shoulder joint, range of motion of, 106, Fig. 65

Skeletal system, 87ff, Figs 49 and 50

—and joints, 88, Fig. 50

—threefold division of, 87

Skin

—location of sense organs in, 291, Fig. 209

—as organ of thermoregulation, 288, Fig. 207

—senses, 286–93

Skull

—base of, 348–49, 376, Figs 243A and 244

—braincase (calvarium), 78, Fig. 43

—evolution of, 75, Fig. 40

—formative principles in, 374–76, Fig. 263

—as a metamorphosis of the torso and limb skeleton, 345–59

—of the newborn, 341, Fig. 237

—postnatal development of, 66, 340–43, Figs 35 and 235–38

—sutures of, 100, 101, Fig. 60A

Skullcap/calvarium, 339–42, 344, 356, 373–75ff, 376, Figs 236–38 and 263

Smell, organ and sense of, 282–85, Figs 202–5

Solar plexus, 301–2, 308, Figs 216 and 220

Somites, 52, Fig. 27

Space

—perception of, 273–75, Fig. 195, Table 24

—problem of, 408

—and time, 35–36

Speech

—centers in the brain, 212–13, Fig. 153

—development of, 80

—and language, 391–92

—organs, evolution of, 211–12, Fig. 150

—organs, relationship to female reproductive organs, 382–84, Fig. 268

—organs of, 211–14, Figs 151–53

Spermatocytes, 38, Fig. 14

Spermatogenesis, 37, Fig. 14

Spermatogenesis and oogenesis, 37, 38

Sperm cells, 37–42, Figs 14, 16 and 18

Spinal cord, 218–19, 221–23, 227, 230, 234–42, Figs 155–56, 158–59, 163–65, 167–69, 171–72, 256 and 366, Table 20

—development of afferent and efferent neurons of, 229, Fig. 163

—embryonic development of, 218, Fig. 155

Spinal nerves, 229, 364, Figs 163 and 256

Spiral principle in biology, 261, Fig. 188

Splanchnocranium, 74

Spleen, 131, 133, 135ff, 136, 137, 139, 140ff, 141–44, 371, Figs 85, 88, 90–92 and 262

—closed circulation of, 142, Fig. 91

—open circulation of, 141, Fig. 90

—red pulp of, 140, 141, Fig. 90

—structure of, 141, Fig. 90

—white pulp of, 140, 142, Fig. 90

Spongy bone, 170–71, 338–40, 358, 372–75, Figs 110, 234, 235 and 263, Table 28

—development of, 338–40ff, Figs 234, 235 and 263

—metamorphosis of, in skull development, 373–76, Fig. 263

Sternum, 90–92

Structural principles in the human body, 26

Sugar, 130, Fig. 83

Sutures, structure and growth of, 100, 101, Fig. 60A

Sympathetic chain, 308

Sympathetic nervous system, 301–4, 306–10ff, 311, 328, Figs 216 and 220, Table 26

Synapses, 227ff, Fig. 160C

Syncytiotrophoblast, 55, 56, Fig. 28

Tactile receptors, types of, 290–91

Talus, 97, Fig. 58A

Tarsus, 97, Fig. 58A

Taste buds, 280–80, Figs 200–201

Teeth, 358–61, Figs 252–54

—occlusion of, 360, Fig. 253

—shapes in human adult, 359, Fig. 252

Temporal (time)

—chronobiological rhythms, 208–11, Figs 147–49, Table 19

—processes, 35, 46, 48, 58

—respiratory rhythm, 206–8

—structure of the body, 35

Temporal bone, 253–54, 357, Figs 181–82 and 251

—and pelvis, 356–58, Fig. 251

Temporomandibular (jaw) joint, 79, 355–56, Fig. 249

Testes, 157, 158, 162, Fig. 102C

—migration of, 158

Thalamus, sensory pathways and, 292, Fig. 210

Thermoreceptors, 288–89, Figs 207–8

Threefoldness. see Functional threefoldness

Thrombocytes, 172, Table 16

Thymus, 325, Fig. 226

Thyroid gland, 323–25, Fig. 226

Tibia, 98, 99, Fig. 59B

Toes, 97, Fig. 58A

Tongue, papillae of the, 280, Fig. 200

Tonsils, 124, 125, 139ff, Fig. 77

Torso

—metameric structure of, 30, 33, Fig. 11

—muscles, dorsal, 109, 110, Figs 70 and 71

—muscles, ventral, 108, Fig. 69

—segments, 29, 30, 31, 89, Fig. 11

—skeleton, development of, 343–45, Fig. 240

Touch, organs of, 289–93, Figs 209–10

Transferrin, 132, Fig. 84

Transverse or horizontal plane, 34, Fig. 9

Trapezius muscle, 110, Fig. 71

Trigeminal nerve, 363–65, Figs 255 and 257

Trophoblast, 50, 55–57, Figs 23, 28 and 29

Tympanic cavity, 252

Ulna, 98, 99, Fig. 59A

Umbilical cord, 59, 60, 121, Figs 30, 31 and 75B

Umbilical vein, 176, 197, Fig. 140

Up-down dimension, 28ff

Upper abdomen/labyrinth metamorphosis, 370–72

Uprightness, 391

Ureter, 149ff, 153, 158, 162, Fig. 99

Urinary system, 145–49ff

Uterus, 150, 158–59, Figs 103B and 103C

—relationship to speech organs, 382–84, Fig. 268B

Vagus nerve, 307, 310, Fig. 220

Vallate papillae, 280–81, Figs 200–201

Valve plane of the heart, 194, Fig. 137B

Vascular development, stages of, 171, Fig. 111

Ventricle, 176, 177, 179, 181, 183, 185, 188, 189, 191–93, 195–98, Figs 115, 118, 119, 121–23, 128, 129, 132 and 134–38

Ventricular musculature, 193, Fig. 136

Vertebrae, structure of, 346, Fig. 241

Vertebral metamorphosis, 346–51, Figs 241–45

Vertebrate evolution. see Evolution

Vertebrate groups, 69, Table 11

Vestibular apparatus, 242ff. see also balance, organ of

Visceral senses, 297–98

Viscerocranium, 74

Visual centers of the brain, 7–8, 269–70, Figs 4 and 193

Visual cortex, maturation of, 393, Fig. 271B

Visual process, 269–76

Warmth or temperature, sense of, 286–89, Figs 206–8

Wolffian duct, 150, 153, 158, 162, Figs 97–99 and 102

Yolk sac, 50, Fig. 23

Zygote, 39ff, 43, 46, 48

About the Author

Johannes W. Rohen (b. 1921) studied medicine at the universities of Cologne, Freiburg, Breslau, Danzig, and finally Tübingen, where he was awarded his doctorate in 1946. Tübingen was also where he began his scientific career, which focused on researching the physiology of the eye, especially as it relates to the problem of glaucoma. In 1953 he qualified as a lecturer at the University of Mainz in the fields of anatomy and embryology. He accepted the Benninghoff chair of anatomy at the University of Marburg/Lahn in 1964 and a call to the University of Erlangen-Nürnberg in 1974. He retired in 1989. Professor Rohen is the author of many textbooks, which reflect his standing as one of the founders of functional anatomy.

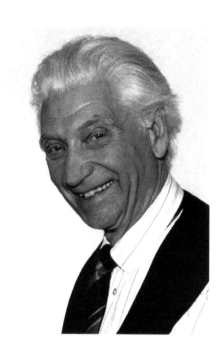

To date, the following books by Johannes Rohen are available in English:

1) J. W. Rohen, *Practical Anatomy, Regional and Clinical*. Schattauer Verlag, Stuttgart, New York, 1973.

2) C. Yokochi, J. W. Rohen, and E. Lurie Weinreb, *Photographic Anatomy of the Human Body*. Igaku-Shoin, Tokyo, New York, 3rd edit., 1989.

3) J. W. Rohen, *Functional Morphology of Receptor Cells*. Internat. Symposium, Tokyo, 1975. Fr. Steiner Verlag, Wiesbaden, 1979.

4) W. G. Müller, and J. W. Rohen, *Biochemical and Morphological Aspects of Ageing*. Fr. Steiner Verlag, Wiesbaden, 1981.

5) J. W. Rohen, Chamber Angle, *Functional Anatomy, Physiology, and Pathology in Glaucoma*. Thieme Verlag, Stuttgart, 1978.

6) E. Lütjen-Drecoll, and J. W. Rohen, *Atlas of Anatomy, The Functional Systems of the Human Body*. Williams and Wilkins, Baltimore, 1998.

7) J. W. Rohen, C. Yokochi, E. Lütjen-Drecoll, *Color Atlas of Anatomy, A Photographic Study of the Human Body*. Lippincott, Williams and Wilkens, 6th edit., 2006.